WHO Classification of Tumou

MW00984149

Head and Neck Tumours

Part A

WHO Classification of Tumours Editorial Board

International Agency for Research on Cancer

World Health
Organization

Suggested citation

WHO Classification of Tumours Editorial Board. Head and neck tumours.
Lyon (France): International Agency for Research on Cancer; 2024.
(WHO classification of tumours series, 5th ed.; vol. 9).
https://publications.iarc.who.int/629.

Sales, rights, and permissions

Print copies are distributed by WHO Press, World Health Organization, 20 Avenue Appia, 1211 Geneva 27, Switzerland
Tel.: +41 22 791 3264; Fax: +41 22 791 4857; email: bookorders@who.int; website: https://whobluebooks.iarc.who.int/

To purchase IARC publications in electronic format, see the IARC Publications website (https://publications.iarc.who.int).

Requests for permission to reproduce or translate IARC publications – whether for sale or for non-commercial distribution – should be submitted through the IARC Publications website (https://publications.iarc.who.int/Rights-And-Permissions).

Third-party materials

If you wish to reuse material from this work that is attributed to a third party, such as figures, tables, or boxes, it is your responsibility to determine whether permission is needed for that reuse and to obtain permission from the copyright holder. See *Sources*, pages 712–719. The risk of claims resulting from infringement of any third-party-owned component in the work rests solely with the user.

The contributors of all images in which the patient may be identifiable have affirmed that the appropriate informed consent has been obtained for the use of said images in this publication.

General disclaimers

The designations employed and the presentation of the material in this publication do not imply the expression of any opinion whatsoever on the part of WHO or contributing agencies concerning the legal status of any country, territory, city, or area, or of its authorities, or concerning the delimitation of its frontiers or boundaries. Dotted and dashed lines on maps represent approximate border lines for which there may not yet be full agreement.

The mention of specific companies or of certain manufacturers' products does not imply that they are endorsed or recommended by WHO or contributing agencies in preference to others of a similar nature that are not mentioned. Errors and omissions excepted, the names of proprietary products are distinguished by initial capital letters.

All reasonable precautions have been taken by WHO to verify the information contained in this publication. However, the published material is being distributed without warranty of any kind, either expressed or implied. The responsibility for the interpretation and use of the material lies with the reader. In no event shall WHO or contributing agencies be liable for damages arising from its use.

First print run (10 000 copies)

Updated corrigenda can be found at https://publications.iarc.who.int

IARC Library Cataloguing-in-Publication Data

Names: WHO Classification of Tumours Editorial Board.
Title: Head and neck tumours / edited by WHO Classification of Tumours Editorial Board.
Description: Fifth edition. | Lyon: International Agency for Research on Cancer, 2024. | Series: World Health Organization classification of tumours.
| Includes bibliographical references and index.
Identifiers: ISBN 9789283245148 (pbk.) | ISBN 9789283245155 (ebook)
Subjects: MESH: Head and Neck Neoplasms. | Odontogenic Tumors.
Classification: NLM WE 707

The WHO classification of head and neck tumours presented in this book
reflects the views of the WHO Classification of Tumours Editorial Board
that convened via video conference 14–16 June 2021,
as well as subsequent consultation.

The WHO Classification of Tumours Editorial Board

For the complete list of all contributors and their affiliations, see pages 701–711.

For the complete list of all contributors and their affiliations, see pages 701–711.

WHO Classification of Tumours
Head and Neck Tumours

Edited by	The WHO Classification of Tumours Editorial Board
IARC Editors	Subasri Armon
	Ian A. Cree
	Anil Felix Angelo Fonseca
	Daphne Fonseca
	Gabrielle Goldman-Lévy
	Dilani Lokuhetty
	Valerie A. White
Project Assistant	Asiedua Asante
Assistant	Anne-Sophie Bres
Production Editor	Jessica Cox
Copy Editing	Julia Slone-Murphy
Principal Information Assistant	Alberto Machado
Information Assistant	Catarina Marques
Layout	Meaghan Fortune
Printed by	Omnibook
	74370 Argonay, France
Publisher	International Agency for Research on Cancer (IARC)
	25 Av. Tony Garnier, CS 90627
	69366 Lyon, CEDEX 07, France

Contents

Please note that the contents of this volume have been split into two parts for publication in print: Part A (in this book) and Part B (in the accompanying book).

List of abbreviations

2D, 3D	two-dimensional, three-dimensional
AIDS	acquired immunodeficiency syndrome
AR	androgen receptor
CI	confidence interval
CMV	cytomegalovirus
CNS	central nervous system
CT	computed tomography
dDNA	denatured deoxyribonucleic acid
DNA	deoxyribonucleic acid
EAC	external auditory canal
EBV	Epstein–Barr virus
ER	estrogen receptor
ESR	erythrocyte sedimentation rate
ETP	early T-precursor
FDC	follicular dendritic cell
FDG	18F-fluorodeoxyglucose
FDOPA	18F-L-dihydroxyphenylalanine
FISH	fluorescence in situ hybridization
FNA	fine-needle aspiration
FNAB	fine-needle aspiration biopsy
FNAC	fine-needle aspiration cytology
GFAP	glial fibrillary acidic protein
H&E	haematoxylin and eosin stain
HCV	hepatitis C virus
HIV	human immunodeficiency virus
HPV	human papillomavirus
HRS cell	Hodgkin/Reed–Sternberg cell
HRS-like cell	Hodgkin/Reed–Sternberg–like cell
IARC	International Agency for Research on Cancer
ICD	International Classification of Diseases
ICD-11	International Classification of Diseases, 11th revision
ICD-O	International Classification of Diseases for Oncology
Ig	immunoglobulin
IQ	intelligence quotient
IRSG	Intergroup Rhabdomyosarcoma Study Group
kDa	kilodalton
KSHV/HHV8	Kaposi sarcoma–associated herpesvirus / human herpesvirus 8
long ncRNA	long non-coding ribonucleic acid
LP cell	lymphocyte-predominant cell
M:F ratio	male-to-female ratio
MCPyV	Merkel cell polyomavirus
MIM number	Mendelian Inheritance in Man number
MITF	melanocyte-inducing transcription factor
MRI	magnetic resonance imaging
mRNA	messenger ribonucleic acid
N:C ratio	nuclear-to-cytoplasmic ratio
NK cell	natural killer cell
NOS	not otherwise specified
NSAID	non-steroidal anti-inflammatory drug
NSE	neuron-specific enolase
Pap	Papanicolaou stain
PAS staining	periodic acid–Schiff staining
PCR	polymerase chain reaction
PET	positron emission tomography
PET-CT	positron emission tomography–computed tomography
PR	progesterone receptor
RNA	ribonucleic acid
RT-PCR	reverse transcription polymerase chain reaction
SEER Program	Surveillance, Epidemiology, and End Results Program
SNP	single-nucleotide polymorphism
TNM	tumour, node, metastasis
UV	ultraviolet

Foreword

The WHO Classification of Tumours, published as a series of books (also known as the WHO Blue Books) and now as a website (https://tumourclassification.iarc.who.int), is an essential tool for standardizing diagnostic practice worldwide. It also serves as a vehicle for the translation of cancer research into practice. The diagnostic criteria and standards that make up the classification are underpinned by evidence evaluated and debated by experts in the field. About 200 authors and editors participate in the production of each volume, and they give their time freely to this task. We are very grateful for their help; it is a remarkable international team effort of great significance to both patients and their doctors.

This volume, like the rest of the fifth edition, has been led by the WHO Classification of Tumours Editorial Board, composed of standing and expert members. The standing members, who have been nominated by pathology organizations, are the equivalent of the series editors of previous editions. The expert members for each volume, equivalent to the volume editors of previous editions, are selected on the basis of informed bibliometric analysis and advice from the standing members. The diagnostic process is increasingly multidisciplinary, and we are delighted that several radiology and clinical experts have joined us to address specific needs.

The most conspicuous change to the format of the books in the fifth edition is that tumour types common to multiple systems are dealt with together – so there are typically separate chapters on mesenchymal tumours, melanocytic tumours, haematolymphoid tumours, and neuroendocrine tumours. There is also a chapter on genetic tumour syndromes. Genetic disorders are of increasing importance to diagnosis in individual patients, and the study of these disorders has undoubtedly informed our understanding of tumour biology and behaviour over the past decade.

We have attempted to take a more systematic approach to the multifaceted nature of tumour classification; each tumour type is described on the basis of its localization, clinical features, epidemiology, etiology, pathogenesis, histopathology, diagnostic molecular pathology, staging, and prognosis and prediction. We have also included information on macroscopic appearance and cytology, as well as essential and desirable diagnostic criteria. This standardized, modular approach makes it easier for the books to be accessible online, and it also enables us to call attention to areas in which there is little information, and where serious gaps in our knowledge remain to be addressed.

Table A Approximate number of fields per 1 mm^2 based on the field diameter and its corresponding area

Field diameter (mm)	Field area (mm^2)	Approximate number of fields per 1 mm^2
0.40	0.126	8
0.41	0.132	8
0.42	0.138	7
0.43	0.145	7
0.44	0.152	7
0.45	0.159	6
0.46	0.166	6
0.47	0.173	6
0.48	0.181	6
0.49	0.188	5
0.50	0.196	5
0.51	0.204	5
0.52	0.212	5
0.53	0.221	5
0.54	0.229	4
0.55	0.237	4
0.56	0.246	4
0.57	0.255	4
0.58	0.264	4
0.59	0.273	4
0.60	0.283	4
0.61	0.292	3
0.62	0.302	3
0.63	0.312	3
0.64	0.322	3
0.65	0.332	3
0.66	0.342	3
0.67	0.352	3
0.68	0.363	3
0.69	0.374	3

The organization of the WHO Blue Books content now follows the normal progression from benign to malignant – a break with the fourth edition, but one we hope will be welcome.

Most volumes are still organized by anatomical site (digestive system, breast, soft tissue and bone, etc.), and each tumour type is listed within a taxonomic classification that follows the format below, which helps to structure the books in a systematic manner:

Site: e.g. head and neck

    Category: e.g. nasopharyngeal tumours

        Family (class): e.g. carcinomas

            Type: e.g. nasopharyngeal carcinoma

                Subtype: e.g. non-keratinizing squamous cell carcinoma

The issue of whether a given tumour type represents a distinct entity rather than a subtype continues to exercise pathologists, and it is the topic of many publications in the literature. We continue to deal with this issue on a case-by-case basis, but we believe there are inherent rules that can be applied. For example, tumours in which multiple histological patterns contain shared truncal mutations are clearly of the same type, despite the differences in their appearance. Equally, genetic heterogeneity within the same tumour type may have implications for treatment. A small shift in terminology in the fifth edition is that the term "variant" in reference to a specific kind of tumour has been wholly superseded by "subtype", in an effort to more clearly differentiate this meaning from that of "variant" in reference to a genetic alteration.

Another important change in this edition of the WHO Classification of Tumours series is the conversion of mitotic count from the traditional denominator of 10 HPF to a defined area expressed in mm^2 {969}. This serves to standardize the true area over which mitoses are enumerated, because different microscopes have high-power fields of different sizes. This change will also be helpful for anyone reporting using digital systems. The approximate number of fields per 1 mm^2 based on the field diameter and its corresponding area is presented in Table A.

We are continually working to improve the consistency and standards within the classification. In addition to having moved to the International System of Units (SI) for all mitotic counts, we have standardized genomic nomenclature by using Human Genome Variation Society (HGVS) notation. This includes the recent move in fusion gene notation to the separation of involved genes by a double colon (e.g. *BCR::ABL1*) {604}. We have also standardized our use of units of length, adopting the convention used by the International Collaboration on Cancer Reporting (https://www.iccr-cancer.org/) and the UK Royal College of Pathologists (https://www.rcpath.org/), so that the size of tumours is now given exclusively in millimetres (mm) rather than centimetres (cm). This is clearer, in our view, and avoids the use of decimal points – a common source of medical errors.

The WHO Blue Books are much appreciated by pathologists of all types, and they are of increasing importance to practitioners of other clinical disciplines involved in cancer management, as well as to researchers. We, along with the entire editorial board, certainly hope that the series will continue to meet the need for standards in diagnosis and to facilitate the translation of diagnostic research into practice worldwide. It is particularly important that cancers continue to be classified and diagnosed according to the same standards internationally so that patients can benefit from multicentre clinical trials, as well as from the results of local trials conducted on different continents.

Dr Ian A. Cree
Former Head, WHO Classification of Tumours Programme
International Agency for Research on Cancer

Dr Dilani Lokuhetty
Head, WHO Classification of Tumours Programme
International Agency for Research on Cancer

ICD-O topographical coding of head and neck tumours

The ICD-O topography codes for the main anatomical sites covered in this volume are as follows {1482}:

C00–C14 Lip, oral cavity, and pharynx

C00 Lip
C00.0 External upper lip
C00.1 External lower lip
C00.2 External lip, NOS
C00.3 Mucosa of upper lip
C00.4 Mucosa of lower lip
C00.5 Mucosa of lip, NOS
C00.6 Commissure of lip
C00.8 Overlapping lesion of lip
C00.9 Lip, NOS

C01 Base of tongue
C01.9 Base of tongue, NOS

C02 Other and unspecified parts of tongue
C02.0 Dorsal surface of tongue, NOS
C02.1 Border of tongue
C02.2 Ventral surface of tongue, NOS
C02.3 Anterior two thirds of tongue, NOS
C02.4 Lingual tonsil
C02.8 Overlapping lesion of tongue
C02.9 Tongue, NOS

C03 Gum
C03.0 Upper gum
C03.1 Lower gum
C03.9 Gum, NOS

C04 Floor of mouth
C04.0 Anterior floor of mouth
C04.1 Lateral floor of mouth
C04.8 Overlapping lesion of floor of mouth
C04.9 Floor of mouth, NOS

C05 Palate
C05.0 Hard palate
C05.1 Soft palate, NOS
C05.2 Uvula
C05.8 Overlapping lesion of palate
C05.9 Palate, NOS

C06 Other and unspecified parts of mouth
C06.0 Cheek mucosa
C06.1 Vestibule of mouth
C06.2 Retromolar area
C06.8 Overlapping lesion of other and unspecified parts of mouth
C06.9 Mouth, NOS

C07 Parotid gland
C07.9 Parotid gland

C08 Other and unspecified major salivary glands
C08.0 Submandibular gland
C08.1 Sublingual gland
C08.8 Overlapping lesion of major salivary glands
C08.9 Major salivary gland, NOS

C09 Tonsil
C09.0 Tonsillar fossa
C09.1 Tonsillar pillar
C09.8 Overlapping lesion of tonsil
C09.9 Tonsil, NOS

C10 Oropharynx
C10.0 Vallecula
C10.1 Anterior surface of epiglottis
C10.2 Lateral wall of oropharynx
C10.3 Posterior wall of oropharynx
C10.4 Branchial cleft
C10.8 Overlapping lesion of oropharynx
C10.9 Oropharynx, NOS

C11 Nasopharynx
C11.0 Superior wall of nasopharynx
C11.1 Posterior wall of nasopharynx
C11.2 Lateral wall of nasopharynx
C11.3 Anterior wall of nasopharynx
C11.8 Overlapping lesion of nasopharynx
C11.9 Nasopharynx, NOS

C12 Piriform sinus
C12.9 Piriform sinus

C13 Hypopharynx
C13.0 Postcricoid region
C13.1 Hypopharyngeal aspect of aryepiglottic fold
C13.2 Posterior wall of hypopharynx
C13.8 Overlapping lesion of hypopharynx
C13.9 Hypopharynx, NOS

C14 Other and ill-defined sites in lip, oral cavity, and pharynx
C14.0 Pharynx, NOS
C14.2 Waldeyer ring
C14.8 Overlapping lesion of lip, oral cavity, and pharynx

C30–C39 Respiratory system and intrathoracic organs
C30 Nasal cavity and middle ear
> C30.0 Nasal cavity
> C30.1 Middle ear

C31 Accessory sinuses
> C31.0 Maxillary sinus
> C31.1 Ethmoid sinus
> C31.2 Frontal sinus
> C31.3 Sphenoid sinus
> C31.8 Overlapping lesion of accessory sinuses
> C31.9 Accessory sinus, NOS

C32 Larynx
> C32.0 Glottis
> C32.1 Supraglottis
> C32.2 Subglottis
> C32.3 Laryngeal cartilage
> C32.8 Overlapping lesion of larynx
> C32.9 Larynx, NOS

C40–C41 Bones, joints, and articular cartilage
C41 Bones, joints, and articular cartilage of other and unspecified sites
> C41.0 Bones of skull and face and associated joints
> C41.1 Mandible
> C41.2 Vertebral column
> C41.8 Overlapping lesion of bones, joints, and articular cartilage

C44 Skin
> C44.0 Skin of lip, NOS
> C44.1 Eyelid
> C44.2 External ear
> C44.3 Skin of other and unspecified parts of face
> C44.4 Skin of scalp and neck
> C44.8 Overlapping lesion of skin

C47 Peripheral nerves and autonomic nervous system
> C47.0 Peripheral nerves and autonomic nervous system of head, face, and neck

C49 Connective, subcutaneous, and other soft tissues
> C49.0 Connective, subcutaneous, and other soft tissues of head, face, and neck

C76 Other and ill-defined sites
> C76.0 Head, face, or neck, NOS

C77 Lymph nodes
> C77.0 Lymph nodes of head, face, and neck

C80 Unknown primary site
> C80.9 Unknown primary site

ICD-O morphological coding: Introduction

The ICD-O coding system uses a topography (T) code and a morphology (M) code together, but these are presented in separate lists for ease of use. Behaviour is coded /0 for benign tumours; /1 for unspecified, borderline, or uncertain behaviour; /2 for carcinoma in situ and grade III intraepithelial neoplasia; /3 for malignant tumours, primary site; and /6 for malignant tumours, metastatic site. Behaviour code /6 is not generally used by cancer registries. For various reasons, the ICD-O morphology terms may not always be identical to the entity names used in the WHO classification, but they should be sufficiently similar to avoid confusion. The designation "NOS" ("not otherwise specified") is provided to make coding possible when subtypes exist but exact classification may not be possible in small biopsies or certain other scenarios. Therefore, it is usual to have "NOS" even when a more specific alternative term is listed in ICD-O.

ICD-O coding of nasal, paranasal, and skull base tumours

ICD-O-3.2   ICD-O label (subtypes are indicated in grey text, with the label indented);
              Please note that the WHO classification of tumour types is more readily reflected in the table of contents

Hamartomas
Respiratory epithelial adenomatoid hamartoma
    Chondro-osseous respiratory epithelial hamartoma
Seromucinous hamartoma
Nasal chondromesenchymal hamartoma

Respiratory epithelial lesions
    Sinonasal papillomas
8121/1   Sinonasal papilloma, inverted
8121/1   Sinonasal papilloma, oncocytic
8121/0   Sinonasal papilloma, exophytic

Carcinomas
8071/3   Squamous cell carcinoma, keratinizing, NOS
8086/3   HPV-independent squamous cell carcinoma
8052/3   Papillary squamous cell carcinoma
8051/3   Verrucous carcinoma
8074/3   Spindle cell squamous cell carcinoma
8075/3   Acantholytic squamous cell carcinoma
8560/3   Adenosquamous carcinoma
8051/3   Carcinoma cuniculatum
8072/3   Squamous cell carcinoma, non-keratinizing, NOS
8085/3   HPV-associated squamous cell carcinoma
8072/3   *DEK::AFF2* squamous cell carcinoma
8023/3   NUT carcinoma
    SWI/SNF complex–deficient sinonasal carcinoma
8044/3   SMARCB1-deficient sinonasal carcinoma
8044/3   SMARCB1-deficient sinonasal adenocarcinoma
8044/3   SMARCA4-deficient sinonasal carcinoma
8082/3   Lymphoepithelial carcinoma
8020/3   Sinonasal undifferentiated carcinoma
9081/3   Teratocarcinosarcoma
8483/3   HPV-related multiphenotypic sinonasal carcinoma

Adenocarcinomas
8144/3   Intestinal-type adenocarcinoma
8140/3   Adenocarcinoma, NOS
8140/3   Renal cell–like sinonasal adenocarcinoma

Mesenchymal tumours of the sinonasal tract
9160/0	Angiofibroma, NOS
8824/0	Myopericytoma
9045/3	Biphenotypic sinonasal sarcoma
9370/3	Chordoma
9370/3	Conventional chordoma
9371/3	Chondroid chordoma
9372/3	Poorly differentiated chordoma
9372/3	Dedifferentiated chordoma

Other sinonasal tumours
9310/0	Ameloblastoma, NOS
9351/1	Adamantinomatous craniopharyngioma
9530/0	Meningioma, NOS
9531/0	Meningothelial meningioma
9533/0	Psammomatous meningioma
9522/3	Olfactory neuroblastoma

These morphology codes are from the International Classification of Diseases for Oncology, third edition, second revision (ICD-O-3.2) {2020}. Behaviour is coded /0 for benign tumours; /1 for unspecified, borderline, or uncertain behaviour; /2 for carcinoma in situ and grade III intraepithelial neoplasia; /3 for malignant tumours, primary site; and /6 for malignant tumours, metastatic site. Behaviour code /6 is not generally used by cancer registries.

This classification is modified from the previous WHO classification, taking into account changes in our understanding of these lesions.

n/a, not available (provisional entity).

* Codes marked with an asterisk were approved by the IARC/WHO Committee for ICD-O at its meeting in July 2022, or during subsequent consultation.

† Labels marked with a dagger have undergone a change in terminology of a previous code.

ICD-O coding of nasopharyngeal tumours

Hamartomas

    Hairy polyp
    Salivary gland anlage tumour

Carcinomas

8260/3   Low-grade nasopharyngeal papillary adenocarcinoma
8070/3   Nasopharyngeal carcinoma
8071/3   Squamous cell carcinoma, keratinizing, NOS
8072/3   Squamous cell carcinoma, non-keratinizing, NOS
8083/3   Basaloid squamous cell carcinoma

These morphology codes are from the International Classification of Diseases for Oncology, third edition, second revision (ICD-O-3.2) {2020}. Behaviour is coded /0 for benign tumours; /1 for unspecified, borderline, or uncertain behaviour; /2 for carcinoma in situ and grade III intraepithelial neoplasia; /3 for malignant tumours, primary site; and /6 for malignant tumours, metastatic site. Behaviour code /6 is not generally used by cancer registries.

This classification is modified from the previous WHO classification, taking into account changes in our understanding of these lesions.

n/a, not available (provisional entity).

* Codes marked with an asterisk were approved by the IARC/WHO Committee for ICD-O at its meeting in July 2022, or during subsequent consultation.

† Labels marked with a dagger have undergone a change in terminology of a previous code.

ICD-O coding of hypopharyngeal, laryngeal, tracheal, and parapharyngeal tumours

ICD-O-3.2   ICD-O label (subtypes are indicated in grey text, with the label indented);
                   Please note that the WHO classification of tumour types is more readily reflected in the table of contents

Precursor lesions
8052/0   Squamous papilloma
8060/0   Squamous papillomatosis
                Laryngeal and hypopharyngeal epithelial dysplasia
8077/0   Squamous intraepithelial neoplasia, low grade
8077/2   Squamous intraepithelial neoplasia, high grade
8070/2   Squamous cell carcinoma in situ, NOS

Squamous cell carcinomas
8070/3   Squamous cell carcinoma, NOS
8051/3   Verrucous carcinoma, NOS
8070/3   Hybrid verrucous carcinoma
8083/3   Basaloid squamous cell carcinoma
8052/3   Papillary squamous cell carcinoma
8074/3   Squamous cell carcinoma, spindle cell
8560/3   Adenosquamous carcinoma
8082/3   Lymphoepithelial carcinoma

Mesenchymal tumours unique to the hypopharynx, larynx, trachea, and parapharyngeal space
Laryngeal cartilaginous tumours
9220/0   Chondroma
9220/3   Chondrosarcoma
9242/3   Clear cell chondrosarcoma
9243/3   Dedifferentiated chondrosarcoma

These morphology codes are from the International Classification of Diseases for Oncology, third edition, second revision (ICD-O-3.2) {2020}. Behaviour is coded /0 for benign tumours; /1 for unspecified, borderline, or uncertain behaviour; /2 for carcinoma in situ and grade III intraepithelial neoplasia; /3 for malignant tumours, primary site; and /6 for malignant tumours, metastatic site. Behaviour code /6 is not generally used by cancer registries.

This classification is modified from the previous WHO classification, taking into account changes in our understanding of these lesions.

n/a, not available (provisional entity).

* Codes marked with an asterisk were approved by the IARC/WHO Committee for ICD-O at its meeting in July 2022, or during subsequent consultation.

† Labels marked with a dagger have undergone a change in terminology of a previous code.

ICD-O coding of salivary gland tumours

ICD-O-3.2   ICD-O label (subtypes are indicated in grey text, with the label indented);
                  Please note that the WHO classification of tumour types is more readily reflected in the table of contents

Non-neoplastic epithelial lesions
Nodular oncocytic hyperplasia
Lymphoepithelial sialadenitis

Benign epithelial tumours
8940/0	Pleomorphic adenoma
8940/3*	Metastasizing pleomorphic adenoma
8940/0	Oncocytic pleomorphic adenoma
8147/0	Basal cell adenoma
8147/0	Membranous basal cell adenoma
8561/0	Warthin tumour
8561/0	Infarcted/metaplastic Warthin tumour
8290/0	Oncocytoma
8290/0	Clear cell oncocytoma
8982/0	Myoepithelioma
8149/0	Canalicular adenoma
8440/0	Cystadenoma
8450/0	Papillary cystadenoma
8440/0	Oncocytic cystadenoma
8470/0	Mucinous cystadenoma
8503/0	Intraductal papilloma
8406/0	Sialadenoma papilliferum
8563/0	Lymphadenoma
8563/0	Sebaceous lymphadenoma
8563/0	Non-sebaceous lymphadenoma
8410/0	Sebaceous adenoma
	Intercalated duct adenoma and hyperplasia
8503/0	Striated duct adenoma
8140/0	Sclerosing polycystic adenoma
8052/0	Keratocystoma

Malignant epithelial tumours
8430/3	Mucoepidermoid carcinoma
9270/3	Central intraosseous mucoepidermoid carcinoma
8200/3	Adenoid cystic carcinoma
8550/3	Acinic cell carcinoma
8502/3	Secretory carcinoma
8502/3	Microsecretory adenocarcinoma
8525/3	Polymorphous adenocarcinoma
8525/3	Polymorphous adenocarcinoma, conventional subtype
8525/3	Polymorphous adenocarcinoma, cribriform subtype (cribriform adenocarcinoma of the salivary glands)
8310/3	Hyalinizing clear cell carcinoma
8147/3	Basal cell adenocarcinoma
8500/2	Intraductal carcinoma
8500/2	Intercalated duct intraductal carcinoma
8500/2	Apocrine intraductal carcinoma
8500/2	Oncocytic intraductal carcinoma
8500/2	Mixed intraductal carcinoma
8500/3	Salivary duct carcinoma
8033/3	Sarcomatoid salivary duct carcinoma
8481/3	Mucin-rich salivary duct carcinoma
8265/3	Micropapillary salivary duct carcinoma
8500/3	Basal-like salivary duct carcinoma
8290/3	Oncocytic salivary duct carcinoma

| ICD-O-3.2 | ICD-O label (subtypes are indicated in grey text, with the label indented); |
| Please note that the WHO classification of tumour types is more readily reflected in the table of contents |

8982/3	Myoepithelial carcinoma
8562/3	Epithelial-myoepithelial carcinoma
8480/3	Mucinous adenocarcinoma
8407/3	Sclerosing microcystic adenocarcinoma
8941/3	Carcinoma ex pleomorphic adenoma
8980/3	Carcinosarcoma
8410/3	Sebaceous adenocarcinoma
8082/3	Lymphoepithelial carcinoma
8070/3	Squamous cell carcinoma, NOS
8974/1	Sialoblastoma
8140/3	Adenocarcinoma, NOS
8290/3	Oncocytic adenocarcinoma
8144/3	Intestinal-type adenocarcinoma

Mesenchymal tumours specific to the salivary glands
8850/0	Sialolipoma
8850/0	Oncocytic lipoadenoma

These morphology codes are from the International Classification of Diseases for Oncology, third edition, second revision (ICD-O-3.2) {2020}. Behaviour is coded /0 for benign tumours; /1 for unspecified, borderline, or uncertain behaviour; /2 for carcinoma in situ and grade III intraepithelial neoplasia; /3 for malignant tumours, primary site; and /6 for malignant tumours, metastatic site. Behaviour code /6 is not generally used by cancer registries.

This classification is modified from the previous WHO classification, taking into account changes in our understanding of these lesions.

n/a, not available (provisional entity).

* Codes marked with an asterisk were approved by the IARC/WHO Committee for ICD-O at its meeting in July 2022, or during subsequent consultation.

† Labels marked with a dagger have undergone a change in terminology of a previous code.

ICD-O coding of oral cavity and mobile tongue tumours

ICD-O-3.2   ICD-O label (subtypes are indicated in grey text, with the label indented);
                 Please note that the WHO classification of tumour types is more readily reflected in the table of contents

Non-neoplastic lesions
        Necrotizing sialometaplasia
        Multifocal epithelial hyperplasia
        Oral melanoacanthoma

Epithelial tumours
Papillomas
8052/0   Squamous papilloma
           Condyloma acuminatum
           Verruca vulgaris

Oral potentially malignant disorders and oral epithelial dysplasia
        Oral potentially malignant disorders
        Proliferative verrucous leukoplakia
        Submucous fibrosis
8077/0   Low-grade squamous intraepithelial lesion
8077/2   High-grade squamous intraepithelial lesion
8085/0   HPV-associated oral epithelial dysplasia, low grade
8085/2   HPV-associated oral epithelial dysplasia, high grade

Squamous cell carcinomas
8070/3   Squamous cell carcinoma
8074/3   Spindle cell squamous cell carcinoma
8083/3   Basaloid squamous cell carcinoma
8075/3   Acantholytic squamous cell carcinoma
8560/3   Adenosquamous carcinoma
8052/3   Papillary squamous cell carcinoma
8082/3   Lymphoepithelial carcinoma
8051/3   Verrucous carcinoma, NOS
8051/3   Carcinoma cuniculatum

Tumours of uncertain histogenesis
        Congenital granular cell epulis
9580/0   Granular cell tumour, NOS
9580/3   Granular cell tumour, malignant
8982/0   Ectomesenchymal chondromyxoid tumour
9363/1   Melanotic neuroectodermal tumour, NOS
9363/3   Melanotic neuroectodermal tumour, malignant

These morphology codes are from the International Classification of Diseases for Oncology, third edition, second revision (ICD-O-3.2) {2020}. Behaviour is coded /0 for benign tumours; /1 for unspecified, borderline, or uncertain behaviour; /2 for carcinoma in situ and grade III intraepithelial neoplasia; /3 for malignant tumours, primary site; and /6 for malignant tumours, metastatic site. Behaviour code /6 is not generally used by cancer registries.

This classification is modified from the previous WHO classification, taking into account changes in our understanding of these lesions.

n/a, not available (provisional entity).

* Codes marked with an asterisk were approved by the IARC/WHO Committee for ICD-O at its meeting in July 2022, or during subsequent consultation.

† Labels marked with a dagger have undergone a change in terminology of a previous code.

ICD-O coding of oropharyngeal tumours

ICD-O-3.2   ICD-O label (subtypes are indicated in grey text, with the label indented);
Please note that the WHO classification of tumour types is more readily reflected in the table of contents

Benign oropharyngeal lesions
        Hamartomatous polyps

Epithelial tumours
Squamous cell carcinoma

Code	Label
8085/3	Squamous cell carcinoma, HPV-associated
8085/3	Non-keratinizing squamous cell carcinoma, HPV-associated
8085/3	Keratinizing squamous cell carcinoma, HPV-associated
8085/3	Papillary squamous cell carcinoma, HPV-associated
8085/3	Adenosquamous carcinoma, HPV-associated
8085/3	Ciliated adenosquamous carcinoma, HPV-associated
8085/3	Lymphoepithelial carcinoma, HPV-associated
8085/3	Spindle cell / sarcomatoid squamous cell carcinoma, HPV-associated
8085/3	Basaloid squamous cell carcinoma, HPV-associated
8086/3	Squamous cell carcinoma, HPV-independent
8086/3	Keratinizing squamous cell carcinoma, HPV-independent
8086/3	Verrucous carcinoma, HPV-independent
8086/3	Basaloid squamous cell carcinoma, HPV-independent
8086/3	Papillary squamous cell carcinoma, HPV-independent
8086/3	Spindle cell / sarcomatoid squamous cell carcinoma, HPV-independent
8086/3	Adenosquamous carcinoma, HPV-independent
8086/3	Lymphoepithelial carcinoma, HPV-independent

These morphology codes are from the International Classification of Diseases for Oncology, third edition, second revision (ICD-O-3.2) {2020}. Behaviour is coded /0 for benign tumours; /1 for unspecified, borderline, or uncertain behaviour; /2 for carcinoma in situ and grade III intraepithelial neoplasia; /3 for malignant tumours, primary site; and /6 for malignant tumours, metastatic site. Behaviour code /6 is not generally used by cancer registries.

This classification is modified from the previous WHO classification, taking into account changes in our understanding of these lesions.

n/a, not available (provisional entity).

* Codes marked with an asterisk were approved by the IARC/WHO Committee for ICD-O at its meeting in July 2022, or during subsequent consultation.

† Labels marked with a dagger have undergone a change in terminology of a previous code.

ICD-O coding of odontogenic and maxillofacial bone tumours

ICD-O-3.2 ICD-O label (subtypes are indicated in grey text, with the label indented);
Please note that the WHO classification of tumour types is more readily reflected in the table of contents

Cysts of the jaw

Radicular cyst
   Residual cyst (residual radicular cyst)
Inflammatory collateral cysts
   Paradental cyst
   Mandibular buccal bifurcation cyst
Surgical ciliated cyst
Nasopalatine duct cyst
Gingival cysts
Dentigerous cyst
   Eruption cyst
Orthokeratinized odontogenic cyst
Lateral periodontal cyst
   Botryoid odontogenic cyst
Calcifying odontogenic cyst
Glandular odontogenic cyst
Odontogenic keratocyst

Odontogenic tumours

Benign epithelial odontogenic tumours

9300/0	Adenomatoid odontogenic tumour
9312/0	Squamous odontogenic tumour
9340/0	Calcifying epithelial odontogenic tumour
9340/0	Clear cell calcifying epithelial odontogenic tumour
9340/0	Cystic/microcystic calcifying epithelial odontogenic tumour
9340/0	Non-calcifying / Langerhans cell–rich calcifying epithelial odontogenic tumour
9310/0	Ameloblastoma, unicystic
9310/0	Luminal ameloblastoma, unicystic
9310/0	Intraluminal ameloblastoma, unicystic
9310/0	Mural ameloblastoma, unicystic
9310/0	Ameloblastoma, extraosseous/peripheral
9310/0	Ameloblastoma, NOS
9310/0	Follicular ameloblastoma
9310/0	Plexiform ameloblastoma
9310/0	Acanthomatous ameloblastoma
9310/0	Granular cell ameloblastoma
9310/0	Basal cell ameloblastoma
9310/0	Desmoplastic ameloblastoma
9310/0	Adenoid ameloblastoma
9310/3	Ameloblastoma, metastasizing

Benign mixed epithelial and mesenchymal odontogenic tumours

9280/0	Odontoma, NOS
9280/0	Complex odontoma
9280/0	Compound odontoma
	Primordial odontogenic tumour
9330/0	Ameloblastic fibroma
9302/0	Dentinogenic ghost cell tumour

Benign mesenchymal odontogenic tumours

9321/0	Odontogenic fibroma, NOS
9321/0	Odontogenic fibroma, amyloid subtype
9321/0	Odontogenic fibroma, granular cell subtype
9321/0	Hybrid odontogenic fibroma with central giant cell granuloma
9273/0	Cementoblastoma
9274/0	Cemento-ossifying fibroma
9320/0	Odontogenic myxoma

Malignant odontogenic tumours

9270/3	Sclerosing odontogenic carcinoma
9270/3	Ameloblastic carcinoma
9341/3	Clear cell odontogenic carcinoma
9302/3	Ghost cell odontogenic carcinoma
9270/3	Primary intraosseous carcinoma, NOS
9342/3	Odontogenic carcinosarcoma
9330/3	Odontogenic sarcomas
9330/3	Ameloblastic fibrosarcoma
9330/3	Ameloblastic fibrodentinosarcoma
9330/3	Ameloblastic fibro-odontosarcoma

Giant cell lesions and bone cysts

	Central giant cell granuloma
	Peripheral giant cell granuloma
	Cherubism
9260/0	Aneurysmal bone cyst
	Simple bone cyst

Bone and cartilage tumours

Fibro-osseous tumours and dysplasias

	Cemento-osseous dysplasia
	Periapical cemento-osseous dysplasia
	Focal cemento-osseous dysplasia
	Florid cemento-osseous dysplasia
	Familial florid cemento-osseous dysplasia
	Segmental odontomaxillary dysplasia
8818/0	Fibrous dysplasia
8818/0	Monostotic fibrous dysplasia
8818/0	Polyostotic fibrous dysplasia
8818/0	Craniofacial fibrous dysplasia
9262/0	Juvenile trabecular ossifying fibroma
9262/0	Psammomatoid ossifying fibroma
	Familial gigantiform cementoma

Benign maxillofacial bone and cartilage tumours

9180/0	Osteoma
9180/0	Surface (periosteal) osteoma
9180/0	Central (endosteal) osteoma
9210/0	Osteochondroma
9200/1	Osteoblastoma, NOS
9230/0	Chondroblastoma, NOS
9241/0	Chondromyxoid fibroma
8823/1	Desmoplastic fibroma

ICD-O-3.2   ICD-O label (subtypes are indicated in grey text, with the label indented);
                Please note that the WHO classification of tumour types is more readily reflected in the table of contents

Malignant maxillofacial bone and cartilage tumours
9180/3   Osteosarcoma, NOS
9186/3   Conventional osteosarcoma
9185/3   Small cell osteosarcoma
9183/3   Telangiectatic osteosarcoma
9187/3   Low-grade central osteosarcoma
9192/3   Parosteal osteosarcoma
9193/3   Periosteal osteosarcoma
9194/3   High-grade surface osteosarcoma
9184/3   Radiation-induced osteosarcoma
                The chondrosarcoma family of tumours
9222/3   Chondrosarcoma, grade 1
9220/3   Chondrosarcoma, grade 2
9220/3   Chondrosarcoma, grade 3
9221/3   Periosteal chondrosarcoma
9243/3   Dedifferentiated chondrosarcoma
9242/3   Clear cell chondrosarcoma
9240/3   Mesenchymal chondrosarcoma
8900/3   Rhabdomyosarcoma with *TFCP2* rearrangement

These morphology codes are from the International Classification of Diseases for Oncology, third edition, second revision (ICD-O-3.2) {2020}. Behaviour is coded /0 for benign tumours; /1 for unspecified, borderline, or uncertain behaviour; /2 for carcinoma in situ and grade III intraepithelial neoplasia; /3 for malignant tumours, primary site; and /6 for malignant tumours, metastatic site. Behaviour code /6 is not generally used by cancer registries.

This classification is modified from the previous WHO classification, taking into account changes in our understanding of these lesions.

n/a, not available (provisional entity).

* Codes marked with an asterisk were approved by the IARC/WHO Committee for ICD-O at its meeting in July 2022, or during subsequent consultation.

† Labels marked with a dagger have undergone a change in terminology of a previous code.

ICD-O coding of ear tumours

ICD-O-3.2   ICD-O label (subtypes are indicated in grey text, with the label indented);
                   Please note that the WHO classification of tumour types is more readily reflected in the table of contents

Tumours of the external auditory canal
	Chondrodermatitis nodularis chronica helicis
	Cystic chondromalacia
9180/0	Osteoma, NOS
8420/0	Ceruminous adenoma
8420/0	Ceruminous pleomorphic adenoma
8420/0	Ceruminous syringocystadenoma papilliferum
8420/3	Ceruminous adenocarcinoma
8420/3	Ceruminous adenoid cystic carcinoma
8420/3	Ceruminous mucoepidermoid carcinoma
8070/3	Squamous cell carcinoma, NOS

Tumours of the middle and inner ear
	Otosclerosis
	Clinical otosclerosis
	Histological otosclerosis
	Cholesteatoma
	Congenital cholesteatoma
	Acquired cholesteatoma
8121/0	Middle ear papilloma
8121/1	Inverted sinonasal-type papilloma
8121/0	Oncocytic sinonasal-type papilloma
8121/0	Exophytic sinonasal-type papilloma
9560/0	Schwannoma, NOS
9560/0	Ancient schwannoma
9560/0	Cellular schwannoma
9560/0	Plexiform schwannoma
9560/0	Epithelioid schwannoma
9560/0	Microcystic/reticular schwannoma
8240/3*	Middle ear neuroendocrine tumour
8140/3	Endolymphatic sac tumour
8070/3	Squamous cell carcinoma, NOS
8260/3	Middle ear adenocarcinoma

These morphology codes are from the International Classification of Diseases for Oncology, third edition, second revision (ICD-O-3.2) {2020}. Behaviour is coded /0 for benign tumours; /1 for unspecified, borderline, or uncertain behaviour; /2 for carcinoma in situ and grade III intraepithelial neoplasia; /3 for malignant tumours, primary site; and /6 for malignant tumours, metastatic site. Behaviour code /6 is not generally used by cancer registries.

This classification is modified from the previous WHO classification, taking into account changes in our understanding of these lesions.

n/a, not available (provisional entity).

* Codes marked with an asterisk were approved by the IARC/WHO Committee for ICD-O at its meeting in July 2022, or during subsequent consultation.

† Labels marked with a dagger have undergone a change in terminology of a previous code.

ICD-O coding of soft tissue tumours

ICD-O-3.2   ICD-O label (subtypes are indicated in grey text, with the label indented);
Please note that the WHO classification of tumour types is more readily reflected in the table of contents

Adipocytic tumours
8850/0	Lipoma, NOS
8857/0	Atypical spindle cell / pleomorphic lipomatous tumour
8850/1	Atypical lipomatous tumour
8851/3	Liposarcoma, well-differentiated, NOS
8858/3	Dedifferentiated liposarcoma
8852/3	Myxoid liposarcoma
8854/3	Pleomorphic liposarcoma

Fibroblastic and myofibroblastic tumours
8828/0	Nodular fasciitis
8828/0	Intravascular fasciitis
8828/0	Cranial fasciitis
8821/1	Desmoid-type fibromatosis
8815/0	Solitary fibrous tumour, benign
8815/1	Solitary fibrous tumour, NOS
8815/1	Lipomatous solitary fibrous tumour
8815/1	Giant cell–rich solitary fibrous tumour
8815/3	Solitary fibrous tumour, malignant
8825/3	Low-grade myofibroblastic sarcoma
8825/1	Inflammatory myofibroblastic tumour
8825/1	Epithelioid inflammatory myofibroblastic sarcoma

Vascular tumours
9120/0	Haemangioma, NOS
9131/0	Capillary haemangioma
9121/0	Cavernous haemangioma
9131/0	Lobular capillary haemangioma
9125/0	Epithelioid haemangioma
9125/0	Cellular epithelioid haemangioma
9125/0	Atypical epithelioid haemangioma
9170/0	Lymphangioma, NOS
9170/0	Mixed lymphangioma
9173/0	Cystic lymphangioma
9173/0	Microcystic lymphangioma
9173/0	Macrocystic lymphangioma
9133/3	Epithelioid haemangioendothelioma, NOS
9133/3	Epithelioid haemangioendothelioma with *WWTR1::CAMTA1* fusion
9133/3	Epithelioid haemangioendothelioma with *YAP1::TFE3* fusion
9140/3	Kaposi sarcoma
9140/3	Classic indolent Kaposi sarcoma
9140/3	Endemic African Kaposi sarcoma
9140/3	AIDS-associated Kaposi sarcoma
9140/3	Iatrogenic Kaposi sarcoma
9120/3	Angiosarcoma

Pericytic (perivascular) tumours
8824/0	Myopericytoma

Smooth muscle tumours
8890/0	Leiomyoma, NOS
8894/0	Angioleiomyoma
8897/1	EBV-associated smooth muscle tumour
8897/1	Smooth muscle tumour of uncertain malignant potential
8890/3	Leiomyosarcoma, NOS

Skeletal muscle tumours

8900/0	Rhabdomyoma, NOS
8904/0	Adult-type rhabdomyoma
8903/0	Fetal-type rhabdomyoma
8900/3	Rhabdomyosarcoma, NOS
8910/3	Embryonal rhabdomyosarcoma
8912/3	Spindle cell rhabdomyosarcoma
8920/3	Alveolar rhabdomyosarcoma
8901/3	Pleomorphic rhabdomyosarcoma

Chondro-osseous tumours

9220/0	Chondroma, NOS
9220/0	Chondroblastoma-like soft tissue chondroma

Peripheral nerve sheath tumours

Neurofibroma

9540/0	Neurofibroma, NOS
9540/0	Ancient neurofibroma
9540/0	Cellular neurofibroma
9550/0	Plexiform neurofibroma
9540/0	Atypical neurofibroma

Schwannoma

9560/0	Schwannoma, NOS
9560/0	Ancient schwannoma
9560/0	Cellular schwannoma
9560/0	Plexiform schwannoma
9560/0	Epithelioid schwannoma
9560/0	Microcystic reticular schwannoma

Neuromas

	Traumatic neuroma
9570/0	Solitary circumscribed neuroma
	MEN2B-mucosal neuroma
	Oral pseudoperineurioma
	PIK3CA-related overgrowth spectrum–associated neuromas

Malignant peripheral nerve sheath tumour

9540/3	Malignant peripheral nerve sheath tumour, NOS
9542/3	Epithelioid malignant peripheral nerve sheath tumour

ICD-O-3.2   ICD-O label (subtypes are indicated in grey text, with the label indented);
              Please note that the WHO classification of tumour types is more readily reflected in the table of contents

Tumours of uncertain differentiation

8990/0	Phosphaturic mesenchymal tumour, NOS
8990/3	Phosphaturic mesenchymal tumour, malignant
8840/0	Myxoma, NOS
9231/3	Extraskeletal myxoid chondrosarcoma
9040/3	Synovial sarcoma, NOS
9041/3	Synovial sarcoma, monophasic
9043/3	Synovial sarcoma, biphasic
9040/3	Synovial sarcoma, poorly differentiated
9150/3	*GLI1*-altered soft tissue tumour
8805/3	Undifferentiated sarcoma
8801/3	Spindle cell sarcoma, undifferentiated
8802/3	Pleomorphic sarcoma, undifferentiated
8803/3	Round cell sarcoma, undifferentiated

Undifferentiated small round cell sarcomas of bone and soft tissue

9364/3	Ewing sarcoma
9364/3	Adamantinoma-like Ewing sarcoma

These morphology codes are from the International Classification of Diseases for Oncology, third edition, second revision (ICD-O-3.2) {2020}. Behaviour is coded /0 for benign tumours; /1 for unspecified, borderline, or uncertain behaviour; /2 for carcinoma in situ and grade III intraepithelial neoplasia; /3 for malignant tumours, primary site; and /6 for malignant tumours, metastatic site. Behaviour code /6 is not generally used by cancer registries.

This classification is modified from the previous WHO classification, taking into account changes in our understanding of these lesions.

n/a, not available (provisional entity).

* Codes marked with an asterisk were approved by the IARC/WHO Committee for ICD-O at its meeting in July 2022, or during subsequent consultation.

† Labels marked with a dagger have undergone a change in terminology of a previous code.

ICD-O coding of haematolymphoid proliferations and neoplasia

ICD-O-3.2   ICD-O label (subtypes are indicated in grey text, with the label indented);
                 Please note that the WHO classification of tumour types is more readily reflected in the table of contents

Reactive haematolymphoid and related lesions
	Reactive lymphoid hyperplasia
9680/1	EBV-positive mucocutaneous ulcer
9760/1*	IgG4-related disease

Myeloid tumours
9930/3	Myeloid sarcoma

B-cell lymphomas
9699/3	Extranodal marginal zone lymphoma
9673/3	Mantle cell lymphoma
9690/3	Follicular lymphoma
9690/3	Paediatric-type follicular lymphoma
9698/3	Large B-cell lymphoma with *IRF4* rearrangement
9680/3	Diffuse large B-cell lymphoma, NOS
9687/3	Burkitt lymphoma, NOS
9687/3	Endemic Burkitt lymphoma
9687/3	Sporadic Burkitt lymphoma
9687/3	Immunodeficiency-associated Burkitt lymphoma
9731/3	Plasmacytoma of bone
9735/3	Plasmablastic lymphoma

T/NK-cell tumours
9837/3	T-lymphoblastic leukaemia/lymphoma
9837/3	Cortical T-lymphoblastic leukaemia/lymphoma
9837/3	Medullary T-lymphoblastic leukaemia/lymphoma
9837/3	Early thymic precursor T-lymphoblastic leukaemia/lymphoma
9718/1	Primary mucosal CD30-positive T-cell lymphoproliferative disorder
9719/3	Extranodal NK/T-cell lymphoma
9719/3	Nasal lymphoma, involving the nasal and/or paranasal region
9719/3	Extranasal lymphoma, arising from the skin, gastrointestinal tract, testis, or soft tissue

Hodgkin lymphoma
9650/3	Classic Hodgkin lymphoma, NOS
9663/3	Classic Hodgkin lymphoma, nodular sclerosis
9652/3	Classic Hodgkin lymphoma, mixed cellularity
9651/3	Classic Hodgkin lymphoma, lymphocyte-rich
9653/3	Classic Hodgkin lymphoma, lymphocyte depletion
9659/3	Hodgkin lymphoma, nodular lymphocyte-predominant type

ICD-O-3.2   ICD-O label (subtypes are indicated in grey text, with the label indented);
Please note that the WHO classification of tumour types is more readily reflected in the table of contents

Histiocytic and dendritic cell tumours

9749/1	Juvenile xanthogranuloma
9749/3	Erdheim–Chester disease
9749/3	Rosai–Dorfman–Destombes disease†
9751/1	Langerhans cell histiocytosis, NOS
9751/1	Single-system Langerhans cell histiocytosis, with one organ/system involved (unifocal or multifocal)
9751/1	Multisystem Langerhans cell histiocytosis, with two or more organs/systems involved
9751/3	Langerhans cell histiocytosis, disseminated
9758/3	Follicular dendritic cell sarcoma
9758/3	EBV-positive inflammatory follicular dendritic cell sarcoma

---

These morphology codes are from the International Classification of Diseases for Oncology, third edition, second revision (ICD-O-3.2) {2020}. Behaviour is coded /0 for benign tumours; /1 for unspecified, borderline, or uncertain behaviour; /2 for carcinoma in situ and grade III intraepithelial neoplasia; /3 for malignant tumours, primary site; and /6 for malignant tumours, metastatic site. Behaviour code /6 is not generally used by cancer registries.

This classification is modified from the previous WHO classification, taking into account changes in our understanding of these lesions.

n/a, not available (provisional entity).

* Codes marked with an asterisk were approved by the IARC/WHO Committee for ICD-O at its meeting in July 2022, or during subsequent consultation.

† Labels marked with a dagger have undergone a change in terminology of a previous code.

ICD-O coding of melanocytic tumours

ICD-O-3.2	ICD-O label (subtypes are indicated in grey text, with the label indented); Please note that the WHO classification of tumour types is more readily reflected in the table of contents

8720/3	Mucosal melanoma
8745/3	Desmoplastic mucosal melanoma
8746/3	Mucosal lentiginous melanoma
8721/3	Nodular melanoma

These morphology codes are from the International Classification of Diseases for Oncology, third edition, second revision (ICD-O-3.2) (2020). Behaviour is coded /0 for benign tumours; /1 for unspecified, borderline, or uncertain behaviour; /2 for carcinoma in situ and grade III intraepithelial neoplasia; /3 for malignant tumours, primary site; and /6 for malignant tumours, metastatic site. Behaviour code /6 is not generally used by cancer registries.

This classification is modified from the previous WHO classification, taking into account changes in our understanding of these lesions.

n/a, not available (provisional entity).

* Codes marked with an asterisk were approved by the IARC/WHO Committee for ICD-O at its meeting in July 2022, or during subsequent consultation.

† Labels marked with a dagger have undergone a change in terminology of a previous code.

ICD-O coding of tumours and tumour-like lesions of the neck and lymph nodes

ICD-O-3.2   ICD-O label (subtypes are indicated in grey text, with the label indented);
             Please note that the WHO classification of tumour types is more readily reflected in the table of contents

Cysts and cyst-like lesions
              Ranula
                    Simple or oral ranula
                    Plunging or cervical ranula
              Lymphoepithelial cyst
              Branchial cleft cyst
              Thyroglossal duct cyst
              Dermoid and teratoid cysts

Other tumours of the neck and lymph nodes
              Branchioma
8010/3   Heterotopia-associated carcinoma
8010/3   Thyroid carcinoma
8010/3   Salivary carcinoma
8010/6   Carcinoma, metastatic, NOS

These morphology codes are from the International Classification of Diseases for Oncology, third edition, second revision (ICD-O-3.2) {2020}. Behaviour is coded /0 for benign tumours; /1 for unspecified, borderline, or uncertain behaviour; /2 for carcinoma in situ and grade III intraepithelial neoplasia; /3 for malignant tumours, primary site; and /6 for malignant tumours, metastatic site. Behaviour code /6 is not generally used by cancer registries.

This classification is modified from the previous WHO classification, taking into account changes in our understanding of these lesions.

n/a, not available (provisional entity).

* Codes marked with an asterisk were approved by the IARC/WHO Committee for ICD-O at its meeting in July 2022, or during subsequent consultation.

† Labels marked with a dagger have undergone a change in terminology of a previous code.

ICD-O coding of germ cell tumours

ICD-O-3.2   ICD-O label (subtypes are indicated in grey text, with the label indented);
Please note that the WHO classification of tumour types is more readily reflected in the table of contents

Germ cell tumours of the head and neck

9080/0	Mature teratoma
9080/3	Immature teratoma
9084/3	Teratoma with somatic-type malignancy
9064/3	Germinoma
9070/3	Embryonal carcinoma
9071/3	Yolk sac tumour
9100/3	Choriocarcinoma
9085/3	Mixed germ cell tumour

These morphology codes are from the International Classification of Diseases for Oncology, third edition, second revision (ICD-O-3.2) {2020}. Behaviour is coded /0 for benign tumours; /1 for unspecified, borderline, or uncertain behaviour; /2 for carcinoma in situ and grade III intraepithelial neoplasia; /3 for malignant tumours, primary site; and /6 for malignant tumours, metastatic site. Behaviour code /6 is not generally used by cancer registries.

This classification is modified from the previous WHO classification, taking into account changes in our understanding of these lesions.

n/a, not available (provisional entity).

* Codes marked with an asterisk were approved by the IARC/WHO Committee for ICD-O at its meeting in July 2022, or during subsequent consultation.

† Labels marked with a dagger have undergone a change in terminology of a previous code.

ICD-O coding of neuroendocrine neoplasms and paraganglioma

ICD-O-3.2   ICD-O label (subtypes are indicated in grey text, with the label indented);
                 Please note that the WHO classification of tumour types is more readily reflected in the table of contents

Neuroendocrine neoplasms
Neuroendocrine tumours
8240/3	Neuroendocrine tumour, NOS
8240/3	Neuroendocrine tumour, grade 1
8249/3	Neuroendocrine tumour, grade 2
8249/3	Neuroendocrine tumour, grade 3
8272/3	Pituitary neuroendocrine tumour (PitNET), NOS / pituitary adenoma, NOS
8272/3	Somatotroph PitNET
8271/3	Lactotroph PitNET
8280/3	Mammosomatotroph PitNET
8272/3	Thyrotroph PitNET
8272/3	Mature plurihormonal PIT1-lineage PitNET
8280/3	Acidophil stem cell PitNET
8272/3	Immature PIT1-lineage PitNET
8272/3	Corticotroph PitNET
8272/3	Gonadotroph PitNET
8272/3	Plurihormonal PitNET
8272/3	Null cell PitNET
8272/3	PitNET with metastasis (formerly pituitary carcinoma)[†]

Neuroendocrine carcinomas
8041/3	Small cell carcinoma
8045/3	Combined small cell carcinoma
8013/3	Large cell neuroendocrine carcinoma
8247/3	Merkel cell carcinoma

Paraganglion tumours
8693/3*	Head and neck paraganglioma
8693/3	Composite paraganglioma
8692/3	Carotid body paraganglioma
8693/3	Vagal paraganglioma
8690/3	Middle ear paraganglioma
8693/3	Laryngeal paraganglioma

These morphology codes are from the International Classification of Diseases for Oncology, third edition, second revision (ICD-O-3.2) {2020}. Behaviour is coded /0 for benign tumours; /1 for unspecified, borderline, or uncertain behaviour; /2 for carcinoma in situ and grade III intraepithelial neoplasia; /3 for malignant tumours, primary site; and /6 for malignant tumours, metastatic site. Behaviour code /6 is not generally used by cancer registries.

This classification is modified from the previous WHO classification, taking into account changes in our understanding of these lesions.

n/a, not available (provisional entity).

* Codes marked with an asterisk were approved by the IARC/WHO Committee for ICD-O at its meeting in July 2022, or during subsequent consultation.

[†] Labels marked with a dagger have undergone a change in terminology of a previous code.

TNM staging of head and neck tumours

Head and Neck Tumours

Introductory Notes
The following sites are included:
- Lip and oral cavity
- Pharynx: oropharynx (p16 negative and p16 positive), nasopharynx, hypopharynx
- Larynx: supraglottis, glottis, subglottis
- Nasal cavity and paranasal sinuses (maxillary and ethmoid sinus)
- Unknown primary carcinoma – cervical nodes
- Malignant melanoma of upper aerodigestive tract
- Major salivary glands

Carcinomas arising in minor salivary glands of the upper aerodigestive tract are classified according to the rules for tumours of their anatomic site of origin, e.g. oral cavity.

Each site is described under the following headings:
- Rules for classification with the procedures for assessing T, N, and M categories; additional methods may be used when they enhance the accuracy of appraisal before treatment
- Anatomical sites and subsites where appropriate
- Definition of the regional lymph nodes
- TNM clinical classification
- pTNM pathological classification
- Stage

Regional Lymph Nodes
Midline nodes are considered ipsilateral nodes.

TNM staging of carcinomas of the lip and oral cavity

Lip and Oral Cavity
(ICD-O-3 C00, C02-06)

Rules for Classification
The classification applies only to carcinomas of the vermilion surfaces of the lips and of the oral cavity, including those of minor salivary glands. There should be histological confirmation of the disease.

The following are the procedures for assessing T, N, and M categories:

T categories	Physical examination and imaging
N categories	Physical examination and imaging
M categories	Physical examination and imaging

Anatomical Sites and Subsites
Lip (C00)
1. External upper lip (vermilion border) (C00.0)
2. External lower lip (vermilion border) (C00.1)
3. Commissures (C00.6)

Oral Cavity (C02.0-C02.3, C02.9, C03-C06)*
1. Buccal mucosa
   a) Mucosa of upper and lower lips (C00.3, 4)
   b) Cheek mucosa (C06.0)
   c) Retromolar areas (C06.2)
   d) Buccoalveolar sulci, upper and lower (vestibule of mouth) (C06.1)
2. Upper alveolus and gingiva (upper gum) (C03.0)
3. Lower alveolus and gingiva (lower gum) (C03.1)
4. Hard palate (C05.0)
5. Tongue*
   a) Dorsal surface and lateral borders anterior to vallate papillae (anterior two-thirds) (C02.0, 1)
   b) Inferior (ventral) surface (C02.2)
6. Floor of mouth (C04)

Note
* Lingual tonsil (C02.4) is classified in the oropharynx.

Regional Lymph Nodes
The regional lymph nodes are the cervical nodes.

TNM Clinical Classification
T – Primary Tumour
TX	Primary tumour cannot be assessed
T0	No evidence of primary tumour
Tis	Carcinoma in situ
T1	Tumour 2 cm or less in greatest dimension and 5 mm or less depth of invasion*
T2	Tumour 2 cm or less in greatest dimension and more than 5 mm depth of invasion or tumour more than 2 cm but not more than 4 cm in greatest dimension and depth of invasion no more than 10 mm

T3	Tumour more than 2 cm but not more than 4 cm in greatest dimension and depth of invasion more than 10 mm or tumour more than 4 cm in greatest dimension and not more than 10 mm depth of invasion
T4a	*(Lip and oral cavity)* Tumour more than 4 cm in greatest dimension and more than 10 mm depth of invasion or *(Lip)* Tumour invades through cortical bone, inferior alveolar nerve, floor of mouth, or skin (of the chin or the nose) *(Oral cavity)* Tumour invades through the cortical bone of the mandible or maxilla or involves the maxillary sinus, or invades the skin of the face
T4b	*(Lip and oral cavity)* Tumour invades masticator space, pterygoid plates, or skull base, or encases internal carotid artery

Note
* Superficial erosion alone of bone/tooth socket by gingival primary is not sufficient to classify a tumour as T4a.

N – Regional Lymph Nodes
NX	Regional lymph nodes cannot be assessed
N0	No regional lymph node metastasis
N1	Metastasis in a single ipsilateral lymph node, 3 cm or less in greatest dimension without extranodal extension
N2	Metastasis described as:
	N2a Metastasis in a single ipsilateral lymph node, more than 3 cm but not more than 6 cm in greatest dimension without extranodal extension
	N2b Metastasis in multiple ipsilateral lymph nodes, none more than 6 cm in greatest dimension, without extranodal extension
	N2c Metastasis in bilateral or contralateral lymph nodes, none more than 6 cm in greatest dimension, without extranodal extension
N3a	Metastasis in a lymph node more than 6 cm in greatest dimension without extranodal extension
N3b	Metastasis in a single or multiple lymph nodes with clinical extranodal extension*

Notes
* The presence of skin involvement or soft tissue invasion with deep fixation/tethering to underlying muscle or adjacent structures or clinical signs of nerve involvement is classified as clinical extranodal extension.
Midline nodes are considered ipsilateral nodes.

M – Distant Metastasis
M0	No distant metastasis
M1	Distant metastasis

pTNM Pathological Classification
The pT categories correspond to the clinical T categories.

pN – Regional Lymph Nodes
Histological examination of a selective neck dissection specimen will ordinarily include 10 or more lymph nodes. Histological examination of a radical or modified radical neck dissection specimen will ordinarily include 15 or more lymph nodes.

pNX Regional lymph nodes cannot be assessed
pN0 No regional lymph node metastasis
pN1 Metastasis in a single ipsilateral lymph node, 3 cm or less in greatest dimension without extranodal extension
pN2 Metastasis described as:
  pN2a Metastasis in a single ipsilateral lymph node, 3 cm or less in greatest dimension with extranodal extension *or* more than 3 cm but not more than 6 cm in greatest dimension without extranodal extension
  pN2b Metastasis in multiple ipsilateral lymph nodes, none more than 6 cm in greatest dimension, without extranodal extension
  pN2c Metastasis in bilateral or contralateral lymph nodes, none more than 6 cm in greatest dimension, without extranodal extension
pN3a Metastasis in a lymph node more than 6 cm in greatest dimension without extranodal extension
pN3b Metastasis in a lymph node more than 3 cm in greatest dimension with extranodal extension or, multiple ipsilateral, or any contralateral or bilateral node(s) with extranodal extension

pM – Distant Metastasis*
pM1 Distant metastasis microscopically confirmed

Note
* pM0 and pMX are not valid categories.

Stage

Stage			
Stage 0	Tis	N0	M0
Stage I	T1	N0	M0
Stage II	T2	N0	M0
Stage III	T3	N0	M0
	T1,T2,T3	N1	M0
Stage IVA	T4a	N0,N1	M0
	T1,T2,T3,T4a	N2	M0
Stage IVB	Any T	N3	M0
	T4b	Any N	M0
Stage IVC	Any T	Any N	M1

TNM staging of carcinomas of the pharynx (oropharynx, nasopharynx, hypopharynx)

Pharynx
(ICD-O-3 C01, C02.4, C05.1-2, C09, C10.0, 2-3, 9, C11-13)

Rules for Classification
The classification applies only to carcinomas. There should be histological confirmation of the disease.

Changes to the seventh edition for carcinoma of the nasopharynx and the introduction of a separate classification for p16-positive oropharyngeal cancer are based on the recommendations referenced.[1,2]

The following are the procedures for assessing T, N, and M categories:

T categories   Physical examination, endoscopy and imaging
N categories   Physical examination and imaging
M categories   Physical examination and imaging

Anatomical Sites and Subsites
Oropharynx (ICD-O-3 C01, C02.4, C05.1-2, C09.0-1, 9, C10.0, 10.9, 2-3)
1. Anterior wall (glossoepiglottic area)
   a) Base of tongue (posterior to the vallate papillae or posterior third) (C01)
   b) Vallecula (C10.0)
   c) Lingual tonsil (C02.4)
2. Lateral wall (C10.2)
   a) Tonsil (C09.9)
   b) Tonsillar fossa (C09.0) and tonsillar (faucial) pillars (C09.1)
   c) Glossotonsillar sulci (tonsillar pillars) (C09.1)
3. Posterior wall (C10.3)
4. Superior wall
   a) Inferior surface of soft palate (CO5.1)
   b) Uvula (CO5.2)

Nasopharynx (C11)
1. Posterosuperior wall: extends from the level of the junction of the hard and soft palates to the base of the skull (C11.0, 1)
2. Lateral wall: including the fossa of Rosenmüller (C11.2)
3. Inferior wall: consists of the superior surface of the soft palate (C11.3)

Note
The margin of the choanal orifices, including the posterior margin of the nasal septum, is included with the nasal fossa.

Hypopharynx (C12, C13)
1. Pharyngo-oesophageal junction (postcricoid area) (C13.0): extends from the level of the arytenoid cartilages and connecting folds to the inferior border of the cricoid cartilage, thus forming the anterior wall of the hypopharynx
2. Piriform sinus (C12.9): extends from the pharyngoepiglottic fold to the upper end of the oesophagus. It is bounded laterally by the thyroid cartilage and medially by the hypopharyngeal surface of the aryepiglottic fold (C13.1) and the arytenoid and cricoid cartilages
3. Posterior pharyngeal wall (C13.2): extends from the superior level of the hyoid bone (or floor of the vallecula) to the level of the inferior border of the cricoid cartilage and from the apex of one piriform sinus to the other

Regional Lymph Nodes
The regional lymph nodes are the cervical nodes.

TNM Clinical Classification
T – Primary Tumour
TX   Primary tumour cannot be assessed
T0   No evidence of primary tumour
Tis   Carcinoma in situ

Oropharynx
p16-negative cancers of the oropharynx or oropharyngeal cancers without a p16 immunohistochemistry performed.
T1   Tumour 2 cm or less in greatest dimension
T2   Tumour more than 2 cm but not more than 4 cm in greatest dimension
T3   Tumour more than 4 cm in greatest dimension or extension to lingual surface of epiglottis
T4a   Tumour invades any of the following: larynx*, deep/extrinsic muscle of tongue (genioglossus, hyoglossus, palatoglossus, and styloglossus), medial pterygoid, hard palate, or mandible
T4b   Tumour invades any of the following: lateral pterygoid muscle, pterygoid plates, lateral nasopharynx, skull base; or encases carotid artery

Note
* Mucosal extension to lingual surface of epiglottis from primary tumours of the base of the tongue and vallecula does not constitute invasion of the larynx.

Oropharynx – p16-Positive Tumours
Tumours that have positive p16 immunohistochemistry overexpression.

T1   Tumour 2 cm or less in greatest dimension
T2   Tumour more than 2 cm but not more than 4 cm in greatest dimension
T3   Tumour more than 4 cm in greatest dimension or extension to lingual surface of epiglottis
T4   Tumour invades any of the following: larynx*, deep/extrinsic muscle of tongue (genioglossus, hyoglossus, palatoglossus, and styloglossus), medial pterygoid, hard palate, mandible*, lateral pterygoid muscle, pterygoid plates, lateral nasopharynx, skull base; or encases carotid artery

Note
* Mucosal extension to lingual surface of epiglottis from primary tumours of the base of the tongue and vallecula does not constitute invasion of the larynx.

Hypopharynx
T1   Tumour limited to one subsite of hypopharynx (see above) and/or 2 cm or less in greatest dimension
T2   Tumour invades more than one subsite of hypopharynx or an adjacent site, or measures more than 2 cm but not more than 4 cm in greatest dimension, without fixation of hemilarynx
T3   Tumour more than 4 cm in greatest dimension, or with fixation of hemilarynx or extension to oesophageal mucosa
T4a   Tumour invades any of the following: thyroid/cricoid cartilage, hyoid bone, thyroid gland, oesophagus, central compartment soft tissue*
T4b   Tumour invades prevertebral fascia, encases carotid artery, or invades mediastinal structures

Note
* Central compartment soft tissue includes prelaryngeal strap muscles and subcutaneous fat.

Nasopharynx
T1   Tumour confined to nasopharynx, or extends to oropharynx and/or nasal cavity without parapharyngeal involvement
T2   Tumour with extension to parapharyngeal space and/or infiltration of the medial pterygoid, lateral pterygoid, and/or prevertebral muscles
T3   Tumour invades bony structures of skull base, cervical vertebra, pterygoid structures, and/or paranasal sinuses
T4   Tumour with intracranial extension and/or involvement of cranial nerves, hypopharynx, orbit, parotid gland and/or infiltration beyond the lateral surface of the lateral pterygoid muscle

N – Regional Lymph Nodes
Oropharynx – p16-Negative and Hypopharynx
NX   Regional lymph nodes cannot be assessed
N0   No regional lymph node metastasis
N1   Metastasis in a single ipsilateral lymph node, 3 cm or less in greatest dimension without extranodal extension
N2   Metastasis described as:
    N2a   Metastasis in a single ipsilateral lymph node more than 3 cm but not more than 6 cm in greatest dimension without extranodal extension
    N2b   Metastasis in multiple ipsilateral lymph nodes, none more than 6 cm in greatest dimension, without extranodal extension
    N2c   Metastasis in bilateral or contralateral lymph nodes, none more than 6 cm in greatest dimension, without extranodal extension
N3a   Metastasis in a lymph node more than 6 cm in greatest dimension without extranodal extension
N3b   Metastasis in a single or multiple lymph nodes with clinical extranodal extension*

Notes
* The presence of skin involvement or soft tissue invasion with deep fixation/tethering to underlying muscle or adjacent structures or clinical signs of nerve involvement is classified as clinical extranodal extension.
Midline nodes are considered ipsilateral nodes.

Oropharynx – p16-Positive
NX   Regional lymph nodes cannot be assessed
N0   No regional lymph node metastasis
N1   Unilateral metastasis, in lymph node(s), all 6 cm or less in greatest dimension
N2   Contralateral or bilateral metastasis in lymph node(s), all 6 cm or less in greatest dimension
N3   Metastasis in lymph node(s) greater than 6 cm in dimension

Note
Midline nodes are considered ipsilateral nodes.

Nasopharynx
NX   Regional lymph nodes cannot be assessed
N0   No regional lymph node metastasis
N1   Unilateral metastasis, in cervical lymph node(s), and/or unilateral or bilateral metastasis in retropharyngeal lymph nodes, 6 cm or less in greatest dimension, above the caudal border of cricoid cartilage
N2   Bilateral metastases in cervical lymph nodes, 6 cm or less in greatest dimension, above the caudal border of cricoid cartilage
N3   Metastasis in cervical lymph node(s) greater than 6 cm in dimension and/or extension below the caudal border of cricoid cartilage

Note
Midline nodes are considered ipsilateral nodes.

M – Distant Metastasis

M0   No distant metastasis
M1   Distant metastasis

pTNM Pathological Classification

The pT categories correspond to the T categories.

pN – Regional Lymph Nodes

Histological examination of a selective neck dissection specimen will ordinarily include 10 or more lymph nodes. Histological examination of a radical or modified radical neck dissection specimen will ordinarily include 15 or more lymph nodes.

Oropharynx – p16-Negative and Hypopharynx

pNX   Regional lymph nodes cannot be assessed
pN0   No regional lymph node metastasis
pN1   Metastasis in a single ipsilateral lymph node, 3 cm or less in greatest dimension without extranodal extension
pN2   Metastasis described as:
    pN2a   Metastasis in a single ipsilateral lymph node, 3 cm or less in greatest dimension with extranodal extension or more than 3 cm but not more than 6 cm in greatest dimension without extranodal extension
    pN2b   Metastasis in multiple ipsilateral lymph nodes, none more than 6 cm in greatest dimension, without extranodal extension
    pN2c   Metastasis in bilateral or contralateral lymph nodes, none more than 6 cm in greatest dimension, without extranodal extension
pN3a Metastasis in a lymph node more than 6 cm in greatest dimension without extranodal extension
pN3b Metastasis in a lymph node more than 3 cm in greatest dimension with extranodal extension or, multiple ipsilateral, or any contralateral or bilateral node(s) with extranodal extension

Oropharynx – p16-Positive

pNX   Regional lymph nodes cannot be assessed
pN0   No regional lymph node metastasis
pN1   Metastasis in 1 to 4 lymph node(s)
pN2   Metastasis in 5 or more lymph node(s)

Nasopharynx

The pN categories correspond to the N categories

pM – Distant Metastasis*

pM1   Distant metastasis microscopically confirmed

Note
* pM0 and pMX are not valid categories.

Stage (Oropharynx – p16-Negative and Hypopharynx)

Stage 0	Tis	N0	M0
Stage I	T1	N0	M0
Stage II	T2	N0	M0
Stage III	T3	N0	M0
	T1,T2,T3	N1	M0
Stage IVA	T1,T2,T3	N2	M0
	T4a	N0,N1,N2	M0
Stage IVB	T4b	Any N	M0
	Any T	N3	M0
Stage IVC	Any T	Any N	M1

Stage (Oropharynx – p16-Positive)

Clinical

Stage 0	Tis	N0	M0
Stage I	T1,T2	N0,N1	M0
Stage II	T1,T2	N2	M0
	T3	N0,N1,N2	M0
Stage III	T1,T2,T3	N3	M0
	T4	Any N	M0
Stage IV	Any T	Any N	M1

Pathological

Stage 0	Tis	N0	M0
Stage I	T1,T2	N0,N1	M0
Stage II	T1,T2	N2	M0
	T3,T4	N0,N1	M0
Stage III	T3,T4	N2	M0
Stage IV	Any T	Any N	M1

Stage (Nasopharynx)

Stage 0	Tis	N0	M0
Stage I	T1	N0	M0
Stage II	T1	N1	M0
	T2	N0,N1	M0
Stage III	T1,T2	N2	M0
	T3	N0,N1,N2	M0
Stage IVA	T4	N0,N1,N2	M0
	Any T	N3	M0
Stage IVB	Any T	Any N	M1

References

1   Pan JJ, Ng WT, Zong J F, et al. Proposal for the 8th edition of the AJCC/UICC staging system for nasopharyngeal cancer in the era of intensity-modulated radiotherapy. *Cancer* 2016; 122: 546–558.
2   O'Sullivan B, Huang SH, Su J, et al. A proposal for UICC/AJCC pre-treatment TNM staging for HPV-related oropharyngeal cancer by the International Collaboration on Oropharyngeal Cancer Network for Staging (ICON-S): A comparative multi-centre cohort study. *Lancet Oncol* 2016; 17: 440–451.

TNM staging of carcinomas of the larynx

Larynx
(ICD-O-3 C32.0-2, C10.1)

Rules for Classification
The classification applies only to carcinomas. There should be histological confirmation of the disease.

The following are the procedures for assessing T, N, and M categories:

T categories	Physical examination, laryngoscopy, and imaging
N categories	Physical examination and imaging
M categories	Physical examination and imaging

Anatomical Sites and Subsites
1. Supraglottis (C32.1)
   a) Suprahyoid epiglottis [including tip, lingual (anterior) (C10.1), and laryngeal surfaces] } *Epilarynx (including marginal zone)*
   b) Aryepiglottic fold, laryngeal aspect
   c) Arytenoid
   d) Infrahyoid epiglottis } *Supraglottis excluding epilarynx*
   e) Ventricular bands (false cords)
2. Glottis (C32.0)
   a) Vocal cords
   b) Anterior commissure
   c) Posterior commissure
3. Subglottis (C32.2)

Regional Lymph Nodes
The regional lymph nodes are the cervical nodes.

TNM Clinical Classification
T – Primary Tumour
TX Primary tumour cannot be assessed
T0 No evidence of primary tumour
Tis Carcinoma in situ

Supraglottis
T1 Tumour limited to one subsite of supraglottis with normal vocal cord mobility
T2 Tumour invades mucosa of more than one adjacent subsite of supraglottis or glottis or region outside the supraglottis (e.g. mucosa of base of tongue, vallecula, medial wall of piriform sinus) without fixation of the larynx
T3 Tumour limited to larynx with vocal cord fixation and/or invades any of the following: postcricoid area, pre-epiglottic space, paraglottic space, and/or inner cortex of thyroid cartilage
T4a Tumour invades through the thyroid cartilage and/or invades tissues beyond the larynx, e.g. trachea, soft tissues of neck including deep/extrinsic muscle of tongue (genioglossus, hyoglossus, palatoglossus, and styloglossus), strap muscles, thyroid, or oesophagus
T4b Tumour invades prevertebral space, encases carotid artery, or mediastinal structures

Glottis
T1 Tumour limited to vocal cord(s) (may involve anterior or posterior commissure) with normal mobility
   T1a Tumour limited to one vocal cord
   T1b Tumour involves both vocal cords
T2 Tumour extends to supraglottis and/or subglottis, and/or with impaired vocal cord mobility
T3 Tumour limited to larynx with vocal cord fixation and/or invades paraglottic space, and/or inner cortex of the thyroid cartilage
T4a Tumour invades through the outer cortex of the thyroid cartilage, and/or invades tissues beyond the larynx, e.g. trachea, soft tissues of neck including deep/extrinsic muscle of tongue (genioglossus, hyoglossus, palatoglossus, and styloglossus), strap muscles, thyroid, oesophagus
T4b Tumour invades prevertebral space, encases carotid artery, or mediastinal structures

Subglottis
T1 Tumour limited to subglottis
T2 Tumour extends to vocal cord(s) with normal or impaired mobility
T3 Tumour limited to larynx with vocal cord fixation
T4a Tumour invades cricoid or thyroid cartilage and/or invades tissues beyond the larynx, e.g. trachea, soft tissues of neck including deep/extrinsic muscle of tongue (genioglossus, hyoglossus, palatoglossus, and styloglossus), strap muscles, thyroid, oesophagus
T4b Tumour invades prevertebral space, encases carotid artery, or mediastinal structures

N – Regional Lymph Nodes
NX Regional lymph nodes cannot be assessed
N0 No regional lymph node metastasis
N1 Metastasis in a single ipsilateral lymph node, 3 cm or less in greatest dimension without extranodal extension
N2 Metastasis described as:
   N2a Metastasis in a single ipsilateral lymph node, more than 3 cm but not more than 6 cm in greatest dimension without extranodal extension
   N2b Metastasis in multiple ipsilateral lymph nodes, none more than 6 cm in greatest dimension, without extranodal extension
   N2c Metastasis in bilateral or contralateral lymph nodes, none more than 6 cm in greatest dimension, without extranodal extension
N3a Metastasis in a lymph node more than 6 cm in greatest dimension without extranodal extension
N3b Metastasis in a single or multiple lymph nodes with clinical extranodal extension*

Notes
* The presence of skin involvement or soft tissue invasion with deep fixation/tethering to underlying muscle or adjacent structures or clinical signs of nerve involvement is classified as clinical extranodal extension.
Midline nodes are considered ipsilateral nodes.

M – Distant Metastasis

M0   No distant metastasis
M1   Distant metastasis

pTNM Pathological Classification

The pT categories correspond to the clinical T categories.

pN – Regional Lymph Nodes

Histological examination of a selective neck dissection specimen will ordinarily include 10 or more lymph nodes. Histological examination of a radical or modified radical neck dissection specimen will ordinarily include 15 or more lymph nodes.

pNX   Regional lymph nodes cannot be assessed
pN0   No regional lymph node metastasis
pN1   Metastasis in a single ipsilateral lymph node, 3 cm or less in greatest dimension without extranodal extension
pN2   Metastasis described as:

     pN2a   Metastasis in a single ipsilateral lymph node, 3 cm or less in greatest dimension with extranodal extension *or* more than 3 cm but not more than 6 cm in greatest dimension without extranodal extension

     pN2b   Metastasis in multiple ipsilateral lymph nodes, none more than 6 cm in greatest dimension, without extranodal extension

     pN2c   Metastasis in bilateral or contralateral lymph nodes, none more than 6 cm in greatest dimension, without extranodal extension

pN3a   Metastasis in a lymph node more than 6 cm in greatest dimension without extranodal extension
pN3b   Metastasis in a lymph node more than 3 cm in greatest dimension with extranodal extension or multiple ipsilateral, or any contralateral or bilateral node(s) with extranodal extension

pM – Distant Metastasis*

pM1   Distant metastasis microscopically confirmed

Note
* pM0 and pMX are not valid categories.

Stage

Stage	T	N	M
Stage 0	Tis	N0	M0
Stage I	T1	N0	M0
Stage II	T2	N0	M0
Stage III	T3	N0	M0
	T1,T2,T3	N1	M0
Stage IVA	T4a	N0,N1	M0
	T1,T2,T3,T4a	N2	M0
Stage IVB	T4b	Any N	M0
	Any T	N3	M0
Stage IVC	Any T	Any N	M1

TNM staging of carcinomas of the nasal cavity and paranasal sinuses

Nasal Cavity and Paranasal Sinuses
(ICD-O-3 C30.0, C31.0-1)

Rules for Classification
The classification applies only to carcinomas. There should be histological confirmation of the disease.

The following are the procedures for assessing T, N, and M categories:

T categories	Physical examination and imaging
N categories	Physical examination and imaging
M categories	Physical examination and imaging

Anatomical Sites and Subsites
1. Nasal cavity (C30.0)
   - Septum
   - Floor
   - Lateral wall
   - Vestibule
2. Maxillary sinus (C31.0)
3. Ethmoid sinus (C31.1)
   - Left
   - Right

Regional Lymph Nodes
The regional lymph nodes are the cervical nodes.

TNM Clinical Classification
T – Primary Tumour
TX   Primary tumour cannot be assessed
T0   No evidence of primary tumour
Tis   Carcinoma in situ

Maxillary Sinus
T1   Tumour limited to the mucosa with no erosion or destruction of bone
T2   Tumour causing bone erosion or destruction, including extension into the hard palate and/or middle nasal meatus, except extension to posterior wall of maxillary sinus and pterygoid plates
T3   Tumour invades any of the following: bone of posterior wall of maxillary sinus, subcutaneous tissues, floor or medial wall of orbit, pterygoid fossa, or ethmoid sinuses
T4a   Tumour invades any of the following: anterior orbital contents, skin of cheek, pterygoid plates, infratemporal fossa, cribriform plate, sphenoid or frontal sinuses
T4b   Tumour invades any of the following: orbital apex, dura, brain, middle cranial fossa, cranial nerves other than maxillary division of trigeminal nerve (V2), nasopharynx, or clivus

Nasal Cavity and Ethmoid Sinus
T1   Tumour restricted to one subsite of nasal cavity or ethmoid sinus, with or without bony invasion
T2   Tumour involves two subsites in a single site or extends to involve an adjacent site within the nasoethmoidal complex, with or without bony invasion
T3   Tumour extends to invade the medial wall or floor of the orbit, maxillary sinus, palate, or cribriform plate
T4a   Tumour invades any of the following: anterior orbital contents, skin of nose or cheek, minimal extension to anterior cranial fossa, pterygoid plates, sphenoid or frontal sinuses
T4b   Tumour invades any of the following: orbital apex, dura, brain, middle cranial fossa, cranial nerves other than V2, nasopharynx, or clivus

N – Regional Lymph Nodes
NX   Regional lymph nodes cannot be assessed
N0   No regional lymph node metastasis
N1   Metastasis in a single ipsilateral lymph node, 3 cm or less in greatest dimension without extranodal extension
N2   Metastasis described as:
- N2a   Metastasis in a single ipsilateral lymph node, more than 3 cm but not more than 6 cm in greatest dimension without extranodal extension
- N2b   Metastasis in multiple ipsilateral lymph nodes, none more than 6 cm in greatest dimension, without extranodal extension
- N2c   Metastasis in bilateral or contralateral lymph nodes, none more than 6 cm in greatest dimension, without extranodal extension

N3a   Metastasis in a lymph node more than 6 cm in greatest dimension without extranodal extension
N3b   Metastasis in a single or multiple lymph nodes with clinical extranodal extension*

Notes
* The presence of skin involvement or soft tissue invasion with deep fixation/tethering to underlying muscle or adjacent structures or clinical signs of nerve involvement is classified as clinical extranodal extension.
Midline nodes are considered ipsilateral nodes.

M – Distant Metastasis
M0   No distant metastasis
M1   Distant metastasis

pTNM Pathological Classification
The pT categories correspond to the clinical T categories.

The information presented here has been excerpted from the 2017 *TNM classification of malignant tumours*, eighth edition {589,4534}. © 2017 UICC.
A help desk for specific questions about the TNM classification is available at https://www.uicc.org/tnm-help-desk.

pN – Regional Lymph Nodes

Histological examination of a selective neck dissection specimen will ordinarily include 10 or more lymph nodes. Histological examination of a radical or modified radical neck dissection specimen will ordinarily include 15 or more lymph nodes.

pNX Regional lymph nodes cannot be assessed
pN0 No regional lymph node metastasis
pN1 Metastasis in a single ipsilateral lymph node, 3 cm or less in greatest dimension without extranodal extension
pN2 Metastasis described as:
    pN2a Metastasis in a single ipsilateral lymph node, 3 cm or less in greatest dimension with extranodal extension *or* more than 3 cm but not more than 6 cm in greatest dimension without extranodal extension
    pN2b Metastasis in multiple ipsilateral lymph nodes, none more than 6 cm in greatest dimension, without extranodal extension
    pN2c Metastasis in bilateral or contralateral lymph nodes, none more than 6 cm in greatest dimension, without extranodal extension
pN3a Metastasis in a lymph node more than 6 cm in greatest dimension without extranodal extension
pN3b Metastasis in a lymph node more than 3 cm in greatest dimension with extranodal extension or multiple ipsilateral, or any contralateral or bilateral node(s) with extranodal extension

pM – Distant Metastasis*

pM1 Distant metastasis microscopically confirmed

Note
* pM0 and pMX are not valid categories.

Stage

Stage	T	N	M
Stage 0	Tis	N0	M0
Stage I	T1	N0	M0
Stage II	T2	N0	M0
Stage III	T3	N0	M0
	T1,T2,T3	N1	M0
Stage IVA	T1,T2,T3	N2	M0
	T4a	N0,N1,N2	M0
Stage IVB	T4b	Any N	M0
	Any T	N3	M0
Stage IVC	Any T	Any N	M1

TNM staging of unknown primary carcinoma – cervical nodes

Unknown Primary – Cervical Nodes

Rules for Classification

There should be histological confirmation of squamous cell carcinoma with lymph node metastases but without an identified primary carcinoma. Histological methods should be used to identify EBV and HPV/p16-related tumours. If there is evidence of EBV, the nasopharyngeal classification is applied. If there is evidence of HPV and positive immunohistochemistry p16 overexpression, the p16-positive oropharyngeal classification is applied.

TNM Clinical Classification

EBV or HPV/p16 negative or unknown

T – Primary Tumour

T0   No evidence of primary tumour

N – Regional Lymph Nodes

N1   Metastasis in a single lymph node, 3 cm or less in greatest dimension without extranodal extension

N2   Metastasis described as:

  N2a   Metastasis in a single lymph node, more than 3 cm but not more than 6 cm in greatest dimension without extranodal extension

  N2b   Metastasis in multiple ipsilateral lymph nodes, none more than 6 cm in greatest dimension, without extranodal extension

  N2c   Metastasis in bilateral lymph nodes, none more than 6 cm in greatest dimension, without extranodal extension

N3a   Metastasis in a lymph node more than 6 cm in greatest dimension without extranodal extension

N3b   Metastasis in a single or multiple lymph nodes with clinical extranodal extension*

M – Distant Metastasis

M0   No distant metastasis

M1   Distant metastasis

pTNM Pathological Classification

There is no pT category.

pN – Regional Lymph Nodes

Histological examination of a selective neck dissection specimen will ordinarily include 10 or more lymph nodes. Histological examination of a radical or modified radical neck dissection specimen will ordinarily include 15 or more lymph nodes.

pN1   Metastasis in a single lymph node, 3 cm or less in greatest dimension without extranodal extension

pN2   Metastasis described as:

  pN2a   Metastasis in a single lymph node, 3 cm or less in greatest dimension with extranodal extension *or* more than 3 cm but not more than 6 cm in greatest dimension without extranodal extension

  pN2b   Metastasis in multiple ipsilateral lymph nodes, none more than 6 cm in greatest dimension, without extranodal extension

  pN2c   Metastasis in bilateral lymph nodes, none more than 6 cm in greatest dimension, without extranodal extension

pN3a Metastasis in a lymph node more than 6 cm in greatest dimension without extranodal extension

pN3b Metastasis in a lymph node more than 3 cm in greatest dimension with extranodal extension or multiple ipsilateral, or any contralateral, or bilateral node(s) with extranodal extension

pM – Distant Metastasis*

pM1   Distant metastasis microscopically confirmed

Note

* pM0 and pMX are not valid categories.

Stage

Stage			
Stage III	T0	N1	M0
Stage IVA	T0	N2	M0
Stage IVB	T0	N3	M0
Stage IVC	T0	N1,N2,N3	M1

TNM Clinical Classification

HPV/p16 positive

T – Primary Tumour

T0   No evidence of primary tumour

N – Regional Lymph Nodes

N1   Unilateral metastasis, in cervical lymph node(s), all 6 cm or less in greatest dimension

N2   Contralateral or bilateral metastasis in cervical lymph node(s), all 6 cm or less in greatest dimension

N3   Metastasis in cervical lymph node(s) greater than 6 cm in dimension

pTNM Pathological Classification
There is no pT category.

pN – Regional Lymph Nodes
Histological examination of a selective neck dissection specimen will ordinarily include 10 or more lymph nodes. Histological examination of a radical or modified radical neck dissection specimen will ordinarily include 15 or more lymph nodes.

pN1   Metastasis in 1 to 4 lymph node(s)
pN2   Metastasis in 5 or more lymph nodes

Stage
Clinical

Stage I	T0	N1	M0
Stage II	T0	N2	M0
Stage III	T0	N3	M0
Stage IV	T0	N1,N2,N3	M1

Pathological

Stage I	T0	N1	M0
Stage II	T0	N2	M0
Stage IV	T0	N1,N2	M1

TNM Clinical Classification
EBV positive
T – Primary Tumour
T0   No evidence of primary tumour

N – Regional Lymph Nodes (Nasopharynx)
N1   Unilateral metastasis, in cervical lymph node(s), and/or unilateral or bilateral metastasis in retropharyngeal lymph nodes, 6 cm or less in greatest dimension, above the caudal border of cricoid cartilage
N2   Bilateral metastasis in cervical lymph node(s), 6 cm or less in greatest dimension, above the caudal border of cricoid cartilage
N3   Metastasis in cervical lymph node(s) greater than 6 cm in dimension and/or extension below the caudal border of cricoid cartilage

Note
Midline nodes are considered ipsilateral nodes.

M – Distant Metastasis
M0   No distant metastasis
M1   Distant metastases

pTNM Pathological Classification
The pT and pN categories correspond to the T and N categories. Histological examination of a selective neck dissection specimen will ordinarily include 10 or more lymph nodes. Histological examination of a radical or modified radical neck dissection specimen will ordinarily include 15 or more lymph nodes.

pM – Distant Metastasis*
pM1   Distant metastasis microscopically confirmed

Note
* pM0 and pMX are not valid categories.

Stage

Stage II	T0	N1	M0
Stage III	T0	N2	M0
Stage IVA	T0	N3	M0
Stage IVB	T0	N1,N2,N3	M1

TNM staging of mucosal melanoma of the upper aerodigestive tract

Malignant Melanoma of Upper Aerodigestive Tract
(ICD-O-3 C00-06, C10-14, C30-32)

Rules for Classification
The classification applies only to mucosal malignant melanomas of the head and neck region, i.e. of the upper aerodigestive tract. There should be histological confirmation of the disease and division of cases by site.

The following are the procedures for assessing T, N, and M categories:

T categories	Physical examination and imaging
N categories	Physical examination and imaging
M categories	Physical examination and imaging

Regional Lymph Nodes
The regional lymph nodes are those appropriate to the site of the primary tumour.

TNM Clinical Classification
T – Primary Tumour
TX   Primary tumour cannot be assessed
T0   No evidence of primary tumour
T3   Tumour limited to the epithelium and/or submucosa (mucosal disease)
T4a Tumour invades deep soft tissue, cartilage, bone, or overlying skin
T4b Tumour invades any of the following: brain, dura, skull base, lower cranial nerves (IX, X, XI, XII), masticator space, carotid artery, prevertebralspace, mediastinal structures

Note
Mucosal melanomas are aggressive tumours; therefore, T1 and T2 are omitted as are stages I and II.

N – Regional Lymph Nodes
NX   Regional lymph nodes cannot be assessed
N0   No regional lymph node metastasis
N1   Regional lymph node metastasis

M – Distant Metastasis
M0   No distant metastasis
M1   Distant metastasis

pTNM Pathological Classification
The pT and pN categories correspond to the T and N categories.

pN0 Histological examination of a regional lymphadenectomy specimen will ordinarily include 6 or more lymph nodes. If the lymph nodes are negative, but the number ordinarily examined is not met, classify as pN0.

pM – Distant Metastasis*
pM1 Distant metastasis microscopically confirmed

Note
* pM0 and pMX are not valid categories.

Stage

Stage			
Stage III	T3	N0	M0
Stage IVA	T4a	N0	M0
	T3,T4a	N1	M0
Stage IVB	T4b	Any N	M0
Stage IVC	Any T	Any N	M1

TNM staging of carcinomas of the major salivary glands

Major Salivary Glands
(ICD-O-3 C07, C08)

Rules for Classification
The classification applies only to carcinomas of the major salivary glands. Tumours arising in minor salivary glands (mucus-secreting glands in the lining membrane of the upper aerodigestive tract) are not included in this classification but at their anatomic site of origin, e.g. lip. There should be histological confirmation of the disease.

The following are the procedures for assessing T, N, and M categories:

T categories	Physical examination and imaging
N categories	Physical examination and imaging
M categories	Physical examination and imaging

Anatomical Sites
- Parotid gland (C07.9)
- Submandibular (submaxillary) gland (C08.0)
- Sublingual gland (C08.1)

Regional Lymph Nodes
The regional lymph nodes are the cervical nodes.

TNM Clinical Classification
T – Primary Tumour
TX	Primary tumour cannot be assessed
T0	No evidence of primary tumour
Tis	Carcinoma in situ
T1	Tumour 2 cm or less in greatest dimension without extraparenchymal extension*
T2	Tumour more than 2 cm but not more than 4 cm in greatest dimension without extraparenchymal extension*
T3	Tumour more than 4 cm and/or tumour with extraparenchymal extension*
T4a	Tumour invades skin, mandible, ear canal, and/or facial nerve
T4b	Tumour invades base of skull, and/or pterygoid plates, and/or encases carotid artery

Note
* Extraparenchymal extension is clinical or macroscopic evidence of invasion of soft tissues or nerve, except those listed under T4a and T4b. Microscopic evidence alone does not constitute extraparenchymal extension for classification purposes.

N – Regional Lymph Nodes
NX	Regional lymph nodes cannot be assessed
N0	No regional lymph node metastasis
N1	Metastasis in a single ipsilateral lymph node, 3 cm or less in greatest dimension without extranodal extension
N2	Metastasis described as:
N2a	Metastasis in a single ipsilateral lymph node, more than 3 cm but not more than 6 cm in greatest dimension without extranodal extension
N2b	Metastasis in multiple ipsilateral lymph nodes, none more than 6 cm in greatest dimension, without extranodal extension
N2c	Metastasis in bilateral or contralateral lymph nodes, none more than 6 cm in greatest dimension, without extranodal extension
N3a	Metastasis in a lymph node more than 6 cm in greatest dimension without extranodal extension
N3b	Metastasis in a single or multiple lymph nodes with clinical extranodal extension*

Notes
* The presence of skin involvement or soft tissue invasion with deep fixation/tethering to underlying muscle or adjacent structures or clinical signs of nerve involvement is classified as clinical extranodal extension.
Midline nodes are considered ipsilateral nodes.

M – Distant Metastasis
M0	No distant metastasis
M1	Distant metastasis

pTNM Pathological Classification
The pT categories correspond to the clinical T categories.

pN – Regional Lymph Nodes
Histological examination of a selective neck dissection specimen will ordinarily include 10 or more lymph nodes. Histological examination of a radical or modified radical neck dissection specimen will ordinarily include 15 or more lymph nodes.

pNX Regional lymph nodes cannot be assessed
pN0 No regional lymph node metastasis
pN1 Metastasis in a single ipsilateral lymph node, 3 cm or less in greatest dimension without extranodal extension
pN2 Metastasis described as:

    pN2a Metastasis in a single ipsilateral lymph node, 3 cm or less in greatest dimension with extranodal extension *or* more than 3 cm but not more than 6 cm in greatest dimension without extranodal extension

    pN2b Metastasis in multiple ipsilateral lymph nodes, none more than 6 cm in greatest dimension, without extranodal extension

    pN2c Metastasis in bilateral or contralateral lymph nodes, none more than 6 cm in greatest dimension, without extranodal extension

pN3a Metastasis in a lymph node more than 6 cm in greatest dimension without extranodal extension
pN3b Metastasis in a lymph node more than 3 cm in greatest dimension with extranodal extension or multiple ipsilateral, or any contralateral, or bilateral node(s) with extranodal extension

pM – Distant Metastasis*

pM1 Distant metastasis microscopically confirmed

Note

* pM0 and pMX are not valid categories.

Stage

Stage			
Stage 0	Tis	N0	M0
Stage I	T1	N0	M0
Stage II	T2	N0	M0
Stage III	T3	N0	M0
	T1,T2,T3	N1	M0
Stage IVA	T1,T2,T3	N2	M0
	T4a	N0,N1,N2	M0
Stage IVB	T4b	Any N	M0
	Any T	N3	M0
Stage IVC	Any T	Any N	M1

TNM staging of skin carcinoma of the head and neck

Skin Carcinoma of the Head and Neck

(ICD-O-3 C44.0, C44.2-4)

Rules for Classification

The classification applies only to cutaneous carcinomas of the head and neck region excluding the eyelid and excluding Merkel cell carcinoma and malignant melanoma. There should be histological confirmation of the disease.

The following are the procedures for assessing T, N, and M categories:

T categories	Physical examination and imaging
N categories	Physical examination and imaging
M categories	Physical examination and imaging

Anatomical Sites

The following sites are identified by ICD-O-3 topography rubrics:
- Lip (excluding vermilion surface) (C44.0)
- External ear (C44.2)
- Other and unspecified parts of face (C44.3)
- Scalp and neck (C44.4)

TNM Clinical Classification

T – Primary Tumour

TX	Primary tumour cannot be identified
T0	No evidence of primary tumour
Tis	Carcinoma in situ
T1	Tumour 2 cm or less in greatest dimension
T2	Tumour > 2 cm and ≤ 4 cm in greatest dimension
T3	Tumour > 4 cm in greatest dimension or minor bone erosion or perineural invasion or deep invasion*
T4a	Tumour with gross cortical bone/marrow invasion
T4b	Tumour with skull base or axial skeleton invasion including foraminal involvement and/or vertebral foramen involvement to the epidural space

Note
* Deep invasion is defined as invasion beyond the subcutaneous fat or > 6 mm (as measured from the granular layer of adjacent normal epidermis to the base of the tumour); perineural invasion for T3 classification is defined as clinical or radiographic involvement of named nerves without foramen or skull base invasion or transgression.

N – Regional Lymph Nodes

NX	Regional lymph nodes cannot be assessed
N0	No regional lymph node metastasis
N1	Metastasis in a single ipsilateral lymph node, 3 cm or less in greatest dimension without extranodal extension
N2	Metastasis described as:

	N2a	Metastasis in a single ipsilateral lymph node more than 3 cm but not more than 6 cm in greatest dimension without extranodal extension
	N2b	Metastasis in multiple ipsilateral lymph nodes, none more than 6 cm in greatest dimension, without extranodal extension
	N2c	Metastasis in bilateral or contralateral lymph nodes, none more than 6 cm in greatest dimension, without extranodal extension

N3a	Metastasis in a lymph node more than 6 cm in greatest dimension without extranodal extension
N3b	Metastasis in a single or multiple lymph nodes with clinical extranodal extension*

Note
* The presence of skin involvement or soft tissue invasion with deep fixation/tethering to underlying muscle or adjacent structures or clinical signs of nerve involvement is classified as clinical extranodal extension.

M – Distant Metastasis

M0	No distant metastasis
M1	Distant metastasis

pTNM Pathological Classification

The pT categories correspond to the clinical T categories.

pN – Regional Lymph Nodes

Histological examination of a selective neck dissection specimen will ordinarily include 10 or more lymph nodes. Histological examination of a radical or modified radical neck dissection specimen will ordinarily include 15 or more lymph nodes.

The information presented here has been excerpted from the 2017 *TNM classification of malignant tumours*, eighth edition {589,4534}. © 2017 UICC. A help desk for specific questions about the TNM classification is available at https://www.uicc.org/tnm-help-desk.

pNX Regional lymph nodes cannot be assessed
pN0 No regional lymph node metastasis
pN1 Metastasis in a single ipsilateral lymph node, 3 cm or less
     in greatest dimension without extranodal extension
pN2 Metastasis described as:
     pN2a Metastasis in a single ipsilateral lymph node, less
           than 3 cm in greatest dimension with extranodal
           extension or, more than 3 cm but not more than
           6 cm in greatest dimension without extranodal
           extension
     pN2b Metastasis in multiple ipsilateral lymph nodes,
           none more than 6 cm in greatest dimension,
           without extranodal extension
     pN2c Metastasis in bilateral or contralateral lymph
           nodes, none more than 6 cm in greatest
           dimension, without extranodal extension
pN3a Metastasis in a lymph node more than 6 cm in greatest
     dimension without extranodal extension
pN3b Metastasis in a lymph node more than 3 cm in greatest
     dimension with extranodal extension or multiple ipsilateral,
     or any contralateral or bilateral node(s) with extranodal
     extension

pM – Distant Metastasis*
pM1 Distant metastasis microscopically confirmed

Note
* pM0 and pMX are not valid categories.

Stage

Stage			
Stage 0	Tis	N0	M0
Stage I	T1	N0	M0
Stage II	T2	N0	M0
Stage III	T3	N0	M0
	T1,T2,T3	N1	M0
Stage IVA	T1,T2,T3	N2,N3	M0
	T4	Any N	M0
Stage IVB	Any T	Any N	M1

TNM staging of melanoma of the skin

Malignant Melanoma of Skin
(ICD-O-3 C44, C51.0, C60.9, C63.2)

Rules for Classification
There should be histological confirmation of the disease.
The following are the procedures for assessing N and M categories:

N categories	Physical examination and imaging
M categories	Physical examination and imaging

Regional Lymph Nodes
The regional lymph nodes are those appropriate to the site of the primary tumour.

TNM Clinical Classification
T – Primary Tumour
The extent of the tumour is classified after excision; see pT, below.

N – Regional Lymph Nodes
NX   Regional lymph nodes cannot be assessed
N0   No regional lymph node metastasis
N1   Metastasis in one regional lymph node or intralymphatic regional metastasis without nodal metastases
    N1a   Only microscopic metastasis (clinically occult)
    N1b   Macroscopic metastasis (clinically apparent)
    N1c   Satellite or in-transit metastasis without regional nodal metastasis
N2   Metastasis in two or three regional lymph nodes or intralymphatic regional metastasis with lymph node metastases
    N2a   Only microscopic nodal metastasis
    N2b   Macroscopic nodal metastasis
    N2c   Satellite or in-transit metastasis with only one regional nodal metastasis
N3   Metastasis in four or more regional lymph nodes, or matted metastatic regional lymph nodes, or satellite(s) or in-transit metastasis with metastasis in two or more regional lymph node(s)
    N3a   Only microscopic nodal metastasis
    N3b   Macroscopic nodal metastasis
    N3c   Satellite(s) or in-transit metastasis with two or more regional nodal metastasis

Note
Satellites are tumour nests or nodules (macro- or microscopic) within 2 cm of the primary tumour. In-transit metastasis involves skin or subcutaneous tissue more than 2 cm from the primary tumour but not beyond the regional lymph nodes.

M – Distant Metastasis
M0   No distant metastasis
M1   Distant metastasis*
    M1a   Skin, subcutaneous tissue or lymph node(s) beyond the regional lymph nodes
    M1b   Lung
    M1c   Other non-central nervous system sites
    M1d   Central nervous system

Notes
* Suffixes for M category:
(0) lactic dehydrogenase (LDH) – not elevated
(1) LDH – elevated
so that M1a(1) is metastasis in skin, subcutaneous tissue, or lymph node(s) beyond the regional lymph nodes with elevated LDH.
No suffix is used if LDH is not recorded or unspecified.

pTNM Pathological Classification
pT – Primary Tumour
pTX   Primary tumour cannot be assessed*
pT0   No evidence of primary tumour
pTis   Melanoma in situ (Clark level I)

Note
* pTX includes shave biopsies and curettage that do not fully assess the thickness of the primary.

pT1   Tumour 1 mm or less in thickness
    pT1a   Less than 0.8 mm in thickness without ulceration
    pT1b   Less than 0.8 mm in thickness with ulceration or 0.8 mm or more but no more than 1 mm in thickness, with or without ulceration
pT2   Tumour more than 1 mm but not more than 2 mm in thickness
    pT2a   without ulceration
    pT2b   with ulceration
pT3   Tumour more than 2 mm but not more than 4 mm in thickness
    pT3a   without ulceration
    pT3b   with ulceration
pT4   Tumour more than 4 mm in thickness
    pT4a   without ulceration
    pT4b   with ulceration

pN – Regional Lymph Nodes
The pN categories correspond to the N categories.

pN0   Histological examination of a regional lymphadenectomy specimen will ordinarily include 6 or more lymph nodes. If the lymph nodes are negative, but the number ordinarily examined is not met, classify as pN0. Classification based solely on sentinel node biopsy without subsequent axillary lymph node dissection is designated (sn) for sentinel node, e.g. (p)N1(sn).

pM – Distant Metastasis*
pM1 Distant metastasis microscopically confirmed

Note
* pM0 and pMX are not valid categories.

Clinical Stage

Stage 0	pTis	N0	M0
Stage IA	pT1a	N0	M0
Stage IB	pT1b	N0	M0
	pT2a	N0	M0
Stage IIA	pT2b	N0	M0
	pT3a	N0	M0
Stage IIB	pT3b	N0	M0
	pT4a	N0	M0
Stage IIC	pT4b	N0	M0
Stage III	Any pT	N1,N2,N3	M0
Stage IV	Any pT	Any N	M1

Pathological Stage^

Stage 0	pTis	N0	M0
Stage I	pT1	N0	M0
Stage IA	pT1a	N0	M0
	pT1b	N0	M0
Stage IB	pT2a	N0	M0
Stage IIA	pT2b	N0	M0
	pT3a	N0	M0
Stage IIB	pT3b	N0	M0
	pT4a	N0	M0
Stage IIC	pT4b	N0	M0
Stage III	Any pT	N1,N2,N3	M0
Stage IIIA	pT1a,T1b,T2a	N1a,N2a	M0
Stage IIIB	pT1a,T1b,T2a	N1b,N1c,N2b	M0
	pT2b–T3a	N1,N2a,N2b	M0
Stage IIIC	pT1a,T1b,T2a,T2b,T3a	N2c,N3	M0
	pT3b,T4a	N1,N2,N3	M0
	pT4b	N1,N2	M0
Stage IIID	pT4b	N3	M0
Stage IV	Any pT	Any N	M1

Note
* If lymph nodes are identified with no apparent primary, the stage is as below:

Stage IIIB	pT0	N1b,N1c	M0
Stage IIIC	pT0	N2b,N2c,N3b,N3c	M1

TNM staging of Merkel cell carcinoma of the skin

Merkel Cell Carcinoma of Skin
(ICD-O-3 C44.0-9, C63.2)

Rules for Classification
The classification applies only to Merkel cell carcinomas. There should be histological confirmation of the disease.

The following are the procedures for assessing T, N, and M categories:

T categories	Physical examination
N categories	Physical examination and imaging
M categories	Physical examination and imaging

Regional Lymph Nodes
The regional lymph nodes are those appropriate to the site of the primary tumour.

TNM Clinical Classification
T – Primary Tumour
TX   Primary tumour cannot be assessed
T0   No evidence of primary tumour
Tis   Carcinoma in situ
T1   Tumour 2 cm or less in greatest dimension
T2   Tumour more than 2 cm but not more than 5 cm in greatest dimension
T3   Tumour more than 5 cm in greatest dimension
T4   Tumour invades deep extradermal structures, i.e. cartilage, skeletal muscle, fascia or bone

N – Regional Lymph Nodes
NX   Regional lymph nodes cannot be assessed
N0   No regional lymph node metastasis
N1   Regional lymph node metastasis
N2   In-transit metastasis *without* lymph node metastasis
N3   In-transit metastasis *with* lymph node metastasis

Note
In-transit metastasis: a discontinuous tumour distinct from the primary lesion and located between the primary lesion and the draining regional lymph nodes or distal to the primary lesion.

M – Distant Metastasis
M0   No distant metastasis
M1   Distant metastasis
      M1a   Skin, subcutaneous tissues or non-regional lymph node(s)
      M1b   Lung
      M1c   Other site(s)

pTNM Pathological Classification
The pT category correspond to the T category.

pN – Regional Lymph Nodes
pN0   Histological examination of a regional lymphadenectomy specimen will ordinarily include 6 or more lymph nodes. If the lymph nodes are negative, but the number ordinarily examined is not met, classify as pN0.
pNX   Regional lymph nodes cannot be assessed
pN0   No regional lymph node metastasis
pN1   Regional lymph node metastasis
      pN1a(sn)   Microscopic metastasis detected on sentinel node biopsy
      pN1a   Microscopic metastasis detected on node dissection
      pN1b   Macroscopic metastasis (clinically apparent)
pN2   In-transit metastasis without lymph node metastasis
pN3   In-transit metastasis with lymph node metastasis

Note
In-transit metastasis: a discontinuous tumour distinct from the primary lesion and located between the primary lesion and the draining regional lymph nodes or distal to the primary lesion.

pM – Distant Metastasis*
pM1   Distant metastasis microscopically confirmed

Note
* pM0 and pMX are not valid categories.

Clinical Stage

Stage 0	Tis	N0	M0
Stage I	T1	N0	M0
Stage IIA	T2,T3	N0	M0
Stage IIB	T4	N0	M0
Stage III	Any T	N1,N2,N3	M0
Stage IV	Any T	Any N	M1

Pathological Stage

Stage 0	Tis	N0	M0
Stage I	T1	N0	M0
Stage IIA	T2,T3	N0	M0
Stage IIB	T4	N0	M0
Stage IIIA	T0	N1b	M0
	T1,T2,T3,T4	N1a,N1a(sn)	M0
Stage IIIB	T1,T2,T3,T4	N1b,N2,N3	M0
Stage IV	Any T	Any N	M1

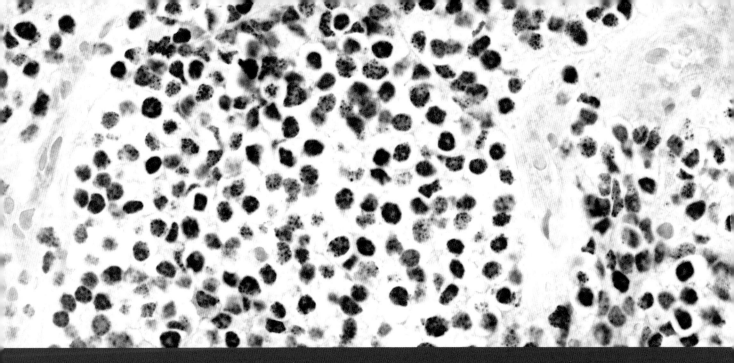

1

Nasal, paranasal, and skull base tumours

Edited by: Bishop JA, Loney EL, Thompson LDR

Nasal, paranasal, and skull base tumours: Introduction

Bishop JA
Thompson LDR

The sinonasal tract (including the nasal cavity, paranasal sinuses, and skull base) has always been an anatomical region in which a remarkable diversity of neoplasms can develop. It is because of this broad coverage that a taxonomic classification must be very focused to include entities that either develop in these sites exclusively (i.e. olfactory neuroblastoma) or develop anywhere in the head and neck but account for a significant proportion of disease in this location. Furthermore, some entities are considered in this chapter because they are potential candidates in the differential diagnosis with other lesions and should be mentioned. As such, squamous cell carcinoma is included in this chapter, but only keratinizing and non-keratinizing types, which predominate in this region, whereas subtypes (acantholytic, adenoid, basaloid, spindle cell, papillary, verrucous, adenosquamous, carcinoma cuniculatum), which rarely occur in the sinonasal tract, are covered more thoroughly in other chapters (occurring more commonly in the larynx, oral cavity, nasopharynx, and oropharynx). One of the most significant differences between the fourth and fifth editions is the exclusive coverage in their own chapters of the soft tissue tumours, haematolymphoid proliferations and neoplasms, melanocytic tumours, metastatic tumours to the head and neck, and most significantly, neuroendocrine neoplasms (NENs, including paraganglioma). Accordingly, aside from olfactory neuroblastoma, neuroendocrine tumours (NETs) and neuroendocrine carcinomas (NECs, small cell and large cell types) are not discussed in this chapter other than in the differential diagnosis context. Bone tumours, including fibro-osseous lesions, occur in the sinonasal tract but are covered in the chapter on odontogenic and maxillofacial bone tumours, where histological overlap and tumour centring are more likely to be problematic. There are always exceptions to rules; hence, tumours that develop exclusively (sinonasal glomangiopericytoma, biphenotypic sinonasal sarcoma, sinonasal angiofibroma) or predominantly (chordoma, meningioma, craniopharyngioma) in the sinonasal tract are covered in this chapter rather than in general topic chapters.

New entities in this edition include HPV-related multiphenotypic sinonasal carcinoma (provisionally included as HPV-related carcinoma with adenoid cystic–like features in the fourth edition) and SWI/SNF complex–deficient sinonasal carcinoma (provisionally included as SMARCB1-deficient sinonasal carcinoma in the fourth edition). The SWI/SNF complex–deficient sinonasal carcinomas constitute a group of tumours defined by inactivation of one of the SWI/SNF complex genes and include SMARCB1-deficient sinonasal carcinoma, SMARCB1-deficient sinonasal adenocarcinoma, and SMARCA4-deficient sinonasal carcinoma. A subset of teratocarcinosarcomas also exhibit *SMARCA4* loss but are considered separately because of the tumour's unique histological features and because *SMARCA4* loss is not always present. Developing and emerging entities include the IDH-mutant sinonasal malignancies, which are high-grade sinonasal tract neoplasms presently classified predominantly as sinonasal undifferentiated carcinoma but also sometimes as NEC, sinonasal adenocarcinoma, or even olfactory neuroblastoma. In future editions, these tumours may be better categorized separately as IDH-mutant sinonasal malignancies {1609}. Along similar lines, *DEK::AFF2* squamous cell carcinoma is an emerging category presently covered as a subtype of non-keratinizing squamous cell carcinoma, sometimes showing a deceptively bland histological appearance {473,3740,2418}. With additional experience, *DEK::AFF2* squamous cell carcinoma may be recognized as a distinct entity. A few specific fusions and mutations have been identified in non–intestinal-type sinonasal adenocarcinomas, but these alterations are not yet sufficiently well defined as to warrant separate categorization. In the context of worldwide global access to certain testing modalities (immunohistochemical and genetic studies), the tumours of the sinonasal tract, for the most part, are still defined by their histological features, utilizing ancillary testing to narrow the diagnosis when required for differences in treatment and prognostication.

Improvements in imaging studies continue to guide diagnosis and management. To wit, for the first time, this edition of the WHO classification included a radiologist as a member of the writing team to incorporate pertinent imaging findings into the classification as a multidisciplinary approach to meaningful diagnosis and patient management.

Respiratory epithelial adenomatoid hamartoma

Bullock MJ
Baněčková M
Wenig BM

Definition

Respiratory epithelial adenomatoid hamartoma (REAH) is an overgrowth of surface epithelium–derived medium-sized, ciliated glands surrounded by thickened basement membrane.

ICD-O coding

None

ICD-11 coding

None

Related terminology

Not recommended: glandular hamartoma.

Subtype(s)

Chondro-osseous respiratory epithelial (CORE) hamartoma

Localization

Most REAHs occur in the nasal cavity, particularly in the posterior septum and olfactory clefts {4786,2528,696}, sometimes secondarily involving the ethmoid labyrinth {1553}. Less common sites include the lateral nasal wall, middle meatus, and turbinates; rare sites are the nasopharynx, maxillary sinus, and frontal sinus. Bilateral lesions are frequent {4786,696}.

Clinical features

Patients may present with nasal obstruction (most commonly), anosmia, headache, and epistaxis, often with longstanding chronic rhinosinusitis.

Imaging

Imaging studies may demonstrate olfactory cleft expansion without bone erosion {4786,1803,2528,696}.

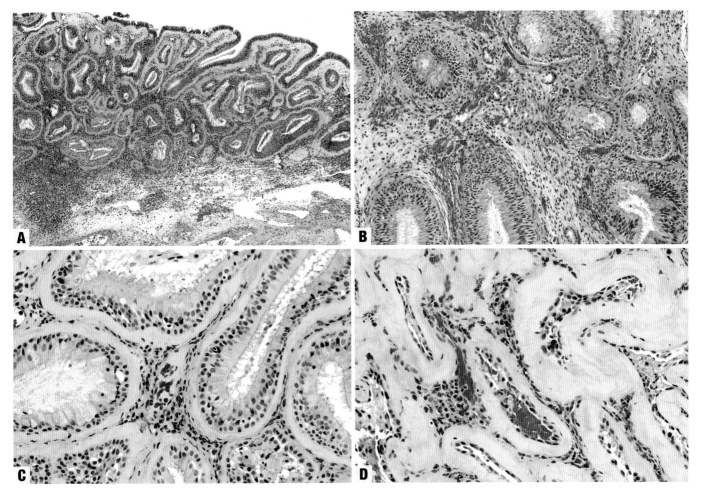

Fig. 1.01 Respiratory epithelial adenomatoid hamartoma. **A** Polypoid mass consisting of elongated or ovoid glands, descending from the surface. **B** In most cases, collections of small seromucinous glands are also noted between the larger glands. **C** Glands are lined by ciliated epithelium with mucinous cells, enveloped by thick, hyalinized stroma. There is intervening chronic inflammation. **D** Marked stromal hyalinization with flattening of the epithelium is common.

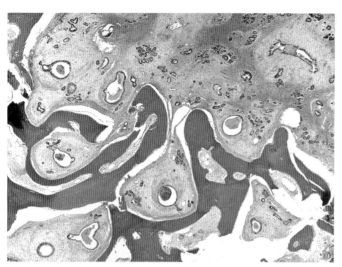

Fig. 1.02 Respiratory epithelial adenomatoid hamartoma, chondro-osseous and respiratory epithelial subtype. This lesion consists of a proliferation of small surface-type and seromucinous glands, associated with spicules of mature lamellar bone.

Epidemiology
Predominantly affected are adults, and there is a male predominance. Patients of a wide age range are affected, with a median age at presentation in the sixth decade of life {4786,2528,3912}.

Etiology
REAH commonly arises in association with allergy and sinonasal inflammatory disorders, suggesting a relationship to central compartment atopic disease {3912}.

Pathogenesis
Increased fractional allelic loss (31%) has been reported, raising the possibility that REAH is a neoplasm rather than a hamartoma {3352}. Other studies have explored the clonal nature of sinonasal hamartomas (REAH, seromucinous hamartoma, or combined) {330} but without documenting a clonal origin for pure REAH. Tryptase-producing mast cells and metalloproteinase expression have been implicated in REAH development {1553}.

Macroscopic appearance
REAHs are polypoid or exophytic with a rubbery consistency, tan-white to reddish-brown, and as large as 60 mm in greatest dimension {696}.

Histopathology
REAH consists of a polypoid proliferation of medium-sized, elongated to rounded, branching glands that expand from the surface epithelium downward into the stroma. They are separated by varying amounts of oedematous or fibrous stroma, usually with chronic inflammation. The epithelium is of the pseudostratified, ciliated type and frequently shows mucinous metaplasia, which can be extensive, resulting in glands dilated by mucin. The epithelium may be atrophic, with a flattened appearance to the limited cell layers. The glands are typically surrounded by thickened, brightly eosinophilic basement membrane {4786}. There is often a limited proliferation of small seromucinous glands in between or budding from the end of typical REAH glands. In large numbers, these may produce a hamartoma with combined features of REAH and seromucinous hamartoma {2271}. Associated findings include hyperplasia or squamous metaplasia of the surface epithelium, or a background of chronic rhinosinusitis and polyps. REAH may be isolated or (rarely) associated with inverted sinonasal papilloma or solitary fibrous tumour {4786}.

Subtype
Chondro-osseous respiratory epithelial (CORE) hamartoma is a subtype of REAH. In addition to the glandular component (less prominent than in REAHs), CORE hamartomas have an admixture of cartilaginous and/or osseous trabeculae that are intimately associated with the glandular proliferation {1405,1348, 3477,1333,1023}. A spectrum of chondro-osseous differentiation can be found, from cases manifesting immature-appearing mesenchyme in which cartilaginous plates display a zonal phenomenon resembling endochondral ossification in fetal skeletal development to cases with well-developed bony trabeculae in a myxoid to fibrous stroma.

Histochemistry
PAS highlights the thickened basement membrane.

Immunohistochemistry
The epithelium of REAH stains for CK7, MUC4, and CK8/18, but not for CK5/6, CK20, CDX2, or SATB2 {330}. The basal layer is intact and stains for p63 and p40; a basal layer is lacking in the small (seromucinous) gland component {1553}. There is no EBV association {1938}.

Differential diagnosis
The differential diagnosis includes an inflammatory polyp, inverted papilloma, biphenotypic sinonasal sarcoma, and low-grade non–intestinal-type sinonasal adenocarcinoma.

Cytology
Not clinically relevant

Diagnostic molecular pathology
None

Essential and desirable diagnostic criteria
Essential: surface epithelial origin; ciliated glands; retained basal layer; thickened basement membrane; displaced normal elements.

Staging
Not applicable

Prognosis and prediction
Recurrence is rare after complete excision {4786,2528,1553}.

Seromucinous hamartoma

Weinreb I
Ambrosini-Spaltro A
Skalova A

Definition
Seromucinous hamartoma (SH) is a benign proliferation of small eosinophilic glands arising in the sinonasal tract.

ICD-O coding
None

ICD-11 coding
None

Related terminology
Not recommended: microglandular adenosis of the nose; glandular hamartoma; serous hamartoma.

Subtype(s)
None

Localization
SH arises in the nasal cavity and paranasal sinuses, typically in the posterior nasal septum and nasopharynx {4475}.

Clinical features
The most common symptoms are nasal obstruction, purulent rhinorrhoea, and epistaxis {1956,2516}. Endoscopically, a papillomatous lesion is usually seen, sometimes with concurrent inflammatory nasal polyps {2271}.

Imaging
SH is well defined and homogeneous on both CT and MRI {1066}.

Epidemiology
SH is rare. It has an equal sex distribution, with a wide age range (11–86 years) at presentation {4761,164,2271,1940}.

Etiology
Unknown

Pathogenesis
One case harboured an *EGFR::ZNF267* gene fusion, and another case displayed monoclonality by AR X-chromosome inactivation assay, supporting the hypothesis of a neoplastic process {330}. Mitochondrial DNA revealed a slightly increased mutation rate mainly in heteroplasmy, consistent with a benign neoplasm {164}.

Macroscopic appearance
SH presents as a polypoid mass, ranging from 4 to 60 mm {4761}.

Histopathology
SH is a polypoid lesion lined by respiratory ciliated epithelium, with many small eosinophilic glands in the stroma, resembling microglandular adenosis of the breast {4761,164,2271,1940}. SH displays a lobular or horizontal distribution, with no infiltrative growth. Tubules are small and uniform, and they may contain an amorphous eosinophilic material; they are lined by epithelial cuboidal cells with small nuclei, without mitoses. Myoepithelial/basal cells are absent, or only focally present {1407}, but basal lamina around tubules is discernible. The tubules may be seen between native bony elements, but no true destructive infiltration is seen. No complex architectural patterns have been identified, such as exophytic growth, papillary architecture, or gland fusion.

The small glands of SH are sometimes combined with cystic structures lined by respiratory epithelium and p63-positive basal cells, more characteristic of respiratory epithelial adenomatoid hamartoma. Mixed forms exist as well.

Cytology
Not clinically relevant

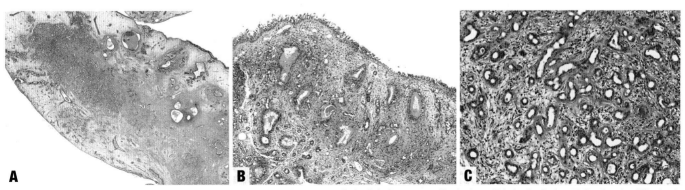

Fig. 1.03 Seromucinous hamartoma. **A** The lesion is polypoid and contains many small glands in the stroma, with a horizontal/lobular distribution. **B** Small eosinophilic glands may be admixed with cystic structures lined by respiratory epithelium. **C** Glands are small, eosinophilic, and uniform, and they may contain an amorphous eosinophilic material. Basal lamina around tubules is discernible.

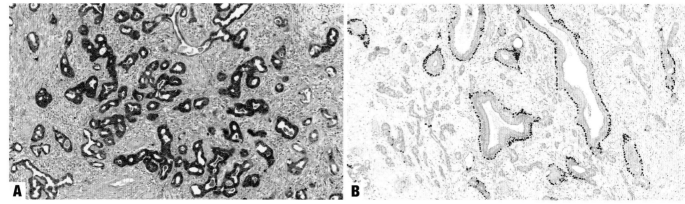

Fig. 1.04 Seromucinous hamartoma. **A** Glands are immunoreactive for S100. **B** p63-positive basal cells are absent around small glands but are evident around cystic structures lined by respiratory epithelium.

Diagnostic molecular pathology

Not clinically relevant

Essential and desirable diagnostic criteria

Essential: a monotonous proliferation of small tubules without atypia; absent/rare myoepithelial/basal cells; discernible basal lamina; no infiltrative pattern; no papillary architecture or gland fusion.

Staging

Not applicable

Prognosis and prediction

Recurrences are rare after complete excision {4761}.

Nasal chondromesenchymal hamartoma

Thompson LDR
Hill DA

Definition
Nasal chondromesenchymal hamartoma (NCMH) is a benign mesenchymal sinonasal tract tumour composed of cysts lined by respiratory epithelium associated with nodules of cartilage and a variably myxoid spindle cell stroma.

ICD-O coding
None

ICD-11 coding
2E90.6 & XH2P15 Benign neoplasm of nasopharynx & Mesenchymal hamartoma

Related terminology
Not recommended: chondroid hamartoma; nasal hamartoma; congenital mesenchymoma.

Subtype(s)
None

Localization
Frequently bilateral (~25%), tumours involve the paranasal sinuses (mostly ethmoid) and nasal cavity, sometimes with skull base extension {2902,3590,2870}.

Clinical features
Symptoms are nonspecific, with a mass identified {2902,3351, 3590,4230,2870}. Patients may have a history of other neoplasms associated with *DICER1* pathogenic variants {3590, 1165,4230,3932}.

Imaging
Imaging studies show a complex, solid and cystic, heterogeneous soft tissue mass, frequent calcification, and associated bone erosion {2902,4717,1703,2319}.

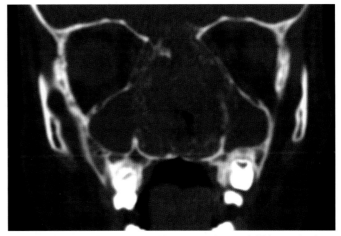

Fig. 1.05 Nasal chondromesenchymal hamartoma. A coronal CT image showing a destructive sinonasal tract mass with intracranial extension.

Epidemiology
Fewer than 1% of patients with pleuropulmonary blastoma have NCMH {3590}. There is a wide age range, but most patients are aged < 1 year (mean: 10 years). There is a male predominance.

Etiology
NCMH is associated with *DICER1* pathogenic variants {3590, 397}.

Pathogenesis
Like other neoplasms in *DICER1* syndrome, NCMH shows biallelic, loss-of-function, and missense RNase IIIb mutations in *DICER1*. This combination of mutations is expected to alter expression of microRNAs important in regulating the cell cycle and limiting differentiation {3590,3602,3933,1703}.

Macroscopic appearance
Polypoid, fleshy soft tissue masses

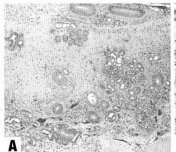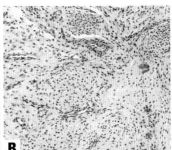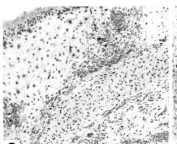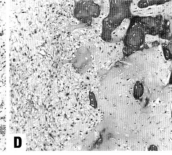

Fig. 1.06 Nasal chondromesenchymal hamartoma. **A** Low-power view shows immature cartilage and stroma in a background of minor mucoserous glands. **B** Intermediate-power view demonstrating immature islands of cartilage in a cellular background stroma. **C** High-power view shows immature cartilage in a cellular stroma showing mild nuclear pleomorphism. Extravasated erythrocytes are noted, with focal cystic changes. **D** Bone, immature cartilage, and a cellular spindled cell stroma are noted in this hamartoma.

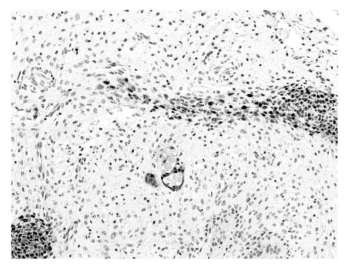

Fig. 1.07 Nasal chondromesenchymal hamartoma. S100 strongly highlights the nuclei and cytoplasm of the cartilaginous portions of the hamartoma. (The minor mucoserous gland is a good internal control.)

Histopathology

NCMH is composed of epithelial cysts lined by respiratory epithelium associated with nodules of immature to mature cartilage with a rim of spindled cells set in a loose, myxoid to spindled cell stroma. Focal osteoclast-like giant cells may be seen in the stroma near erythrocyte-filled spaces, resembling aneurysmal bone cyst {2902,4027,3351,3590}. A fibro-osseous proliferation with ossicles or trabeculae of immature (woven) bone can be seen {1935}. Concurrent sinonasal papilloma and chronic rhinosinusitis may be seen.

Immunohistochemistry
The cartilage is highlighted with S100 or SOX9 immunohistochemistry, and SMA highlights stromal myofibroblasts {3351, 1935}.

Differential diagnosis
The differential diagnosis includes sinonasal tract hamartomas, biphenotypic sinonasal sarcoma, and embryonal rhabdomyosarcoma (which can be seen in *DICER1* syndrome).

Cytology
Not clinically relevant

Diagnostic molecular pathology
When NCMH is diagnosed, germline *DICER1* genetic testing is suggested {3933}.

Essential and desirable diagnostic criteria
Essential: cysts lined by respiratory epithelium associated with nodules of immature to mature cartilage within a bland spindled cell stroma.
Desirable: biallelic *DICER1* pathogenic variants in selected cases.

Staging
Not applicable

Prognosis and prediction
Local recurrences may occur with incomplete excision (~25%) {2902,2870,3153}. Rare malignant transformation has been reported {2631}.

Sinonasal papilloma, inverted

Udager AM
McHugh JB
Mehrad M
Pai S
Stelow EB

Definition
Inverted sinonasal papilloma (ISP) is a benign epithelial neoplasm of ectodermally derived sinonasal epithelium showing inverted non-destructive growth into the stroma.

ICD-O coding
8121/1 Sinonasal papilloma, inverted

ICD-11 coding
2F00.Y & XH7YQ5 Other specified benign neoplasm of middle ear or respiratory system & Squamous cell papilloma, inverted

Related terminology
Not recommended: inverted Schneiderian papilloma; inverting papilloma; endophytic papilloma.

Subtype(s)
None

Localization
ISP usually involves the lateral nasal cavity wall and/or paranasal sinuses (most commonly ethmoid or maxillary); it may rarely occur on the nasal septum {3530,1979,2243,2491,4659,2923}. ISP rarely involves the lacrimal sac, middle ear, nasopharynx, and/or pharynx {4659,4781,4278,4426}.

Clinical features
Patients with ISP typically present with unilateral nasal obstruction and may also manifest with rhinorrhoea, epistaxis, facial pain / sinus pressure, headache, anosmia, and/or epiphora {3530,1979,2491,4659}.

Imaging
Imaging studies document a mass centred around the middle meatus, often with bone remodelling {3998,2075,2195}. Imaging is not definitive for ISP, but there are a number of features that are highly suggestive, including an origin from the lateral wall of the nasal cavity (with associated focal osteitis at this site on CT), lobulated shape, cerebriform (columnar) pattern on T2-weighted and postcontrast T1-weighted MRI, plateau enhancement on time–intensity curves (early peak and sustained high signal), and relatively high apparent diffusion coefficient values in keeping with benign disease. ISP usually causes bone thinning and remodelling on CT but can occasionally be locally aggressive. The combination of columnar enhancement and absent bone erosion allows for the confident discrimination of ISP from malignant sinonasal tumours {2846,4911}.

Epidemiology
ISP constitutes 47–73% of all sinonasal papillomas {1979,348, 2975,2171}. Although ISP is the most common type of sinonasal papilloma, it is still relatively uncommon overall, with an

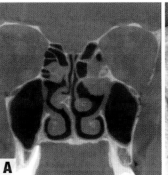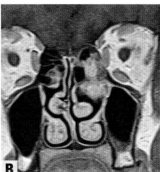

Fig. 1.08 Sinonasal papilloma, inverted. **A** Coronal bone window CT showing focal osteitis with hyperostosis in the left lateral nasal wall, a classic feature of inverted sinonasal papilloma arising from this site. **B** Coronal postcontrast T1-weighted MRI demonstrates an enhancing lobulated soft tissue mass confined to the nasal cavity.

estimated incidence of 0.2–1.5 cases per 100 000 person-years; reported incidence rates are higher in White people than in people of Asian descent {620,3340,4000,3250}. It typically occurs in older adults (peak incidence in the sixth decade of life) but may rarely be observed in children; there is a marked male predilection (M:F ratio: ~3–5:1) {3530,1979,2491,4659}.

Etiology
ISP may be associated with various occupational and/or industrial exposures; however, its relationship to tobacco smoke exposure remains uncertain {3530,2800,1078,3999}. Whereas historical studies documented HPV DNA (both low- and high-risk subtypes) in subsets of ISP and ISP-associated sinonasal carcinomas {4318,387,4316,4315}, modern RNA in situ hybridization analyses of ISP and ISP-associated sinonasal carcinomas have demonstrated a consistent lack of high-risk HPV E6/E7 transcripts, despite the presence of low-risk HPV E6/E7 transcripts in a subset of cases {3744,2923}. Furthermore, molecular profiling studies demonstrated somatic *EGFR* mutations in as many as 88% of ISPs and 77% of ISP-associated sinonasal carcinomas {4527,4694,2923}. The vast majority of *EGFR* mutations are frame-preserving indels in exon 20, although mutations in exon 6 or 19 occur in a small subset {4527,599}. Somatic *EGFR* mutations and low-risk HPV infection are mutually exclusive in ISP and ISP-associated sinonasal carcinoma, suggesting that they are essential alternative oncogenic mechanisms {4526,2923}.

Pathogenesis
Oncogenic hotspot mutations in *EGFR* exons 19 or 20 stimulate tumour growth via constitutive EGFR (HER1) activity and downstream activation of the MAPK and PI3K/AKT pathways {4923}. In HPV-associated ISPs, low-risk HPV infection is transcriptionally active, generating corresponding E6 and E7 transcripts {2923}. Malignant progression of ISP to sinonasal carcinoma is

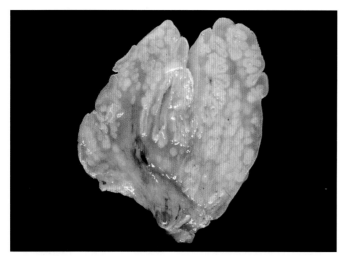

Fig. 1.09 Sinonasal papilloma, inverted. Gross image of the cut surface, showing visible endophytic tan nests/ribbons within a pale, oedematous stroma.

associated with deleterious *TP53* and/or *CDKN2A* alterations {599}.

Macroscopic appearance

ISP has a polypoid gross appearance with a convoluted cerebriform surface and typically demonstrates broad attachment to the underlying mucosa {4659,3240}.

Histopathology

ISP is a non-invasive epithelial neoplasm with predominantly endophytic growth {1979,4659}. Tumours comprise nests and/or ribbons of hyperplastic immature squamous epithelium (formerly transitional epithelium) within oedematous hypocellular stroma. The nests are rounded with an intact basement membrane. Prominent transmigrating intraepithelial neutrophilic inflammation is a characteristic feature. Scattered admixed ciliated or mucous columnar cells may be present superficially, and irritative changes may include increased squamous maturation, overlying keratosis, and/or underlying fibrosis. Low-risk HPV-associated ISPs may have a thickened epithelium with koilocyte-like cells, clear cell change, and binucleation, as well as verrucoid growth with limited involvement of the underlying

subepithelial stroma {2923}. Rare papillomas have overlapping features of inverted and oncocytic sinonasal papilloma {4694}.

Epithelial dysplasia is uncommon in ISP and may manifest in keratinizing and/or non-keratinizing forms {1979,3250}. Keratinizing epithelial dysplasia is similar to that observed in the oral cavity or larynx and may include hyperkeratosis, squamous dysmaturation, pleomorphism, and/or increased mitotic activity. Non-keratinizing epithelial dysplasia may resemble non-keratinizing squamous cell carcinoma (NKSCC) and include loss of transmigrating intraepithelial neutrophilic inflammation, basaloid morphology, conspicuous cytological atypia, and/or increased mitotic activity. Although there is no consensus grading system for dysplasia in ISP, it is important to recognize and report severe dysplasia / carcinoma in situ when present {3250}.

Differential diagnosis

Given its distinct differences in etiology and clinical behaviour, the most important differential diagnosis for ISP is NKSCC. Although both tumours may demonstrate an endophytic growth pattern, NKSCC frequently has a basaloid appearance, conspicuous pleomorphism and/or mitotic activity, atypical mitoses, predominantly exophytic growth, and/or a lack of transmigrating intraepithelial neutrophilic inflammation. Furthermore, although NKSCC is often positive for high-risk HPV by RNA in situ hybridization for high-risk HPV E6/E7 transcripts, ISP is consistently negative {3744,2923}.

Cytology

Not clinically relevant

Diagnostic molecular pathology

None

Essential and desirable diagnostic criteria

Essential: predominantly endophytic non-destructive growth; ribbons/nests of hyperplastic, immature squamous epithelium; transmigrating intraepithelial neutrophilic inflammation.

Staging

There is no applicable Union for International Cancer Control (UICC) / American Joint Committee on Cancer (AJCC) TNM

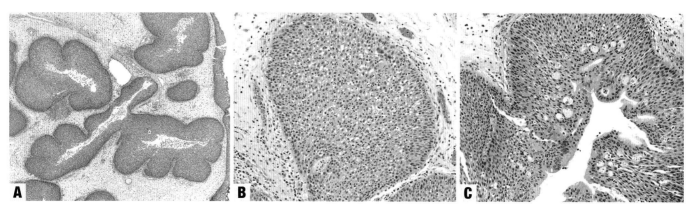

Fig. 1.10 Sinonasal papilloma, inverted. **A** Low-power photomicrograph showing the characteristic predominantly endophytic growth pattern. **B** High-power photomicrograph showing an endophytic nest of hyperplastic immature squamous epithelium with transmigrating intraepithelial neutrophilic inflammation characteristic of this entity. **C** High-power photomicrograph highlighting scattered superficial ciliated and mucous columnar cells.

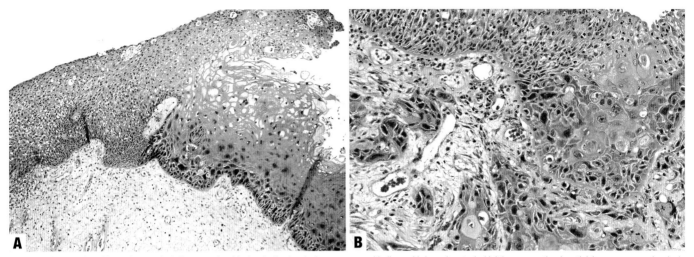

Fig. 1.11 Sinonasal papilloma, inverted. **A** An example with dysplasia. Atypical squamous epithelium with hyperkeratosis (right), representing keratinizing squamous dysplasia arising in a sinonasal papilloma, inverted (left). **B** An example with keratinizing squamous cell carcinoma. There are infiltrating irregular nests of atypical squamous epithelial cells involving the subepithelial stroma, representing keratinizing squamous cell carcinoma arising in association with a sinonasal papilloma, inverted.

classification, but the Krouse clinical staging system (T1–T4) classifies ISP by anatomical location, tumour extent, and presence of concurrent malignancy {2393}.

Prognosis and prediction

Reported recurrence rates vary widely for ISP – particularly when historical cohorts are considered – and depend on a number of clinical factors, including surgical approach (higher with non-endoscopic techniques), tumour anatomical location (higher for frontal and anterior maxillary sinus tumours), and Krouse stage (higher for T3 tumours than for T2 tumours) {637, 2287,2673,3019}. According to a large multicentre study and meta-analysis, the overall estimated recurrence rate for ISP is 12–16% {2287,2673}.

Malignant transformation – either synchronous or metachronous – develops at a rate of about 2–4% according to large longitudinal and multicentre studies {2287,3250}, rather than at the higher rates reported by referral centres. The vast majority of ISP-associated sinonasal carcinomas are keratinizing or nonkeratinizing squamous cell carcinomas; however, other types of malignancies have been reported, including sinonasal undifferentiated carcinoma {3319}. Although ISP-associated mucoepidermoid carcinomas have been rarely reported, they probably represent adenosquamous carcinomas {3250}. Cigarette smoke

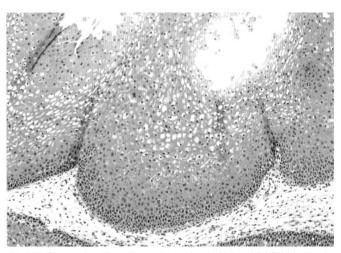

Fig. 1.12 Sinonasal papilloma, inverted, associated with low-risk HPV infection. Intermediate-power photomicrograph highlighting the verrucoid growth and thickened epithelium with koilocyte-like cells, increased clear cell change, and binucleation.

exposure is a risk factor for ISP malignant progression {1911}, and recent evidence suggests that low-risk HPV infection in ISP may be associated with an increased risk of malignant progression {4526,2923}.

Sinonasal papilloma, oncocytic

Udager AM
McHugh JB
Mehrad M
Pai S
Stelow EB

Definition

Oncocytic sinonasal papilloma (OSP) is a benign epithelial neoplasm of ectodermally derived sinonasal epithelium showing multilayered oncocytic cuboidal to columnar epithelium.

ICD-O coding

8121/1 Sinonasal papilloma, oncocytic

ICD-11 coding

2F00.Y & XH17Q9 Other specified benign neoplasm of middle ear or respiratory system & Papilloma, NOS

Related terminology

Not recommended: oncocytic Schneiderian papilloma; cylindrical cell papilloma; columnar cell papilloma; Ringertz papilloma.

Subtype(s)

None

Localization

OSP involves the lateral wall of the nasal cavity and/or paranasal sinuses (most commonly the maxillary sinus) and may also rarely involve other head and neck sites, including the middle ear {1979,348,4781,2196,2644,4426}.

Clinical features

Patients with OSP typically present with unilateral nasal obstruction and may also manifest rhinorrhoea, epistaxis, and/or anosmia {348,2196}.

Imaging

Imaging studies document a mass centred around the middle meatus, often with bone remodelling {2196,1031,4911}. OSP appears similar to inverted sinonasal papilloma (ISP) on imaging, but studies have shown three distinctive features that may be helpful: T1-weighted high signal, multiple mucinous cystic foci, and a lack of focal osteitis {4911}.

Epidemiology

OSPs constitute 3–19% of all sinonasal papillomas {1979, 2171,2196}, estimated to have an incidence of 0.05 cases per 100 000 person-years {620}. They typically occur in older adults (peak incidence in the sixth to seventh decades of life), are rare in patients aged < 30 years, and have an equal sex distribution {2196,2644}.

Etiology

There are no confirmed risk factors. HPV infection is not an etiological factor {619,4526}.

Pathogenesis

Oncogenic hotspot mutations in *KRAS* exon 2 or 3 stimulate tumour growth via constitutive KRAS activity and downstream activation of the MAPK and PI3K/AKT pathways {3637,2797}. Malignant progression of OSP to sinonasal carcinoma is associated with deleterious *TP53* and *CDKN2A* mutations {599}.

Macroscopic appearance

OSP has a papillary and/or polypoid gross appearance; tumours can be very large (> 100 mm) but are typically < 50 mm {348}.

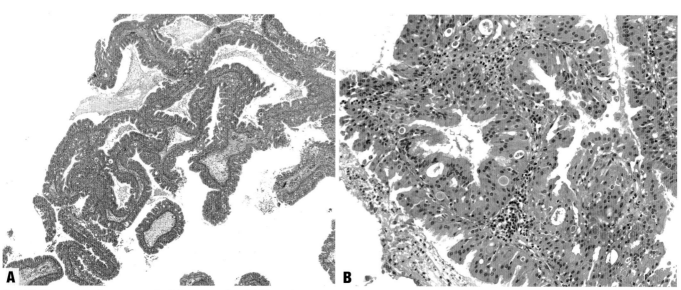

Fig. 1.13 Sinonasal papilloma, oncocytic. **A** Low-power view highlighting the mixed exophytic and endophytic growth pattern. **B** High-power view showing the characteristic oncocytic cuboidal to columnar cells and intraepithelial microcysts with mucin and/or neutrophilic microabscesses.

Histopathology

OSP is a non-invasive papillary epithelial neoplasm with mixed exophytic and endophytic growth {1979,348}. Tumours comprise multiple layers of cuboidal to columnar cells with abundant oncocytic cytoplasm, slightly enlarged and irregular but centrally placed nuclei, and small nucleoli. Scattered admixed ciliated or mucous columnar cells may be present superficially. Intraepithelial neutrophilic inflammation is common, whereas microcysts with mucin and/or neutrophilic microabscesses are characteristic. Epithelial dysplasia is uncommon in OSP but may manifest as increased nuclear atypia and/or mitotic activity {2171,4730,4426}.

Cytology

Not clinically relevant

Diagnostic molecular pathology

None

Essential and desirable diagnostic criteria

Essential: mixed exophytic and endophytic growth pattern; oncocytic cells with cuboidal to columnar morphology; intraepithelial microcysts with mucin and/or neutrophilic microabscesses.

Staging

None

Prognosis and prediction

Reported recurrence rates vary widely – from 6% to 40% of tumours in large studies with long-term follow-up – and these observed differences are probably multifactorial in origin, including tumour anatomical location (higher for paranasal sinus tumours) and surgical approach (higher with non-endoscopic techniques) {2196,2644}.

Malignant transformation – either synchronous or metachronous – occurs in 3–17% of OSPs {2171,2215,2196}; the vast majority of these tumours are keratinizing or non-keratinizing squamous cell carcinomas, but other types of malignancies have been reported (rarely), including adenocarcinoma, small cell carcinoma, and sinonasal undifferentiated carcinoma {2798,5012}. OSP-associated mucoepidermoid carcinomas

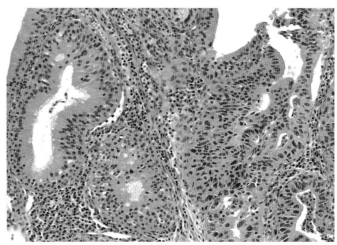

Fig. 1.14 Sinonasal papilloma, oncocytic, with dysplasia. There is increased nuclear atypia and mitotic activity (right half of image) characteristic of dysplasia.

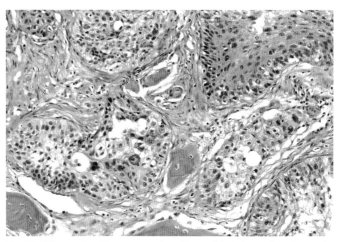

Fig. 1.15 Sinonasal papilloma, oncocytic, with associated sinonasal carcinoma. Infiltrating nests of atypical squamous epithelial cells involve bone, corresponding to a sinonasal carcinoma arising in association with sinonasal papilloma, oncocytic.

have been reported {2171}; however, according to contemporary criteria, they most likely represent adenosquamous carcinomas.

Sinonasal papilloma, exophytic

Stelow EB
McHugh JB
Mehrad M
Pai S
Udager AM

Definition
Exophytic sinonasal papilloma is a benign sinonasal tract epithelial neoplasm composed of broad papillary fronds with delicate fibrovascular cores covered by a maturing multilayered epithelium.

ICD-O coding
8121/0 Sinonasal papilloma, exophytic

ICD-11 coding
2F00.Y & XI I0TP8 Other specified benign neoplasm of middle ear or respiratory system & Sinonasal papilloma, exophytic

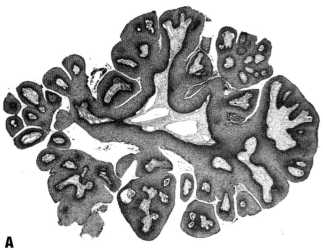

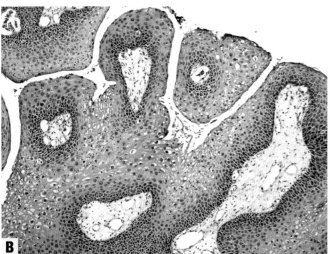

Fig. 1.16 Sinonasal papilloma, exophytic. **A** The lesion is exophytic and covered by a maturing multilayered squamous epithelium. **B** Maturing squamous epithelium with superficial koilocytes lines these finger-like projections. Scattered transmigrating intraepithelial neutrophils are seen.

Related terminology
Not recommended: Schneiderian papilloma, exophytic type; fungiform papilloma; everted papilloma; transitional cell papilloma; septal papilloma; Ringertz tumour.

Subtype(s)
None

Localization
Exophytic sinonasal papillomas usually arise on the lower anterior nasal septum {620,1605}. As they enlarge, they may secondarily involve the lateral nasal wall, but they rarely originate there. Involvement of the paranasal sinuses is extremely rare. Bilateral lesions are exceptional {620,1605}.

Clinical features
Typical presenting symptoms include epistaxis and unilateral nasal obstruction caused by a mass lesion. Endoscopy aids in defining the site and extent of disease, but imaging is unnecessary.

Epidemiology
These tumours are 2–10 times as common in male patients as female patients, and they typically occur in individuals aged 20–50 years (range: 2–87 years) {889,4650}.

Etiology
The majority of these tumours harbour low-risk HPV (mostly types 6 and 11) {619,4316}.

Pathogenesis
Unknown

Macroscopic appearance
The tumours present as papillary or warty, grey, pink, or tan growths attached to the nasal septum by a relatively broad base. They range in size up to about 20 mm.

Histopathology
Exophytic sinonasal papillomas are composed of papillary fronds with fibrovascular cores covered by a proliferative, multilayered epithelium that is 5–20 cells thick. The epithelium varies from squamous to ciliated pseudostratified columnar (respiratory), or it may be transitional between the two. Scattered mucocytes and intraepithelial neutrophils are common. Surface keratinization is absent or scant, unless irritated by trauma or dried by air. Mitoses are rare and not atypical. Unless infected or irritated, the stroma contains few inflammatory cells. Malignant change in exophytic papilloma is extremely rare {889,371}.

Differential diagnosis

Exophytic papillomas must be distinguished from cutaneous keratinizing squamous papilloma (which is much more common in the nasal vestibule), inverted sinonasal papilloma, and papillary squamous cell carcinoma.

Cytology
Not clinically relevant

Diagnostic molecular pathology
None

Essential and desirable diagnostic criteria
Essential: proliferative, exophytic, and papillary growth; lined by a multilayered sinonasal-type epithelium; no high-grade squamous dysplasia; no inverted or destructive infiltrative growth.

Staging
Not applicable

Prognosis and prediction
Local recurrence rates are 22–50%; recurrence is associated with inadequate excision {889,620}. Malignant transformation is extremely rare {3250,505}.

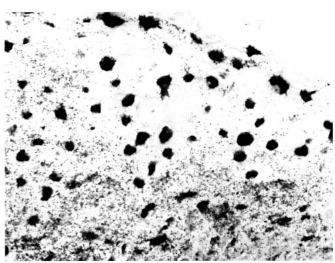

Fig. 1.17 Sinonasal papilloma, exophytic. Most exophytic sinonasal papillomas harbour low-risk HPV, demonstrated here by RNA in situ hybridization for HPV types 6 and 11.

Keratinizing squamous cell carcinoma

Bell D
Jain D
Sandison A
Yamamoto H

Definition

Sinonasal keratinizing squamous cell carcinoma (KSCC) is an epithelial malignancy originating from surface epithelium with squamous differentiation and keratin production.

ICD-O coding

8071/3 Squamous cell carcinoma, keratinizing, NOS
8086/3 HPV-independent squamous cell carcinoma
8052/3 Papillary squamous cell carcinoma
8051/3 Verrucous carcinoma
8074/3 Spindle cell squamous cell carcinoma
8075/3 Acantholytic squamous cell carcinoma
8560/3 Adenosquamous carcinoma
8051/3 Carcinoma cuniculatum

ICD-11 coding

2C20.4 & XH4CR9 Squamous cell carcinoma of nasal cavity & Squamous cell carcinoma, keratinizing, NOS
2C22.1 & XH4CR9 Squamous cell carcinoma of accessory sinuses & Squamous cell carcinoma, keratinizing, NOS

Related terminology

Not recommended: squamous cell carcinoma NOS; conventional squamous cell carcinoma; epidermoid carcinoma.

Subtype(s)

HPV-independent squamous cell carcinoma; papillary squamous cell carcinoma; verrucous carcinoma; spindle cell squamous cell carcinoma; acantholytic squamous cell carcinoma; adenosquamous carcinoma; carcinoma cuniculatum

Localization

The maxillary antrum, lateral nasal wall, and sphenoid sinuses are the most commonly affected sites, whereas the nasal septum, nasal floor, and frontal and sphenoid sinuses are less frequently involved. KSCC is the most common malignancy of the nasal vestibule {64}.

Clinical features

Patients present with nonspecific nasal obstruction, facial pain, rhinorrhoea, and epistaxis {2589}. Tumours grow by local extension, infiltrating the neighbouring structures {2589}. Lymph node metastases are rare.

Imaging

Imaging studies demonstrate an aggressive soft tissue–density mass with poorly defined, irregular to spiculated margins, often with bone destruction, and documentation of distant metastatic disease or multifocal primaries {3632,1226,2517,2521,1496}.

Epidemiology

KSCC represents as many as 45–50% of sinonasal tract malignancies {4519,1208,2051,1227}. The M:F ratio is 2:1, and the majority arise in patients aged > 50 years {4519,1208,2051, 1227}.

Etiology

Occupational hazards explain some KSCC risk as well as the male predominance. Long exposures to nickel, chrome, arsenic, formaldehyde, welding fumes, leather dust, glues, and various textile-related compounds are attributed to tumorigenesis in as many as 30% of cases {1227}. A clear association between KSCC and cigarette smoking has been documented {2589}.

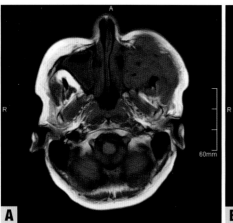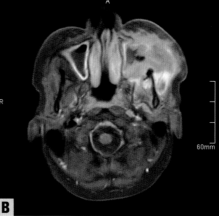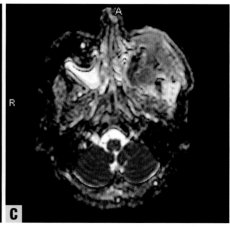

Fig. 1.18 Keratinizing squamous cell carcinoma. T1-weighted axial MRI (**A**), fat-suppressed T1-weighted axial MRI (**B**), and axial apparent diffusion coefficient map (**C**) demonstrate a large tumour centred on the left maxillary sinus, extending into the soft tissues of the cheek, masticator space, and retromaxillary fat, involving the pterygoid process and pterygomaxillary region. Note the tumour's low apparent diffusion coefficient value (**C**), consistent with a highly cellular mass.

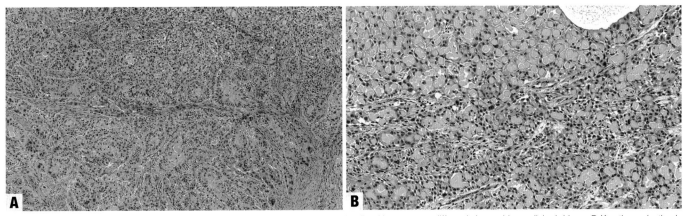

Fig. 1.19 Keratinizing squamous cell carcinoma. **A** Proliferation of malignant epithelial cells with squamous differentiation and intercellular bridges. **B** Keratin production is frequent.

Chronic sinonasal inflammation is considered a predisposing factor.

Pathogenesis

KSCC originates in the sinonasal mucosa from areas of pre-existing squamous metaplasia. About 60% of KSCCs arising from inverted papillomas present synchronously {3250,2589}. Aside from KSCC ex sinonasal papilloma, squamous dysplasia / carcinoma in situ is uncommon in adjacent mucosa.

The genomic landscape of KSCC is poorly defined, with reports of *TP53* mutations, p53 expression alterations, microsatellite instability, chromosomal aberrations {2766}, *EGFR* mutations {3880}, and alterations in *PTEN*, *CDKN2A*, and *KMT2D* {1}. Approximately 20% of sinonasal KSCCs harbour an *EGFR* mutation, and most of them are associated with inverted papilloma {4526,3880,1914}. High microsatellite instability is very rare. Sinonasal KSCC is much less likely to harbour high-risk HPV infection than non-keratinizing squamous cell carcinoma {2095}.

Macroscopic appearance

Nonspecific, similar to KSCC at other sites

Histopathology

KSCC shows infiltrative proliferations of malignant epithelial cells with squamous differentiation in the form of glassy eosinophilic cytoplasm, intercellular bridges, and frequent keratin production. Differentiation degree, cellular pleomorphism, and mitotic activity account for three grades (well-/moderately/poorly differentiated). Well-differentiated KSCC is uncommon. Moderately or poorly differentiated KSCCs constitute the majority. Special types, such as papillary, verrucous, spindle cell, acantholytic, and adenosquamous carcinomas, as well as carcinoma cuniculatum, each constitute a small percentage of tumours (and are more extensively discussed in the larynx and oral sections).

Immunohistochemistry

Immunohistochemistry is seldom required, but pancytokeratin, p40, p63, and CK5/6 are usually identified.

Differential diagnosis

The primary differential diagnosis is with sinonasal papilloma, necrotizing sialometaplasia, pseudoepitheliomatous hyperplasia, and verrucous hyperplasia; other spindled cell neoplasms would be considered in the spindle cell squamous cell carcinoma category.

Cytology

Smears show plentiful dispersed spindle, polygonal, and tadpole cells, showing varying degrees of keratinization with dense light-blue (Giemsa stain) or orangeophilic (Pap) cytoplasm, as well as relatively cohesive tissue fragments of similar cells with well-defined dense cytoplasm. Nuclei vary from various stages of pyknosis in the keratinized cells to more open, large, often centrally placed nuclei with coarse chromatin and prominent nucleoli. There is often a large amount of keratinous debris in the background, with or without a granulomatous reaction {1835}.

Diagnostic molecular pathology

Not clinically relevant

Essential and desirable diagnostic criteria

Essential: malignant epithelial cells with squamous differentiation and keratinization.
Desirable: positivity for p40 immunostain (in selected cases).

Staging

Staging follows the eighth edition of the Union for International Cancer Control (UICC) / American Joint Committee on Cancer (AJCC) TNM staging system.

Prognosis and prediction

Although the incidence is decreasing, 5-year overall survival rates are about 50% {205,3855,1227}. The 5-year relative survival rate for patients with nasal cavity KSCC is 74.5%, compared with 35% for maxillary and ethmoid sinus KSCC and < 30% for frontal and sphenoid KSCC {1227}. Although tumours with PDL1 expression show improved outcomes for the oropharynx, oral cavity, and larynx {2766}, studies in sinonasal KSCC are still ongoing {3703,3620}.

Non-keratinizing squamous cell carcinoma

Rooper LM
Ihrlcr S
Kiss K
Lewis JS Jr
Westra W
Yamamoto H

Definition

Non-keratinizing squamous cell carcinoma (NKSCC) is an epithelial malignancy of sinonasal surface origin that shows histological and immunohistochemical evidence of squamous differentiation but has no or minimal keratinization.

ICD-O coding

8072/3 Squamous cell carcinoma, non-keratinizing, NOS
8085/3 HPV-associated squamous cell carcinoma
8072/3 *DEK::AFF2* squamous cell carcinoma

ICD-11 coding

2C20.4 & XH6705 Squamous cell carcinoma of nasal cavity & Squamous cell carcinoma, large cell, non-keratinizing, NOS
2C22.1 & XH6705 Squamous cell carcinoma of accessory sinuses & Squamous cell carcinoma, large cell, non-keratinizing, NOS

Related terminology

Not recommended: Schneiderian carcinoma, transitional cell carcinoma, cylindrical cell carcinoma.

Subtype(s)

HPV-associated squamous cell carcinoma; *DEK::AFF2* squamous cell carcinoma

Localization

Sinonasal NKSCC most commonly arises in the nasal cavity or maxillary sinuses {2592,4519,205,3855}.

Clinical features

Patients present with mass effect, including nasal obstruction, epistaxis, and pain. Paranasal sinus tumours present at a higher stage than nasal cavity tumours {4519,205}.

Imaging

Imaging studies cannot accurately differentiate NKSCC from keratinizing squamous cell carcinoma (SCC) and in both cases demonstrate an aggressive soft tissue lesion with bony destruction of adjacent sinus walls, most frequently arising from the maxillary sinus, followed by ethmoid air cells and the nasal cavity. Because many present at an advanced stage, invasion of the orbit, infratemporal fossa, and skull base is frequently observed. A combination of postcontrast CT and MRI is helpful to accurately delineate tumour extension through bone and soft tissues. Intratumoural necrosis is commonly seen in larger lesions, with average solid tumour apparent diffusion coefficient values of 0.95×10^{-3} mm^2/s {2616,2224}.

Epidemiology

NKSCC accounts for 20–48% of sinonasal SCCs, while recognizing the historical overlap with papillary and basaloid patterns {1247,474,2473,2589}. Tumours most frequently arise in the sixth to seventh decades of life, and there is a male predominance {3711,3327,1247,474}.

Etiology

Like other sinonasal SCCs, NKSCC has a weak association with tobacco use {2694}. High-risk HPV is implicated in 20–62% of all sinonasal SCCs in North America and Europe and 7–21% in Asia. Specifically, 36–58% of NKSCCs are HPV-associated {1247,137,474,2473,2601,2449,869,2095,920,2305,3917}.
HPV16 is relatively less common in the sinonasal tract than in the oropharynx, representing 41–82% of HPV-associated cases {474,2449,2305,2868}. Only rare EBV-positive NKSCCs have been reported {2575}, and about 15% of carcinomas ex sinonasal papilloma are NKSCC {346,3250}.

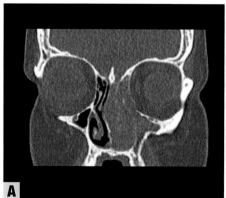 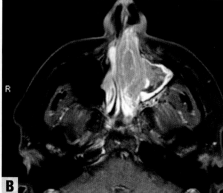 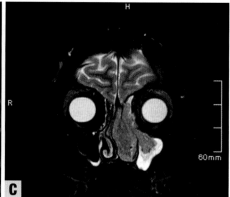

Fig. 1.20 Non-keratinizing squamous cell carcinoma. **A** Coronal CT (bone window) shows a large soft-tissue lesion filling the left nasal cavity, with attenuation of the left lamina papyracea. **B** Postcontrast fat-suppressed T1-weighted axial MRI shows linear cerebriform enhancement, suggesting that this non-keratinizing squamous cell carcinoma may have arisen from inverted papilloma. **C** Coronal short-tau inversion recovery (STIR) MRI shows clear differentiation between the soft tissue tumour (intermediate signal) extending into the left maxillary sinus and the retained sinus secretions (high signal).

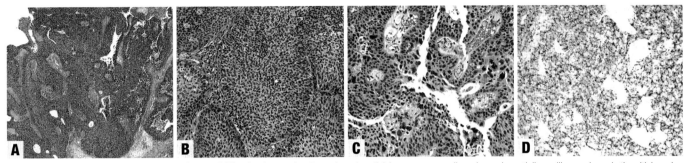

Fig. 1.21 Non-keratinizing squamous cell carcinoma. **A** The classic growth pattern of non-keratinizing squamous cell carcinoma is partially papillary and exophytic, with invasion as broad, pushing, smooth-edged ribbons. This pattern is reminiscent of inverted papilloma, but non-keratinizing squamous cell carcinoma is much more basophilic, owing to the high N:C ratios of the neoplastic cells. **B** Nested and lobulated growth of cells with high N:C ratios and no keratinization, with peripheral palisading and minimal stromal desmoplasia. **C** Predominantly papillary growth can be seen in a subset of tumours, and cytological atypia can vary widely. **D** HPV-associated squamous cell carcinoma is a subtype of non-keratinizing squamous cell carcinoma defined by the presence of transcriptionally active high-risk HPV, highlighted here by RNA in situ hybridization.

Pathogenesis

The molecular underpinnings of sinonasal NKSCC have not been comprehensively characterized, although those sequenced show similar molecular profiles to other head and neck SCCs {2709,2694,892,2095,1914}. Transcriptional activity is identified in HPV-associated NKSCC via p16 overexpression combined with PCR positivity or RNA in situ hybridization {474, 2473,2449,3744}. Nearly half of HPV-negative NKSCCs tested have been shown to harbour recurrent fusions between the *DEK* gene on chromosome 6p22.3 and the *AFF2* gene on chromosome Xq28 {4921,4466,473,3740,2418}, which probably represent oncogenic drivers.

Macroscopic appearance

Tumours can be endophytic or exophytic and have a friable white-tan surface with haemorrhage and necrosis. Tumours are typically large and bulky.

Histopathology

NKSCC is arranged in expansile nests, lobules, or ribbons that display a pushing pattern of invasion with a smooth stromal interface and minimal associated desmoplastic response, despite often deep and destructive growth. A subset shows predominantly papillary architecture with extensive (sometimes complete) surface growth and colonization of adjacent flat surface epithelium {2107,2589}. Invasive growth, as classically defined for SCC in other anatomical sites, is not necessary in mass-forming tumours. Tumour cells have a high N:C ratio, a columnar basal layer with peripheral palisading, and a more flattened superficial layer, and they lack significant keratinization. Cytological atypia is highly variable, ranging from minimal to pronounced, but grading is not applied. Mitotic rates also vary widely, and necrosis may occasionally be seen.

Subtypes

HPV-associated SCC is a subtype of sinonasal NKSCC defined by the presence of transcriptionally active high-risk HPV. The majority of these tumours demonstrate otherwise classic NKSCC morphology, although a minority of HPV-associated sinonasal carcinomas represent keratinizing, basaloid, or adenosquamous subtypes {1247,474,2473,2601,2449,3917}.

DEK::AFF2 squamous cell carcinoma is an emerging subtype of NKSCC defined by recurrent *DEK::AFF2* fusions {4921, 4466,473,2418}. They demonstrate complex exophytic and

endophytic growth, with broad papillary fronds and anastomosing lobules lined by transitional epithelium with amphophilic to eosinophilic cytoplasm. The presence of strikingly monotonous round to oval nuclei, surface or intraepithelial discohesion, and frequent tumour-infiltrating neutrophils or lymphocytes may help differentiate them from other NKSCCs. *DEK::AFF2* squamous cell carcinoma shows substantial morphological overlap with tumours reported as low-grade papillary sinonasal (Schneiderian) carcinoma {2594,2076,598,682,5001,3793}, and recent data suggest that many, if not most, of these tumours also harbour *DEK::AFF2* fusions {2418}.

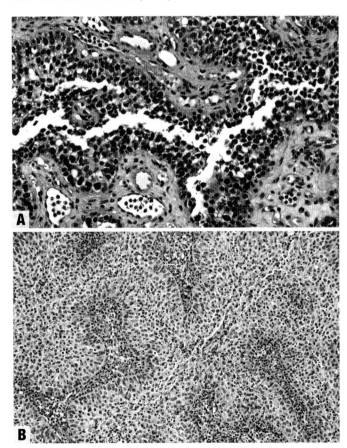

Fig. 1.22 Non-keratinizing squamous cell carcinoma, *DEK::AFF2* subtype. **A** Confluent exophytic and endophytic growth with surface epithelial discohesion and strikingly monotonous oval nuclei. **B** Dense tumour-infiltrating neutrophils are frequently seen.

Immunohistochemistry

NKSCCs are diffusely positive for cytokeratins, particularly high-molecular-weight cocktails such as CK5/6 and 34βE12 (CK903), and for p63 and p40 {762,4453}. They are negative for synaptophysin, chromogranin, INSM1, S100, NUT, and CD99, with intact SMARCB1 (INI1) and SMARCA4 (BRG1) {4817,468, 466,3743,3752}.

Differential diagnosis

Although some NKSCCs were historically classified as basaloid SCC, this subtype should be restricted to tumours with nested architecture, prominent basement membrane deposition, and comedonecrosis. Although inverted growth in NKSCC may be reminiscent of inverted papilloma, definitive synchronous or metachronous benign sinonasal papilloma must be present for a designation of carcinoma ex sinonasal papilloma. *DEK::AFF2* squamous cell carcinomas can overlap with benign sinonasal papillomas because of their bland cytology, but they demonstrate more irregular stromal interfaces and complex architecture. HPV-related multiphenotypic sinonasal carcinoma displays basaloid areas similar to NKSCC but also demonstrates ductal and/or myoepithelial differentiation. Several other sinonasal tumours with squamous differentiation are now regarded as distinct entities, including NUT carcinoma, adamantinoma-like Ewing sarcoma, and SWI/SNF complex–deficient sinonasal carcinoma. Other sinonasal carcinomas lack squamous differentiation by immunohistochemistry but are unique tumours, such as sinonasal undifferentiated carcinoma and neuroendocrine carcinoma (NEC).

Cytology

Smears show predominantly large sheets and tissue fragments consisting of cells with well-defined dense cytoplasm, lacking keratinization, with large pleomorphic nuclei with coarse chromatin and one or more prominent pleomorphic nucleoli. Necrosis and variable keratinous debris are seen in the background.

Diagnostic molecular pathology

Although routine HPV testing is not recommended in sinonasal NKSCC, it can occasionally be helpful for diagnostic purposes. If used, HPV-specific testing such as in situ hybridization or PCR must be performed, because p16 has poor specificity in sinonasal tumours {4663,474,136,218}. *DEK::AFF2* fusions can be confirmed via RNA sequencing or *DEK* FISH.

Essential and desirable diagnostic criteria

Essential: morphological and/or immunohistochemical evidence of squamous differentiation; no to minimal keratinization; active exclusion of mimics, such as NUT carcinoma, SMARCB1-deficient sinonasal carcinoma, and adamantinoma-like Ewing sarcoma.

Staging

Staging follows the eighth edition of the Union for International Cancer Control (UICC) / American Joint Committee on Cancer (AJCC) TNM staging system.

Prognosis and prediction

Although specific outcomes of NKSCC are unknown, sinonasal SCC overall has a 5-year survival rate of approximately 60% {3711,4442,4519,205,3855}. Although single-institution and large database studies have often shown better prognosis in HPV-associated tumours, the benefit has not translated in clinical practice {1247,137,474,2473,2601,2449,869,2282,2095, 3293,920,141,2305,3917}. In limited experience, *DEK::AFF2* squamous cell carcinomas showed frequent local recurrence, and 25% of patients died of disease {3740}.

NUT carcinoma

French CA
Minato H
Stelow EB

Definition
NUT carcinoma is an epithelial malignancy with a relatively monotonous appearance, genetically defined by a rearrangement of the nuclear protein in testis (NUT) gene *NUTM1*.

ICD-O coding
8023/3 NUT carcinoma

ICD-11 coding
2C20 & XH1YY4 Malignant neoplasms of nasal cavity & Carcinoma, undifferentiated, NOS
2C22 & XH1YY4 Malignant neoplasms of accessory sinuses & Carcinoma, undifferentiated, NOS

Related terminology
Not recommended: nuclear protein in testis carcinoma; NUT midline carcinoma; NUT-rearranged carcinoma; t(15;19) carcinoma; carcinoma with t(15;19) translocation; aggressive t(15;19)-positive carcinoma; midline lethal carcinoma; midline carcinoma of children and young adults with NUT rearrangement.

Subtype(s)
None

Localization
Head and neck primary sites constitute about 40% of NUT carcinomas {769}. Most head and neck cases affect the sinonasal tract (57%), and others affect the nasopharynx (6%) or major salivary glands (4%) {768,41,4695}. Rare cases involve the orbit, pharynx, or larynx {5047,373,1182,768,1827,730}.

Clinical features
Patients with NUT carcinoma present with symptoms caused by a rapidly growing mass. In the sinonasal tract, this manifests as nasal obstruction, pain, headache, epistaxis, and nasal

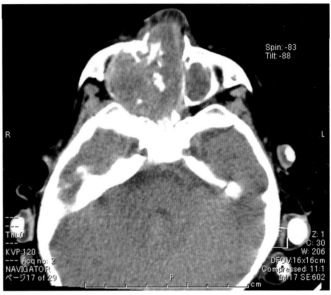

Fig. 1.23 NUT carcinoma. Axial non-contrast CT shows a destructive soft tissue mass containing coarse foci of calcification centred on the right nasal cavity / ethmoid air cells.

discharge, and ocular symptoms (proptosis, diplopia) may be seen {489,2808}. NUT carcinoma commonly spreads by local invasion and by lymphatic and haematogenous metastasis {373,768,2539,769}. NUT carcinoma presents with neck lymph node metastases in 33% of cases, and with distant metastases in 13% {768}. Bone metastases are observed early, and multiorgan dissemination is seen later in the disease course {4602,3568,3015}.

Imaging
Imaging studies reveal extensive local destructive invasion into neighbouring structures such as bone, sinus, orbit, or brain {489,2808,2539}.

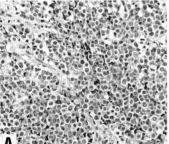
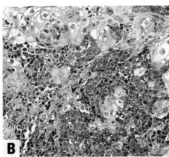
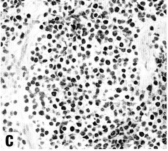
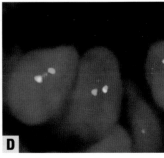

Fig. 1.24 NUT carcinoma. **A** Sheet-like growth pattern of round, medium-sized, monomorphic cells with distinct nucleoli and vesicular open chromatin. The glycogenated, clear cytoplasm gives the cells a fried egg–like appearance. Single cell necrosis and frequent mitoses are seen. **B** Abrupt, keratinized squamous differentiation is a characteristic feature, seen in 33% of cases. **C** Diffuse nuclear staining with the NUT monoclonal antibody (clone C52B1). The speckled pattern of staining is characteristic. **D** FISH demonstrates *BRD4* rearrangement by the splitting apart of red and green DNA probes flanking the *BRD4* genomic locus. Demonstration by FISH of *BRD4* and *NUTM1* break-apart indicates a *BRD4::NUT* fusion.

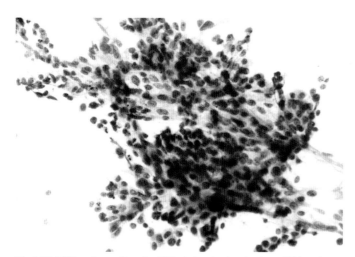

Fig. 1.25 NUT carcinoma. Pap of an FNA of a head and neck primary NUT carcinoma reveals some spindling of medium-sized monomorphic cells with delicate cytoplasm and distinct nucleoli.

Epidemiology

NUT carcinoma is reported to account for as many as 18% of poorly differentiated carcinomas of the upper aerodigestive tract and about 1% of all head and neck carcinomas {1467, 4213,2539}. The sexes are equally affected over a very broad age range but with a median of 24 years {1467,4213,1466,769}.

Etiology

Unknown

Pathogenesis

NUT carcinoma is characterized by chromosomal translocation and fusion of the *NUTM1* gene to *BRD4*, t(15;19)(q14;p13.1) (in 78%); genes coding for BRD4-interacting proteins, such as *BRD3* (9q34.2) (15%), *NSD3* (8p11.23) (6%), and other genes (*ZNF532, ZNF592*) (2%); or unidentified gene(s) (7%) {1468, 1470,1469,97,4047}. NUT-fusion oncoproteins, most commonly BRD4::NUT, act as single drivers of NUT carcinoma that

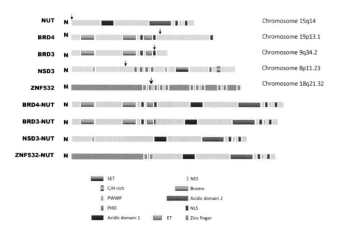

Fig. 1.26 NUT carcinoma. Schematic of predicted NUT fusions and respective wildtype proteins. Arrows indicate breakpoints. PWWP, proline-tryptophan-tryptophan-proline domain; PHD, plant homeodomain; SET, Su(var)3–9, enhancer of zeste, and trithorax domain; C/H rich, cysteine/histidine–rich domain; NLS, nuclear localization signal; NES, nuclear export signal; Bromo, bromodomain; ET, extraterminal domain.

function by blocking differentiation and maintaining proliferation {1468,1470,4713,1469}.

Macroscopic appearance

NUT carcinoma presents as an exophytic, ulcerated, necrotic mass {4602}.

Histopathology

NUT carcinoma typically shows sheets and nests of small to intermediate-sized undifferentiated cells with a monomorphic appearance. The cells have evenly sized nuclei with irregular outlines, vesicular chromatin, and prominent nucleoli. The cytoplasm varies from pale eosinophilic to basophilic. A characteristic feature of the sheet-like growth pattern is the even spacing of cells, often with separation between cells, and a lack of nuclear moulding. A neutrophilic infiltrate is common. There is brisk mitotic activity, and necrosis is often present. NUT carcinomas demonstrate characteristic abrupt foci of keratinization in about one third of cases {769}. Definitive glandular differentiation is not seen, but mesenchymal differentiation can occur, both in primary sites and in metastatic sites {1093,3015}. Histological features alone are not specific for NUT carcinoma.

Immunohistochemistry

NUT carcinoma is positive for NUT (usually in a speckled nuclear pattern) in 87% of cases, using a highly specific monoclonal NUT antibody {1729}. With the exception of weak staining in some germ cell tumours, staining with this antibody is highly specific for NUT carcinoma {1729}. Cytokeratins are positive in the majority of cases, although a subset are negative {5040}. Most cases show nuclear staining for p63; however, p40 staining is less consistent and is not a reliable marker of NUT carcinoma or other, rarer, *NUTM1*-rearranged malignancies {4453, 2876}. Occasional NUT carcinomas can stain for chromogranin, synaptophysin, or thyroid transcription factor 1 (TTF1), but these have only been reported in thoracic, not head and neck, primaries {5034,1961}. NUT carcinomas often stain for CD34, which may lead to a misdiagnosis of acute leukaemia {1467}. Ki-67 expression is high.

Differential diagnosis

NUT carcinoma must be considered in the differential diagnosis of poorly differentiated carcinomas of the head and neck, including poorly differentiated squamous cell carcinoma, sinonasal undifferentiated carcinoma, and SWI/SNF complex–deficient sinonasal carcinoma {4213,1093,468,43}, along with conventional / adamantinoma-like Ewing sarcoma, neuroendocrine carcinomas (NECs), and olfactory neuroblastoma {1467,466}.

Cytology

Smears usually appear hypercellular with large numbers of round to oval nuclei with intermediate-sized cells with a high N:C ratio and a narrow rim of cytoplasm. The nuclei are monomorphic with pale, fine, evenly dispersed chromatin and single discrete small nucleoli. Occasional small syncytial tissue fragments can be present with nuclear moulding resembling neuroendocrine differentiation, and mitoses are prominent. Considerable karyorrhectic debris and variable lymphocytes are seen in the granular background. Squamous differentiation is usually not seen {414,5040,2328,470}.

Diagnostic molecular pathology

Demonstration of *NUTM1* rearrangement is required, such as by positive immunostaining for nuclear NUT expression in > 50% of nuclei, which achieves 100% specificity and 87% sensitivity {1729}. In the remaining cases, cytogenetic analysis, in situ hybridization, RT-PCR, or next-generation sequencing may be necessary {1129,4047,4228}.

Essential and desirable diagnostic criteria

Essential: demonstration of *NUTM1* rearrangement (immunohistochemistry or a molecular technique) in a monotonous, undifferentiated epithelioid malignancy.

Desirable (in selected cases): demonstration of the NUT carcinoma–related *NUTM1*-fusion partner gene to distinguish NUT carcinoma from other rare *NUTM1*-rearranged neoplasms of either cutaneous or bone / soft tissue origin.

Staging

Staging follows the eighth edition of the Union for International Cancer Control (UICC) / American Joint Committee on Cancer (AJCC) TNM staging system.

Prognosis and prediction

NUT carcinoma is an extremely aggressive cancer, having a median survival time of 6.5 months across all molecular subsets and anatomical sites {769}. Head and neck patients with non-*BRD4::NUTM1* fusions (*BRD3::NUTM1* or *NSD3::NUTM1*) have significantly better survival (median overall survival time:

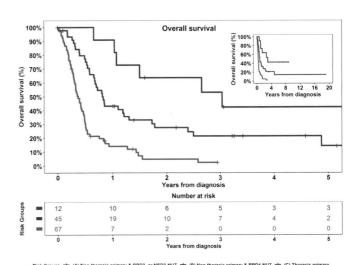

Fig. 1.27 NUT carcinoma. Kaplan–Meier overall survival curves of NUT carcinoma patient risk groups defined on the basis of anatomical location and *NUTM1* fusion partner.

36.5 months) than those with *BRD4::NUTM1* fusions (median overall survival time: 10 months), independent of metastatic disease extent at presentation. Overall survival is significantly lower in the presence of metastasis but not significantly correlated with age or sex {769}.

SWI/SNF complex–deficient sinonasal carcinoma

Agaimy A
Bal MM
Jain D
Mittal N
Rooper LM
Ud Din N

Definition
SWI/SNF complex–deficient sinonasal carcinomas are poorly differentiated to undifferentiated epithelial malignancies defined by the loss of one SWI/SNF complex subunit (either SMARCB1 or SMARCA4) without histological features allowing classification into another specific entity.

ICD-O coding
8044/3 SMARCB1-deficient sinonasal carcinoma
8044/3 SMARCB1-deficient sinonasal adenocarcinoma
8044/3 SMARCA4-deficient sinonasal carcinoma

ICD-11 coding
2C20 & XH1YY4 Malignant neoplasms of nasal cavity & Carcinoma, undifferentiated, NOS
2C22 & XH1YY4 Malignant neoplasms of accessory sinuses & Carcinoma, undifferentiated, NOS

Related terminology
Acceptable: SMARCB1-deficient undifferentiated sinonasal carcinoma; SMARCA4-deficient undifferentiated sinonasal carcinoma.

Subtype(s)
SMARCB1-deficient sinonasal carcinoma; SMARCB1-deficient sinonasal adenocarcinoma; SMARCA4-deficient sinonasal carcinoma.

Localization
The paranasal sinuses, especially the ethmoid sinuses, are most often involved by SMARCB1-deficient carcinoma, whereas SMARCB1-deficient adenocarcinoma and SMARCA4-deficient carcinoma predominantly involve the nasal cavity and less frequently involve contiguous or multiple sites {43,3991,46}.

Clinical features
Most patients present with locally advanced disease (T4), including involvement of the orbit and skull base. Symptoms are nonspecific (nasal obstruction, sinusitis, epistaxis, and headache) and are related to obstruction of the sinonasal cavities with frequent orbital complications {43,2145,3991,46}.

Imaging
Imaging studies document extensive invasion, often into nearby structures {43}.

Epidemiology
SWI/SNF complex–deficient carcinomas constitute 1–3% of sinonasal carcinomas and 3–20% of tumours diagnosed as sinonasal undifferentiated carcinoma {47,468}. SMARCB1-deficient carcinoma is rare {47,468,43}, with even fewer cases of SMARCB1-deficient adenocarcinoma and SMARCA4-deficient

carcinoma {4983,3991,46}. SMARCB1-deficient carcinomas affect patients ranging in age from 11 to 89 years, with a peak in the sixth decade of life. SMARCA4-deficient carcinoma occurs at a lower median age of 44 years (range: 20–67 years). SWI/SNF complex–deficient carcinomas show a male predominance {43,46}.

Etiology
Unknown

Pathogenesis
Inactivation of the respective SWI/SNF complex gene represents the central driver event and probably the sole genetic alteration in these tumours {43,3991,46,1144}. For SMARCB1-deficient carcinomas, biallelic (homozygous) deletions of the SMARCB1 gene are detected by FISH in two thirds of cases {43}. Inactivating SMARCB1 gene mutations have been detected by sequencing, but the sensitivity of next-generation sequencing panels to detect the deletions is unclear. For SMARCA4-deficient carcinomas, biallelic inactivation of SMARCA4 is the consequence of loss-of-function (mainly truncating) mutations {2099}. Loss of additional SWI/SNF subunits (mainly SMARCA2) is seen in a few cases {43,46}. These tumours lack the IDH mutations characteristic of many sinonasal undifferentiated carcinomas {1143, 2099,1148,46}.

Macroscopic appearance
SWI/SNF complex–deficient carcinomas present as diffusely infiltrating, soft, fragile, necrotic masses with a variable polypoid component associated with extensive ulceration and necrosis.

Histopathology
SMARCB1-deficient carcinomas display a monomorphic, predominantly basaloid (60%) or plasmacytoid/rhabdoid (33%) cell morphology. In basaloid cases, rhabdoid cells may be present but are usually focal. Cell spindling is rare. Unequivocal squamous cells, prominent glandular features, and surface epithelial dysplasia are absent. Secondary diffuse or pagetoid surface spread may mimic dysplasia and carcinoma in situ.

SMARCB1-deficient adenocarcinoma predominantly displays an oncocytoid/plasmacytoid cell pattern with prominent gland formation (well-formed tubules, cribriforming, intracellular and/or intraluminal mucin). Different patterns of yolk sac tumours are seen focally in 25% of cases and may rarely be the predominant pattern. The tumour cells are uniformly high-grade with severe nuclear pleomorphism, brisk mitotic activity, and foci of tumour necrosis {3991}.

SMARCA4-deficient carcinomas are histologically undifferentiated, composed of large epithelioid anaplastic cells in nests and trabeculae reminiscent of sinonasal undifferentiated carcinoma. Rhabdoid and basaloid cells are encountered less

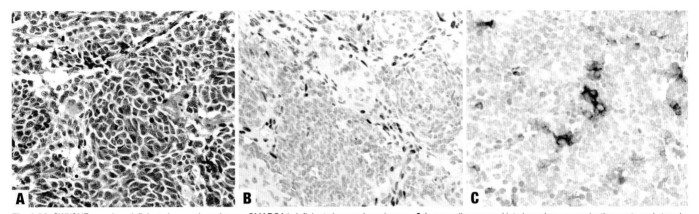

Fig. 1.28 SWI/SNF complex–deficient sinonasal carcinoma: SMARCA4-deficient sinonasal carcinoma. **A** Large cells arranged into irregular communicating nests and strands, with a vaguely neuroendocrine appearance. **B** Complete loss of SMARCA4 limited to the neoplastic cells. **C** Focal synaptophysin reactivity is common in SMARCA4-deficient sinonasal carcinoma.

frequently. They lack squamous and glandular differentiation histologically. Abortive rosettes may be seen.

Immunohistochemistry
SMARCB1-deficient carcinoma: Tumour cells are positive with pancytokeratins (97%), and variably positive for CK5 (64%), p63 or p40 (55%), and CK7 (48%). Focal and weak neuroendocrine marker expression may occur (8–18%) {43,2145}. Complete

SMARCB1 (INI1) loss is required; rarely, co-loss of SMARCA2 is seen, but SMARCA4 is not lost {468,43}.
SMARCB1-deficient adenocarcinoma: By immunohistochemistry, in addition to loss of SMARCB1, CK7 expression (83%) and variable p40 (33%), CK20 (25%), and CDX2 (27%) are seen {3991}. Variable reactivity for yolk sac tumour markers is observed irrespective of the presence or absence of overtly yolk sac tumour–like foci {3991}.

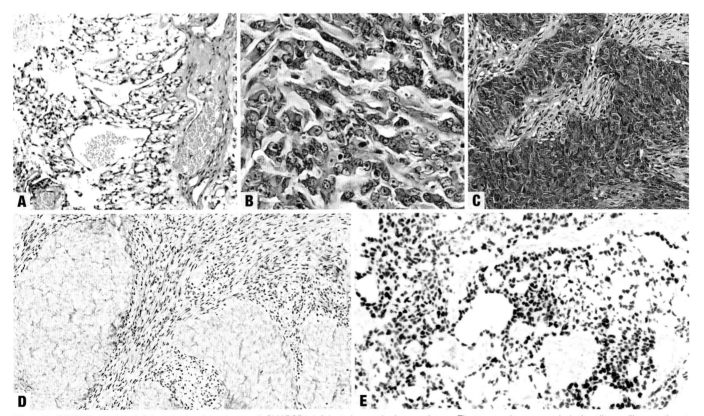

Fig. 1.29 SWI/SNF complex–deficient sinonasal carcinoma. **A** SMARCB1-deficient sinonasal adenocarcinoma. The tumour shows an exclusively yolk sac–like growth pattern. **B** SMARCB1-deficient carcinoma. High-grade tumour cells with a rhabdoid morphology. **C** SMARCB1-deficient carcinoma. Anastomosing islands of tumour cells with vesicular nuclei, conspicuous nucleoli, and moderate amounts of cytoplasm. **D** SMARCB1-deficient carcinoma. On immunohistochemistry, the tumour cells show loss of SMARCB1 staining, whereas the stromal cells, endothelial cells, and lymphocytes retain nuclear expression. **E** SMARCB1-deficient sinonasal adenocarcinoma. Diffuse SALL4 expression in a tumour with a yolk sac–like growth pattern.

SMARCA4-deficient carcinoma: These tumours lack squamous and glandular differentiation by immunohistochemistry. Tumour cells are reactive for pancytokeratin and (rarely) CK7, but they are negative for CK5, p40, and p16. Focal reactivity for synaptophysin (90%), chromogranin A (40%), and CD56 (60%) is observed. Loss of SMARCA4 (BRG1) is definitional, rarely accompanied by co-loss of SMARCA2, but SMARCB1 is retained {46,39}.

No viral association (HPV and EBV) has been reported. NUT immunohistochemistry is consistently negative.

Differential diagnosis

Although some sinonasal teratocarcinosarcomas are SMARCA4-deficient, they are distinguished from SMARCA4-deficient carcinoma by the presence of sarcomatoid and teratoid tumour elements.

Cytology

Cellular smears show loosely cohesive sheets of relatively monomorphic polygonal or plasmacytoid epithelioid cells with large round to oval nuclei, small single nucleoli, occasional nuclear pseudoinclusions, and eccentric granular cytoplasm. Occasional larger cells with large nuclei are present. Mitotic figures and background necrosis are seen, but there is no stromal matrix and no squamous or glandular differentiation {119,111}.

Diagnostic molecular pathology

Not clinically relevant

Essential and desirable diagnostic criteria

Essential: sinonasal tract location; undifferentiated carcinoma with SMARCB1 (INI1) or SMARCA4 (BRG1) loss but no features of other entities; unequivocal gland formation and/or yolk sac tumour–like features are required for the adenocarcinoma subtype.

Desirable: presence of rhabdoid cells; yolk sac–like features for the adenocarcinoma variant.

Staging

Staging follows the eighth edition of the Union for International Cancer Control (UICC) / American Joint Committee on Cancer (AJCC) TNM staging system.

Prognosis and prediction

SWI/SNF complex–deficient sinonasal carcinomas are highly aggressive, with more than half of all patients dying within 2 years. Mortality seems higher for SMARCA4-deficient cases than for others {43,46}.

Sinonasal lymphoepithelial carcinoma

Hsieh MS
Stevens TM

Definition
Lymphoepithelial carcinoma (LEC) is an undifferentiated-appearing carcinoma arising within the sinonasal tract showing an associated prominent non-neoplastic lymphoplasmacytic cell infiltrate, strongly associated with EBV.

ICD-O coding
8082/3 Lymphoepithelial carcinoma

ICD-11 coding
2C20.4 & XH1E40 Squamous cell carcinoma of nasal cavity & Lymphoepithelial carcinoma
2C22.1 & XH1E40 Squamous cell carcinoma of accessory sinuses & Lymphoepithelial carcinoma

Related terminology
Not recommended: lymphoepithelioma-like carcinoma; primary sinonasal nasopharyngeal-type undifferentiated carcinoma.

Subtype(s)
None

Localization
LEC affects the nasal cavity and less commonly the paranasal sinuses {5057,3792,4339}. The sinonasal tract location defines LEC as a distinct entity from nasopharyngeal carcinoma {2070}.

Clinical features
Patients usually have nasal obstruction, bloody nasal discharge, facial swelling, and/or pain {2070,2130,4339}. An advanced tumour with skull base invasion may cause cranial nerve palsy {2070,4779}.

Imaging
Imaging studies document tumour site and extent {3121,4339, 525}.

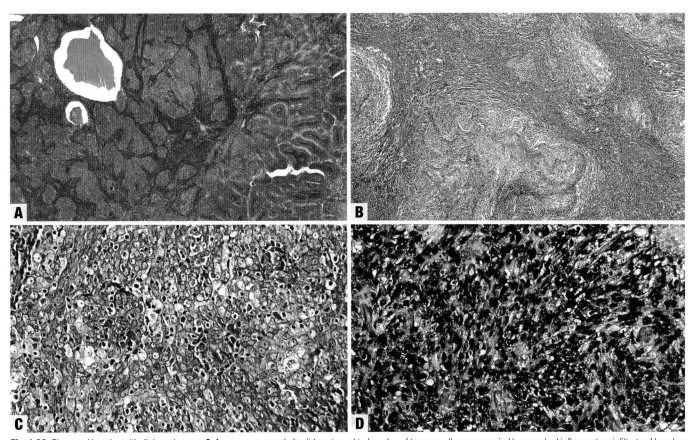

Fig. 1.30 Sinonasal lymphoepithelial carcinoma. **A** A mass composed of solid nests and trabeculae of tumour cells accompanied by a marked inflammatory infiltrate of lymphocytes and plasma cells. **B** Thick, fibrous bands separating tumour islands can be observed. **C** Tumour cells show large nuclei, vesicular chromatin, prominent nucleoli, indistinct cell borders, and an associated inflammatory infiltrate of lymphocytes and plasma cells. **D** Most cases are positive for EBV-encoded small RNA (EBER) by in situ hybridization.

Epidemiology

Tumours are more common in men (M:F ratio: 2–3:1) in their fifth to seventh decade of life (median: 58 years) {5057,2070,4779}, with an increased incidence in patients from regions where nasopharyngeal carcinoma has a high prevalence, e.g. southeastern Asia {2575,5057,2070}.

Etiology

Sinonasal LEC is strongly associated with EBV infection, especially in endemic areas {2575,5057,2070}.

Pathogenesis

Unknown

Macroscopic appearance

Sinonasal LEC presents with an irregular or polypoid mass that may have erosion and haemorrhagic surfaces {3792,2308}.

Histopathology

Tumours are composed of a syncytium of large cells arranged in lobules, nests, trabeculae, or cords, and associated with a rich lymphoplasmacytic infiltrate, which can be florid, obscuring the tumour cells. The malignant cells typically have large round nuclei, vesicular chromatin, prominent nucleoli, and poorly defined cell borders (a syncytial pattern); occasional tumour cell spindling may be encountered. Necrosis or keratinization is typically absent {2070,3792,4779}. In some cases, thick fibrous septa separating tumour islands may be observed. Extracellular amyloid deposits may be present.

Immunohistochemistry

Tumour cells are positive for cytokeratins and usually positive for squamous markers such as p40, p63, and CK5/6; they are negative for neuroendocrine, lymphoid, and melanocytic markers. p16 is usually negative or patchy and weak {4779}. Sinonasal LECs are typically reactive for EBV-encoded small RNA (EBER) by in situ hybridization {5057,2070,4779}, but rare cases may be EBER-negative {2130,3792}.

Differential diagnosis

Tumours must be separated from sinonasal undifferentiated carcinoma, nasopharyngeal carcinoma, oropharyngeal carcinoma, SMARCB1-deficient carcinoma, NUT carcinoma, neuroendocrine carcinoma (NEC), melanoma, lymphoma, and undifferentiated pleomorphic sarcoma, among others.

Cytology

Smears show irregular tissue fragments of epithelial cells with spindle or epidermoid cytoplasm that can be poorly defined, and large highly pleomorphic nuclei, in an often prominent and obscuring lymphoplasmacytic background. Lymphocytes can infiltrate the epithelium. The epithelial component resembles non-keratinizing nasopharyngeal carcinoma.

Diagnostic molecular pathology

Most cases will demonstrate EBV by in situ hybridization.

Essential and desirable diagnostic criteria

Essential: syncytial clusters of crowded, large, undifferentiated cells in an intimate relationship with the lymphoplasmacytic infiltrate; cytokeratin immunoreactivity; exclusion of a nasopharyngeal/oropharyngeal primary.

Desirable: EBER in situ hybridization (especially in endemic cases).

Staging

Staging follows the eighth edition of the Union for International Cancer Control (UICC) / American Joint Committee on Cancer (AJCC) TNM staging system.

Prognosis and prediction

Sinonasal LEC appears to metastasize to cervical lymph nodes (15–25%) less frequently than nasopharyngeal carcinoma {2130}, while distant metastasis are exceptional {2070,4339}. Sinonasal LEC prognosis is favourable even with cervical lymph node metastasis, but survival data are limited by disease rarity {3792,4779}.

Sinonasal undifferentiated carcinoma

Jo VY
Agaimy A
Franchi A
Ud Din N

Definition

Sinonasal undifferentiated carcinoma (SNUC) is a malignant epithelial tumour without any identifiable line of differentiation (including squamous, glandular, and neuroendocrine) and is a diagnosis of exclusion.

ICD-O coding

8020/3 Sinonasal undifferentiated carcinoma

ICD-11 coding

2C20 & XH1YY4 Malignant neoplasms of nasal cavity & Carcinoma, undifferentiated, NOS
2C22 & XH1YY4 Malignant neoplasms of accessory sinuses & Carcinoma, undifferentiated, NOS

Related terminology

None

Subtype(s)

None

Localization

SNUCs most often present as very large masses involving multiple sinonasal tract sites, with the exact site of origin being difficult to determine {4890}. As many as 60% show invasion into adjacent structures, including the orbital apex, skull base, and brain {3677}. Despite the large primary tumour size, nodal metastases are uncommon, occurring in 10–30% of cases {816,3677,1683,4856}.

Clinical features

Common presenting symptoms are nasal obstruction, sinusitis, epistaxis, and/or headache {4890,4856}. With orbital involvement, patients may experience diplopia or other visual symptoms, proptosis, and periorbital swelling {4890}.

Imaging

Destructive tumours with poorly defined margins are seen radiographically {3527}.

Epidemiology

SNUC is rare, accounting for about 3–5% of all sinonasal carcinomas {2694}. The median patient age is between 50 and 60 years, with a wide age range affected {3677,734}. Most patients are male (60–70%) {3677,734}.

Etiology

Unknown

Pathogenesis

IDH2 hotspot mutations are identified in a significant subset of cases (33–85%) {2099,1143,3031,3702}. *IDH2* p.R172S is most common; others include p.R172M, p.R172T, p.R172G, and p.R172K. Rarely, *IDH1* mutations are reported {3031}. IDH-mutant SNUC demonstrates a hypermethylator phenotype, and DNA methylation–based profiling studies show that IDH-mutant sinonasal malignancies constitute a distinct group from IDH-wildtype tumour types {1148}. Given the varied sensitivity and specificity of mutant IDH1/2 immunohistochemistry, sequencing-based methods are most reliable for identifying IDH-mutant SNUC.

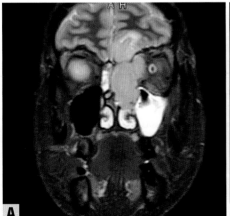 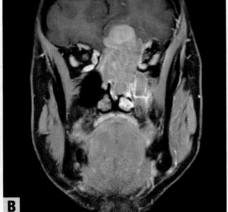 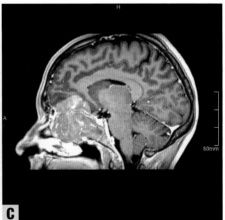

Fig. 1.31 Sinonasal undifferentiated carcinoma . MRI shows a large tumour mass centred on the left ethmoid air cells, with orbital and intracranial extension. **A** This coronal short-tau inversion recovery (STIR) image demonstrates an intermediate-signal tumour, high-signal secretions in the obstructed left maxillary sinus, and vasogenic oedema in the left frontal lobe. **B** This coronal postcontrast fat-suppressed T1-weighted image shows the extent of the tumour and its proximity to the left optic nerve. **C** This sagittal postcontrast T1-weighted image shows extension across the cribriform plate into the anterior cranial fossa and involvement of the sphenoid sinus.

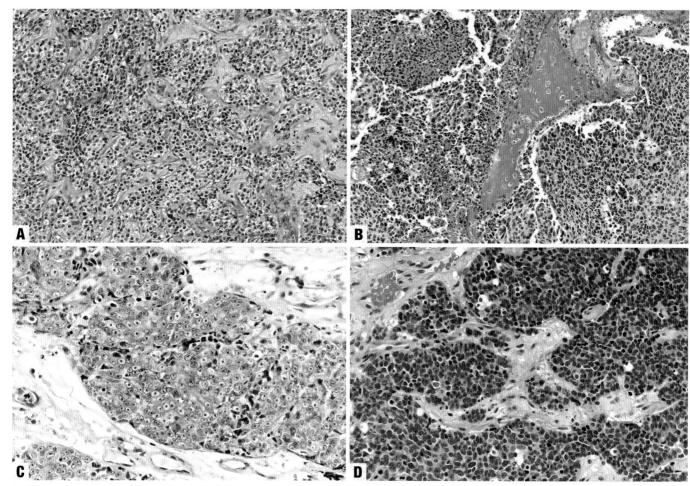

Fig. 1.32 Sinonasal undifferentiated carcinoma. **A** Lobules, trabeculae, and nests of malignant epithelial cells. **B** Invasion into bone by tumour cells and abundant necrosis. **C** Undifferentiated tumour cell population showing a high N:C ratio, an open or vesicular chromatin pattern, and prominent nucleoli. **D** Tumour showing more basaloid morphology.

Macroscopic appearance

Tumours are usually large (> 40 mm) at presentation and show a fungating endoscopic appearance.

Histopathology

SNUC is composed of sheets, lobules, nests, and trabeculae of malignant cells with enlarged round nuclei, varying amounts

of cytoplasm, and well-defined cell borders. Tumour cell nuclei are hyperchromatic or vesicular, with open to vesicular chromatin and prominent nucleoli. Some examples may appear basaloid with tumour cells that have higher N:C ratios. Despite its high-grade morphology, SNUC has a characteristically uniform appearance, with a relatively consistent nuclear size and shape. By definition, there is no squamous or glandular differentiation, and surface squamous dysplasia is absent.

Immunohistochemistry

By immunohistochemistry, SNUC is positive for cytokeratins (pancytokeratin, AE1/AE3, CAM5.2, OSCAR, and CK18) and occasionally for CK7. Notably, CK5/6 and p40 are negative, while patchy nonspecific p63 reactivity may be seen {4085}. SNUC can show very focal or patchy synaptophysin and chromogranin reactivity {725,816}, but the histological features of neuroendocrine carcinoma (NEC) are absent. Differentiation-specific markers, including CD45, S100, SOX10, and desmin are negative. SNUC may show positivity for p16; however, this does not reflect transcriptionally active high-risk HPV infection {4663,1683}. Immunohistochemistry for mutation-specific IDH1/2 (both multispecific and monoclonal mutant IDH antibodies) identifies a proportion of SNUC with IDH mutations including most with R172S, although it lacks sensitivity for the full range of IDH mutations {3031,1145,1146}. Presently, no

Fig. 1.33 Sinonasal undifferentiated carcinoma. IDH2 p.R172S showing granular cytoplasmic staining for a multispecific antibody for mutant IDH1/2 p.R132/172 (clone MsMab-1).

morphological or immunohistochemical differences between IDH-mutant and IDH-wildtype SNUCs are recognized {1143, 3031,3702}.

Differential diagnosis
The differential diagnosis for SNUC is broad, and because it is a diagnosis of exclusion, other entities must be excluded with a thorough histological and immunohistochemical evaluation, directed to exclude squamous, glandular, neuroendocrine, salivary, olfactory, melanocytic, and haematolymphoid differentiation.

Cytology
Smears are hypercellular, showing predominantly single dispersed cells and scattered cohesive tissue fragments with stripped, naked nuclei and necrotic debris in the background. Tumour cells are intermediate in size, with a high N:C ratio, a small amount of poorly defined cytoplasm, and irregular large pleomorphic nuclei that may appear moulded and crushed and have easily identifiable nucleoli. There are frequent intracytoplasmic vacuoles including signet ring–like cells, but mucin is absent. Occasional mitotic figures and abundant karyorrhectic debris are seen {413}.

Diagnostic molecular pathology
Although IDH mutations define a subset of SNUC, identification is not required for diagnosis.

Essential and desirable diagnostic criteria
Essential: a high-grade tumour with cytokeratin-positive tumour cells; no histological or immunohistochemical evidence of any specific line of differentiation; all histological mimics (see above) excluded.
Desirable: verification of IDH mutation status (in selected cases).

Staging
Staging follows the eighth edition of the Union for International Cancer Control (UICC) / American Joint Committee on Cancer (AJCC) TNM staging system.

Prognosis and prediction
SNUC is a highly aggressive malignancy with a poor prognosis {3677}. SEER data analyses revealed a median overall survival time of 22.1 months, and 3-, 5-, and 10-year survival rates of 44.3%, 34.9%, and 31.3%, respectively {3677,734}. *IDH2* mutations have been associated with better disease-specific survival {3702}.

Teratocarcinosarcoma

Rooper LM
Agaimy A
Bal MM
Jain D

Mittal N
Ud Din N
Wenig BM

Definition
Teratocarcinosarcoma (TCS) is a malignant sinonasal tract neoplasm with mixed epithelial, mesenchymal, and primitive neuroepithelial elements.

ICD-O coding
9081/3 Teratocarcinosarcoma

ICD-11 coding
2C20.Y & XH2RK1 Other specified malignant neoplasm of nasal cavity & Carcinosarcoma, embryonal

Related terminology
Not recommended: malignant teratoma; teratocarcinoma; teratoid carcinosarcoma; blastoma; mixed olfactory neuroblastoma–craniopharyngioma.

Subtype(s)
None

Localization
Most cases of TCS are centred in the superior aspect of the nasal cavity, with frequent extension into the ethmoid, maxillary, or sphenoid sinuses {4152,1818}.

Clinical features
Presenting symptoms result from mass effect and include nasal obstruction, epistaxis, and headache, and they are usually of short duration {4152}. Cervical lymph node metastases are rarely seen {1818}, but distant metastases may occur {4267, 1343}.

Epidemiology
TCS tends to affect adults (median age: 50 years); approximately 80% of patients are male {4152,764}.

Etiology
No risk factors or tumour predisposition syndrome associations are known.

Pathogenesis
Recurrent molecular driver alterations have been documented, particularly biallelic inactivation of *SMARCA4* and activating *CTNNB1* mutation {463,3752}.

Macroscopic appearance
Tumours generally have a variable grey-tan fleshy to reddish-brown haemorrhagic appearance, with areas of necrosis.

Histopathology
TCS is composed of mixed epithelial, mesenchymal, and neuroepithelial elements. The epithelial components can include both squamous epithelium, which may be keratinizing or non-keratinizing, and glandular structures, which can be simple or stratified and can include mucinous or ciliated cells. Frequently, the squamous and glandular elements have a clear cell appearance, reminiscent of fetal tissues. The mesenchymal components are most often composed of nondescript hypercellular fascicles of spindle cells, but areas of overt smooth muscle or of rhabdomyoblastic, adipocytic, cartilaginous, or osteoblastic differentiation can be seen. Both the epithelial and mesenchymal components can show variable cytological atypia, ranging from relatively bland to overtly malignant appearances. The neuroepithelial component consists of primitive epithelioid cells

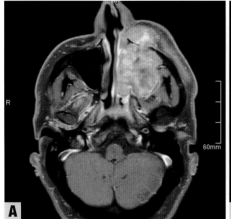
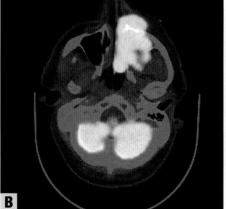
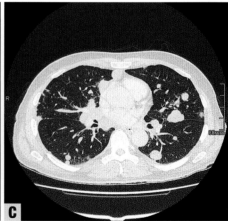

Fig. 1.34 Teratocarcinosarcoma. **A** Axial postcontrast fat-suppressed MRI showing an aggressive soft tissue mass centred on the left maxillary sinus extending through all bony margins into the nasal cavity, cheek, and retromaxillary fat. **B** Avid FDG uptake was demonstrated on PET-CT. **C** Despite treatment, the patient rapidly developed multiple lung lesions consistent with metastases, as seen in this axial CT image.

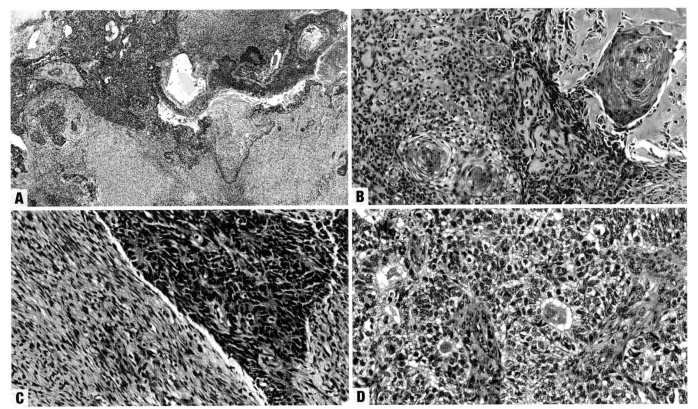

Fig. 1.35 Teratocarcinosarcoma. **A** Mixed epithelial, mesenchymal, and primitive neuroepithelial elements. **B** Intermixed squamous epithelium with a fetal-like clear cell appearance and spindle cells embedded in chondroid and osseous matrix. **C** Primitive neuroepithelium with abundant rosette formation surrounded by hypercellular fascicles of spindle cells. **D** Primitive neuroepithelium with transition to gland-like structures.

with large, hyperchromatic nuclei arranged in nests and sheets with a patchy neurofibrillary background and rosette formation {4152,1343,3752}. In some instances, the primitive neuroepithelial component may undergo neuronal maturation after chemotherapy {2160}.

Immunohistochemistry
The immunoprofile of TCS corresponds to its constituent elements, with consistent strong positivity for cytokeratin in epithelial elements and weak positivity in neuroepithelial elements; reactivity for desmin in rhabdomyosarcomatous elements (which may only be identified immunohistochemically); staining for CK5/6, p63, and p40 in squamous components; and expression of the neuroendocrine markers synaptophysin, chromogranin A, and INSM1 in the neuroepithelial elements {1343, 3743}. Markers of germ cell derivation, including PLAP, SALL4, AFP, and hCG, are negative {1818,3364}. Approximately 80% of cases show some degree of SMARCA4 (BRG1) loss, with complete loss in as many as 70% of cases {3752}. A subset of cases display aberrant nuclear β-catenin localization {463}.

Differential diagnosis
The admixture of various tissue elements in TCS is unique for the diagnosis, but it can show overlap with a wide range of other sinonasal tumours, including olfactory neuroblastoma, squamous cell carcinoma, adenocarcinoma, neuroendocrine carcinomas (NECs), and various sarcomas when not all components are sampled. Immunohistochemistry for SMARCA4 or β-catenin

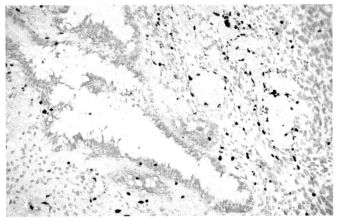

Fig. 1.36 Teratocarcinosarcoma. Loss of SMARCA4 in tumour elements including glands and neuroepithelium, with retained expression in blood vessels.

can support the diagnosis in such cases. SMARCA4-deficient sinonasal carcinoma may overlap with TCS in limited samples but frequently shows a large cell epithelioid or rhabdoid cell pattern that is absent in TCS {46}.

Cytology
Not clinically relevant

Diagnostic molecular pathology
Not clinically relevant

Essential and desirable diagnostic criteria

Essential: sinonasal tract location; an admixture of epithelial, mesenchymal, and primitive neuroepithelial elements.

Desirable: fetal-like clear cell appearance in epithelial components; SMARCA4 loss and/or nuclear β-catenin expression (in selected cases).

Staging

Staging follows the eighth edition of the Union for International Cancer Control (UICC) / American Joint Committee on Cancer (AJCC) TNM staging system.

Prognosis and prediction

TCS is an aggressive tumour that shows frequent local recurrences within the first 2 years {622}. However, more recent 5-year survival rates are > 50% {764}.

HPV-related multiphenotypic sinonasal carcinoma

Bishop JA
Hang JF
Kiss K
Rupp NJ
Westra W

Definition

HPV-related multiphenotypic sinonasal carcinoma (HMSC) is an epithelial neoplasm exhibiting features of both surface-derived and minor salivary gland–derived elements, harbouring transcriptionally active HPV.

ICD-O coding

8483/3 HPV-related multiphenotypic sinonasal carcinoma

ICD-11 coding

2C20 & XH1YY4 Malignant neoplasms of nasal cavity & Carcinoma, undifferentiated, NOS

2C22 & XH1YY4 Malignant neoplasms of accessory sinuses & Carcinoma, undifferentiated, NOS

Related terminology

Acceptable: HPV-associated multiphenotypic sinonasal carcinoma.

Not recommended: HPV-related carcinoma with adenoid cystic–like features.

Subtype(s)

None

Localization

The vast majority of HMSCs affect the nasal cavity (89%) with a predilection for the turbinate, with or without concurrent paranasal sinus involvement. Rare cases affect the sinuses exclusively {478,189,1762,467,486}.

Clinical features

Most patients present with obstruction and epistaxis. Tumours are nearly always localized to the sinonasal tract at presentation {478,189,1762,467,486}.

Epidemiology

HMSC typically affects adults (mean age: 54 years), with a slight female predominance {478,189,1762,467,486}.

Etiology

By definition, HMSC harbours high-risk HPV, most commonly type 33 (~80%), and occasionally type 35, 16, 52, 56, or 82 {26, 486,3786,4732}. Because HPV16 is uncommon, HPV assays must include other types, especially type 33. *MYB* rearrangements are not identified by FISH {467}. Origin from a terminal excretory duct at its transition with surface epithelium may explain mixed lines of phenotypic differentiation {486}.

Pathogenesis

Unknown

Macroscopic appearance

HMSC grossly appears as a tan-white, often polypoid mass.

Histopathology

"Multiphenotypic" refers to multiple lines of cellular differentiation encountered in any single HMSC. Tumours typically grow in solid sheets, lobules, and cribriform nests as basaloid cells, reminiscent of solid adenoid cystic carcinoma. The salivary gland–type features are supported by the presence of both ductal and myoepithelial components. The myoepithelial cells are typically basaloid with varying degrees of spindling, plasmacytoid change, or clear cell change within a myxohyaline stroma, whereas the scattered ducts, variable in number and sometimes subtle, are more eosinophilic. Occasionally, these dual components are arranged as an inner luminal ductal layer surrounded by an outer peripheral layer of cleared myoepithelial cells, resembling epithelial-myoepithelial carcinoma. Squamous differentiation often takes the form of high-grade squamous dysplasia of the surface epithelium. Less frequently, the invasive component can demonstrate areas of overt squamous differentiation with keratin production. Bizarre pleomorphism,

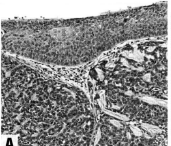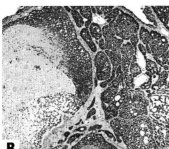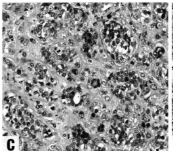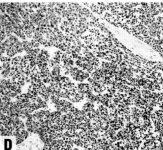

Fig. 1.37 HPV-related multiphenotypic sinonasal carcinoma. **A** The invasive basaloid tumour (bottom) is often accompanied by high-grade squamous dysplasia of the overlying surface epithelium (top). **B** The tumour typically grows as solid and cribriform nests, with frequent myxohyaline stroma and necrosis. **C** The predominant myoepithelial-type cells are basaloid with clear cell change, with scattered eosinophilic ducts (centre). The tumour is pleomorphic and mitotically active. **D** The tumour, by definition, harbours high-risk HPV, here demonstrated by RNA in situ hybridization. HPV33 is the most frequently associated type.

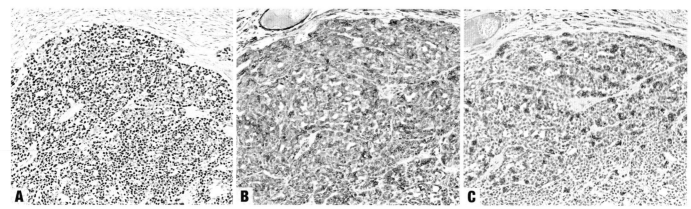

Fig. 1.38 HPV-related multiphenotypic sinonasal carcinoma. Myoepithelial markers like p40 (**A**) and SMA (**B**) show an abluminal staining pattern in the myoepithelial tumour cells. **C** KIT (CD117) highlights the tumour ducts, in a staining pattern that is the inverse of the myoepithelial cell marker pattern.

sarcomatoid transformation, and heterologous cartilaginous differentiation is rare. HMSC typically exhibits high-grade cellular features in addition to a high mitotic index and tumour necrosis. Bone invasion is common, but perineural or lymphovascular invasion is not.

Immunohistochemistry
HMSC usually exhibits both ductal and myoepithelial differentiation, which can be demonstrated by immunostaining for p40, p63, SMA, and calponin (myoepithelial); KIT (CD117) (ductal); and S100 and SOX10 (both cell types). MYB immunohistochemistry and *MYB* RNA in situ hybridization are also usually positive, despite the lack of *MYB* rearrangements {3993,3748}. HMSC is positive for p16 and high-risk HPV by direct HPV assays such as RNA in situ hybridization. Negative p16 immunohistochemistry helps exclude the tumour, but p16 immunopositivity is a poor HPV surrogate in this tumour {218}.

Differential diagnosis
Unlike true adenoid cystic carcinomas, HMSC is restricted to the sinonasal tract in all reported cases, is often associated with surface squamous dysplasia, and harbours HPV, requiring direct HPV-specific testing. Furthermore, HMSC does not harbour the *MYB*, *MYBL1*, and/or *NFIB* fusions that characterize most adenoid cystic carcinomas. In contrast to squamous cell carcinoma, basaloid squamous cell carcinoma, and adenosquamous carcinoma, HMSC shows myoepithelial differentiation by histology and immunohistochemistry, albeit that SOX10

may be coexpressed in basaloid squamous cell carcinoma {3749}.

Cytology
Not clinically relevant

Diagnostic molecular pathology
High-risk HPV must be demonstrated by in situ hybridization or PCR-based techniques, specifically to include HPV33.

Essential and desirable diagnostic criteria
Essential: a carcinoma composed of basaloid type cells; high-risk HPV by HPV-specific assay (not p16 alone); myoepithelial differentiation by immunohistochemistry.
Desirable: sinonasal tract location; ductal differentiation; overlying squamous dysplasia.

Staging
Staging follows the eighth edition of the Union for International Cancer Control (UICC) / American Joint Committee on Cancer (AJCC) TNM staging system.

Prognosis and prediction
HMSC has paradoxically indolent behaviour despite a typically high-grade histological appearance. Local recurrences are common (about one third of cases), including some late recurrences, but distant metastases are rare (5%) {3993,486,3717}. Regional spread and tumour-related death are exceptional.

Intestinal-type sinonasal adenocarcinoma

Franchi A
Leivo I
Patil A
Vivanco B

Definition
Intestinal-type sinonasal adenocarcinoma (ITAC) is a gland-forming malignant epithelial neoplasm of the sinonasal tract that is morphologically similar to primary intestinal adenocarcinoma.

ICD-O coding
8144/3 Intestinal-type adenocarcinoma

ICD-11 coding
2C20.0 & XH0349 Adenocarcinoma of nasal cavity & Adeno-carcinoma, intestinal type
2C22.0 & XH0349 Adenocarcinoma of accessory sinuses & Adenocarcinoma, intestinal type

Related terminology
Not recommended: colloid-type adenocarcinoma; colonic-type adenocarcinoma; enteric-type adenocarcinoma.

Subtype(s)
None

Localization
ITAC is thought to originate from the olfactory cleft {2055}, and most cases are localized in the ethmoid sinus or nasal cavity. The maxillary sinus is affected in a minority of cases, usually in patients without occupational exposure. ITAC invades the osseous structures and may spread to other sinuses, the orbit, and the skull base. Bilateral extension is seen in about 10% of cases {2055,867,658}.

Clinical features
Presentation includes unilateral nasal obstruction, epistaxis, and rhinorrhoea. Patients with advanced-stage tumours present with pain, exophthalmos, diplopia, headache, and facial contour changes {867,2695}. Anosmia is an initial symptom in a subset {1566}.

Imaging
Imaging studies show a poorly defined, enhancing sinonasal tract mass and are used to document destructive extension into the orbit or skull base {3632,2712}.

Epidemiology
Geographical regional incidence variation is noted {4952}, with Europe reporting 0.24 cases in men and 0.04 cases in women per 100 000 person-years {457}, and the USA reporting 4.4 cases per 100 000 person-years {2283}. There is a marked male predominance. The peak age is in the fifth and sixth decades of life.

Etiology
An occupational etiology is identified, with exposure to wood dusts, especially from hardwood species such as oak and beech, and also leather dusts, often with prolonged exposure (> 30 years) and a long latency (> 40 years) {2891}. Other associated occupational exposures suggested include textile manufacturing and exposure to cork, chrome, nickel, formaldehyde, solvents, tannins, and pesticides {2891,1456,528,458,1778, 1160,3440,140}.

Pathogenesis
ITAC is thought to develop through intestinal metaplasia of the sinonasal epithelium, observed adjacent to invasive ITAC {4644, 1459}. Chronic inflammation, possibly induced by occupational agents, is thought to play an important role in the pathogenesis {1902}. The molecular mechanisms of tumour development are beginning to be explained. The genetic alterations in ITAC are partially similar to those observed in colorectal adenocarcinoma {4102}. *TP53* is the most frequently mutated gene (40–50%) {3482,1901,3470}; *APC*, *KRAS*, and *BRAF* mutations are present in a minor subset {1463,2708,1543,1454,4102}. High levels of EGFR (HER1) expression and gene amplification are reported in a subset {1453,1543}, while overexpression of c-Met (MET) {3597} and nuclear β-catenin expression are frequently present {3473,1126}. Next-generation sequencing has identified recurrent somatic sequence variants in *PIK3CA*, *APC*, *ATM*, *KRAS*, *NF1*, *LRP1B*, *BRCA1*, *ERBB3*, *CTNNB1*, *NOTCH2*, and *CDKN2A* {3850}. These variants mainly affect the PI3K, MAPK/ERK, WNT, and DNA repair signalling pathways {3850}.

Macroscopic appearance
ITACs appear as large, polypoid, papillary, or nodular lesions. They are friable, sometimes haemorrhagic, or (uncommonly) gelatinous or mucoid.

Histopathology
ITACs show a morphological spectrum similar to that of gastrointestinal primary adenocarcinomas. They extensively infiltrate the submucosa and bone and may show perineural invasion. Stromal tissues are loose and fibrovascular, often containing abundant chronic inflammation. They consist of proliferations of dysplastic columnar cells with interspersed goblet cells, forming papillae and glands. Paneth cells and endocrine cells are also present in varying proportions. Differentiation varies from very well differentiated to poorly differentiated tumours classified as papillary, colonic, solid, or mixed. Well-differentiated ITACs predominately show a papillary or tubulopapillary architecture and consist of elongated outgrowths lined by atypical intestinal-type cells. Sometimes atypia may be difficult to appreciate, but nuclear changes that appear at least adenomatous are the rule. Nuclei are cigar-shaped, hyperchromatic, and enlarged. As ITACs become poorly differentiated, tubular

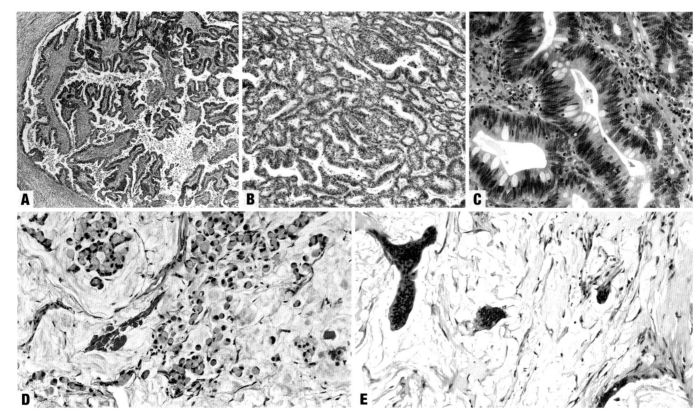

Fig. 1.39 Intestinal-type sinonasal adenocarcinoma. **A** A well-differentiated tumour showing a papillary architecture with fibrovascular cores lined by dysplastic columnar epithelium. **B** A moderately differentiated tumour with a tubular arrangement of neoplastic cells. **C** This tumour consists of a proliferation of dysplastic columnar cells, with interspersed goblet cells. Numerous Paneth cells with granular eosinophilic cytoplasm are also visible in this example. **D** This mucinous tumour has a signet-ring morphology. **E** This mucinous tumour consists of small groups of neoplastic cells dispersed within abundant mucus.

and papillary structures are replaced by nested, cribriform, and solid growths. Mitotic figures are frequent, and central comedonecrosis is usually present. A minority of cases (20–25%) show abundant mucus, resulting in two different growth patterns: alveolar spaces partially lined by and containing glands or strips of attenuated epithelium rich in goblet cells, with the strips suspended like ribbons within mucus lakes and sometimes forming small cribriform structures; or, less commonly, mucous lakes containing signet-ring cells. Some tumours have a mixed growth pattern, appearing both papillary/tubular and mucinous.

Histochemistry
Histochemical stains show intracytoplasmic, intraluminal, and/or extracellular mucicarmine; and diastase-resistant, PAS-positive material.

Immunohistochemistry
Neoplastic cells express pancytokeratins, are variably reactive for CK7 and CEA, and are mostly positive for CK20. ITACs are also positive for CDX2, villin, MUC2, and SATB2 {1455,2249, 4118}. In addition, there is variable expression of neuroendocrine markers {3598,2558}.

Differential diagnosis
The differential diagnosis between ITAC and non–intestinal-type sinonasal adenocarcinomas is made on morphological grounds, aided by immunohistochemistry. Metastatic gastrointestinal tumours must be excluded by clinical and/or imaging findings.

Mucoepidermoid and adenosquamous carcinomas show squamous differentiation, which is absent in ITAC. A mucocele lacks pleomorphism, necrosis, and brisk mitotic activity.

Cytology
Primary tumours are not usually aspirated, but smears of cervical lymph node or distant metastases show large stripped nuclei, columnar cells, and sometimes signet-ring cells with prominent mucin vacuoles seen singly or in small tissue fragments in a background of a variable amount of mucin and granular necrotic debris {4084}. The features are diagnostic of adenocarcinoma, but ancillary tests on cell blocks are required.

Diagnostic molecular pathology
Not clinically relevant

Essential and desirable diagnostic criteria
Essential: atypical intestinal-type columnar cells forming papillae, tubules, or cribriform and solid structures; exclusion of gastrointestinal primary metastasis.
Desirable: abundant extracellular or intracellular mucus; immunolabelling for markers of intestinal differentiation (in selected cases).

Staging
Staging follows the eighth edition of the Union for International Cancer Control (UICC) / American Joint Committee on Cancer (AJCC) TNM staging system.

Prognosis and prediction

Sinonasal ITAC is a high-grade malignancy, with frequent local recurrences (30–60%), associated with a poor prognosis when there is skull base, orbit, and/or dural invasion {867,1160,1386}. Additional negative prognostic factors are local recurrence, distant metastases, and positive surgical margins {867,658,3212, 1386}. Lymph node and distant metastases are infrequently detected (1–5% and 5–10% of patients, respectively) {867,658, 651,1161}. Stage is more significant than tumour grade or type {2891,209,651,1160,3661,2713,2283}. Still, well-differentiated papillary ITAC tends to have an indolent behaviour, whereas mucinous and poorly differentiated tumours have poorer outcomes {1458,3212}. Tumour budding seems to be an adverse prognostic factor in ITAC {2771}. By comparative genomic hybridization, subgroups of ITAC with distinct genetic signatures and copy-number alterations, and with clinical outcomes independent from disease stage or histological subtype, have been identified {2713}. The median time to recurrence is 25–30 months {867,658}. The 5-year survival rate is 50–84% and the 10-year survival rate is 30–50% {867,658,651,3212,1160,3661}.

Non–intestinal-type sinonasal adenocarcinoma

Stelow EB
Laco J
Leivo I
Skalova A

Definition

Non–intestinal-type sinonasal adenocarcinoma (SNAC) is a sinonasal tract gland-forming malignancy lacking intestinal-type features and characteristics of salivary gland–specific tumour entities.

ICD-O coding

8140/3 Adenocarcinoma, NOS
8140/3 Renal cell–like sinonasal adenocarcinoma

ICD-11 coding

2C20.0 & XH74S1 Adenocarcinoma of nasal cavity & Adenocarcinoma, NOS
2C22.0 & XH74S1 Adenocarcinoma of paranasal sinuses & Adenocarcinoma, NOS

Related terminology

Not recommended: terminal tubulus adenocarcinoma; tubulopapillary low-grade adenocarcinoma; low-grade adenocarcinoma; seromucinous adenocarcinoma.

Subtype(s)

Renal cell–like sinonasal adenocarcinoma

Localization

The majority (64%) of low-grade SNACs (LG-SNACs) arise in the nasal cavity (frequently the middle turbinate), and 20% arise in the ethmoid sinus {1819,2106}. The remaining tumours affect the other individual sinuses or expand to involve multiple subsites. Approximately half of all high-grade SNACs (HG-SNACs) are locally advanced at presentation and involve multiple sinonasal tract sites {1819,4214}.

Clinical features

Patients with LG-SNACs present most commonly with obstruction {3189,4109}, and less commonly with epistaxis and pain. Patients with HG-SNACs present with obstruction, epistaxis, pain, deformity, and proptosis {1819}.

Imaging

On imaging, LG-SNACs present as solid masses, filling the nasal cavity and/or paranasal sinuses. HG-SNACs show a more destructive appearance, with osseous involvement and direct extension into the orbit and skull base.

Epidemiology

LG-SNACs are uncommon, show no sex predilection {1819, 3189,2106}, and affect a broad age range (9–89 years), with a peak in the sixth decade of life. HG-SNACs are rare, show a male predominance, and occur over a wide age range with a similar peak {1819,4214}.

Etiology

The etiology is unknown for LG-SNAC. Rare HG-SNACs have been associated with high-risk HPV or sinonasal papillomas {4214}. Exposure to carcinogens such as wood or other dusts and solvents may be related to the development of some HG-SNACs {867,529}.

Pathogenesis

Some LG-SNACs harbour fusions, such as *ETV6::NTRK3/RET* {194,191,4173,330}, and others have *CTNNB1* mutations {4634}. Rare *BRAF* mutations have been reported {1454}, whereas *KRAS* mutations arc not seen. The molecular underpinnings of HG-SNAC are still unknown.

Macroscopic appearance

Non-intestinal SNACs may appear red and polypoid or raspberry-like and firm {2320}.

Histopathology

Tumours are histologically separated by grade.

LG-SNACs have predominantly papillary and/or tubular (glandular) features with complex growth, including back-to-back (cribriform) glands with little intervening stroma {1819,2106, 2320}. A single layer of uniform mucinous cuboidal to columnar epithelial cells lines the structures. These cells have eosinophilic cytoplasm and uniform, basally located nuclei. Mitotic figures are rare and necrosis is not seen. Invasive growth, including within the submucosa as well as into bone, may be present. Calcospherites and squamous morules are sometimes seen {1819, 4634}. Occasional tumours have more dilated glands {2320, 3189}.

HG-SNACs show much more diversity in their histology {1819, 4214}. Many have a predominantly solid growth with occasional glandular structures and/or individual mucocytes. Some have a nested growth and are destructively infiltrative into bone. Numerous mitotic figures are seen with necrosis (individual-cell and confluent).

Subtype

Occasional SNACs are composed predominantly of clear cells, reminiscent of renal cell carcinoma {4242,4021,2401,4967}. These tumours have been referred to as sinonasal renal cell–like adenocarcinomas. The tumours are composed of monomorphic cuboidal to columnar glycogen-rich clear cells that lack mucin production. The cellular cytoplasm may be crystal clear or slightly eosinophilic. Intranuclear inclusions are common. Perineural invasion, lymphovascular invasion, necrosis, and severe pleomorphism are absent, and the overall histological impression is that of a low-grade neoplasm.

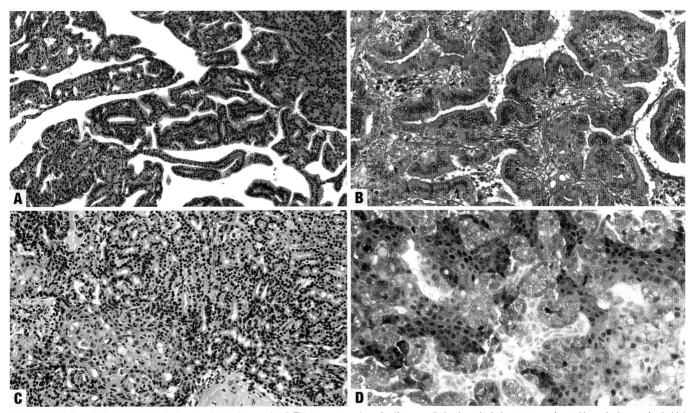

Fig. 1.40 Non–intestinal-type sinonasal adenocarcinoma, low-grade. **A** The tumour consists of uniform small glands and tubular structures formed by a single row of cuboidal or columnar cells and displays a papillary growth pattern. Most papillae are simple and composed of a loose fibrovascular core and bland-looking epithelium arranged in one row or in a bilayered pattern. Some papillae are more complex, with a branching pattern. **B** The tumour cells are uniform, with regular rounded nuclei with finely granular chromatin and abundant eosinophilic cytoplasm. **C** The tumour is composed of closely packed tubules with occasional squamous morules. **D** Occasional cases exhibit abnormal nuclear localization with β-catenin immunohistochemistry.

Histochemistry

In most SNACs, intraluminal mucin or material that gives a diastase-resistant positive reaction with PAS can be identified. In HG-SNACs, cells with intracytoplasmic mucin or diastase-resistant PAS positivity may be present.

Immunohistochemistry

The tumours express cytokeratins (typically CK7 and infrequently focal CK20) {4214}. Squamous antigens such as p40 are typically not expressed or are expressed only focally {4109}.

Markers of intestinal differentiation, such as CDX2, SATB2, and MUC2, may be focally present but are usually absent {715, 4214,4118}. Tumour cells may also express DOG1, SOX10, and S100 {3605}. HG-SNACs can focally express neuroendocrine antigens {4214}. Renal cell–like adenocarcinomas express CAIX and CD10 but do not express PAX8 or RCCm {4021}. β-Catenin and mismatch repair protein expression is wildtype in HG-SNACs {4939}, although a subset of LG-SNACs (often tubular with squamous morules) will show nuclear localization of β-catenin {4634}. Overexpression of p53 may be seen {4109}.

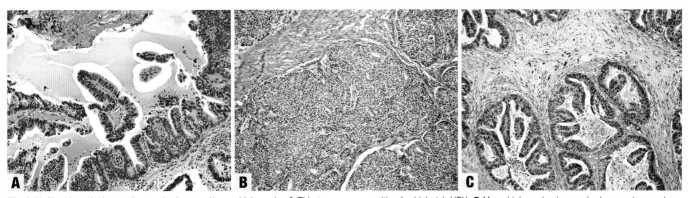

Fig. 1.41 Non–intestinal-type sinonasal adenocarcinoma, high-grade. **A** This tumour was positive for high-risk HPV. **B** Many high-grade sinonasal adenocarcinomas have nests and ribbons of tumour cells intermixed with smaller glands or rosettes. **C** This tumour is composed of small cysts with papillae projecting into them.

Cytology

The cytology of SNAC has not yet been reported in the cytopathology literature. The cytological features are expected to be similar to those of intestinal-type sinonasal adenocarcinoma.

Diagnostic molecular pathology

Not clinically relevant

Essential and desirable diagnostic criteria

Essential: a gland-forming sinonasal tract malignancy with no intestinal phenotype or features of a specific salivary gland neoplasm.

Staging

Staging follows the eighth edition of the Union for International Cancer Control (UICC) / American Joint Committee on Cancer (AJCC) TNM staging system.

Prognosis and prediction

Approximately 25% of LG-SNACs recur, although only 6% of patients die from their tumours, usually owing to a lack of local control {1819,2106,3189}. Patients with HG-SNACs fare worse {1819}, with most dying from the disease within 5 years. Occasional HG-SNACs metastasize locally and distally. The reported

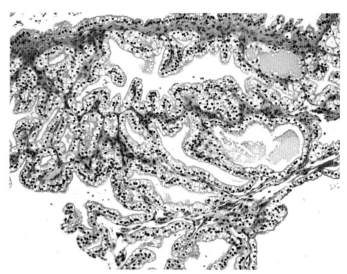

Fig. 1.42 Non–intestinal-type sinonasal adenocarcinoma, renal cell–like subtype. The tumour consists of a tubulopapillary proliferation of polygonal cells with optically clear cytoplasm and small, uniform, round nuclei.

cases of renal cell–like adenocarcinoma have neither recurred nor metastasized {4242,4021,2401,4967}.

Sinonasal tract angiofibroma

Thompson LDR
Agaimy A
Jo VY

Definition
Sinonasal tract angiofibroma is a locally aggressive, variably cellular fibrovascular neoplasm.

ICD-O coding
9160/0 Angiofibroma, NOS

ICD-11 coding
2F00.Y & XA43C9 & XA43C9 & XH1JJ2 Other specified benign neoplasm of middle ear or respiratory system & Nasal cavity & Accessory sinuses & Angiofibroma, NOS

Related terminology
Not recommended: angiofibroma; juvenile nasopharyngeal angiofibroma.

Subtype(s)
None

Localization
Tumours arise from the posterolateral wall of the roof of the nasal cavity or lateral nasopharynx {3173,4984,510}.

Clinical features
The classic triad of nasal obstruction, epistaxis, and sinonasal/nasopharyngeal mass is seen in many patients, often over a prolonged symptom duration {510,2280}. Biopsy is contraindicated because of potentially profuse bleeding. With tumour progression, facial deformity, deafness, diplopia, and proptosis may be seen {3173,4984}.

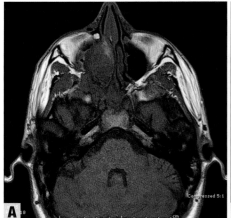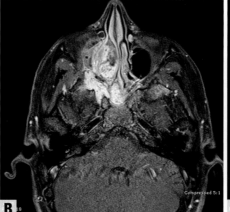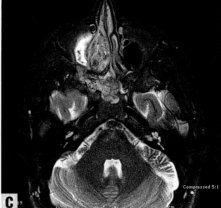

Fig. 1.43 Sinonasal tract angiofibroma. Axial T1-weighted MRI (**A**), postcontrast fat-saturated/suppressed T1-weighted MRI (**B**), and T2-weighted MRI (**C**) images demonstrating a highly vascular soft tissue lesion in the right nasal cavity, with involvement and widening of the pterygopalatine fossa – a common finding on cross-sectional imaging. Note internal low-signal foci on the T2-weighted image denoting flow voids, as well as extension on postcontrast imaging into the pterygoid canal (Vidian canal).

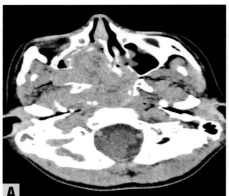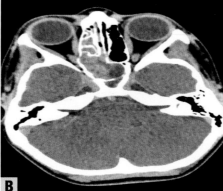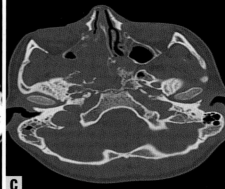

Fig. 1.44 Sinonasal tract angiofibroma. Axial postcontrast CT images. **A** A large heterogeneous, avidly enhancing soft tissue mass in the right nasal cavity involving a grossly expanded pterygopalatine fossa, filling the postnasal space and extending into adjacent parapharyngeal and masticator spaces. **B** Involvement of the right sphenoid sinus and intracranial extension into the right cavernous sinus. **C** Gross erosion of the right central skull base (pterygoid process and margins of the sphenoid sinus).

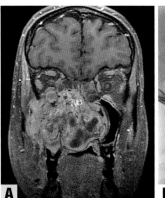
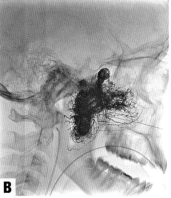

Fig. 1.45 Sinonasal tract angiofibroma. **A** T1-weighted coronal MRI shows a large central destructive neoplasm. Although it is a benign tumour, it can reach a large size and be locally aggressive. **B** Fluoroscopic angiography documents the vascular nature of the tumour, while also allowing for presurgical embolization.

Imaging

Imaging studies {198,749,3630,3307,4154,2280} reveal a highly vascular soft tissue mass, often with internal flow voids on T2-weighted MRI, typically involving and widening the pterygopalatine fossa with anterior bowing of the posterior wall of the adjacent maxillary antrum (Holman–Miller sign, considered pathognomonic) {3173,4984}. Bone destruction and intracranial extension may be seen {3173,2883,510,2564}. Preoperative angiography and embolization are often performed to reduce intraoperative haemorrhage {503}.

Epidemiology

Sinonasal angiofibroma is rare, with an annual incidence of 0.37 cases per 100 000 at-risk population {1600,4984,510}. The tumour develops exclusively in adolescent boys and young men {3173,4836,510,3852}, and if it is identified in a female patient, she should be evaluated for testicular feminization.

Etiology

Hormone dependency is correlated with tumour growth at puberty onset and strong AR expression {3173,4836,1977,3852}.

Pathogenesis

Somatic mutations in the gene encoding β-catenin (*CTNNB1*) arc seen in 75% of tumours, although immunohistochemical nuclear localization of β-catenin is seen in most tumours {15}. These findings and the increased incidence in patients with familial adenomatous polyposis support the importance of aberrant WNT signalling as a common event in these tumours {4776}. Gain of the X chromosome and loss of the Y chromosome have been documented {3914,606}.

Macroscopic appearance

Polypoid to lobulated tumours can be as large as 220 mm (average: 40 mm).

Histopathology

There are numerous blood vessels of various sizes, from slit-like capillaries to irregularly dilated and branching vessels. The vascular walls may be thin to focally or continuously thickened and muscular. No elastic tissue is identified in the vessels except in the feeding arteries. The stroma is composed of bipolar or stellate fibroblastic cells with plump, vesicular, spindled nuclei and indistinct nucleoli. Isolated multinucleated stellate stromal giant cells may be seen. Mitoses are inconspicuous. The stromal cellularity varies from loose and oedematous to densely collagenized. Mast cells are common. Embolized tumours show areas of necrosis and intravascular foreign material. AR blocker–treated tumours are hypocellular with increased stromal collagen {1551}.

Immunohistochemistry

By immunohistochemistry, stromal cells show strong nuclear expression of AR and β-catenin, while vascular markers highlight the vessels and SMA stains the smooth muscle vascular walls {1977,15,3852}. EBV and KSHV/HHV8 are absent {674}.

Cytology

Not clinically relevant

Diagnostic molecular pathology

Not clinically relevant

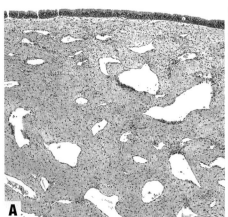
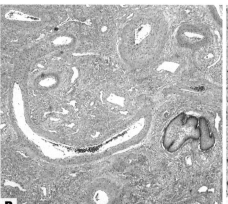
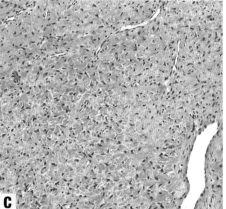

Fig. 1.46 Sinonasal tract angiofibroma. **A** The surface epithelium is unremarkable, overlying a variably cellular vascular neoplasm. Patulous vessels with and without smooth muscle walls are noted. **B** Several vessel types are set within a fibrocollagenous stroma. There is embolic material, a finding noted after embolization. **C** The stroma may be quite cellular, with fibroblastic cells set within a collagenized stroma.

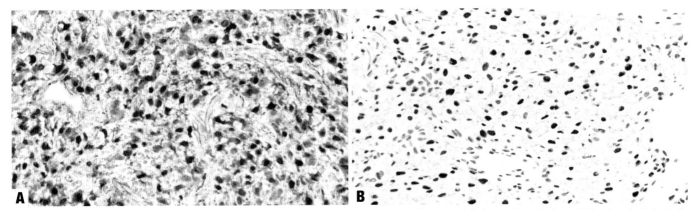

Fig. 1.47 Sinonasal tract angiofibroma. **A** The stromal cells show a strong and diffuse nuclear reaction for β-catenin by immunohistochemistry. **B** The stromal spindled cells show a strong and diffuse nuclear reaction for AR by immunohistochemistry.

Essential and desirable diagnostic criteria

Essential: male patient; posterior nasal cavity / nasopharynx location; numerous vessel types and sizes, some with muscular walls; stromal stellate fibroblasts with variably collagenized stroma.

Desirable: stromal cell nuclear β-catenin and AR immunoreactivity.

Staging

Radiographic and clinical staging systems are used to guide treatment and determine recurrence risk {749,4154,198,3630, 3307,2280}.

Prognosis and prediction

The course is characterized by recurrence (sometimes multiple) in 5–25% of cases {510,2280,2564}. Prognosis depends on the size and extent of the tumour and the completeness of surgical resection {4154,2883}. Rare examples of sarcomatous transformation after radiation have been reported {4836}. Spontaneous regression after puberty may rarely occur {4836}.

Sinonasal glomangiopericytoma

Thompson LDR
Jun S-Y
Lai CK

Definition
Glomangiopericytoma is a sinonasal soft tissue tumour showing perivascular myoid differentiation, usually associated with *CTNNB1* mutations.

ICD-O coding
8824/0 Myopericytoma

ICD-11 coding
2F00.Y & XA43C9 & XA3523 & XH2HE9 Other specified benign neoplasm of middle ear or respiratory system & Nasal cavity & Paranasal sinuses & Myopericytoma

Related terminology
Not recommended: sinonasal-type haemangiopericytoma; sinonasal haemangiopericytoma; intranasal myopericytoma.

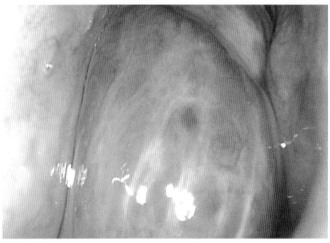

Fig. 1.48 Sinonasal glomangiopericytoma. This endoscopic view demonstrates a polypoid, non-translucent, fleshy, pink-red mass filling the nasal cavity.

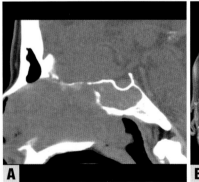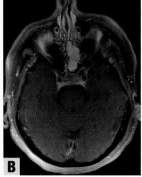

Fig. 1.49 Sinonasal glomangiopericytoma. **A** CT shows a large, polypoid, soft tissue–density mass filling the nasal cavity and extending into the nasopharynx. **B** T1-weighted, fat-suppressed, postcontrast axial MRI shows an enhancing mass within the nasal cavity and adjacent sinuses.

Subtype(s)
None

Localization
Unilateral nasal cavity involvement (turbinate and septum) is most common (< 5% bilateral), with frequent extension into paranasal sinuses (usually the ethmoid and maxillary sinuses); rarely, there is isolated paranasal sinus involvement {935,1250, 710,4419,3402}.

Clinical features
Most patients present with nasal obstruction and/or epistaxis and other nonspecific findings {935,1250,710,4419}. There is rare association with severe oncogenic osteomalacia {710, 3815,562,2519,3402}.

Imaging
Imaging studies show a destructive polypoid mass often accompanied by bone erosion, frequently with concurrent sinusitis {4419,941,4394,4277}.

Epidemiology
Glomangiopericytomas account for about 1% of all sinonasal tract neoplasms {4419}. Identified from infancy to old age, there is a peak in the sixth to seventh decades of life. There is a slight female predilection {935,1220,710,4419,3402}.

Etiology
Unknown

Pathogenesis
Key molecular drivers are recurrent missense mutations within *CTNNB1* exon 3, consisting of somatic single-nucleotide substitutions clustering at positions 32–45 (most commonly codon 33) of the glycogen serine kinase-3 β-phosphorylation (GSK3β) region. The affected region corresponds to the recognition site of the β-catenin destruction complex, which prevents β-catenin phosphorylation and proteasomal degradation, leading to aberrant nuclear translocation and accumulation of β-catenin. Subsequent *CCND1* upregulation and overexpression of cyclin D1 ultimately leads to oncogenic activation {2479,1739,4303,2370, 3256}. Tumours lack the *NAB2::STAT6* fusion of solitary fibrous tumour {1173}, the *MIR143*::NOTCH fusion of glomus tumour {3087}, and the *GLI1* fusions or amplification of *GLI1*-altered soft tissue tumours {1000,1001,4885}.

Macroscopic appearance
Intact tumours are polypoid, non-translucent, soft, oedematous, fleshy masses that are beefy-red to grey-pink. Cut surfaces appear sponge-like to solid with oedematous and/or haemorrhagic areas. Tumours can be as large as 140 mm, but average 30 mm {1250,4419,3402}.

Histopathology

Tumours are unencapsulated but well delineated within the sub-mucosa, separated from a generally intact surface epithelium by a tumour-free zone. The diffuse, patternless cellular prolif-eration effaces the normal submucosal elements, although fascicular, storiform, whorled, reticular, and meningothelial-like patterns may be identified. Tumour cells demonstrate a syncy-tial arrangement of spindle-shaped to ovoid cells containing blunt-ended nuclei with coarse nuclear chromatin and slightly eosinophilic to clear cytoplasm. There is a complex, ramifying vascular network of thin-walled capillary-sized to large patulous staghorn vessels, with characteristic peritheliomatous hyalini-zation. Limited mitotic figures without atypical forms and mild nuclear pleomorphism are seen, but there is usually no tumour necrosis. Extravasated erythrocytes, mast cells, and eosinophils are seen in nearly all tumours. Rarely, tumour giant cells, lipo-matous change, extramedullary haematopoiesis, and collision tumours (solitary fibrous tumour, respiratory epithelial adeno-matoid hamartoma) are reported {4419,37}. Concurrent inflam-matory sinonasal polyps are frequently present. Rare cases show profound nuclear pleomorphism, atypical and increased mitoses, and tumour necrosis, which are features associated with aggressive behaviour {935,710,2382,2415,3402}.

Immunohistochemistry

Immunohistochemical analyses demonstrate strong tumour cell immunoreactivity for actins (SMA > MSA), nuclear β-catenin, LEF1, cyclin D1, and factor XIIIa. No significant staining is observed for CD31, ERG, D2-40, von Willebrand factor (fac-tor VIII–related antigen), pancytokeratin, STAT6, desmin, S100,

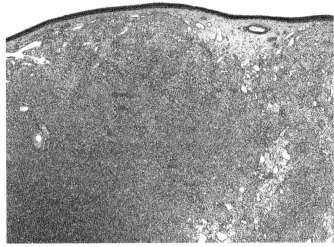

Fig. 1.50 Sinonasal glomangiopericytoma. An intact respiratory lining covers a cellu-lar neoplastic proliferation with short, interlacing fascicles.

SOX10, KIT (CD117), and SATB2 {1220,710,2382,4419,1765, 1173,37,776,1739,1089,3402,49,4436,4303,3256,3857}. CD34 is variably present, clone dependent (absent with clone My10) {4419,3857}.

Differential diagnosis

Several spindle cell tumours are considered in the differential diagnosis for glomangiopericytoma, but it is most commonly distinguished from smooth muscle tumours, solitary fibrous tumour, meningioma, schwannoma, biphenotypic sinonasal

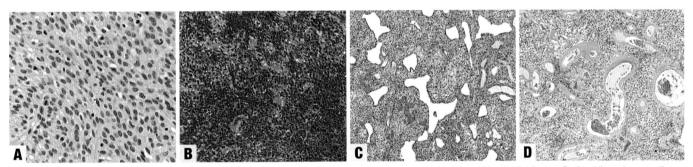

Fig. 1.51 Sinonasal glomangiopericytoma. **A** Tumour cells are isomorphic, with bland, monotonous nuclei with fine chromatin distribution. Eosinophils and mast cells are commonly present. **B** Marked erythrocyte extravasation into the tumour may obscure the true nature of the neoplasm. **C** Open, patulous vessels with a staghorn or antler-like configuration are characteristic of the tumour. **D** A peritheliomatous hyalinization with a patternless proliferation of ovoid to spindled cells is a characteristic finding of the tumour.

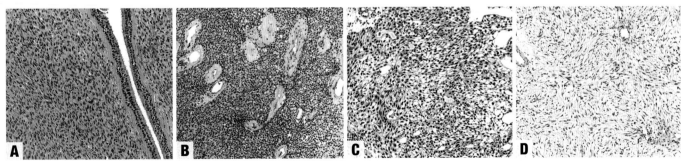

Fig. 1.52 Sinonasal glomangiopericytoma. **A** The spindled cell neoplasm is separated from the surface epithelium by a well-developed zone of fibrosis. **B** Tumours show a variable cellularity, with a high cellularity seen in this tumour. Note the syncytial quality to the neoplastic cells. **C** A reticulated pattern shows open spaces with extravasated erythrocytes along with large, patulous vascular spaces. **D** Cellularity can be quite variable, with this field demonstrating a hypocellular area, where the neoplastic cells are spindled with a cleared cytoplasm.

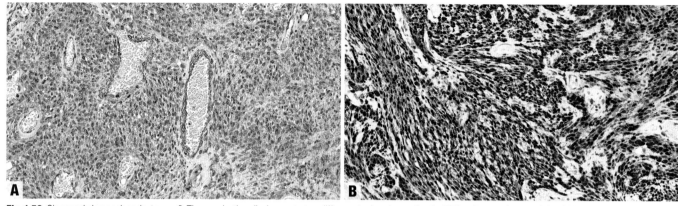

Fig. 1.53 Sinonasal glomangiopericytoma. **A** The neoplastic cells demonstrate a diffuse cytoplasmic reaction for SMA, a feature characteristic of this tumour. **B** The neoplastic cells demonstrate a strong and diffuse nuclear reaction for β-catenin, a reflection of the *CTNNB1* mutation in this tumour (note the negative endothelial nucleus as an internal control).

sarcoma, desmoid-type fibromatosis, and synovial sarcoma by histomorphology and a pertinent immunohistochemical panel.

Cytology
Not clinically relevant

Diagnostic molecular pathology
Identification of mutations in *CTNNB1* may aid in the diagnosis, although this is rarely necessary {2479,1739,42,2101}.

Essential and desirable diagnostic criteria
Essential: an ovoid to spindled syncytium of myoid-type cells within a richly vascularized stroma.
Desirable: peritheliomatous hyalinization; extravasated erythrocytes, mast cells, and eosinophils; immunoreactivity for

actins and nuclear β-catenin, with negativity for STAT6, S100, SOX10, and cytokeratins (in selected cases).

Staging
Not applicable

Prognosis and prediction
Considered a very indolent tumour, especially in patients aged < 60 years {3402}. Recurrences are seen in 20%, often due to incomplete excision {935,1250,1220,710,4419,1646,3402}. Late local recurrence (> 10 years) suggests prolonged clinical follow-up. Features suggestive of aggressive behaviour include tumour size > 50 mm, destructive bone invasion, intracranial extension, profound nuclear pleomorphism, > 4 mitoses/2 mm^2, and tumour necrosis {935,710,2382,4419,2415}.

Biphenotypic sinonasal sarcoma

Le Loarer F
Benzerdjeb N
Jo VY

Definition

Biphenotypic sinonasal sarcoma (BSNS) is a bland spindle cell malignancy demonstrating a neural and myogenic phenotype, exclusively involving the sinonasal tract and usually associated with *PAX3* rearrangement.

ICD-O coding

9045/3 Biphenotypic sinonasal sarcoma

ICD-11 coding

2C20.Y & XH4UM7 Malignant neoplasms of nasal cavity & Sarcoma, NOS

Related terminology

Not recommended: low-grade sinonasal sarcoma with neural and myogenic features.

Subtype(s)

None

Localization

BSNS primarily develops in the nasal cavity and ethmoid sinus, but any sinonasal tract site may be involved {2602,2501}. BSNS often develops locoregional infiltration, including the lamina papyracea, anterior skull base, cribriform plate, orbit, and brain {1488,2659}.

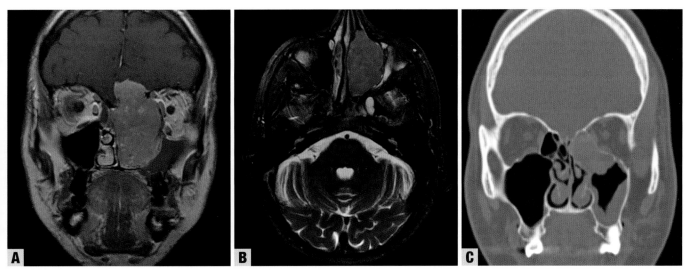

Fig. 1.54 Biphenotypic sinonasal sarcoma. **A** MRI of the left ethmoid air cells shows tumour infiltrating the orbital wall, frontal lobe, and left nasal cavity (coronal view, T1 spin echo signal, with injection of gadolinium). **B** MRI picture of a tumour of the left maxillary sinus infiltrating the left nasal cavity (T2 fast spin echo signal with fat saturation). **C** Coronal CT. The tumour is seen infiltrating the left maxillary sinus, ethmoid sinus, and left nasal cavity.

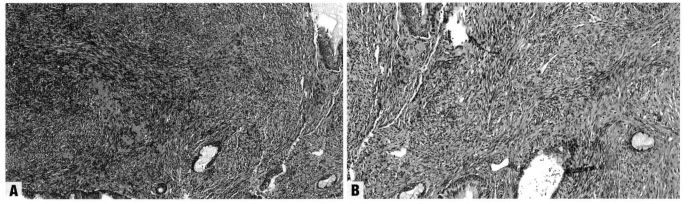

Fig. 1.55 Biphenotypic sinonasal sarcoma. **A** The tumour exhibits a densely cellular spindle cell proliferation forming long fascicles with entrapped epithelial foci. **B** Densely cellular spindle cell proliferations forming long fascicles with entrapped epithelial foci.

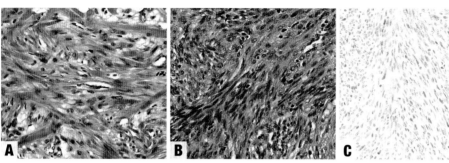

Fig. 1.56 Biphenotypic sinonasal sarcoma. **A** The tumour can occasionally display focal rhabdomyoblastic differentiation. **B** The tumour cells display monotonous elongated nuclei with fine chromatin and low mitotic activity. **C** The tumour cells show heterogeneous nuclear immunoreactivity of rhabdomyoblastic cells for MYOD1. **D** The tumour cells show heterogeneous staining with desmin antibody, which is most often patchy and focal (desmin immunohistochemistry).

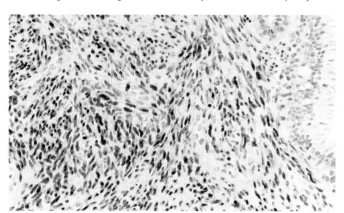

Fig. 1.57 Biphenotypic sinonasal sarcoma. Diffuse nuclear PAX3 staining (using clone 274212).

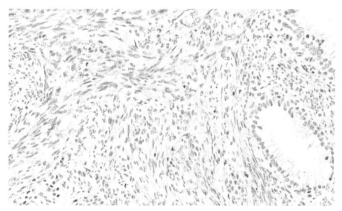

Fig. 1.58 Biphenotypic sinonasal sarcoma. The tumour cells never express SOX10 (SOX10 immunohistochemistry).

Clinical features

BSNS may cause nasal obstruction, pain, epistaxis, rhinorrhoea, or mucocoele. Regional infiltration may cause diplopia or cerebral haemorrhage {1488,2659,1758}.

Imaging

Involved bones show mixed lytic and sclerotic changes on imaging {2998}.

Epidemiology

Patients are adults with a mean age of 53 years (range: 24–85 years) {2602,2501}. There is a notable female predominance {190}.

Etiology

Unknown

Pathogenesis

BSNS is associated with recurrent driver gene fusions, most frequently *PAX3::MAML3* (60%) {1479}. Alternative 3′ partners include *NCOA1*, *NCOA2*, *FOXO1*, and *WWTR1* {4846,1949, 1479,2501}. The fusion deregulates the expression of factors involved in neural development, in particular *NTRK3* {4722}. The translocation may be unbalanced {2105}.

Macroscopic appearance

BSNS is a nonspecific tan-white, firm mass. Tumours are often large, with a median size of 40 mm {2602,2501}.

Histopathology

BSNS is unencapsulated, with an infiltrative growth composed of spindled cells forming medium to long fascicles, often with a herringbone pattern. BSNSs are mostly densely cellular with overlapping nuclei, although they can show variations in cellular density. Tumour cells are uniform, harbouring ovoid or wavy nuclei with fine chromatin dotted with small or inconspicuous nucleoli. Cytoplasm tends to be scant and palely eosinophilic. Rhabdomyoblastic differentiation is uncommon and typically focal when present, and it may be associated with specific fusion-gene partners {1949}. Foci of hyperplastic respiratory epithelium are commonly entrapped within the tumour. Infiltration of bone is common. Mitotic activity is consistently low, mostly < 2 mitoses/mm². Necrosis is not present. Hypocellular fibrous areas and thin-walled haemangiopericytoma-like vessels are common {2105}.

Immunohistochemistry

BSNSs are consistently positive for S100, although staining extent may be heterogeneous. SOX10 is always negative. SMA is consistently positive. Desmin is expressed in half to two thirds of cases {3745}. MYOD1 and myogenin staining is inconsistent and typically patchy or focal when positive. Most cases show nuclear PAX3 staining (using clone 274212) {2105}. Pan-TRK staining is common, as is focal nuclear expression of β-catenin {3745,2146}. Occasional reactivity for calponin, GFAP, cytokeratins, and CD34 has been reported {2105}.

Differential diagnosis

Entities in the differential diagnosis are summarized in Table 1.01, the main mimics being synovial sarcoma, cellular schwannoma, and respiratory epithelial adenomatoid hamartoma.

Table 1.01 Main differential diagnosis of biphenotypic sinonasal sarcoma

Tumour type	Morphology	Immunohistochemistry	Molecular
Cellular schwannoma (benign)	Hyalinized vessels, well delineated, Antoni A and B areas	SOX10+	No *PAX3* fusion
Glomangiopericytoma (benign)	Plump eosinophilic cytoplasm, short fascicles, whorls, haemangiopericytic vessels	β-catenin+, MYOD1−	*CTNNB1* mutation
Solitary fibrous tumour (intermediate malignancy)	Less cellular, short fascicles, collagenous stroma, haemangiopericytic vessels	STAT6+	*STAT6* fusion
Spindle cell tumour with NTRK fusion (intermediate malignancy)	Shorter fascicles, less cellular, fibrous stroma	Pan-TRK+, CD34+/−, S100+/−, MYOD1−, desmin−	*NTRK1/2/3* fusion
Synovial sarcoma (malignant)	Densely cellular	Cytokeratins+, SS18::SSX+	*SS18::SSX1/2/4* fusion
TFCP2-fused rhabdomyosarcoma (malignant)	High-grade (vesicular nuclei, mitosis, necrosis), epithelioid cytomorphology	Cytokeratins+, desmin+, MYOD1+, ALK+	*TFCP2* fusion
MPNST (malignant)	High-grade (mitosis, necrosis), anisokaryosis	S100 and SOX10+ focal, pan-TRK−	Inactivating mutations of PRC2 core components (*EED* or *SUZ12*)

MPNST, malignant peripheral nerve sheath tumour.

Cytology

Not clinically relevant

Diagnostic molecular pathology

FISH with a *PAX3* break-apart probe is helpful to confirm the diagnosis {1479}. Technical failures are mostly related to decalcification, with next-generation sequencing having the advantage of detecting all possible fusion genes. A possibly related tumour of the head and neck with a similar morphology shows a *RREB1::MRTFB* (*MKL2*) fusion {4060,2913}. No fusion is detected in a minority of cases.

Essential and desirable diagnostic criteria

Essential: a monotonous spindle cell proliferation with fascicular architecture with variably high cellular density; reactivity for S100 and myogenic markers (most commonly SMA).
Desirable: confirmation of *PAX3* rearrangement in selected cases.

Staging

Staging follows the eighth edition of the Union for International Cancer Control (UICC) / American Joint Committee on Cancer (AJCC) TNM staging system classification for head and neck soft tissue sarcomas.

Prognosis and prediction

Local recurrences are seen in one third to half of all cases {2366} and may occur years after initial diagnosis {1488}. No distant metastases have been reported.

Chordoma

Flanagan AM
Varlet P

Definition
Chordoma is a primary malignant bone tumour with neoplastic cells recapitulating notochordal differentiation.

ICD-O coding
9370/3 Chordoma
9370/3 Conventional chordoma
9371/3 Chondroid chordoma
9372/3 Poorly differentiated chordoma
9372/3 Dedifferentiated chordoma

ICD-11 coding
2C20.Y & XH9GH0 Malignant neoplasms of nasal cavity & Chordoma, NOS
2C20.Y & XH17D8 Malignant neoplasms of nasal cavity & Chondroid chordoma
2C20.Y & XH7303 Malignant neoplasms of nasal cavity & Dedifferentiated chordoma

Related terminology
None

Subtype(s)
Conventional chordoma; chondroid chordoma; poorly differentiated chordoma; dedifferentiated chordoma

Localization
Approximately 30% present in the skull base and upper mobile spine {2910,3104}.

Clinical features
Pain, a mass lesion, and neurological deficits are noted.

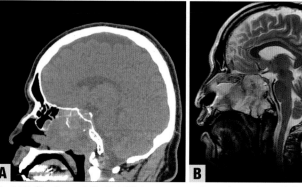

Fig. 1.59 Chordoma. **A** Sagittal CT demonstrates a large, destructive, soft tissue–density mass within the nasopharynx and skull base. **B** This sagittal T2-weighted image shows a hyperintense, destructive, nasopharynx midline mass.

Imaging
Tumours expand bone as large, destructive, lytic midline masses. On MRI, there is a loss of bone-marrow fat (high T1-weighted signal), replaced with intermediate-signal material on T1-weighted images that is T2-hyperintense and demonstrates variable postcontrast enhancement {4296,4724,4197}.

Epidemiology
The incidence of chordoma is 0.08 cases per 100 000 person-years; it is rare in Black patients {1033}. There is a male predominance. All ages are affected, but children / young adults most often present with craniocervical tumours. Poorly differentiated tumours generally present in children and rarely arise in people aged > 30 years {4035}.

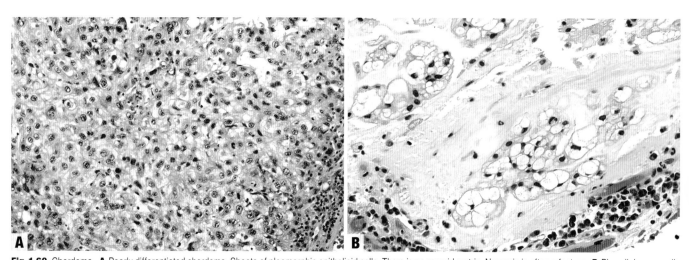

Fig. 1.60 Chordoma. **A** Poorly differentiated chordoma. Sheets of pleomorphic epithelioid cells. There is no myxoid matrix. Necrosis is often a feature. **B** Physaliphorous cells are quite characteristic of chordoma, where there are numerous vacuolations in the cytoplasm that result in a spider-like appearance.

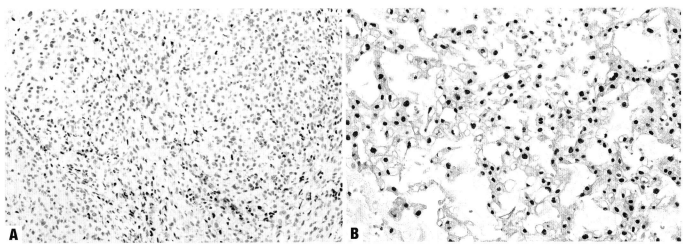

Fig. 1.61 Chordoma. **A** Poorly differentiated chordoma. Characteristic loss of expression of SMARCB1. **B** There is strong, diffuse nuclear expression of brachyury in the neoplastic cells of chordoma.

Etiology

Rarely, there is an autosomal dominant trait resulting from tandem duplication of *TBXT* (encoding brachyury) {2241} or in the setting of tuberous sclerosis with germline alterations in *TSC1* or *TSC2* {2546,998}.

Pathogenesis

Aberrant expression of *TBXT* is implicated in the pathogenesis of chordoma {4662,3181,3909,4373,2776,953}, resulting in the expression of brachyury. Alterations of *PBRM1/SETD2*, encoding members of the SWI/SNF complex, represent the most common events (in 16%) in skull base chordomas, along with homozygous *CDKN2A* deletion {314,954}. In poorly differentiated chordoma, there is homozygous deletion of *SMARCB1*, with loss of protein expression {1794}.

Macroscopic appearance

Chordoma is a bone-destructive, lobular, solid, gelatinous mass expanding into soft tissues.

Histopathology

Conventional chordomas exhibit lobules separated by fibrous septa, composed of large epithelioid cells with bubbly cytoplasm (physaliphorous cells) embedded in an extracellular myxoid or chondroid matrix as cords or nests of cells.

Subtypes

Chondroid chordoma represents a subtype composed predominantly of hyaline cartilage–like extracellular matrix.

The poorly differentiated subtype is composed of solid epithelioid cells with areas of rhabdoid morphology and loss of SMARCB1 immunoreactivity.

Dedifferentiated chordoma is a biphasic tumour in which the dedifferentiated component commonly exhibits features of high-grade sarcoma.

Immunohistochemistry

Neoplastic cells are strongly immunoreactive for cytokeratin, EMA, and brachyury (encoded by *TBXT*), with variable S100, CEA, and GFAP {3259,2485,2103}.

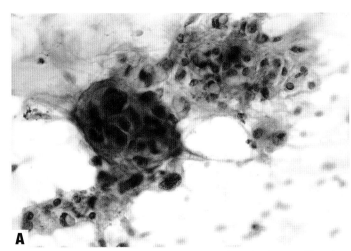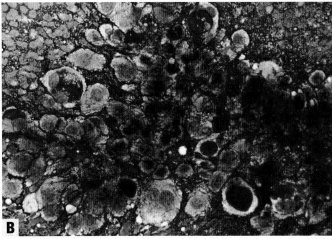

Fig. 1.62 Chordoma. **A** Small groups of cells clustered together in a myxoid-mucinous matrix. Note the large signet ring–like cells along with smaller cells with granular cytoplasm (Pap-stained smear). **B** Cellular smear with large cells containing cytoplasmic vacuoles set within a magenta matrix material (Giemsa).

Differential diagnosis

Tumours are distinguished from chondrosarcoma, carcinoma, meningioma, and myoepithelial tumours.

Cytology

Smears are usually cellular with small polygonal to elongated cells that have granular bluish cytoplasm and round bland nuclei embedded in abundant chondromyxoid magenta matrix (Giemsa). Larger cells with copious finely vacuolated cytoplasm and similar round nuclei are also present and resemble physaliphorous cells {2231,2103}. Binucleated and multinucleated cells and occasional mitoses may be seen.

Diagnostic molecular pathology

Deletion in *SMARCB1* can be detected by FISH in poorly differentiated chordoma {3346A,4034A}.

Essential and desirable diagnostic criteria

Essential: a bone tumour by imaging; lobules of large epithelioid cells embedded in a myxoid/chondroid matrix.

Desirable: brachyury and cytokeratin expression; SMARCB1 loss in the poorly differentiated subtype; brachyury not expressed in the dedifferentiated component.

Staging

Staging follows the eighth edition of the Union for International Cancer Control (UICC) / American Joint Committee on Cancer (AJCC) TNM staging system, with specific reference to bone sarcoma protocols.

Prognosis and prediction

The median overall survival time is 7 years for conventional chordoma, but the prognosis is less favourable for the dedifferentiated and poorly differentiated subtypes {1794,386,4035,5029}.

Sinonasal ameloblastoma

Magliocca K
Betz SJ
Wenig BM

Definition
Sinonasal ameloblastoma (SA) is a benign but locally aggressive extragnathic sinonasal tract epithelial odontogenic neoplasm composed of ameloblast-like cells and stellate reticulum.

ICD-O coding
9310/0 Ameloblastoma, NOS

ICD-11 coding
2E83.0 & XH1SV4 Benign osteogenic tumours of bone or articular cartilage of skull or face & Ameloblastoma, NOS

Related terminology
None

Subtype(s)
None

Localization
SA affects the nasal cavity (septum, lateral wall), paranasal sinuses, or both {3907,4490}.

Clinical features
Patients commonly present with nasal obstruction and/or epistaxis {3907}. With tumour progression, extension into the nasal vestibule {4778,3079} or orbitofacial deformity may develop {4778,3907}.

Imaging
Imaging studies reveal a solid rather than multicystic appearance, with remodelled and/or destroyed sinus bony walls {3079}. Radiographic evidence of an intraosseous maxillary alveolar bone component precludes a diagnosis of SA {3907}.

Epidemiology
SA is very rare, with a strong male predilection. Patients are adults in their sixth to seventh decade of life, notably older than those with its gnathic counterparts {3907,354}.

Etiology
Unknown

Pathogenesis
Although not studied in sinonasal tract tumours, *BRAF* activating mutations are most common in jaw tumours, followed by mutually exclusive RAS mutations {2422,4307,600,1821}, with *SMO* mutation being a common co-occurring mutation {4307, 600}.

Macroscopic appearance
The cut surface is solid with limited cystic change {3907,354}.

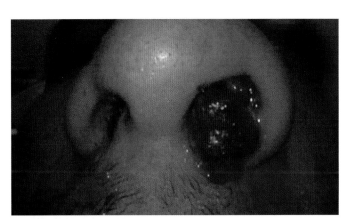

Fig. 1.63 Sinonasal ameloblastoma. Polypoid nasal vestibular projection of sinonasal ameloblastoma.

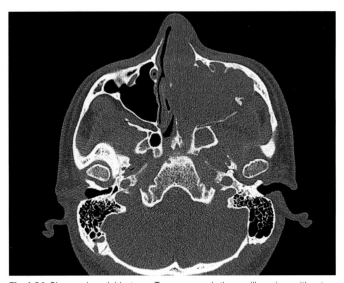

Fig. 1.64 Sinonasal ameloblastoma. Tumour expands the maxillary sinus with extension into the nasal cavity (CT, axial plane).

Histopathology
SA is a basaloid epithelial neoplasm commonly arranged in a plexiform or follicular pattern, with a loosely arranged stellate reticulum–like component centrally. Peripheral cells palisade with reverse polarity and subnuclear vacuolization. Direct surface epithelial continuity may be identified {3907}.

Differential diagnosis
The differential diagnosis includes salivary gland neoplasms, skin basal cell carcinoma, and basaloid squamous cell carcinoma. Craniopharyngioma is separable with clinicoradiographic correlation.

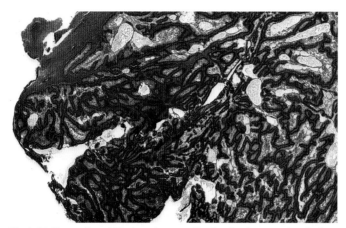

Fig. 1.65 Sinonasal ameloblastoma. Low-magnification view demonstrating plexiform patterned growth.

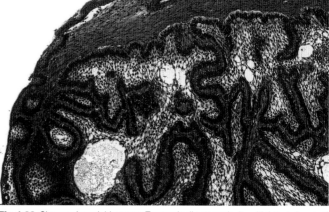

Fig. 1.66 Sinonasal ameloblastoma. Tumour in direct continuity with intact sinonasal surface epithelium (far left).

Cytology

Hypercellular smears show tissue fragments of small basaloid cells with hyperchromatic round nuclei and peripheral palisading, and distinct larger cells with more open chromatin. There may be occasional stromal fragments with spindle cells with elongated nuclei and abundant clear cytoplasm {2875}. Keratin and cholesterol crystals are not seen {4980}.

Diagnostic molecular pathology

Not clinically relevant

Essential and desirable diagnostic criteria

Essential: sinonasal location; radiographic exclusion of jaw origin; ameloblastic-type epithelium with central stellate reticulum–like material.

Staging

Not applicable

Prognosis and prediction

Morbidity depends on tumour size and sites of tumour extension. Local recurrences may occur, but no distant metastases are reported {3907}.

Adamantinomatous craniopharyngioma

Santagata S
Jacques TS
Martinez-Barbera JP
Müller HL

Definition

Adamantinomatous craniopharyngioma is a mixed solid and cystic squamous epithelial tumour with stellate reticulum and wet keratin (ghost cells), characterized by activating *CTNNB1* mutations.

ICD-O coding

9351/1 Adamantinomatous craniopharyngioma

ICD-11 coding

2E83.0 & XH15X9 Benign osteogenic tumours of bone or articular cartilage of skull or face & Craniopharyngioma, adamantinomatous

Related terminology

None

Subtype(s)

None

Localization

Adamantinomatous craniopharyngioma can arise anywhere along the craniopharyngeal canal, with rare presentation in the nasopharynx or sinonasal tract {640,4966,2774,2410, 5024,3814,3372,14,1507,3108}. This section refers to sinonasal tumours; sellar tumours are covered within other volumes {4809,4805}.

Clinical features

Infrasellar craniopharyngioma within the sinonasal tract presents with nonspecific clinical findings, different from the headaches, visual changes, and endocrine deficits of intrasellar or suprasellar tumours {640,4966,2774,2410,5024,3814,3372,14, 1507,3108}.

Imaging

Imaging findings demonstrate cystic masses with prominent calcification and contrast-enhancing walls {421,1867,2774, 3814,3108}.

Epidemiology

Sinonasal tract tumours are extremely rare, with tumours reported in all ages, without a sex predilection {640,4966,4977, 2774,2410,5024,3814,3372,14,1507}.

Etiology

Unknown

Pathogenesis

Although not studied in sinonasal tract sites, craniopharyngiomas are proposed to arise from cellular elements related to the Rathke pouch / hypophysial duct {3108}. Tumours are characterized by activating point mutations in exon 3 of *CTNNB1* (the gene that encodes the WNT signalling pathway regulator β-catenin {1768A,225}) in up to 100% of cases tested using sensitive techniques {2210A,225}, and these mutations are considered clonal driver events {225}. Expression of oncogenic β-catenin in early embryonic precursors and in SOX2+ stem cell populations of the pituitary drive formation of tumours resembling adamantinomatous craniopharyngioma {1550,187}. Furthermore, SOX2+ stem cells may contribute to the formation of epithelial whorls with nuclear localized β-catenin. The whorls are senescent and act as local signalling hubs through the synthesis and secretion of numerous growth factors (e.g. sonic hedgehog, EGF, FGF, TGF-β, BMPs) and inflammatory cytokines and chemokines (e.g. IL-1, IL-6) {635,186,963,1652,964,224,591}. These epithelial whorls are analogous to the enamel knot, a critical signalling centre that controls tooth morphogenesis {224,591}, and they implicate

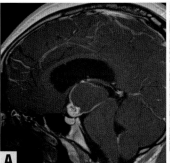
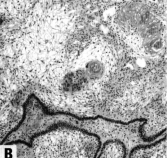
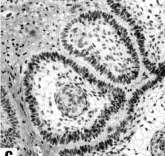
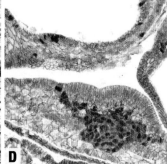

Fig. 1.67 Adamantinomatous craniopharyngioma. **A** Postcontrast T1-weighted MRI shows a suprasellar 37 mm predominantly cystic mass with a thin rim of enhancement extending into the third ventricle. There was a 16 mm region of nodular enhancement inferiorly. This male 18-year-old had a 2-month history of headache, which had become acutely worse with a new onset of nausea and vomiting. The mass demonstrated peripheral calcification on CT. **B** Basal palisading of tumour cells along the tumour–brain interface, epithelial whorls, stellate reticulum, and wet keratin (ghost cells). **C** High-power view of the interface of adamantinomatous craniopharyngioma and brain tissue; Rosenthal fibres are present in the reactive piloid gliosis. **D** Even though mutations in exon 3 of *CTNNB1*, which encodes β-catenin, are clonal and present across the neoplastic epithelium, β-catenin protein only accumulates in the nucleus in a subset of cells, such as those present in epithelial whorls or surrounding wet keratin.

paracrine signalling in tumour formation {963}. Histological and molecular parallels with odontogenic tumours suggest similar cells of origin and similar mechanisms of pathogenesis {431,3439} and explain the occasional presence of teeth in adamantinomatous craniopharyngioma {384}.

Macroscopic appearance
Craniopharyngiomas are solid and cystic. Cyst fluid is dark greenish-brown, often described as machinery oil or crankcase oil. They are frequently calcified.

Histopathology
The tumours consist of epithelium arranged in cords, lobules, ribbons, nodular whorls, and irregular trabeculae. Basal palisading is prominent, and nodules of anucleate, ghost-like squamous cells, termed "wet keratin", are common. Loose microcystic areas of stellate reticulum often intermingle between the wet keratin and more densely arranged areas of tumour epithelium. The cysts are often lined by flattened epithelium. Degenerative changes (fibrosis, calcification) are common, and there may be a xanthogranulomatous reaction to ruptured cyst material. Adamantinomatous craniopharyngioma is regarded as CNS WHO grade 1. Malignant progression is exceedingly rare {3725,4159,3161,4692}; when it does occur, it resembles squamous cell carcinoma and ameloblastic or odontogenic ghost cell carcinoma {3725,2969}.

Immunohistochemistry
Adamantinomatous craniopharyngiomas show nuclear accumulation of β-catenin spatially restricted to small epithelial whorls and found in only a small percentage of cells {636,635, 1662,964,225}.

Differential diagnosis
The differential diagnosis includes papillary craniopharyngioma, xanthogranuloma, Rathke cleft cyst, epidermoid and dermoid cysts, ameloblastoma, and teratocarcinosarcoma.

Cytology
Cytology is not clinically relevant, although the features have been reported intraoperatively {1021,4388,2088}.

Diagnostic molecular pathology
Demonstration of *CTNNB1* mutation may be helpful in selected cases.

Essential and desirable diagnostic criteria
Essential: benign squamous non-keratinizing epithelium; stellate reticulum; wet keratin.
Desirable: nuclear immunoreactivity for β-catenin (in selected cases).

Staging
Not relevant

Prognosis and prediction
Overall survival is excellent, but the extent of disease, whether the tumour is completely removed, and patient age contribute to the reported outcomes {4595,3464,3452,2657,921,3298}. Malignant transformation is not reported in sinonasal tract tumours.

Meningioma of the sinonasal tract, ear, and temporal bone

Gyure KA
Bal MM
Gupta R
Kakkar A
Perry A
Sahm F
Thompson LDR

Definition
Meningioma is a neoplasm of meningothelial/arachnoid cap cells.

ICD-O coding
9530/0 Meningioma, NOS
9531/0 Meningothelial meningioma
9533/0 Psammomatous meningioma

ICD-11 coding
2F00.Y & XH11P5 & XA43C9 & XH11P5 Other specified benign neoplasms of middle ear or respiratory system & Nasal cavity & Accessory sinuses & Meningioma, NOS

Related terminology
None

Subtype(s)
Meningothelial and psammomatous meningiomas are the most common; for other subtypes, please see the WHO classification of CNS tumours {4805}.

Localization
Meningiomas of the head and neck most commonly arise by direct extension of an intracranial lesion, but they may occur ectopically within the sinonasal tract (nasal cavity more often than paranasal sinuses) or ear / temporal bone without any discernible connection to the CNS {4416,3584,4414,3516,3788, 93,2685,2125}. Exclusion of an intracranial primary should be documented before diagnosing ectopic meningioma. Multifocality is commonly present, and tumours are more frequently

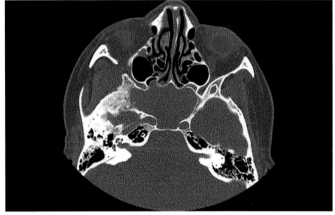

Fig. 1.68 Meningioma of the sinonasal tract. A homogeneous mass is identified within the sphenoid sinus, associated with bone remodelling and hyperostosis, in this CT image.

left-sided {1475,3498,4416,3788}. Rarely, they reach these sites via metastasis from an intracranial tumour.

Clinical features
Symptoms are nonspecific and usually present for years (as long as 15 years; mean: 5 years). These are secondary to mass effects and include nasal obstruction and epistaxis for nasal cavity lesions {1475,1562,3498,4416}, and hearing loss, tinnitus, otitis media, pain, headaches, dizziness, and vertigo for ear / temporal bone lesions {3788,4036,4226}.

Imaging
Imaging studies document the extent, location, and intracranial involvement of the tumour. This is important for meningiomas

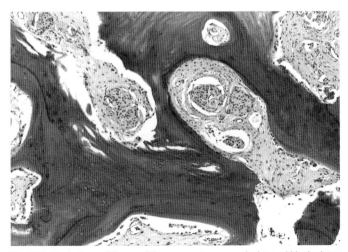

Fig. 1.69 Meningioma of the ear. It is common to see meningioma within the interstices of bone. The tumour frequently grows through the bone from an intracranial primary to present either in the ear or in the sinonasal tract.

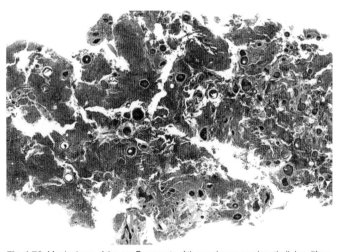

Fig. 1.70 Meningioma of the ear. Fragments of tissue show a meningothelial proliferation associated with innumerable variably sized psammoma bodies.

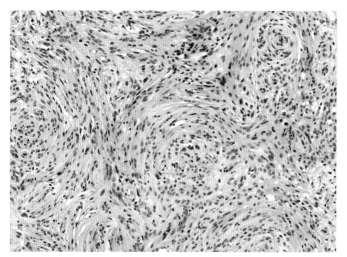

Fig. 1.71 Meningioma of the sinonasal tract. The meningothelial pattern, composed of slightly spindled cells, is seen in this meningothelial meningioma.

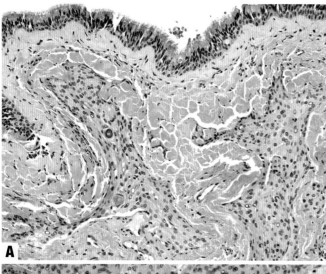

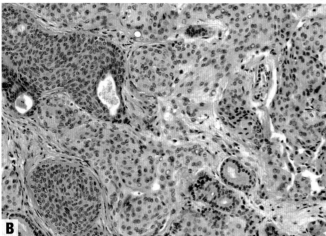

Fig. 1.72 Meningioma of the sinonasal tract. **A** An intact respiratory epithelium is noted above a stromal proliferation of meningothelial cells. Note the small psammoma bodies and well-developed intranuclear cytoplasmic inclusions. **B** The meningothelial proliferation is intimately associated with the surface squamous epithelium and the adjacent minor mucoserous glands. This finding sometimes mimics squamous cell carcinoma. However, the numerous intranuclear cytoplasmic inclusions help with interpretation.

with an en plaque configuration. CT demonstrates a hyperdense mass compared with brain tissue. MRI shows uniform enhancement of the tumour. Calcifications may be seen. Bone invasion is often accompanied by hyperostosis {623,3093,3780,4416, 3024,2630,3036,1673,4726}. Nuclear medicine radiopharmaceutical-labelled scans may identify incidental meningiomas {905,3399}.

Epidemiology

About 20% of intracranial meningiomas extend beyond the cranial cavity (orbit, middle ear, sinonasal tract, skin) {1341, 93,1114}. Primary extracranial meningiomas are rare, accounting for 0.2% of primary sinonasal tract neoplasms {4416} and 2% of all meningiomas. Sinonasal meningiomas account for about a quarter of all primary extracranial meningiomas {3788}. Meningiomas within the head and neck show a slight female predominance (M:F ratio: 1:1.2), with a peak incidence in the fifth decade of life. However, there is a broad age range (9–90 years), with women presenting about a decade later than men (49 vs 37 years) {2259,4416,3584,4414,3788,1989,3574, 4226,93,4031}.

Etiology

Like for intracranial meningiomas, ionizing radiation exposure is a potential etiological factor {1475,1933,4416}, with a long latency period, especially in patients who were very young at the time of exposure or had a high radiation dose {549,548}. Hormones may play a role, given that there is a higher incidence in women of reproductive age and those who use hormone replacement therapy. Hormone receptors, especially PR, are expressed in the tumours; however, a causal role is difficult to prove {690,691,499,426}. There are several genetic predispositions, most commonly neurofibromatosis type 2.

Pathogenesis

Meningiomas are derived from arachnoid cap cells. Extracranial meningiomas are postulated to develop from arachnoidal cells in the proximal sheaths of cranial/spinal nerves and blood vessels where they emerge through skull foramina, from displaced arachnoid cap cells that become detached or entrapped during embryological development in an extracranial location, from a traumatic event or cerebral hypertension that displaces cap cells, or from undifferentiated/multipotential mesenchymal cells {3498,4416,3861,3788}.

Macroscopic appearance

Meningiomas can be as large as 80 mm, with an average size of 30 mm. Tumours are often polypoid and covered by intact epithelium. Bone insinuation is usually present, whether ectopic or by direct extension from an intracranial primary. The tumours are firm to rubbery with granular, gritty cut surfaces related to either psammoma bodies or entrapped bone.

Histopathology

Neoplastic cells are usually intimately blended with an intact respiratory or metaplastic squamous surface epithelium. Cells have an infiltrative appearance, meandering around native minor mucoserous glands and within bone interstices. Remodelled bone may show numerous osteoclasts at the junction with tumour. The cells are arranged in lobules, whorls, and fascicles

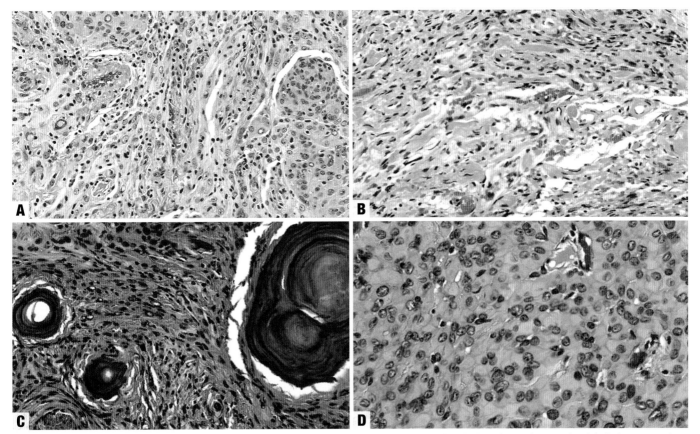

Fig. 1.73 Meningioma. **A** Meningioma of the sinonasal tract. Slight nuclear atypia may be seen in meningothelial meningioma. Intranuclear cytoplasmic inclusions are prominent in this field. **B** Meningioma of the sinonasal tract. Fibrous meningiomas are the most difficult to recognize, because the neoplastic cells take on a spindled appearance within a background of collagen. Special studies are often required to confirm the diagnosis. **C** Meningioma of the ear. The psammomatous subtype of meningioma is seen more commonly in the ear than in the sinonasal tract. There are usually numerous psammoma bodies within the tumour. **D** Meningioma of the ear. The rhabdoid subtype of meningioma has eccentric eosinophilic cytoplasm in cells that show a syncytial architecture. This type of meningioma raises a different differential diagnosis than other subtypes, potentially requiring immunohistochemistry to resolve the diagnosis.

of epithelioid to spindled cells. They have low to intermediate N:C ratios, with slightly eosinophilic to opaque cytoplasm surrounding round to oval, bland, regular nuclei. Nuclei have delicate nuclear chromatin, small nucleoli, and frequent intranuclear clear spaces and cytoplasmic pseudoinclusions {4416}. Psammoma bodies are occasionally present and can be extensive. There are numerous histological subtypes of meningioma {4805}, but meningothelial and psammomatous meningiomas account for the vast majority, while transitional, metaplastic, fibroblastic, and atypical subtypes are occasionally seen. Most tumours in the sinonasal tract correspond to CNS WHO grade 1 lesions {3485,3484,4416,2780}. The association of grade with prognosis is unclear in head and neck tumours.

Immunohistochemistry
Meningiomas are typically immunohistochemically reactive for EMA (often weak and focal), SSTR2A, and MUC4 {40,2942, 4067,2882,4872}. Some subtypes may express cytokeratins, CD34, or S100 {4833,3788,3574,2994,4031,542}. Although variable, PR is usually positive in grade 1 meningiomas {690,4416, 3483}. Ki-67 proliferation index may aid in grading {3486,3788}.

Differential diagnosis
In small samples, the meningothelial and whorled quality of the proliferation may be difficult to detect, raising a differential

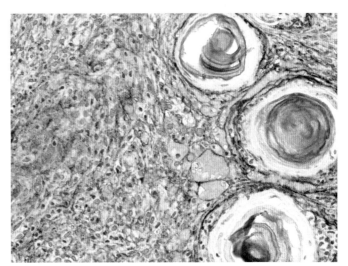

Fig. 1.74 Meningioma of the ear. The neoplastic cells are highlighted by a membranous to cytoplasmic EMA reactivity.

diagnosis that includes epithelioid as well as spindled tumours. Psammoma body–containing lesions may also present a diagnostic challenge. Table 1.02 (p. 106) contains clinical, histological, and immunohistochemical features of entities that may be confused with meningioma.

Table 1.02 Differential diagnosis of ectopic head and neck meningioma

Diagnostic entity	Clinical findings	Histological findings	Immunohistochemistry
Ossifying fibroma	Young patients; mixed radiolucent/radiopaque imaging	Cellular collagenized stroma with calcifications, psammoma bodies, or cementum	n/a
Schwannoma	n/a	Interlacing fascicles, hypercellular and hypocellular areas, perivascular hyalinization, palisaded and wavy-buckled nuclei	Positive: S100, SOX10 Negative: EMA
Leiomyoma	n/a	Spindled bland cells with blunt-ended nuclei showing perinuclear clearing	Positive: desmin, SMA, caldesmon, calponin
Myoepithelioma	n/a	Plasmacytoid to epithelioid or spindled cells in a myxoid background	Positive: epithelial and myoepithelial markers
Sinonasal angiofibroma	Male patients only	Collagenized stroma with stellate cells and haphazard vessels with marked variation in vessel type	Positive: AR and nuclear β-catenin Negative: EMA
Desmoid-type fibromatosis	n/a	Paucicellular lesion with bland spindle cells arranged in long, sweeping fascicles; elongated, thin-walled vessels	Positive: nuclear β-catenin
Glomangiopericytoma	n/a	Syncytium of ovoid to spindled cells with prominent vessels with peritheliomatous hyalinization, admixed eosinophils, and extravasated erythrocytes	Positive: SMA, nuclear β-catenin, CD34 (variable) Negative: EMA, CK7, S100
Paraganglioma	n/a	Nested architecture, cells with basophilic cytoplasm	Positive: chromogranin, synaptophysin, S100 (sustentacular cells)
Solitary fibrous tumour	n/a	Bland, monotonous, spindled cells with variable collagen deposition	Positive: STAT6, CD34, BCL2
Biphenotypic sinonasal sarcoma	n/a	Uniformly bland, cellular, spindled, and fascicular neoplasm with areas of surface epithelial invaginations with destructive growth	Positive: S100 and SMA (variable); nuclear β-catenin Negative: EMA, SOX10
Olfactory neuroblastoma	Ethmoid sinus	Small cells with scant cytoplasm in a fibrillary background with pseudorosettes	Positive: neuroendocrine markers Positive (sustentacular cells): S100, GFAP
Spindle cell squamous cell carcinoma	n/a	Nuclear pleomorphism, surface dysplasia	Positive: p40, p63, CK5/6
Melanoma	n/a	Cytological atypia, cytoplasmic pigmentation, intranuclear cytoplasmic inclusions	Positive: SOX10, HMB45, melan-A Negative: EMA, MUC4
Leiomyosarcoma	n/a	Nuclear pleomorphism, tumour necrosis, increased mitoses, atypical mitoses, lymphovascular invasion and bone destruction	Positive: desmin, SMA

n/a, not applicable.

Cytology

Smears show cohesive tissue fragments of large cells with abundant delicate cytoplasm that may be pulled out and broadly attached to adjacent cells, with oval nuclei showing fine to coarse chromatin, small nucleoli, and scattered intranuclear pseudoinclusions. Whorls may be prominent on intraoperative touch preparations, and psammoma calcifications can be seen. Degenerative changes, with larger nuclei with smudged chromatin and inclusions, and considerable cytoplasm can be seen {4990}.

Diagnostic molecular pathology

None

Essential and desirable diagnostic criteria

Essential: meningothelial or whorled epithelioid cells with low N:C ratios; delicate nuclear chromatin in round nuclei, often with intranuclear cytoplasmic inclusions.

Desirable: immunoreactivity for EMA and/or SSTR2A; lack of melanocytic and haematolymphoid markers.

Staging

Not applicable

Prognosis and prediction

Most meningiomas are slow-growing, indolent tumours. Given the difficulties in obtaining complete excision in this region, recurrences are common (~30%) {3498,3484,4416}. Women and patients aged > 40 years at presentation are more likely to develop recurrence and/or die with the disease. Tumours that have necrosis are associated with a shorter overall patient survival time than those without. Tumours with a higher proliferation index (> 4 mitoses/2 mm^2) have a lower 10-year survival rate than tumours with a lower proliferation index. The best predictor of disease-specific survival is recurrence {4416,3788}.

Olfactory neuroblastoma

Bell D
Classe M
Perez-Ordonez B
Wang BY

Definition
Olfactory neuroblastoma (ONB) is a malignant neuroectodermal neoplasm derived from the specialized sensory olfactory neuroepithelium.

ICD-O coding
9522/3 Olfactory neuroblastoma

ICD-11 coding
2C20.3 Olfactory neuroblastoma

Related terminology
Not recommended: aesthesioneuroblastoma; aesthesioneurocytoma; aesthesioneuroepithelioma; olfactory placode tumour.

Subtype(s)
None

Localization
The anatomical distribution of ONB is confined to the cribriform plate, superior turbinate (concha), and superior half of the nasal septum. The vomeronasal organ (also called Jacobson's organ), sphenopalatine ganglion, olfactory placode, and terminal nerve (also called the ganglion of Loci) are included in the areas of proposed origin. Ectopic tumours within the paranasal sinuses (excluding the ethmoid) are vanishingly rare, except in recurrent tumours, and the diagnosis needs exclusion when the cribriform plate is not involved {3009,4410}.

Clinical features
Nasal obstruction is the most common symptom. Other manifestations of local disease include epistaxis, nasal discharge, and/or pain. Symptoms can also be due to invasion of adjacent

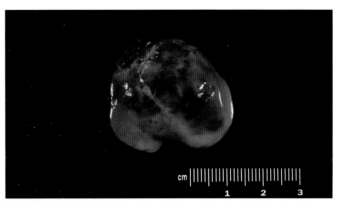
Fig. 1.75 Olfactory neuroblastoma. Gross appearance of a polypoid, red-grey mass.

structures: anosmia (due to extension into the cribriform plate); pain, proptosis, diplopia, and excessive lacrimation (with orbital extension); ear pain and otitis media (Eustachian tube obstruction); or frontal headache (invasion into frontal sinus). Paraneoplastic syndromes (ectopic adrenocorticotrophic hormone or syndrome of inappropriate antidiuretic hormone secretion) are rare {1506}.

Imaging
MRI is better than CT at delineating sinonasal, orbital, and/or intracranial extension, the last of these being a common finding. ONB shows avid homogeneous enhancement with contrast. Bony erosion is better demonstrated by CT, with careful evaluation for erosion of the lamina papyracea, cribriform plate, and fovea ethmoidalis. Peripheral tumour cysts and speckled calcifications are characteristic. Because most ONBs express SSTR, radionucleotide scans (111In-pentetreotide [Octreoscan] {3766, 988} or 68Ga-DOTATATE PET-CT {3766,1512}) may document disease and/or recurrence/metastasis.

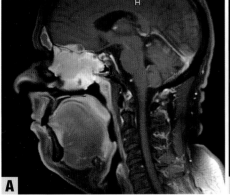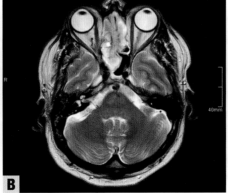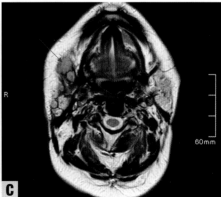
Fig. 1.76 Olfactory neuroblastoma. **A** Postcontrast fat-suppressed T1-weighted sagittal MRI demonstrates intracranial extension and a small, typical, tumoural cyst. **B** T2-weighted axial MRI showing a large soft tissue lesion involving bilateral ethmoid air cells, destroying the intervening bony septum. **C** Four years after treatment, the patient developed multiple metastatic cervical lymph nodes, the largest on the right side at level Ib (arrow).

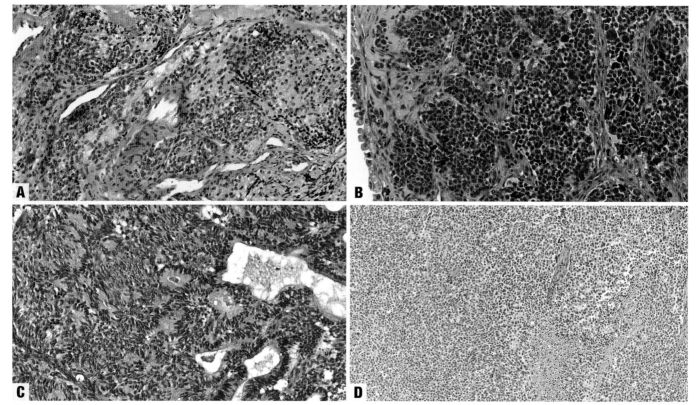

Fig. 1.77 Olfactory neuroblastoma. **A** Hyams grade I tumour showing a lobular architecture and a prominent fibrillary matrix. Homer Wright rosettes are noted. **B** Hyams grade II tumour showing a lobular architecture. Moderate nuclear pleomorphism and occasional mitotic figures are noted. **C** Hyams grade III tumour showing Flexner–Winter-steiner rosettes. **D** Hyams grade IV tumour showing no fibrillary matrix. Mitotic figures are seen. Necrosis is seen.

Epidemiology

ONB has an estimated annual incidence of 0.04 cases per 100 000 people and accounts for approximately 3% of all sinonasal tumours {592}. Patients range in age from 2 to 90 years, with a peak in the fifth and sixth decades of life {592,2077, 3560}. There is a slight male predominance (M:F ratio: 1.2:1); there is no reported racial or familial predilection {2400}.

Etiology

Unknown

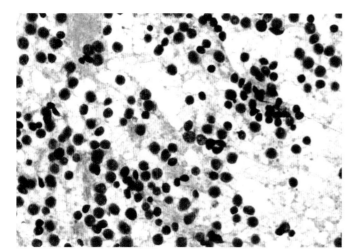

Fig. 1.78 Olfactory neuroblastoma, cytological touch preparation. The nuclei are round with delicate, salt-and-pepper chromatin and small nucleoli.

Pathogenesis

ONB appears to be of neuronal or neural crest origin (neural filaments are present in tumour cells {4499}), and molecular analysis suggests that ONB is derived from immature or progenitor olfactory epithelium cells {684,2970,1651}. Comprehensive genetic profiling studies suggest that ONB is genetically a heterogeneous entity. Although high-frequency recurrent somatic mutations are uncommon, subsets of cases harbour mutations involving *TP53*, *PIK3CA*, *NF1*, and *CDKN2A* {1555}. *FGFR3* and *CCND1* copy-number alterations or amplifications are reported {2497}. Deletions involving dystrophin (*DMD*) suggest a functional role for genes causing hereditary muscular dystrophies in ONB {1522}. Molecular-based subtype classifications have been proposed but are not currently in wide use {666,904}.

Macroscopic appearance

ONB is usually a unilateral, polypoid, glistening, soft, red-grey mass with an intact mucosa; the cut surface is grey-tan to pink-red and hypervascularized. Tumours range from < 10 mm to large masses involving the nasal cavity and intracranial region. Tumours frequently expand into adjacent paranasal sinuses, orbits, and the cranial vault {4410}.

Histopathology

Low-grade ONB forms submucosal, sharply demarcated nests, lobules, or sheets of cells, often separated by a richly vascular stroma. The cells are uniform, with salt-and-pepper nuclear chromatin. ONB is characterized by fibrillary cytoplasm and interdigitating neuronal processes (neuropil), created by a

Table 1.03 Key features and criteria for Hyams grade I, II, III, and IV olfactory neuroblastomas and their corresponding histopathological slides

	Low grade		High grade	
Hyams grade	I	II	III	IV
Architecture	Lobular	Lobular	Lobular	Lobular
Mitotic activity	Absent	Present	Prominent	Marked
Nuclear pleomorphism	Absent	Moderate	Prominent	Marked
Fibrillary matrix	Prominent	Present	Minimal	Absent
Rosettes	HW	HW	FW	FW
Necrosis	Absent	Absent	+/− Present	Common

FW, Flexner–Wintersteiner; HW, Homer Wright.

syncytium of cells. Flexner–Wintersteiner rosettes and Homer Wright pseudorosettes can be seen. High-grade tumours show a more sheet-like growth pattern, with loss of sustentacular cells, greater nuclear pleomorphism, increased mitotic activity, and tumour necrosis. Rosettes by themselves are not diagnostic of ONB, although Homer Wright pseudorosettes with neuropil are nearly pathognomonic in the nasal cavity. The mitotic rate can be variable but is usually low. In situ tumour within the specialized mucosa is rarely seen in clinical material, although it is identified in overlying mucosa in some cases. Calcifications (concretion-like or psammomatous) may be seen, less frequently as the grade increases. Melanin pigment, ganglion cells, rhabdomyoblasts, divergent differentiation as islands of true epithelium (squamous pearls, gland formation), clear cell change, and even metastatic tumours may occasionally be encountered in ONB {2692,3034,1336,366,4310}.

Grading

The most widely used grading system was developed by Hyams et al. {1980} (see Table 1.03). This scheme captures the spectrum of ONB maturation and divides it into four grades – from well differentiated (I, II) to poorly differentiated (III, IV) – based on the tumour architecture, pleomorphism, presence of neurofibrillary matrix and rosettes, mitotic activity, presence of necrosis, and presence of calcifications. This grading scheme has been validated {2216,1521,3795,4331}.

Immunohistochemistry

The typical immunohistochemical profile includes diffuse staining for conventional neuroendocrine markers and S100 reactivity in a typical sustentacular cell pattern. As many as one third of ONBs may react focally for pancytokeratin {3009,1898}. Rarely, cases can be more diffusely positive for epithelial markers, blurring the distinction between ONB and neuroendocrine carcinoma (NEC) or non-intestinal adenocarcinoma {2966}. Ki-67 proliferation index is variable and associated with grade {3009, 4410,903}. Rare desmin or myogenin reactivity is seen in ONB with rhabdomyoblastic differentiation {482}. SSTR2 is consistently expressed in ONB, suggesting a role for somatostatin analogue–based imaging and therapy in this disease {965}.

Differential diagnosis

The differential diagnosis includes many small blue round cell tumours in the sinonasal tract, which must be actively excluded because of management differences.

Box 1.01 Olfactory neuroblastoma staging systems proposed by Kadish {2138}, Morita {3073}, Dulguerov {1198}, and Biller {451}

Kadish stage
- **A** Tumour confined to the nasal cavity
- **B** Tumour involvement of the nasal cavity and paranasal sinuses
- **C** Tumour extends beyond the nasal cavity and paranasal sinuses

Morita modification
- **A** Tumour confined to the nasal cavity
- **B** Tumour involvement of the nasal cavity and paranasal sinuses
- **C** Tumour extends beyond the nasal cavity and paranasal sinuses
- **D** Presence of metastases (regional or distant)

Dulguerov staging system
- **T1** Tumour involves the nasal cavity / paranasal sinuses but spares the sphenoid sinus and superior ethmoid cells
- **T2** Tumour involves the sphenoid sinus and/or the cribriform plate
- **T3** Tumour extends into the orbit or into the anterior cranial fossa, without invasion of the dura
- **T4** Tumour involves the brain
- **N0** No regional lymph node metastases
- **N1** Lymph node metastases present
- **M0** No distant metastases
- **M1** Distant metastasis present

Biller staging system
- **T1** Tumour involves the nasal cavity / paranasal sinuses (excludes the sphenoid)
- **T2** Extension into the orbit and/or cranial cavity
- **T3** Brain involvement but deemed resectable
- **T4** Extensive brain involvement, unresectable tumour
- **N0** No regional lymph node metastases
- **N1** Lymph node metastases present
- **M0** No distant metastases
- **M1** Distant metastasis present

Cytology

Smears are hypercellular, with plentiful stripped nuclei, single cells with high N:C ratios, and a variable number of Homer Wright rosettes with fibrillary cytoplasm and neuropil centrally and a ring of round nuclei with usually smooth outlines, finely granular chromatin, and inconspicuous nucleoli. Paranuclear blue bodies may be seen in the Giemsa stain, in which the neuropil is poorly seen. Some cases show greater nuclear pleomorphism and more mitoses. Necrosis is usually absent {2788, 413,4087}.

Diagnostic molecular pathology

None

Essential and desirable diagnostic criteria

Essential: a tumour originating from and centred around the ethmoid sinus cribriform plate; a small round cell tumour with a lobulated pattern and variable amounts of neuropil; expression of neuroendocrine markers and the presence of S100-positive sustentacular cells (in selected cases).

Staging

Several staging systems have been proposed (see Box 1.01, p. 109), with no system universally accepted. The Kadish system is most commonly used {2138}, but it classifies local disease only; it divides tumours into those that involve the nasal cavity alone (Kadish A), those that extend into the paranasal sinuses (Kadish B), and those that extend beyond the paranasal sinuses (Kadish C) {2138}. Morita modified the Kadish system {3073}, designating as category D those tumours with metastases (regional nodal disease and distant metastasis). The Dulguerov classification system separates patients with and without sphenoid sinus disease, as well as differentiating tumours with intracranial and/ or orbital extension from those with brain parenchymal invasion, while considering lymph node and distant metastasis separately {1198}. The Biller system is based on whether tumours with extension into the brain are amenable to surgery, while segregating those with lymph node and distant metastases {451}. The TNM staging system for paranasal sinus tumours can potentially be applied {1213}, but the biologically unique behaviour of ONB compared with other sinonasal tumours makes the previously mentioned classification systems more prognostic.

Prognosis and prediction

Beyond stage, the histological grade is an essential tool in prognostication and management {2216,2809,4574,410}, with Hyams grade being an accurate predictor of metastasis and overall survival {1663}. Neck metastasis was observed in 18% of high-grade tumours versus 8% of low-grade ONBs. Distant metastasis was noted in 21% of high-grade tumours versus 9% of low-grade tumours. Patients with low-Hyams-grade ONB had 5- and 10-year overall survival rates of 81% and 64%, respectively, compared with 61% and 41%, respectively, for high-Hyams-grade tumours.

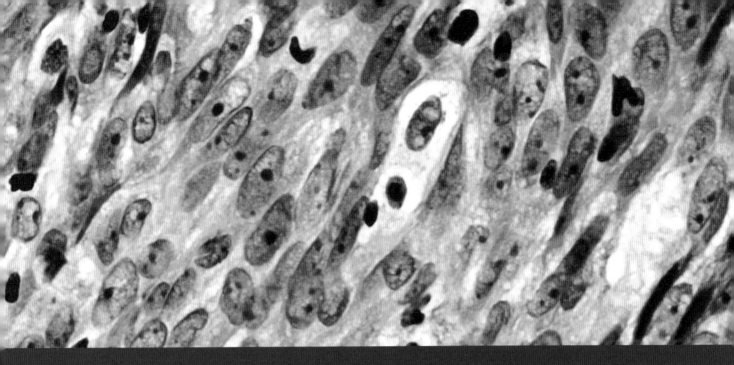

2

Nasopharyngeal tumours

Edited by: Chan JKC, Lewis JS Jr, Tilakaratne WM

Nasopharyngeal tumours: Introduction

Chan JKC

The nasopharynx is the narrow tubular passage behind the nasal cavity. Because the nasopharynx is in close proximity to many different anatomical structures, tumours arising in the adjacent sites can also present clinically as a nasopharyngeal mass; for example, chordoma arising in the clivus. In some cases, it can be difficult to ascertain whether a tumour arises in the nasopharynx or the nasal cavity.

The most common tumour of the nasopharynx is nasopharyngeal carcinoma, which is remarkable for the striking geographical differences in its incidence as well as the near-consistent association with EBV. In addition, a broad range of neoplasms can arise in the nasopharynx, including epithelial, lymphoid, mesenchymal, and neuroendocrine. Rarely, tumours derived from embryonic remnants entrapped in their normal pathway of ascent or descent (ectopic pituitary tumour, craniopharyngioma) can occur.

In this fifth-edition WHO classification of head and neck tumours, tumours not unique to the nasopharynx are covered in the respective generic chapters, including salivary gland tumours, soft tissue tumours, haematolymphoid proliferations and neoplasms, melanocytic tumours, and neuroendocrine neoplasms (NENs). As a result, only a few entities are covered in this chapter on tumours of the nasopharynx:

- Hairy polyp
- Salivary gland anlage tumour
- Low-grade nasopharyngeal papillary adenocarcinoma
- Nasopharyngeal carcinoma

Changes since the fourth edition

Nasopharyngeal carcinoma, including the subtypes, remains unchanged from the previous edition. The main advances are the increase in knowledge on the molecular genetics of nasopharyngeal carcinoma and the adoption of the updated staging system: the eighth edition of the Union for International Cancer Control (UICC) / American Joint Committee on Cancer (AJCC) TNM staging system {3373,2509}.

Nasopharyngeal papillary adenocarcinoma has been renamed "low-grade nasopharyngeal papillary adenocarcinoma" to emphasize the bland morphology and the lack of aggressive behaviour. Salivary gland–type tumours occurring in the nasopharynx, such as adenoid cystic carcinoma, are covered in the chapter on salivary gland tumours. Ectopic pituitary neuroendocrine tumour (PitNET) is covered in the chapter on neuroendocrine neoplasms and paraganglioma, under the designation "ectopic or invasive PitNET / pituitary adenoma". Craniopharyngioma is described in the chapter on nasal, paranasal, and skull base tumours, under the designation "adamantinomatous craniopharyngioma". Chordoma, which typically occurs in the clivus (skull base), is also covered in the same chapter, as is nasopharyngeal angiofibroma ("sinonasal tract angiofibroma").

Haematolymphoid tumours are covered in the chapter on haematolymphoid proliferations and neoplasia. Nasopharyngeal lymphomas account for 2.5% of all extranodal non-Hodgkin lymphomas {1465} and about 15% of all head and neck lymphomas {1283,83,4877}. Diffuse large B-cell lymphoma is the most common type {1311,109,83,4877}. NK- and T-cell lymphomas occur at a higher frequency in Asia than elsewhere, accounting for almost half of all cases in some series {4929, 832}. Other lymphoma types, such as Burkitt lymphoma, follicular lymphoma, mantle cell lymphoma, extranodal marginal zone lymphoma of mucosa-associated lymphoid tissue, and T-lymphoblastic lymphoma, may rarely affect the nasopharynx. Solitary extraosseous plasmacytoma and extramedullary myeloid sarcoma can also occur in the nasopharynx.

Hairy polyp

Schulte JJ
Katabi N

Definition
Hairy polyp is a benign polypoid lesion of the nasopharynx containing both ectodermal and mesodermal elements.

ICD-O coding
None

ICD-11 coding
2E90.6 Benign neoplasm of nasopharynx

Related terminology
Not recommended: dermoid polyp; teratoid polyp; naso(oro) pharyngeal choristoma.

Subtype(s)
None

Localization
Most hairy polyps (60%) arise in the lateral wall of the nasopharynx, but they can also occur in the oropharynx, palate, tongue, lip, and middle ear {2242,226,1207,4389}.

Clinical features
The clinical presentation varies depending on the size, location, and mobility of the lesion. The symptoms include respiratory obstruction, stridor, cough, dyspnoea, feeding and swallowing difficulty, hypersalivation, and vomiting. Rarely, hairy polyp is associated with other congenital abnormalities such as branchial arch anomalies, cleft palate, or Dandy–Walker syndrome {283,1731,68,3695,2276}.

Imaging
Preoperative imaging with CT often shows a smooth polypoid mass with fat attenuation and the presence of a fibrovascular stalk {4869}.

Epidemiology
Hairy polyp is rare, with an incidence rate of 2.5 cases per 100 000 live births. It mostly occurs in neonates and young children and is extremely rare in adults. It has a female predilection, with an M:F ratio of 1:6 {2242,1207,4389,2276}.

Etiology
Unknown

Pathogenesis
Hairy polyp is a manifestation of rare developmental abnormalities. It may be derived from multifunctional tissue with differentiating potentiality forming a choristoma; or it may occur due to malformation of the first and second branchial arches {721, 4389,1939}.

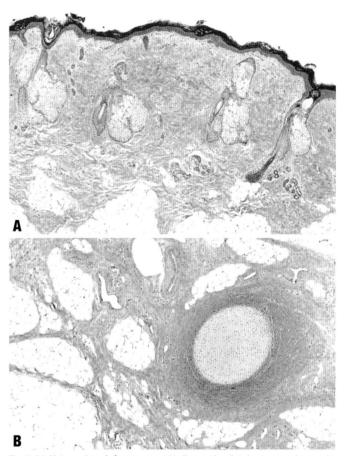

Fig. 2.01 Hairy polyp. **A** Squamous epithelium with pilosebaceous units overlying mesodermal (fibroadipose) tissue. **B** Central portion of a hairy polyp containing mesoderm-derived tissue, including fibroadipose tissue and cartilage.

Macroscopic appearance
Grossly, the hairy polyp is a long, cylindrical structure and the external surface resembles skin. Cut surfaces are solid, without cystic change {4389}.

Histopathology
Hairy polyps are covered by an ectodermal layer characterized by keratinizing squamous epithelium with underlying associated adnexal structures, including hair follicles and sebaceous units. The ectodermal layer overlies various combinations of mesodermal tissue. Fibroadipose tissue is uniformly present, but cartilage, bone, and/or skeletal or smooth muscle is also commonly found {4389}. Rarely, meningothelial, minor salivary gland, or odontogenic elements may be observed {3288,3353}. Endodermal tissue has not been reported as a component of hairy polyp.

Cytology
Not clinically relevant

Diagnostic molecular pathology
Not clinically relevant

Essential and desirable diagnostic criteria
Essential: a polypoid structure with an ectodermal outer layer resembling skin, covering mesodermal tissue; no endodermal tissue should be present.

Staging
Not relevant

Prognosis and prediction
Surgical excision is curative in the majority of cases {2936}.

Salivary gland anlage tumour

Chiosea S
Peters SM

Definition
Salivary gland anlage tumour is a predominantly infantile naso-pharyngeal lesion with biphasic squamoid epithelial and myo-epithelial components continuous with the surface epithelium, resembling developing salivary gland.

ICD-O coding
None

ICD-11 coding
2E90.6 Benign neoplasm of nasopharynx

Related terminology
Not recommended: congenital pleomorphic adenoma.

Subtype(s)
None

Localization
Salivary gland anlage tumours occur in the posterior nasal sep-tum or posterior nasopharyngeal wall.

Clinical features
Patients present with feeding difficulty and respiratory distress due to nasal airway obstruction {1853}. Before birth, salivary gland anlage tumour may be associated with polyhydramnios {3628}.

Epidemiology
Approximately 40 examples of salivary gland anlage tumour have been reported {4233,1077,1853,4660,3041,1851,4457, 1552,2832,3628}. The affected patients are infants (diagnosed by 3 months of age) and there is a male predilection. An in utero case has been reported {3628}.

Etiology
Unknown

Pathogenesis
Whole-exome sequencing of 3 cases showed no plausible driver mutations {3502}, suggestive of a possible hamartoma-tous origin for these tumours.

Macroscopic appearance
Salivary gland anlage tumour is a polypoid to pedunculated, smooth, tan-brown mass with a solid to microcystic cut surface {1853}.

Histopathology
Salivary gland anlage tumour is characterized by a complex network of tubules and ducts. Submucosal ducts and solid and cystic squamous nests with variable keratinization are

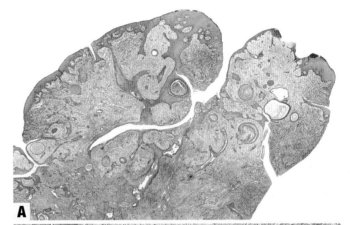

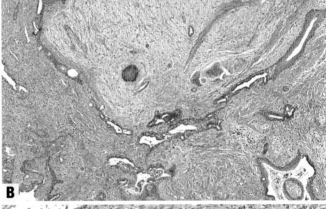

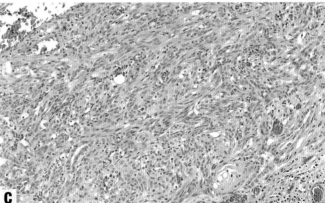

Fig. 2.02 Salivary gland anlage tumour. **A** Polypoid mass with complex squamous proliferation, squamous eddies and myxoid stroma, and ducts connecting to the sur-face. **B** Epithelial tubules and hypocellular myxoid stroma with bland myoepithelial cells. **C** In the core of the polypoid mass, bland-looking spindle cells merge with tu-bules and squamous islands.

continuous with the surface squamous epithelium. The sub-epithelial stroma tends to be hypocellular, with more cellular stromal nodules in the centre of the polyp. Cellular atypia and mitoses are absent {1853}.

Immunohistochemistry
The myoepithelial nature of the stromal cells is confirmed by positive immunohistochemistry for cytokeratins and SMA.

Cytology
Cytological examination is rarely required, but if done, it may reveal cohesive tissue fragments (some with duct-like structures) of uniform cells with small oval nuclei, inconspicuous nucleoli, and sparse cytoplasm with indistinct borders. A component of metaplastic squamous epithelium may be present {521}.

Diagnostic molecular pathology
Not relevant

Essential and desirable diagnostic criteria
Essential: a polypoid lesion with a complex network of ducts and solid-cystic squamous nests, showing continuity with surface squamous epithelium; hypocellular to cellular spindle cell stroma.
Desirable: spindly cells positive for cytokeratins and SMA (in selected cases).

Staging
Not relevant

Prognosis and prediction
There have been no reports of recurrence after excision.

Low-grade nasopharyngeal papillary adenocarcinoma

Wenig BM
Stelow EB

Definition

Low-grade nasopharyngeal papillary adenocarcinoma is a surface-derived malignant glandular neoplasm showing predominant papillary architecture and indolent behaviour.

ICD-O coding

8260/3 Low-grade nasopharyngeal papillary adenocarcinoma

ICD-11 coding

2B6B.Y & XH6LV9 Other specified malignant neoplasms of nasopharynx & Papillary adenocarcinoma, NOS

Related terminology

Acceptable: nasopharyngeal papillary adenocarcinoma.
Not recommended: thyroid-like low-grade nasopharyngeal papillary adenocarcinoma.

Subtype(s)

None

Localization

The tumour may occur anywhere in the nasopharynx but most often involves the posterior nasopharyngeal wall {4789}, the roof of the nasopharynx, and the posterior margin of the nasal septum {2456}.

Clinical features

The most common symptoms are nasal obstruction {4789} and blood-stained rhinorrhoea {2456}.

Epidemiology

The tumour shows no sex predilection and occurs over a wide age range, from the first to the eighth decade of life {4789,2456}.

Etiology

Unknown

Pathogenesis

ROS1::GOPC fusion was reported in 1 case {4700}.

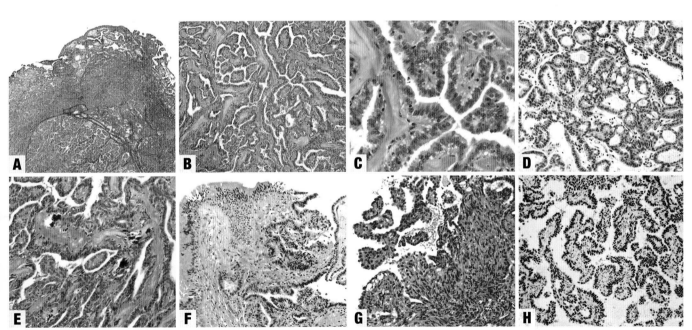

Fig. 2.03 Low-grade nasopharyngeal papillary adenocarcinoma. **A** At low magnification, the tumour is diffusely infiltrative with papillary and glandular growth. **B** Characteristic papillary architecture with fibrovascular cores. **C** The nuclei show features similar to those seen in association with papillary thyroid carcinoma, including nuclear enlargement and elongation with dispersed (very fine) nuclear chromatin, and crowding and overlapping. **D** In conjunction with the papillary architecture, the neoplasm may have focal or more widespread areas of complex glandular growth characterized by a microcystic/cribriform pattern and/or back-to-back glands without intervening stroma. **E** Psammomatoid concretions may be identified, which in association with a papillary architecture and nuclear features would suggest a possible diagnosis of papillary thyroid carcinoma. **F** Transition from normal surface respiratory epithelium to the neoplasm supports a primary origin of this tumour from the nasopharyngeal mucosa and weighs against a possible diagnosis of metastatic papillary thyroid carcinoma. **G** An example showing a prominent component of spindly cells merging with the papillae. The spindly cells exhibit bland-looking nuclei. **H** The neoplasm is diffusely positive for thyroid transcription factor 1 (TTF1), a characteristic finding, but lacks immunoreactivity for thyroglobulin and PAX8.

Macroscopic appearance

Low-grade nasopharyngeal papillary adenocarcinoma is an exophytic, papillary or cauliflower-like lesion with a soft to gritty consistency, measuring from a few millimetres to 40 mm.

Histopathology

This is an unencapsulated neoplasm with papillary and glandular growth patterns. The papillae are complex with arborization and fibrovascular cores. Complex (back-to-back) glandular and cribriform/microcystic architectures are present. The cells vary in appearance from pseudostratified columnar to cuboidal. The nuclei are round to oval with vesicular to optically clear chromatin, indistinct nucleoli, and eosinophilic cytoplasm. Mild to moderate nuclear pleomorphism is seen. Scattered mitotic figures can be seen, but atypical mitoses are not present. Squamous differentiation {3281} and a prominent spindle cell component have been reported {3509,2537}. Psammoma bodies may be present. This tumour has an infiltrative growth into the submucosa. Transition from surface epithelium to carcinoma may be present, supporting a primary nasopharyngeal origin {4789}.

Immunohistochemistry

Diffuse immunoreactivity is seen for cytokeratins and EMA. Thyroid transcription factor 1 (TTF1) staining is positive (including in spindle and squamous cells) but thyroglobulin and PAX8 are negative {689,3281,4700}. EBV-encoded small RNAs (EBERs), p16, p40/p63, S100, and BRAF p.V600E are negative {3509, 3281,2537}. Ki-67 staining consistently shows a low proliferation index (< 5%).

Differential diagnosis

The absence of thyroglobulin and PAX8 and the transition from surface epithelium to carcinoma allow for differentiation from papillary thyroid carcinoma. The complexity of papillary and glandular growth, as well as the extensive involvement of the submucosa, would differentiate the tumour from sinonasal papilloma.

Cytology

Not clinically relevant

Diagnostic molecular pathology

Not relevant

Essential and desirable diagnostic criteria

Essential: complex papillary and glandular growth with infiltration of the submucosa; low-grade cytology.

Desirable: transition from surface epithelium to tumour; TTF1 positivity, and absence of thyroglobulin and PAX8 (in selected cases).

Staging

Staging follows the eighth edition of the Union for International Cancer Control (UICC) / American Joint Committee on Cancer (AJCC) TNM staging system.

Prognosis and prediction

Surgical excision is the treatment of choice and is curative {4789}. This slow-growing tumour has the potential to recur if incompletely excised. Metastatic disease has not been reported.

Nasopharyngeal carcinoma

Chan JKC
Bray F
Lee AWM
Lo KW
Petersson BF
Rajadurai P

Definition
Nasopharyngeal carcinoma (NPC) is a malignant mucosal epithelial neoplasm usually showing evidence of squamous differentiation.

ICD-O coding
8070/3 Nasopharyngeal carcinoma
8071/3 Squamous cell carcinoma, keratinizing, NOS
8072/3 Squamous cell carcinoma, non-keratinizing, NOS
8083/3 Basaloid squamous cell carcinoma

ICD-11 coding
2B6B.0 & XH6705 Squamous cell carcinoma of nasopharynx & Squamous cell carcinoma, keratinizing, NOS
2B6B.0 & XH4CR9 Squamous cell carcinoma of nasopharynx & Squamous cell carcinoma, non-keratinizing, NOS
2B6B.0 & XH3GS1 Squamous cell carcinoma of nasopharynx & Basaloid squamous cell carcinoma

Related terminology
Not recommended: lymphoepithelioma-like carcinoma; lymphoepithelial carcinoma.

Subtype(s)
Keratinizing squamous cell carcinoma; non-keratinizing squamous cell carcinoma; basaloid squamous cell carcinoma

Localization
The commonest site of origin is the lateral wall of the nasopharynx, especially the fossa of Rosenmüller, followed by the superior posterior wall.

Clinical features
The majority of patients present with locoregionally advanced disease. The commonest presentation is a painless enlarging upper neck mass (in as many as 70% of cases); the first echelon includes the retropharyngeal node and the jugulodigastric

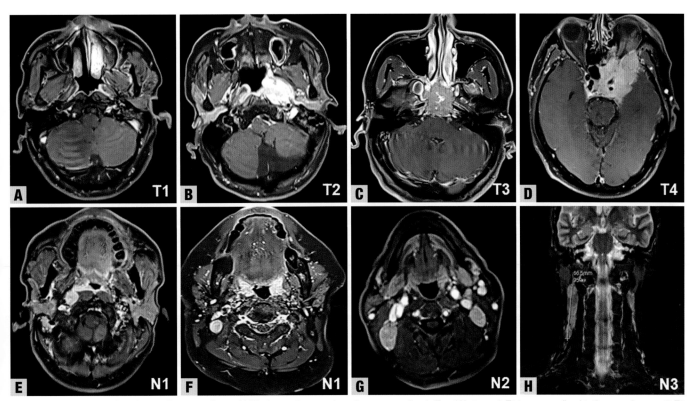

Fig. 2.04 Nasopharyngeal carcinoma. Contrast-enhanced MRI of nasopharyngeal carcinoma, according to T and N stage. **A** T1 tumour confined to the nasopharynx. **B** T2 tumour with extension to adjacent soft tissues (including the parapharyngeal space, pterygoid muscles, and prevertebral muscle). **C** T3 tumour with clivus erosion and invasion into the pterygopalatine fossa and pterygomaxillary fissure. **D** T4 tumour with clivus erosion plus intracranial extension to the cavernous sinus and temporal lobe, with involvement of the ethmoid sinus and orbit. **E** N1 disease with retropharyngeal nodal spread. **F** N1 disease with unilateral cervical nodal metastasis. **G** N2 disease with bilateral cervical nodal metastases ≤ 60 mm in the long axis, above the caudal border of the cricoid cartilage. **H** N3 disease with bilateral bulky nodes (> 60 mm) in the longest diameter and extension below the cricoid cartilage.

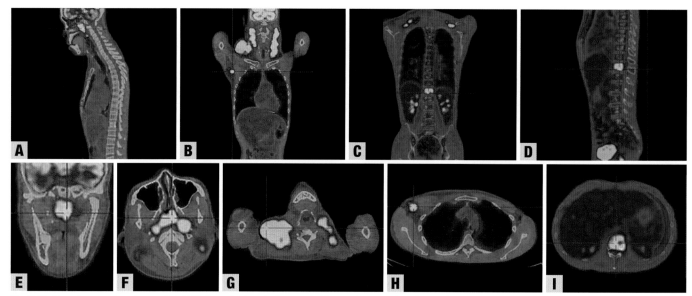

Fig. 2.05 Nasopharyngeal carcinoma. **A–I** PET of a patient newly diagnosed with nasopharyngeal carcinoma. This demonstrates avid FDG uptake by the primary tumour in the nasopharynx, bilateral metastatic cervical lymph nodes, and distant metastases to a right axillary lymph node and L1 vertebral body. Normal uptake is noted in the brain, bladder, and kidneys.

node {4001,1934,4648,2506}. Nearly half of all patients have symptoms related to the presence of a mass in the nasopharynx, such as blood-stained postnasal drip, epistaxis, and nasal obstruction. Aural symptoms related to Eustachian tube blockage include tinnitus, hearing impairment, and serous otitis media. More advanced cases may present with headache due to skull base infiltration, and facial numbness and diplopia due to fifth and sixth cranial nerve involvement. Approximately 5% of patients already have distant metastasis at the time of diagnosis, the commonest sites being bone, lung, liver, and distant lymph nodes {4391}. In endemic areas, 1% of patients with NPC present with dermatomyositis {4390,3457}.

Serology

EBV serology is positive in most patients with non-keratinizing NPC (NK-NPC) {1730}. An IgA antibody against EBV VCA and IgG/IgA against EBV early antigens are commonly used diagnostic tools, with detection rates of 69–93% {1027,746}.

Elevated levels of circulating EBV DNA or RNA, using techniques to detect the BamHI-W region of the EBV genome, EBV-encoded small RNAs (EBERs), or EBNA1 in plasma or serum, can be demonstrated in 85–96% of patients {2699,4052,2654, 745,3210}. Not only is the pretreatment level useful as an independent prognostic factor, but the posttreatment response level is also valuable for adapting subsequent treatment {2655,2741}. Circulating EBV DNA assay is useful for surveillance and early detection of disease relapse, particularly distant metastasis.

Imaging

MRI is widely preferred as the imaging modality of choice in the assessment and staging of NPC, because of its superior soft tissue resolution and ability to visualize perineural extension, bone marrow involvement, and intracranial spread. FDG PET-CT is highly sensitive in detecting distant metastases, small lymph node metastases, and local residual/recurrent disease {1624,4621}.

Epidemiology

NPC is considered a rare malignancy in most parts of the world, with an estimated 133 500 new cases and 80 000 deaths in the year 2020, or about 0.7% and 0.8% of the respective global cancer incidence and mortality burden {4295,1360, 1361}. Age-adjusted incidence rates tend to be < 1–2 cases per 100 000 person-years, although in several regions, rates are much higher, including several provinces in southern China (Guangdong, Zhejiang) and among Inuit populations in Alaska and Canada (Yukon, Nunavut). NPC occurs with a moderately raised incidence in certain populations in northern Africa (Algeria, Tunisia), and in south-eastern Asia (Malaysia, the Philippines, and Thailand) {4752,575}.

The etiology of NPC has been described as enigmatic, with viral, environmental, and genetic components {751}. Although EBV is considered a critical step in disease progression, only a fraction of infected patients develop NPC {1995}. People who migrate from high- to low-risk countries show NPC incidence rates intermediate between those native to their new country of residence and their country of origin, implicating roles for both environmental and host (genetic) factors, possibly in association with EBV. Much of the current understanding of the underlying risk determinants of NPC, including the role of a nitrosamine-rich diet, has arisen from studies of individuals from populations at high to intermediate risk {4962,1865,751}. The age–incidence curves in such populations, the vast majority of which are of the non-keratinizing subtype, exhibit a single peak, with a decline observed at about 50 years {576}, compatible with either viral or carcinogenic exposure early in life (such as from preserved foods), or an exhaustion of the pool of genetically susceptible individuals {1797}. In contrast, in most low-risk populations, the age–incidence curves exhibit a small peak at 15–24 years, with rates steadily increasing to a second peak at 65–74 years, and decreasing thereafter. Keratinizing NPCs (K-NPCs) are predominantly associated with alcohol and cigarette consumption, whereas EBV is the primary risk factor for NK-NPCs {576}.

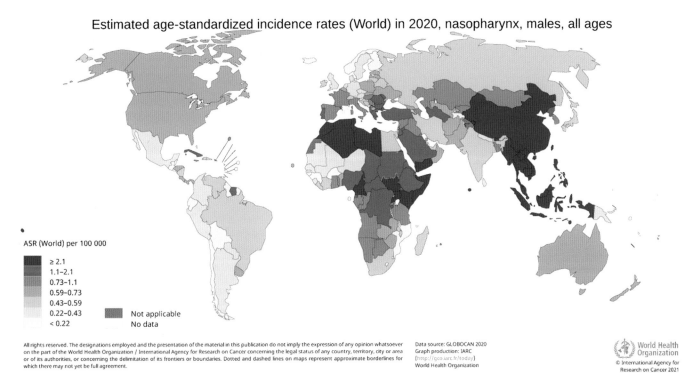

Estimated age-standardized incidence rates (World) in 2020, nasopharynx, males, all ages

ASR (World) per 100 000

- ≥ 2.1
- 1.1–2.1
- 0.73–1.1
- 0.59–0.73
- 0.43–0.59
- 0.22–0.43
- < 0.22
- Not applicable
- No data

Data source: GLOBOCAN 2020
Graph production: IARC
(http://gco.iarc.fr/today)
World Health Organization

World Health Organization
© International Agency for Research on Cancer 2021

Fig. 2.06 Nasopharyngeal carcinoma. Estimated age-standardized incidence rates (ASRs, World Standard Population), per 100 000 person-years, of nasopharyngeal carcinoma in 2020 among males (all ages).

In general, NPC incidence rates have been falling in recent years, an observation attributed to favourable trends in lifestyle and environmental factors, including tobacco control for reducing keratinizing NPC, and changing diet and socioeconomic development for reducing NK-NPC {4367,801,752}. Declining mortality rates are due to advances in diagnostics and chemoradiotherapy strategies {4367,673,801}. However, several studies report an increase in NK-NPC in low-risk populations {248, 233}.

Etiology

A number of etiological factors have been associated with the development of NPC, most consistently EBV {4506,3625, 3433,4508}. This link is strongest with NK-NPC (differentiated and undifferentiated types), whereas viral presence in K-NPC is inconsistent and a subject of controversy {3217,3424}. EBV is present as an early event in the development of NPC; it has been identified in preinvasive neoplasia of the nasopharynx in clonal episomal form, suggesting that NK-NPC is a clonal malignancy derived from a latently EBV-infected progenitor cell {3425,3625}.

Because EBV is a ubiquitous herpesvirus and persists in the human body after infection, the presence of EBV alone is unlikely to be sufficient to result in NPC. Other cofactors and/or carcinogens are likely to be involved in the multistep carcinogenic process of cancer development and progression. Environmental carcinogens such as tobacco smoke, wood dust, and formaldehyde {243}; diet {4963}; preserved foods {4964}; and the consumption of salted fish have been implicated in several studies {1888,3222,244}, particularly in endemic areas.

The remarkable observation of ethnic differences in the prevalence of NPC indicates the importance of genetic susceptibility. Both case–control and genome-wide studies have shown that the risk of developing NPC is strongly linked to variants of MHC class I (HLA-A, HLA-B, HLA-C) loci in Chinese patients {4264,2618}. The association of specific HLA variants/alleles with NPC risk implies a role for immunosurveillance restraining tumour development, possibly due to their different abilities in presenting viral antigens in the EBV-infected nasopharyngeal epithelial cells. The interaction of EBV and inherited genetic factors is supported by the association of two non-synonymous BALF2 gene variants in EBV (162476_C and 163364_T) in patients harbouring specific SNPs at the HLA locus with the higher risk of NPC {4892}. Genome-wide association studies reveal significant links with SNPs in the regions of MDS1-EVI1 (chromosome 3q22), TNFRSF19 (13q12), CDKN2A and/or CDKN2B (9p21), and TERT/CLPTM1L (5p15) loci {400,2688}. Whole-exome sequencing has revealed germline variants of the MST1R gene at chromosome 3p21 in paediatric patients and in patients with early-onset NPC {1007}.

Oncogenic (high-risk) HPV types may play a role in a subset of NPCs {4857}. Similarly to HPV-associated squamous cell carcinomas occurring in the oropharynx, these cancers most frequently show a non-keratinizing histology, and they tend to occur in non-endemic populations and in White people with a history of smoking {3712,4219}. Although the association of HPV with NPC seems to be more common in non-endemic populations, the reported incidence varies greatly between studies (3–35%) {2660,4857}. In endemic areas where the association of NPC with EBV is the rule, the frequency of the association does not appear to be much lower (0% to ~8%) {2660,1952}.

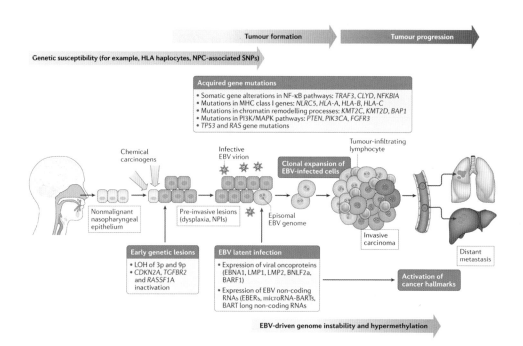

Fig. 2.07 Nasopharyngeal carcinoma (NPC). Exposure to environmental carcinogens induces various genetic lesions (e.g. deletions in chromosomes 3p and 9p) and subsequent inactivation of key tumour suppressor genes (such as *CDKN2A* and *TGFBR2*) that predispose to EBV infection and transformation of nasopharyngeal epithelial cells. In nasopharyngeal epithelial cells persistently infected with EBV, the presence of episomal viral genomes and expression of latency II viral proteins (EBNA1, LMP1, and LMP2) and non-coding RNAs (EBV-encoded small RNAs [EBERs], microRNA-BARTs, and BART long non-coding RNAs) promote genome instability, induce global DNA methylation, and activate virtually all cancer hallmarks. Clonal expansion of EBV-transformed nasopharyngeal epithelial cells leads to the accumulation of multiple genetic and epigenetic events driving NPC progression. The convergence of somatic genomic alterations (e.g. mutations in the proinflammatory NF-κB pathway and in components of antigen presentation machinery) and EBV latent gene expression (e.g. of LMP1 and BNLF2a) modulates the tumour microenvironment and immune escape. Other acquired genetic changes (including alterations of *TP53*, genes involved in chromatin remodelling, and components of the PI3K/MAPK pathway) contribute to tumour progression, occurrence of local recurrences, and distant metastasis {4840}. HLA, human leukocyte antigen; LOH, loss of heterozygosity; MHC, major histocompatibility complex; NPI, nasopharyngeal inlet; SNP, small nucleotide polymorphism.

Pathogenesis

Aside from inherited factors, the interplay between EBV infection and acquired genetic alterations contributes to tumour initiation, promotion, and progression {4508,4505}. Deletions on 3p and 9p appear to be early events in NPC, being found in most dysplastic lesions, even before EBV infection {737, 736}. Inactivation of key tumour suppressor genes in these chromosomal loci (*CDKN2A* [*P16*] on chromosome 9p21.3 and *TGFBR2* on chromosome 3p24.1) has been shown to predispose nasopharyngeal epithelial cells to persistent latent EBV infection initiating malignant transformation and clonal expansion {4507,602}. Expression of EBV-encoded latent proteins (EBNA1, LMP1, LMP2) and non-coding RNAs (EBERs, miR-BARTs) targets multiple cancer hallmarks including inflammation, immune evasion, genomic instability, cell proliferation, and cell survival, driving the progression of NK-NPC {4505}. EBV infection also facilitates epigenetic changes, such as global hypermethylation of the NPC genome {2697,1006,2563,4505}. Genomic sequencing reveals distinctive mutation signatures associated with high APOBEC3 activity, DNA mismatch repair, and homologous recombination repair deficiencies, evidencing virus-driven genomic instability during pathogenesis {2651, 5028,2634}. In addition to the prevalent deletions of *CDKN2A* (*P16*) (43%) that disrupt cell-cycle regulation, acquired genetic alterations activating NF-κB pathways (*TRAF3*, *CYLD*, *NFK-BIA*, *NLRC5*, *LTBR*, *BIRC2/3*) are commonly found in NK-NPC (63%). Along with expression of viral oncoprotein LMP1 (26–33%), genomic aberrations underpin the constitutive activation of NF-κB signalling in almost all cases of NK-NPC, resulting in the induction of various chemokines/cytokines for its distinct proinflammatory phenotype {2634,602}. NPC cells successfully escape the host's innate and adaptive immune responses in a highly inflammatory tumour microenvironment through either viral gene products or acquired genetic alterations. Multiple somatic changes are reported, including inactivating alterations of *TRAF3*, *CYLD*, and type 1 interferon gene cluster, along with the expression of EBV-encoded LMP1, dysregulation of the TLR3/RIG1/IRF3 pathway, and suppression of virus-induced innate immunity. Somatic gene alterations disrupting antigen presentation mechanisms (MHC class I: *NLRC5*, *HLA-A*, *HLA-B*; MHC class II: *CIITA*) contribute to the impairment of T cell–based adaptive immunity in as many as 30% of NK-NPCs {602}. In addition, acquired genomic events commonly alter the chromatin modification machinery (41%; e.g. *KMT2C*, *KMT2D*, *EP300*, *BAP1*), as well as the PI3K/MAPK (49%; e.g. *PTEN*, *PIK3CA*, *NRAS*), NOTCH (20%; e.g. *NOTCH1*, *MAML2*), and TGFB pathways (24%; e.g. *TGFBR2*). Unlike in other head and neck cancers, *TP53* mutations are uncommon in primary tumours (10–20%) but are enriched in advanced disease and recurrences.

Macroscopic appearance

The tumour can produce a smooth bulge, a discrete raised nodule with or without surface ulceration, or a frankly infiltrative exophytic mass. In up to 8% of cases, no grossly visible tumour is identified {2701}.

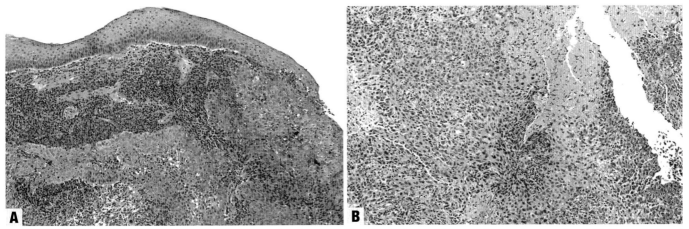

Fig. 2.08 Nasopharyngeal carcinoma, non-keratinizing squamous cell carcinoma, undifferentiated subtype. **A** The nasopharyngeal mucosa shows infiltration by sheets and islands of carcinoma beneath an intact surface epithelium, which shows squamous metaplasia. **B** The ulcerated nasopharyngeal mucosa is infiltrated by sheets of carcinoma cells. Necrosis is present.

Histopathology

Non-keratinizing squamous cell carcinoma

NK-NPC is the commonest subtype of NPC. Nasopharyngeal biopsies vary in appearance, from the presence of a frank tumour with surface ulceration to subtle involvement of the submucosa beneath an intact surface epithelium. The tumour exhibits a variety of architectural patterns, frequently within the same tumour, ranging from solid sheets to irregular islands, trabeculae, and isolated discohesive cells intimately intermingled with variable numbers of lymphocytes and plasma cells.

Classification into undifferentiated and differentiated subtypes has no clinical or prognostic value. The undifferentiated subtype is composed of large neoplastic cells with a syncytial appearance, round to oval vesicular nuclei, and large central nucleoli. The neoplastic cells often appear crowded or even overlapping. They generally have scant amphophilic to eosinophilic cytoplasm. Small foci of primitive squamous differentiation, where

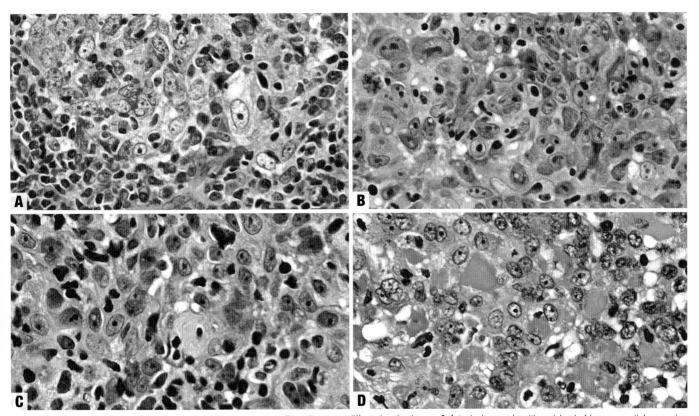

Fig. 2.09 Nasopharyngeal carcinoma, non-keratinizing squamous cell carcinoma, undifferentiated subtype. **A** A typical example with an island of large syncytial-appearing tumour cells with vesicular nuclei and prominent nucleoli. The background is rich in lymphocytes. **B** The large syncytial-appearing tumour cells have vesicular nuclei and large nucleoli. The nuclei commonly appear crowded and overlapping. **C** In undifferentiated nasopharyngeal carcinoma, there can be foci showing subtle squamous differentiation: the tumour cells have more distinct cell borders and a great amount of eosinophilic cytoplasm (lower right). **D** An example with amyloid globules among the carcinoma cells.

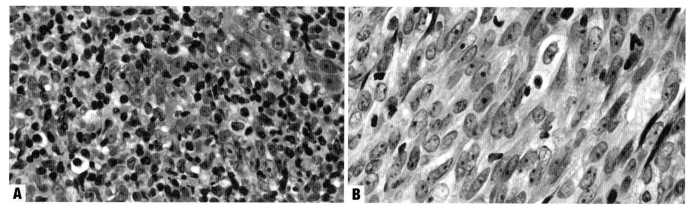

Fig. 2.10 Nasopharyngeal carcinoma, non-keratinizing squamous cell carcinoma, undifferentiated subtype. **A** This example shows a lymphoepithelial carcinoma morphology. Aggregates of syncytial-appearing carcinoma cells with large vesicular nuclei and distinct nucleoli are intimately admixed with many lymphocytes and plasma cells. **B** This example is dominated by spindly tumour cells with indistinct cell borders. The nuclei have fine chromatin and prominent nucleoli.

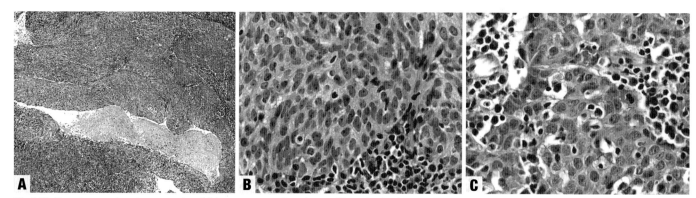

Fig. 2.11 Nasopharyngeal carcinoma, non-keratinizing squamous cell carcinoma, differentiated subtype. **A** The tumour grows in the form of plexiform sheets, showing some resemblance to urothelial carcinoma. **B** The carcinoma cells are polygonal and have a moderate amount of cytoplasm. **C** Compared with the undifferentiated subtype, the carcinoma cells have more distinct cell borders, a greater amount of cytoplasm, and more chromatin-rich nuclei.

groups of tumour cells exhibit more distinct cell borders and a greater amount of lightly eosinophilic cytoplasm, are noted. The malignant cells may be spindly, showing fascicular, whorling, or reticulated growth patterns. The less common differentiated subtype exhibits cellular stratification and pavementing, often with a plexiform growth, reminiscent of urothelial carcinoma. Compared with neoplastic cells of the undifferentiated subtype, the cells are often slightly smaller, cell borders are better defined, the N:C ratio is lower, nuclei are more chromatin-rich, and nucleoli are usually smaller. Vague intercellular bridges may be focally identified, and keratinized cells may rarely be present.

The density of lymphocytes and plasma cells within the tumour is highly variable. When abundant, the inflammatory cells break up the nests and sheets of tumour cells into tiny clusters and/or single cells, making it difficult to recognize the epithelial nature of the neoplasm. The term "lymphoepithelial carcinoma" may be applied for such cases. Some cases may demonstrate abundant eosinophils, neutrophils, or epithelioid granulomas {781,2705,2555,1493}. Desmoplastic stromal reaction is uncommon. In approximately 10% of cases, interspersed intracellular or extracellular small spherical amyloid globules are present {3583}. Other uncommon features include the formation of papillary fronds, clear cell change, intracytoplasmic hyaline globules, accumulation of extracellular oedema fluid or mucosubstances, focal glandular differentiation, and the focal presence of intracytoplasmic mucin {2048,2417,3511,3504, 2270}.

Cervical lymph node metastases show neoplastic cells forming sheets, irregular islands, strands, or dispersed cells. Isolated neoplastic cells may display Reed–Sternberg cell–like features in a mixed inflammatory background, mimicking Hodgkin lymphoma {2559,669}. Epithelioid granulomas (sometimes necrotizing) are present in as many as 20% of cases {2559}. Rarely, the metastatic tumour is completely or partially cystic, simulating metastasis from oropharyngeal carcinoma.

Keratinizing squamous cell carcinoma
K-NPC is an invasive carcinoma showing obvious squamous differentiation, with prominent intercellular bridges and/or various degrees of keratinization, often accompanied by a desmoplastic stroma, similar to conventional keratinizing squamous cell carcinoma at other head and neck sites. K-NPC can arise de novo or as a radiation-associated carcinoma occurring many years after radiation therapy {780,21}.

Basaloid squamous cell carcinoma
Basaloid squamous cell carcinoma, morphologically identical to analogous tumours more commonly occurring in other head and neck sites, has infrequently been reported in the nasopharynx {2559,334,333,4683,3434,3107}. EBV may be positive, especially in high-incidence ethnic groups {4683,3107}.

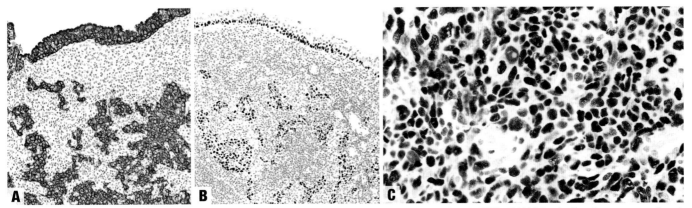

Fig. 2.12 Nasopharyngeal carcinoma, non-keratinizing squamous cell carcinoma. **A** Immunostaining for pancytokeratin (MNF116) highlights the irregular aggregates of carcinoma cells in a lymphoid cell–rich background. **B** Immunostaining for p40 highlights the irregular clusters of carcinoma cells in the nasopharyngeal mucosa. The p40 positivity supports the squamous nature of the carcinoma cells. **C** In situ hybridization for EBV-encoded small RNAs (EBERs) shows positive nuclear labelling of all the tumour cells.

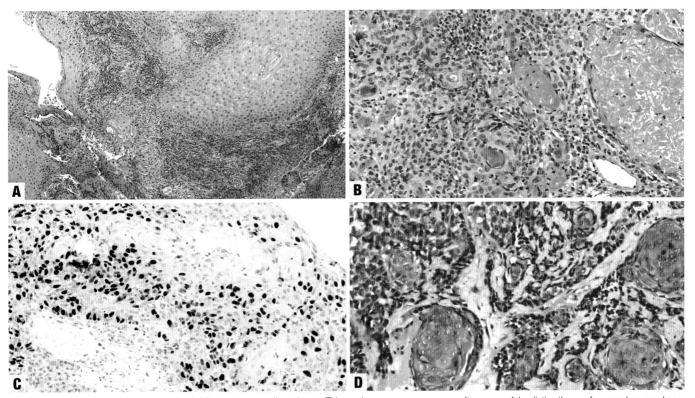

Fig. 2.13 Nasopharyngeal carcinoma. **A** Keratinizing squamous cell carcinoma. This carcinoma arose many years after successful radiation therapy for nasopharyngeal non-keratinizing squamous cell carcinoma (EBV). The carcinoma is very well differentiated, with minimal nuclear atypia or pleomorphism. A diagnosis of malignancy is supported by the presence of stromal invasion. In situ hybridization for EBV-encoded small RNAs (EBERs) is negative (not shown). **B** Keratinizing squamous cell carcinoma. This tumour is morphologically similar to keratinizing squamous cell carcinoma commonly seen in other head and neck sites. **C** Keratinizing squamous cell carcinoma. This case shows association with EBV. In situ hybridization shows labelling of only a proportion of tumour cells, in contrast to the extensive labelling seen in non-keratinizing squamous cell carcinoma. **D** Basaloid squamous cell carcinoma. The tumour comprises nests and festoons of basaloid cells interspersed with variable amounts of hyaline to mucoid stroma. There are foci of abrupt squamous differentiation.

Immunohistochemistry and in situ hybridization

NPC shows strong immunostaining for pancytokeratin and (usually) for high-molecular-weight cytokeratins and p40/p63. It often shows patchy expression of low-molecular-weight cytokeratins, EMA, and desmoglein-3. CK7 and CK20 are negative {1457}. In situ hybridization for EBV (EBER) is positive in practically all cases of NK-NPC but shows variable results in K-NPC and basaloid squamous cell carcinoma. Postirradiation K-NPC is EBV-negative. SOX10 is positive in basaloid NPC {3749}.

Cytology

Smears of involved lymph nodes and other metastatic sites are cellular and show a variable number of irregular crowded tissue fragments and plentiful single cells, in a background of plentiful stripped nuclei, lymphocytes, and plasma cells with apoptotic debris. The tumour cells have high N:C ratios and the cytoplasm is pale and poorly defined in the tissue fragments {747,3042, 2362}. The nuclei are moderately pleomorphic and hyperchromatic (Giemsa stain) or vesicular (Pap), with prominent single nucleoli. Scattered large stripped nuclei with macronucleoli can be seen. The diagnosis can be confirmed by immunostaining for cytokeratins and in situ hybridization for EBER using cell block sections.

Diagnostic molecular pathology
Positive in situ hybridization for EBER may aid in confirming the diagnosis of NPC, in particular for specimens obtained from metastatic sites.

Essential and desirable diagnostic criteria
Non-keratinizing squamous cell carcinoma
Essential: an infiltrative poorly differentiated carcinoma; usually limited evidence of squamous differentiation; variable density of lymphocytes and plasma cells.
Desirable: immunoreactivity for pancytokeratin and positive labelling for EBERs (in problematic biopsies).

Keratinizing squamous cell carcinoma
Essential: an infiltrative squamous cell carcinoma with overt keratinization.

Basaloid squamous cell carcinoma
Essential: an invasive high-grade basaloid carcinoma with a nested growth pattern and frequent comedonecrosis; squamous cell carcinoma component in the form of abrupt keratinization in the basaloid nests, conventional invasive squamous cell carcinoma, or dysplasia / carcinoma in situ in surface epithelium.
Desirable: variable myxoid to hyaline stroma.

Staging
Staging follows the eighth edition of the Union for International Cancer Control (UICC) / American Joint Committee on Cancer (AJCC) TNM staging system. Patients with NPC in Asian centres show the following tumour stage distribution: stage I, 4%; stage II, 20%; stage III, 35%; stage IV, 41% {3373}.

Prognosis and prediction
The stage of presentation is the most important prognostic factor. The validation study for the eighth-edition UICC/AJCC staging system showed that the 5-year overall survival rate for stage I disease was 98%; stage II, 92%; stage III, 83%; and stage IVA, 71% {3373}.

The prognosis depends on multiple factors, including tumour-, host-, and treatment-related factors {2509}. Significant tumour factors include histological type, gross tumour volume, and EBV DNA. Incorporation of pretreatment plasma EBV DNA can refine TNM staging for NK-NPC, especially for identifying poor-risk subgroups among patients with early-stage disease {2540}, this may spare low-risk stage II patients from unnecessary chemotherapy. Significant host factors include age, sex, performance status, comorbidities (particularly for elderly patients), anaemia, and LDH level {4322}. Treatment-related factors affect ultimate survival. Radiotherapy using the best available conformable technique to deliver the cancericidal dose with minimal late damage of adjacent normal structures is fundamental. Addition of the optimal sequence and dose of chemotherapy is needed for all stage III–IVA and high-risk stage II patients for the eradication of micrometastasis and the potentiation of locoregional control {2507,2508,802,3202}.

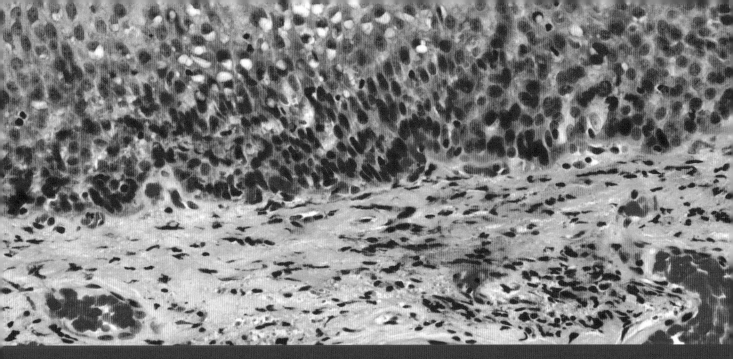

3

Hypopharyngeal, laryngeal, tracheal, and parapharyngeal tumours

Edited by: Gale N, Helliwell T, Wenig BM

Hypopharyngeal, laryngeal, tracheal, and parapharyngeal tumours: Introduction

Gale N
Helliwell T
Thompson LDR

Tumours of the hypopharynx, larynx, and trachea most often originate in the covering epithelium, i.e. squamous cell or respiratory epithelium. Therefore, this chapter primarily focuses on these entities. In a change from the previous edition, tumours not unique to this site (with the exception of cartilage tumours) have been transferred to their corresponding chapters: salivary gland tumours to Chapter 4: *Salivary gland tumours*; soft tissue tumours to Chapter 9: *Soft tissue tumours*; haematolymphoid neoplasms to Chapter 10: *Haematolymphoid proliferations and neoplasia*; melanoma to Chapter 11: *Melanocytic tumours*, neuroendocrine tumours to Chapter 15: *Neuroendocrine neoplasms and paraganglioma*; and metastatic tumours to Chapter 14: *Metastasis*, with a comprehensive table separated into specific anatomical sites. For all listed tumours, particular attention is paid to the practical application of histomorphology, with important differential diagnoses and prognostic factors. Etiology and updated genetic changes are comprehensively reviewed.

Benign tumours are represented only by the most frequent: squamous papilloma. Precursor lesions, usually referred to as dysplasia / squamous intraepithelial lesions, are discussed as a spectrum of histomorphological changes carrying a risk of eventual cancer development. Classification of these lesions remains a challenging and controversial topic. In this chapter, like in the previous edition, a two- to three-tiered system of low-grade and high-grade dysplasia and carcinoma in situ is proposed. NANOG, a stem cell precursor marker, has recently emerged as a new potential diagnostic and prognostic marker for these lesions {1064,1695}. Furthermore, the risk of malignant transformation of laryngeal leukoplakic lesions was reported to be statistically significantly associated with melanoma-associated antigen (MAGEA) expression by immunohistochemical staining and real-time RT-PCR {338}. The central part of this chapter is occupied by conventional squamous cell carcinoma, together with several subtypes (verrucous, papillary, spindle cell, basaloid, adenosquamous, and lymphoepithelial). All entities have specific morphological, genetic, and prognostic characteristics when compared with conventional squamous cell carcinoma.

Squamous papilloma and papillomatosis

Richardson MS
Chernock RD
Gale N

Definition
Squamous papilloma and papillomatosis are benign exophytic squamous epithelial tumours with fibrovascular cores, usually associated with low-risk HPV6 or HPV11 infection.

ICD-O coding
8052/0 Squamous papilloma
8060/0 Squamous papillomatosis

ICD-11 coding
2F00.Y & XA2RH5 & XH50T2 Other specified benign neoplasm of middle ear or respiratory system & Larynx & Squamous papilloma
2F00.Y & XA2RH5 & XH50N3 Other specified benign neoplasm of middle ear or respiratory system & Larynx & Squamous papillomatosis
2F00.1 & XA2RH5 & XH50N3 Recurrent respiratory papillomatosis & Larynx & Squamous papillomatosis

Related terminology
Acceptable: squamous cell papilloma; recurrent respiratory papillomatosis; laryngeal papillomatosis.
Not recommended: juvenile papillomatosis; adult papillomatosis.

Subtype(s)
None

Localization
The distribution of squamous papillomatosis follows a predictable pattern, with the tumours occurring at sites where ciliated and squamous epithelium is juxtaposed. The papillomatosis usually involves the vocal cords and ventricles, followed by transmission to the false cords, epiglottis, subglottic area, hypopharynx, and nasopharynx. Rarely (in 1–3% of cases), the papillomatosis may extend into the lower respiratory tract (trachea, bronchi, and pulmonary parenchyma), which is associated with high mortality {1559,4317,3227}.

Clinical features
The presentation includes progressive hoarseness, stridor, and obstructive airway symptoms associated with growths of exophytic lesions within the larynx.

Epidemiology
Squamous papilloma is the most common benign epithelial tumour of the larynx. Squamous papillomatosis is characterized by multiple contiguous, locally recurrent florid squamous papillomas, although solitary lesions present infrequently. Squamous papillomatosis is a rare disease involving the respiratory tract that occurs in both children and adults. The true incidence and prevalence of squamous papillomatosis are uncertain. The

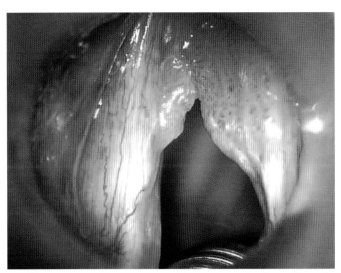

Fig. 3.01 Squamous papilloma, laryngoscopic appearance. Sessile, cauliflower-like masses cover almost two thirds of the right vocal cord and the anterior third of the left vocal cord.

best projected estimates of annual incidence are 4.3 cases per 100 000 children and approximately 1.8 cases per 100 000 adults {1097,672}. The bimodal age distribution demonstrates a first peak in children aged < 5 years (juvenile cases) and a second peak in patients aged 20–40 years (adult cases) {672,2351}. The age of onset of squamous papillomatosis has a trimodal distribution, with peaks at about 7, 35, and 64 years of age {3849}. Squamous papillomatosis is more common in children and is the most aggressive form of the disease, with 25% of cases presenting during infancy {3672,4812}. There is no sex predominance in children, but in adult patients the M:F ratio is 3:2 {1170,1097,3303}. Although the disease is rare, morbidity is notoriously high, with the disease compromising functions such as vocalization, swallowing, and breathing {4813,1559}.

Etiology
HPV6 and HPV11 are the most frequent genotypes (seen in 90% of cases) associated with squamous papillomatosis as well as solitary papillomas {1517,4813}. Integration of low-risk HPV types into the cell genome is an early and common event in the etiology of juvenile and adult recurrent laryngeal papillomas {593}. A minority of cases (4–5%) have coinfection with genotypes HPV6 and HPV11, and fewer cases (3–4%) have coinfection with other HPV genotypes (e.g. 16, 31, 33, 35, and 39) {4813}. The modes of HPV transmission include sexual contact, non-sexual contact, and maternal contact (direct or indirect) {2450}. Most neonatal HPV infection occurs by vertical transmission at birth {4317}. A triad of factors (first-born child, vaginal delivery, and maternal age < 20 years) has been noted to correlate with squamous papillomatosis in children {2202}. An active maternal genital HPV infection at the time of delivery

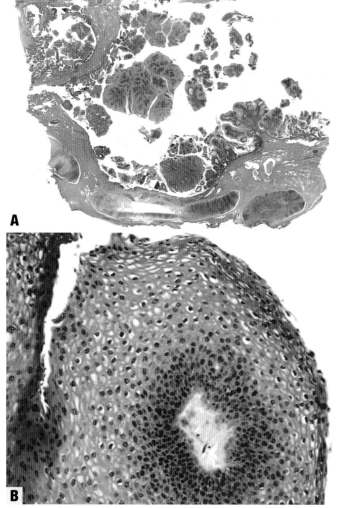

Fig. 3.02 Squamous papilloma and papillomatosis. **A** Squamous papillomatosis, larynx. Friable papillomas line the endolarynx. **B** Squamous cell papilloma of the larynx. High-magnification view of a papilloma branch with pronounced koilocytosis.

increases exposure to a significant viral load, with a high risk of transmitting infection {4317,2450}. Although caesarean section provides a lower risk of transmission, it is not completely protective against infection. In adults, the mode of viral transmission remains unclear; transmission during sexual contact and reactivation of a slowly progressing latent infection from childhood have been suggested {2214,3785,3304}. The unpredictable clinical course of squamous papillomatosis suggests possible host-specific genetic and immunological factors involving the dysregulation of T-lymphocyte activity {2033}. Differences in HPV-specific immune response have been demonstrated between patients with squamous papillomatosis and controls {518,3227,3719,672}.

Pathogenesis

HPVs are double-stranded DNA viruses, differentiated by the genetic sequence of the outer capsid protein L1. The virions replicate within the nuclei of infected host cells {2703}. More than 40 types affect mucosal epithelium, separated into non-oncogenic types (e.g. HPV6 and HPV11) and oncogenic types (e.g. HPV16 and HPV18). Viral infection occurs at the basal epithelium, frequently in zones of the body lined by squamous epithelium with a squamocolumnar transition. The transcripts initiated at major viral promoter sites in oncogenic types are not seen in non-oncogenic types.

Macroscopic appearance

These tumours are intraluminal exophytic, sessile, or pedunculated masses with bosselated surfaces. The papillomas often grow along the airway as a friable cluster and bleed easily with minor trauma.

Histopathology

Squamous papillomas have a complex, thin fibrovascular core covered by hyperplastic squamous epithelium. Parabasal cell hyperplasia is often seen, involving the lower half of the epithelium. Pronounced to subtle koilocytic features are seen in the upper layers of the epithelium. Mitoses present along the basal to mid zones of the epithelium. Premature keratinization of individual epithelial cells contributes to a disorganized appearance. Surface keratinization is minimal. HPV-induced cytological atypia is well recognized. High-grade dysplasia is uncommon, and if it occurs it is typically seen in recurrent disease years after the initial presentation. The histological monitoring of squamous papillomatosis is necessary at every surgical procedure, for the early detection of potentially premalignant epithelial changes.

Immunohistochemistry

Immunohistochemical staining is unnecessary in the diagnosis, but tumour cells are positive for cytokeratins and p40/p63, and negative for p16. In situ hybridization for high-risk HPV is negative. Ki-67 and p53 are of limited utility.

Differential diagnosis

The differential diagnosis may include high-grade dysplasia with papillary or verrucoid features, and papillary squamous cell carcinoma. Distinction can be made on the architectural features of papillomas and their bland cytology.

Cytology

Not clinically relevant

Diagnostic molecular pathology

Specific HPV genotyping is not diagnostically required {3303}, but in situ hybridization can distinguish between episomal and integrated patterns {3303}. Papilloma recurrence in paediatric patients may be more attributable to HPV integration {593}.

Essential and desirable diagnostic criteria

Essential: exophytic multilayered benign squamous cell proliferation; central fibrovascular cores supporting epithelial proliferation.
Desirable: isolated koilocytes; low-risk HPV type (in selected cases).

Staging

Not relevant

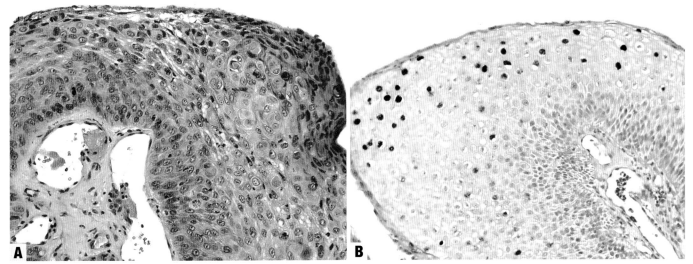

Fig. 3.03 Squamous papilloma and papillomatosis. **A** Squamous cell papillomatosis. Note the high-grade squamous dysplasia present within the surface epithelium of this papillary branch. HPV11 was present. **B** Squamous cell papillomas of the larynx. Positive diffuse in situ hybridization signal for episomal HPV6 and HPV11 within the upper layers of the squamous epithelial lining.

Prognosis and prediction

The clinical course of squamous papillomatosis is unpredictable and ranges from complete remission, to relatively stable lesions, to an aggressive clinical course of rapidly progressive recurrences requiring surgical intervention, and potentially life-threatening respiratory obstruction {1097,2810,4317}. A variety of antivirals and antiangiogenics as adjuvant therapy have not been curative. Early data suggest promising results for adjuvant immunotherapy and therapeutic HPV vaccination {420}. Malignant transformation of squamous papillomatosis into squamous cell carcinoma is reported in 1–4% of cases and occurs primarily in the setting of irradiation, smoking, or another promoter {1097,2214,2158,3304}. Similar findings were detected in a large cohort study of 163 patients with recurrent respiratory papillomatosis, which identified progression to high-grade dysplasia and squamous cell carcinoma in 21.5% and 4.3%, respectively {1610}.

Some studies have found the HPV11 genotype to be the most important risk factor for an aggressive clinical course, but this finding has not been consistently replicated {4813,3303}. HPV11 is more closely associated with a younger age at diagnosis {4813}, and patient age at onset may be prognostic in the paediatric population {611}. Children diagnosed at < 3 years of age are 3.6 times as likely to have > 4 surgeries per year than

children diagnosed at an older age {3672,3303}. In adults, both HPV11 and an observation time of > 10 years have been found to be associated with an aggressive clinical course {3303}. A retrospective sequence analysis of HPV in squamous papillomatosis showed no evidence of strain replacement in 95% of cases during a median follow-up of 4 years, with 1 case having 22 years of follow-up {2351}. These findings indicate that the frequent recurrence of squamous papillomatosis is a consequence of the long-term persistence of the initial HPV genome type. Whether disease severity correlates with specific HPV types has yet to be determined, but some initial reports suggest that there may be significance {934,2810,2019,573}.

The quadrivalent and non-valent vaccines against HPV protect against the most common HPV genotypes (6 and 11) associated with squamous papillomatosis. The effect of these vaccines on HPV infection has resulted in a reported decrease in incidence of squamous papillomatosis, especially where vaccination is a national mandate {672,3249}. Additional research revealed that the quadrivalent HPV vaccine (against HPV types 6, 11, 16, and 18) favourably influences the course of squamous papillomatosis in patients with rapid growth of the papillomas. It significantly prolongs the intervals between surgical procedures and reduces the number of procedures needed in the majority of patients {1891}.

Laryngeal and hypopharyngeal epithelial dysplasia

Zidar N
Fujii S
Gale N
Hernandez-Prera JC
Nadal A

Definition

Laryngeal and hypopharyngeal epithelial dysplasia is a spectrum of architectural and cytological changes of the squamous epithelium of laryngeal, hypopharyngeal, and tracheal mucosa, caused by an accumulation of genetic alterations and associated with an increased risk of progression to invasive squamous cell carcinoma (SCC).

ICD-O coding

8077/0 Squamous intraepithelial neoplasia, low grade
8077/2 Squamous intraepithelial neoplasia, high grade
8070/2 Squamous cell carcinoma in situ, NOS

ICD-11 coding

2F00.Y & XA2RH5 & XH4611 Other specified benign neoplasm of middle ear or respiratory system & Larynx & Squamous intraepithelial neoplasia, grade I

Related terminology

Acceptable: squamous intraepithelial lesion.

Subtype(s)

Low-grade dysplasia; high-grade dysplasia (basaloid subtype and large, spinous cell subtype); carcinoma in situ

Localization

Dysplasia can occur anywhere in the larynx, although it occurs most frequently along one or (less frequently) both vocal cords. The commissures, hypopharynx, and trachea are rarely involved {1518,4360,2132,1495}.

Clinical features

Symptoms and signs are nonspecific and vary according to the site and size of the lesion. In the glottis, symptoms of

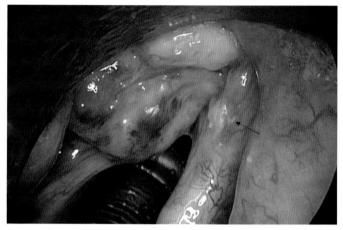

Fig. 3.04 Laryngeal epithelial dysplasia. Laryngoscopic appearance of leukoplakia and squamous cell carcinoma. Endoscopy with white light. The right vocal cord (arrow) is erythematous, with a small focus of leukoplakia anteriorly. The left vocal cord shows exophytic carcinoma of the anterior third infiltrating the sinus of Morgagni and anterior commissure.

dysplasia include voice change and hoarseness, whereas in the supraglottis and subglottis, dysplasia is usually asymptomatic {3264}.

Epidemiology

Dysplasia is mostly seen in adults and affects more men than women, with an M:F ratio as high as 4.6:1 {1516}. This disparity is especially evident after the sixth decade of life. The annual incidence of laryngeal keratosis in the USA has been reported as 10.2 and 2.1 lesions per 100 000 male population and female population, respectively; between 1988 and 2012, 3169 cases of glottic carcinoma in situ (CIS) were reported in the 18-registry SEER database {543,2264}. The annual incidence elsewhere in the world is unknown.

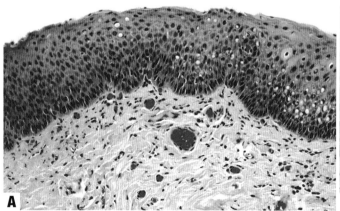
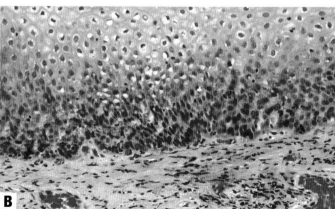

Fig. 3.05 Laryngeal and hypopharyngeal epithelial dysplasia. **A** Laryngeal and hypopharyngeal epithelial dysplasia, low-grade. Augmented basal and parabasal cells, occupying the lower half of the epithelial thickness. **B** Laryngeal epithelial dysplasia, low-grade. Laryngeal mucosa showing architectural disorganization and nuclear hyperchromasia in the lower third of the epithelium, typical of low-grade dysplasia.

Table 3.01 Two- and three-tiered systems for grading dysplasia

Clinical relevance	Extension of epithelial abnormalities	Three-tiered grading system	Two-tiered grading system
Low-risk lesion	Lower half	Low-grade dysplasia/SIL	Low-grade dysplasia/SIL
High-risk lesion	More than lower half	High-grade dysplasia/SIL	High-grade dysplasia/SIL
	Full thickness	Carcinoma in situ	

SIL, squamous intraepithelial lesion.

Etiology

The principal risk factor for laryngeal dysplasia is cigarette smoking, especially in combination with alcohol abuse {3800,4557}. Gastroesophageal reflux disease has been suggested as possible risk factor {2584,912,3980}. High-risk HPV plays a minor role in laryngeal dysplasia development; rare reported cases showed HPV16/18 RNA by in situ hybridization and occurred concurrently with invasive SCC {1203,3063,3359,5013}.

Pathogenesis

Preneoplastic cells are frequently aneuploid {3868,4941}, with chromosomal changes / loss of heterozygosity accumulating at 9p21 (probably targeting *CDKN2A*), 17p13 (*TP53*), 3p26, and 3p14 {3123}. Other molecular alterations consistently detected include cyclin D1 overexpression {3387} and reactivation of telomerase {2740,2739,2684}.

Macroscopic appearance

Laryngeal dysplasia does not have a characteristic macroscopic appearance. Patients may present with leukoplakia (white patch), erythroplakia (red patch), erythroleukoplakia, or chronic laryngitis. It can be a localized or diffuse, flat or exophytic lesion. Macroscopic appearance does not carry any microscopic connotation {1518}.

Narrow-band imaging (applying narrow-band spectrum optical filters to enhance the visualization of mucosal and submucosal blood vessels) may provide useful information: a lack of perpendicular vascular patterns suggests a benign lesion, whereas irregularities of capillary loops and narrow-angled perpendicular vascular patterns point to a high-grade lesion or SCC {1495,4061}.

Histopathology

Several classifications have been devised to represent the spectrum of histological changes and their relation to biological behaviour {2403,1408,4774,1514,2921}. In recent reviews of classification systems of laryngeal dysplasia {1515,1826}, the use of unified terminology including dysplasia / squamous intraepithelial lesion (SIL) has been suggested, with either a two-tiered or a three-tiered grading system (see Table 3.01). A disadvantage of the two-tiered system of grading is a wide category of high-grade dysplasia/SIL (moderate, severe, and CIS), which can be potentially resolved by introducing CIS as the third category.

Lesions previously classified as moderate dysplasia have shown a higher risk of malignant transformation, which supports their inclusion in the high-grade dysplasia/SIL category {4576}. Although the grading of laryngeal dysplasia is subjective to a certain degree, it remains the most important prognostic factor for the biological behaviour of the disease, helping clinicians to offer appropriate treatment {2907,3875,1409}. The diagnosis of laryngeal dysplasia should follow a multidisciplinary approach,

Box 3.01 Morphological criteria for the classification of laryngeal epithelial dysplasia

Low-grade dysplasia/SIL: Changes occupy the lower half of the epithelium

Architectural changes:
- Augmented basal/parabasal cells up to the lower half of the epithelium
- Perpendicular orientation to the basement membrane
- Stratification and maturation are preserved
- Spinous cell layer is retained in the upper half of the epithelium

Cytological changes:
- Minimal cellular atypia
- Basal/parabasal cells: increased cytoplasm, hyperchromatic nuclei, uniformly distributed chromatin
- Regular mitoses in the lower half of the epithelium
- A few dyskeratotic cells may be present

High-grade dysplasia/SIL: Changes occupy more than the lower half of the epithelium

Architectural changes:
- Abnormal maturation
- Keratinizing or non-keratinizing
- Variable degrees of disordered stratification and polarity in up to the entire thickness of epithelium
- Two subtypes: basaloid, with no maturation; large (spinous) cell, with maturation
- Variable degree of irregularly shaped rete (bulbous, downwardly extending)

Cytological changes:
- Cellular and nuclear atypia including marked variation in size and shape
- Marked nuclear hyperchromasia
- Nucleoli increased in number and size
- Increased N:C ratio
- Increased mitoses in up to the entire thickness of the epithelium
- Atypical mitoses may be present
- Dyskeratotic and apoptotic cells may be present within the entire thickness of the epithelium

Carcinoma in situ: Changes occupy the entire thickness of the epithelium

Architectural changes:
- Complete loss of stratification and polarity
- Preserved basement membrane

Cytological changes:
- Severe cellular and nuclear atypia (both qualitatively and quantitatively)
- Atypical mitoses

SIL, squamous intraepithelial lesion.

and pathologists should discuss with their clinicians which system optimizes the treatment decisions for their specific patient populations {1212}.

Morphological features of each grade of dysplasia are described in Box 3.01. Epithelium in laryngeal dysplasia/SIL is usually thickened, but it may be normal or (rarely) atrophic. It may be keratinizing or non-keratinizing; the presence of a surface keratinization is not considered to be an important prognostic factor {4782}. The basement membrane is preserved. The subepithelial stroma may show inflammation, but there is no desmoplastic stromal reaction {5049,2356}.

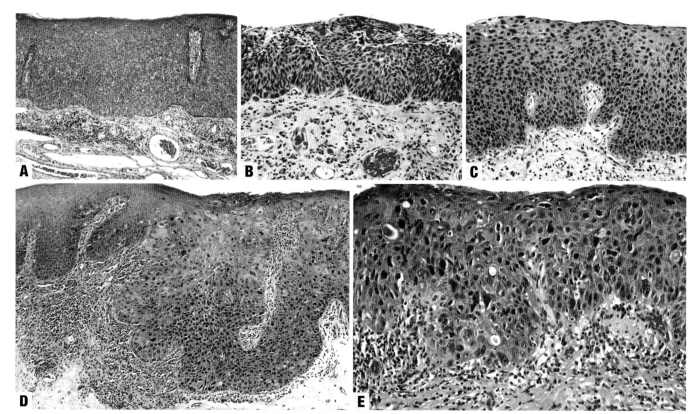

Fig. 3.06 Laryngeal and hypopharyngeal epithelial dysplasia. **A** Laryngeal epithelial dysplasia, high-grade. Laryngeal mucosa showing detail of cytological changes in high-grade dysplasia. **B** High-grade dysplasia of the basaloid subtype with no maturation. Augmented basaloid cells with marked cellular and nuclear atypia occupy almost the entire thickness of the epithelium. **C** High-grade dysplasia of the large, spinous cell type, with maturation. Augmented basaloid and spinous cells with marked cellular and nuclear atypia occupy almost the entire thickness of the epithelium. **D** Laryngeal epithelial dysplasia, carcinoma in situ. Laryngeal mucosa showing marked cytological atypia in keeping with carcinoma in situ. The basement membrane is intact. **E** Carcinoma in situ. There is prominent architectural disorganization, with complete loss of stratification and polarity. Severe cellular and nuclear atypia, mitoses, and apoptotic cells are seen in the entire thickness of the epithelium. The basement membrane is preserved.

Immunohistochemistry

Reliable markers with diagnostic and prognostic value are lacking. Some studies suggested the potential value of p53, p16, Ki-67, EGFR, CK19, and MAGEA, but they are currently not recommended for dysplasia classification {338,1826}.

A stem cell marker, NANOG, has recently emerged as a potential diagnostic and prognostic marker in dysplasia of the head and neck {3721,1064,1695,1694}. Studies have shown that there is no immunohistochemical expression of NANOG in the normal mucosa; weak expression in low-grade dysplasia; and strong expression in high-grade dysplasia, CIS, and SCC. The marked difference in intensity between low- and high-grade dysplasia indicates a potential diagnostic use of NANOG, enabling the distinction between reactive lesions and low-grade dysplasia, and between low- and high-grade dysplasia. However, it does not distinguish between high-grade dysplasia and CIS.

Cytology

Unlike in the uterine cervix, cytopathology has not been used to diagnose and grade dysplasia of the laryngeal epithelium.

Diagnostic molecular pathology

None of the molecular changes are currently of diagnostic or prognostic utility. Expression of members of the MAGEA family is reported to predict malignant transformation in precursor lesions {338}.

Essential and desirable diagnostic criteria

Essential: full-thickness, properly oriented biopsy; appropriate cytological and architectural abnormalities; preserved basement membrane.

Staging

Dysplasia has no staging system. CIS is classified as Tis according to the eighth edition of the Union for International Cancer Control (UICC) / American Joint Committee on Cancer (AJCC) TNM staging system.

Prognosis and prediction

The risk of malignant transformation increases with the degree of laryngeal dysplasia. However, some follow-up studies showed overlapping confidence intervals {2187,4576}. A retrospective follow-up study demonstrated a highly significant difference in the risk of malignant progression between low- and high-grade dysplasia (1.6% and 12.5%, respectively) {1514}. Certain high-grade dysplasias (e.g. CIS) have been associated with an increased progression to invasive growth (40%) and may require more extensive surgery or radiation therapy, depending on the specific site (anterior commissure) and risk factors (alcohol, tobacco) {5011,1518}.

Conventional squamous cell carcinoma

Nadal A
Bishop JA
Brandwein-Weber M
Stenman G
Zidar N

Definition

Conventional squamous cell carcinoma (SCC) is a malignant epithelial tumour with squamous differentiation originating from the mucosal epithelium.

ICD-O coding

8070/3 Squamous cell carcinoma, NOS

ICD-11 coding

2B6C.0 Squamous cell carcinoma of piriform sinus
2B6D.0 Squamous cell carcinoma of hypopharynx and variants
2C23.10 Squamous cell carcinoma of larynx, glottis
2C23.20 Squamous cell carcinoma of larynx, supraglottis
2C23.30 Squamous cell carcinoma of larynx, subglottis
2C24.1 Squamous cell carcinoma of trachea

Related terminology

Not recommended: epidermoid carcinoma.

Subtype(s)

Subtypes are covered in their own separate sections.

Localization

The most affected subsite varies depending on geographical area. Two thirds of cases in the USA are glottic, whereas three quarters of cases in Poland are supraglottic. The subglottis is less commonly affected {4149,4472}. Most hypopharyngeal tumours develop in the piriform sinus. Most tracheal SCCs originate in the intrathoracic segment {1558,4747,5030}.

Clinical features

Hoarseness is the rule for glottic tumours and is also common for supraglottic lesions, usually along with a sore throat {3635}. Dyspnoea is the most common presenting symptom for subglottic and tracheal tumours {1367,4747,5030}. Hypopharyngeal tumours cause dysphagia and odynophagia. One quarter of cases present with a neck mass {4554}. Distant metastases are twice as common in hypopharyngeal tumours as in laryngeal tumours (20% vs 9%) {2647,1202}.

Imaging

Postcontrast CT is the most commonly used imaging modality for evaluating laryngeal cancer, because it avoids the breathing and swallowing artefact often seen on MRI. It also permits the thorax to be staged at the same time. MRI is increasingly used,

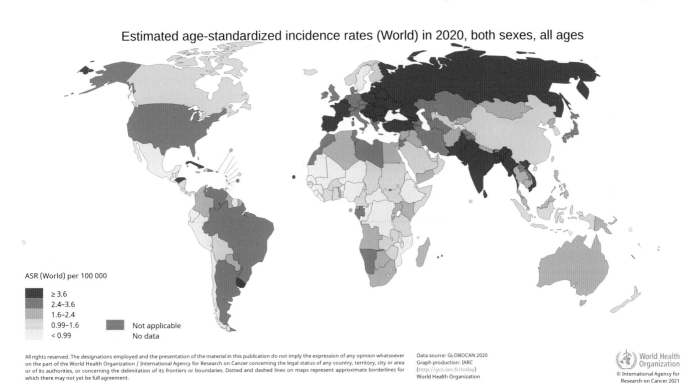

Estimated age-standardized incidence rates (World) in 2020, both sexes, all ages

ASR (World) per 100 000

≥ 3.6
2.4–3.6
1.6–2.4
0.99–1.6
< 0.99

Not applicable
No data

Data source: GLOBOCAN 2020
Graph production: IARC
(http://gco.iarc.fr/today)
World Health Organization

World Health Organization
© International Agency for Research on Cancer 2021

Fig. 3.07 Conventional squamous cell carcinoma. Estimated age-standardized incidence rates (ASRs, World Standard Population), per 100 000 person-years, of laryngeal and hypopharyngeal cancer in 2020 among both sexes (all ages).

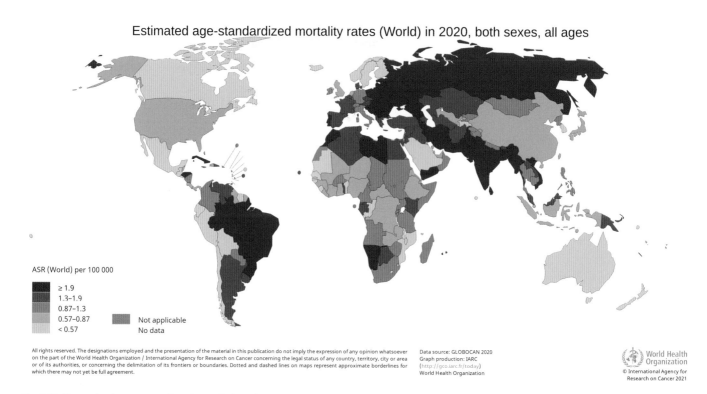

Estimated age-standardized mortality rates (World) in 2020, both sexes, all ages

ASR (World) per 100 000

≥ 1.9
1.3–1.9
0.87–1.3
0.57–0.87
< 0.57

Not applicable
No data

Data source: GLOBOCAN 2020
Graph production: IARC
(http://gco.iarc.fr/today)
World Health Organization

World Health Organization
© International Agency for Research on Cancer 2021

Fig. 3.08 Conventional squamous cell carcinoma. Estimated age-standardized mortality rates (ASRs, World Standard Population), per 100 000 person-years, of laryngeal and hypopharyngeal cancer in 2020 among both sexes (all ages).

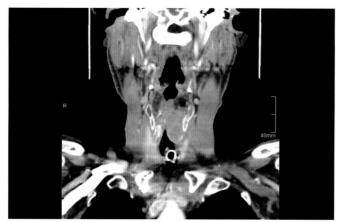

Fig. 3.09 Conventional squamous cell carcinoma. Coronal postcontrast CT of a T4a transglottic laryngeal squamous cell carcinoma. Transglottic extension is demonstrated. Tracheostomy tube in situ.

however, as a problem-solving tool to assess the presence of laryngeal cartilage invasion.

Hypopharyngeal cancer may also be imaged with CT, but MRI is considered by many to be the superior modality, owing to better soft tissue resolution, especially in the evaluation of retropharyngeal and prevertebral tumour extension.

Epidemiology

Laryngeal cancer affects > 1 million individuals worldwide, with > 200 000 new cases every year {1556}. It is the second most common respiratory tract cancer {4058} and accounts for 25% of head and neck cancers {286}. From 1990 to 2017, the annual age-standardized incidence rate of laryngeal cancer decreased, with great variations among regions (> 4 cases per 100 000 person-years in central Europe and the Caribbean vs < 1 case per 100 000 person-years in Andean Latin America) {2656}. It accounts for 0.6% of cancers (1.1% in men and 0.3% in women) {4058} and peaks at 65 years of age {3229}.

The incidence of hypopharyngeal carcinoma is < 1 case per 100 000 person-years. The overall median age at diagnosis is 62.1 years (61.8 years for men, 64 years for women) {2052}. Carcinomas of the piriform sinus and posterior pharyngeal wall occur in men, whereas carcinoma of the postcricoid area is more common in women and occurs in association with sideropenic dysphagia {1825}.

Tracheal tumours are the rarest. Tracheal SCC shows no sex predilection and occurs at a mean age of 64.8 years {1558}.

Etiology

Laryngeal SCC (LSCC) is strongly associated with cigarette smoking (in a dose-dependent manner regarding frequency, duration, and number of pack-years) and with high-volume alcohol intake. Smoking and alcohol drinking have synergistic effects. A mean risk reduction of two thirds is seen after 10 years of quitting smoking {1791,1115}. Glutathione S-transferases are involved in phase II xenobiotic metabolism and provide protection against oxidative stress. The null phenotype of GSTM1 results in an inability to detoxify tobacco-related carcinogens, increasing the risk of developing LSCC {2408,5008}. The GSTT1 null genotype is associated with laryngeal cancer risk in Asians {2619}. In LSCC, the Catalogue Of Somatic Mutations In Cancer (COSMIC) mutation signature 4 (characterized by a high frequency of C>A-G>T transversions) is prominent. This signature is similar to that produced by benzo[α]pyrene (BaP) exposure in cells in vitro and suggests that it arises from

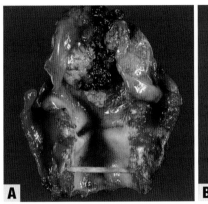
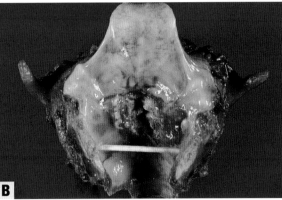
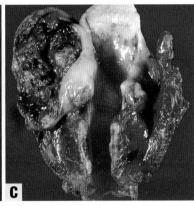

Fig. 3.10 Conventional squamous cell carcinoma, macroscopic appearance. **A** Supraglottic. Exophytic and ulcerated tumour with granular surface of the epiglottis. **B** Glottic. The tumour extends through both vocal cords, affecting the anterior commissure. **C** Hypopharyngeal. Large exophytic and ulcerated tumour involving the left piriform sinus.

the misreplication of DNA damage (adducts) formed by carcinogens from tobacco smoke {100,3528}. The contribution of high-risk HPV is marginal in conventional LSCC {2600,2472, 2305}. Hypopharyngeal cancer is also associated with excess alcohol consumption and tobacco smoking {1825}. Gastroesophageal/laryngopharyngeal reflux is an independent risk factor for the development of LSCC {3406,1217}. Pepsin is considered the etiological agent {4934}. Its relationship with hypopharyngeal carcinoma has not been confirmed in large series {2464,634,1217}. Tracheal SCC is also associated with smoking {1558}.

Pathogenesis

LSCC develops as the result of multiple genetic alterations leading to chromosomal instability and aneuploidy. Microsatellite instability is rare in LSCC {1607,938}. Laryngeal and hypopharyngeal carcinomas have more copy-number alterations than do oral cancers {4034}. More than 50% of tumours harbour p53 mutations {3564}. *CDKN2A* is frequently inactivated in LSCC. Although EGFR (HER1) expression is the rule in head and neck SCC, including laryngeal and hypopharyngeal tumours, as many as 40% express EGFRvIII, leading to a relative inability of blocking monoclonal antibodies to downregulate this receptor {770}. Addition of EGFR inhibitors in laryngeal and hypopharyngeal cancer treatments does not modify overall survival {3214}. *PIK3CA* mutations occur with a low frequency {4271,653} but could predict response to PI3K/AKT/mTOR inhibitor therapy {2056}. MicroRNAs (e.g. let-7 family, miR-7, and miR-206) and long ncRNAs may have a role in the pathogenesis of LSCC {4844,4347,4965,951}.

Macroscopic appearance

Tumours can grow in exophytic or endophytic patterns, or in combinations of these patterns. They are white and firm, and ulceration is common. Supraglottic tumours tend to grow up and forward, invading the prelaryngeal space. Invasion of the different laryngeal subsites sometimes makes it difficult to determine the origin. Some glottic carcinomas grow upwards and may cross the lateral ventricles (so-called transglottic carcinomas, although transglottic is not a site itself). Piriform sinus carcinomas frequently invade the ipsilateral aryepiglottic fold or vocal cords.

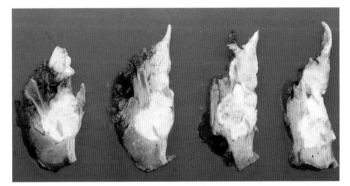

Fig. 3.11 Conventional squamous cell carcinoma infiltrating the thyroid gland. Cross-sections of a glottic carcinoma extending through the supraglottic compartment and thyroid cartilage into the thyroid gland.

Histopathology

Tumour cells grow in irregular nests with evidence of stromal invasion. Squamous differentiation is seen as keratinization with keratin pearls and/or the presence of intercellular bridges. Tumour nests can show maturation: cells are larger at the centre, whereas proliferative activity accumulates at the edges. Cell pleomorphism is variable and used for grading. The stroma shows a desmoplastic reaction, with newly formed extracellular matrix deposition and a variable inflammatory lymphoplasmacytic response. Tumour growth at the invasive front can be expansive, with large cohesive tumour nests; or infiltrative, with small, irregular nests or single cells. The presence of nests composed of ≤ 4 cells is called "budding", but this is not included as a criterion for the grading of differentiation {2734}.

Tumours are traditionally graded according to their similarity to normal squamous epithelium, either in three categories (well differentiated, moderately differentiated, and poorly differentiated) or in four categories (well differentiated, moderately differentiated, poorly differentiated, and undifferentiated), loosely following the Broders criteria. Roughly, grading is done according to the N:C ratio, nuclear morphology, mitotic count, severity of atypia, stromal reaction, and keratinization. Well-differentiated tumours resemble normal epithelium, making the diagnosis of malignancy sometimes more difficult. Poorly differentiated / undifferentiated tumours may be difficult to identify as squamous {55}. Jakobson proposed an improved grading system

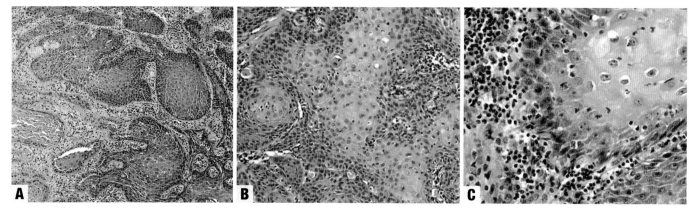

Fig. 3.12 Conventional squamous cell carcinoma, well differentiated. **A** At low magnification, infiltrating nests show squamous maturation resembling normal squamous epithelium. Stromal reaction is light. **B** Cell shape varies according to its position within the nest. At the periphery, the cells are smaller, with higher N:C ratios. At the centre, the cells show large eosinophilic cytoplasm, with low N:C ratios. **C** Nuclei are slightly pleomorphic, with open chromatin. Nucleoli are frequent. Mitoses are sparse and located at the nest margins. Atypical mitoses are not characteristic of well-differentiated tumours.

including mode and stage of invasion, vascular invasion, and lymphoplasmacytic response {2053}. Although there is interobserver variation, grading retains prognostic significance {3987, 1824}.

Perineural invasion affects survival after salvage surgery for laryngeal cancer {1412}, because the perineural plane is a preferential pathway for spread. It is defined as tumour in close proximity to nerve and involving at least one third of its circumference, or tumour cells within any of the three layers of the nerve sheath {2640}, but there is large variability in how to detect and describe it {835}.

Lymphovascular invasion (and surgical resection margin status) is associated with poor overall survival, disease-specific survival, and disease-free survival among patients undergoing salvage total laryngectomy after radiotherapy failure {4504}.

Tumour-infiltrating lymphocytes are strong prognostic factors for both overall survival and disease-free survival, showing a better clinical outcome regardless of the method of assessment {3720}.

Metastatic SCC
Histopathological analysis of neck dissections of clinically node-negative patients reveals occult metastases in 20% of cases. Occult metastases are more frequent in supraglottic tumours

than in glottic tumours, and in advanced (T3–T4) tumours than localized (T1–T2) tumours {4008}.

Extranodal extension is defined as the extension of metastatic tumour (tumour present within the confines of a lymph node and extending through the lymph node capsule) into the surrounding connective tissue, with or without stromal reaction {169}.

Immunohistochemistry
Immunohistochemically, SCCs are usually positive for cytokeratins (e.g. AE1/AE3, CK5, CK5/6, CK14, and CK19) and show nuclear positivity for p63 and p40. CK7, CK20, NUT, CEA, neuroendocrine markers, KIT (CD117), and thyroid transcription factor 1 (TTF1) should be negative.

Differential diagnosis
The differential diagnosis includes other malignant neoplasms with different prognostic significance {2711}, as well as benign conditions such as pseudoepitheliomatous hyperplasia and necrotizing sialometaplasia.

Pseudoepitheliomatous hyperplasia consists of deep, irregular tongues of squamous epithelium mimicking infiltration but lacking cytological atypia and abnormal mitoses. It can be associated with specific diseases such as tuberculosis or other atypical infections {62,4909} or an underlying granular cell

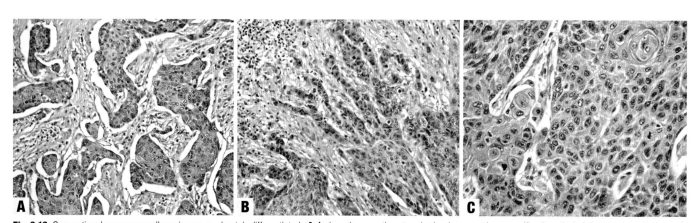

Fig. 3.13 Conventional squamous cell carcinoma, moderately differentiated. **A** An invasive growth pattern is clearly seen at low magnification. **B** An infiltrative growth pattern is evident at the invasive front. **C** At a higher magnification, nuclear atypia is seen, with obvious signs of squamous differentiation (keratinization and intercellular bridges). Mitoses are present in the centre of the nests.

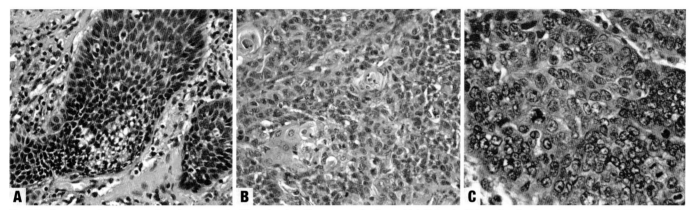

Fig. 3.14 Conventional squamous cell carcinoma, poorly differentiated. **A** The tumour cells show a high N:C ratio. **B** Occasionally, signs of squamous cell differentiation in the form of abrupt and aberrant keratinization can be found. **C** Mitotic count is usually high and includes atypical figures. Nuclear atypia with hyperchromatic nuclei is the rule.

tumour {685,539}. In necrotizing sialometaplasia, deep nests of glandular origin undergo squamous metaplasia; this may also elicit reactive pseudoepitheliomatous hyperplasia {3660,1509}.

Well-differentiated keratinizing and non-keratinizing SCC must be distinguished from verrucous carcinoma and papillary SCC.

Poorly differentiated SCC has a great spectrum of differential diagnostic possibilities. p16 overexpression should not be considered a surrogate for HPV infection, unlike in oropharyngeal carcinomas {2472,4956}. NUT carcinoma shows an abrupt transition between undifferentiated areas and squamous differentiation, and it comprises rather uniform-appearing cells. NUT translocation can be proved by immunohistochemistry, usually in a speckled nuclear pattern, by FISH or RT-PCR {1828}. The differential diagnosis may also include neuroendocrine neoplasms (NENs). These can be identified immunohistochemically with neuroendocrine markers (chromogranin, synaptophysin, INSM1); CD56 should not be considered as evidence of neuroendocrine differentiation. Additional differential diagnostic possibilities are melanoma, which can be distinguished from poorly differentiated SCC by the expression of S100, HMB45, and melan-A; lymphomas, by the presence of CD45 (CLA) and markers of B- and T-cell differentiation; and adenosquamous carcinoma, by the presence of glands and mucin secretion within the tumour cells.

Cytology

Ultrasound-guided FNAC can provide an accurate diagnosis of the primary squamous cell carcinoma, avoiding general anaesthesia and direct laryngoscopic biopsy complications and minimizing the risk of unplanned tracheostomy {3396,75}. The usual keratinizing squamous cell carcinoma can also be diagnosed in cervical lymph node metastases, although some cases may yield extensive keratinous debris.

Diagnostic molecular pathology

Not clinically relevant

Essential and desirable diagnostic criteria

Essential: a malignant epithelial neoplasm with evidence of stromal invasion and squamous differentiation.

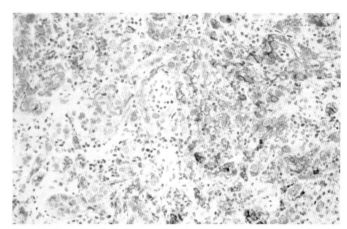

Fig. 3.15 Conventional squamous cell carcinoma. Strong and weak membranous immunohistochemical positivity of PDL1, obtained with the anti-PDL1 22C3 antibody.

Staging

Staging follows the eighth edition of the Union for International Cancer Control (UICC) / American Joint Committee on Cancer (AJCC) TNM staging system.

Prognosis and prediction

The 5-year survival rate for laryngeal cancer is 60.3% in the USA. The site of origin carries prognostic value: glottic tumours show 77% survival at 5 years; supraglottic, 46%; and subglottic, 53%. These figures are related to tumour stage, as most glottic tumours are localized at diagnosis, whereas supraglottic tumours show more frequent regional dissemination due to their richer lymphatic drainage. Nodal status is the single most significant prognostic indicator {553}. Nodal metastases with extranodal extension are associated with worse outcomes than node-negative or node-positive cases without extranodal extension {4727}. Lymph node ratio, calculated as the number of positive lymph nodes divided by the lymph node yield removed through neck dissection, is a valuable prognostic factor for hypopharyngeal and laryngeal tumours {10}. Stage by stage, prognosis in different locations is quite similar {950}. Anterior commissure involvement in T1 glottic tumours is a negative prognostic factor for local recurrence {4512}.

Tumour grading shows controversial results regarding prognosis: whereas a significant prognostic value has been reported

{3987}, prognosis in early-stage laryngeal cancers depends on non-glottic location and T2 (vs T1) stage, but not on histological grade {2530}. Tumour budding predicts distant metastasis and survival {550,2804}. Interobserver variation is the major problem in histological grading. A histological risk model composed of worst pattern of invasion and lymphocytic host response (both at advancing tumour edge) has been proposed, with perineural invasion correlating with local recurrence and overall survival {563}. To date, there is insufficient evidence to include these parameters in the core dataset for pathology reporting {1824}.

Mortality rates differ between the sexes. The prevalence of laryngeal cancer is 25% of head and neck cancers for both men and women, with 28% of head and neck cancer mortality among men and only 12% among women {286}. Mortality is also lower for younger patients (< 40 years) {2620}. Patients with comorbidities have a worse prognosis {3115,1427}.

PDL1-positive tumours show better overall survival. Immune checkpoint inhibitor therapy improves survival in recurrent or metastatic SCC in tumours positive for PDL1, both in tumours with a combined positive score (CPS) of ≥ 1 and in those with CPS ≥ 20 {796,631}.

Adequate surgical margins for glottic cancers are usually limited to 1–2 mm, because in early-stage disease, inadequate margins do not result in worse local control or overall survival {1840,4083}. In advanced laryngeal cancers there are major differences in local control between positive (cut through) and negative (either close [< 5 mm] or clear [≥ 5 mm]) surgical margins {4083}.

The most important prognostic markers in hypopharyngeal carcinomas are the size and extent of local spread, and regional lymph node involvement {1825}. Although the overall prognosis for hypopharyngeal carcinomas is worse than for laryngeal tumours, an improvement in survival has been noted over the past two decades {3195}. Submucosal spread is asymmetrical: larger caudally than laterally, with the shortest spread in the upper direction. This asymmetry could predispose to inadequate margins. Radial clearance < 1 mm is a prognostic factor for overall survival, disease-free survival, and local recurrence-free survival {4083}.

Tracheal SCC has a cumulative survival rate of 48% after 1 year but only 25% after 5 years {1558}.

Verrucous carcinoma of the hypopharynx, larynx, trachea, and parapharyngeal space

Lewis JS Jr
Cardesa A
Helliwell T

Definition

Verrucous carcinoma (VC) is a well-differentiated non-metastasizing squamous cell carcinoma (SCC) that has a spiky keratinized surface and specific architecture, lacks cytological features of malignancy, and is characterized by slow lateral spread and pushing invasion below the level of the adjacent epithelium.

ICD-O coding

8051/3 Verrucous carcinoma, NOS
8070/3 Hybrid verrucous carcinoma

ICD-11 coding

2B6C.0 & XH5PM0 Squamous cell carcinoma of piriform sinus & Verrucous carcinoma, NOS
2B6D.0 & XH5PM0 Squamous cell carcinoma of hypopharynx and variants & Verrucous carcinoma, NOS
2C23.10 & XH5PM0 Squamous cell carcinoma of larynx, glottis & Verrucous carcinoma, NOS
2C23.20 & XH5PM0 Squamous cell carcinoma of larynx, supraglottis & Verrucous carcinoma, NOS
2C23.30 & XH5PM0 Squamous cell carcinoma of larynx, subglottis & Verrucous carcinoma, NOS
2C24.1 & XH5PM0 Squamous cell carcinoma of trachea & Verrucous carcinoma, NOS

Related terminology

Not recommended: Ackerman tumour.

Subtype(s)

Hybrid verrucous carcinoma

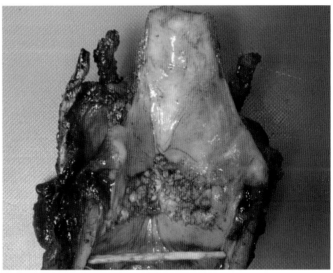

Fig. 3.16 Verrucous carcinoma of the larynx. A large verrucous carcinoma of the true cords from a laryngectomy specimen showing a granular, tan, exophytic mass.

Localization

The larynx is the second most common site of VC in the head and neck, after the oral cavity. Most (~85%) involve the true cords {1365,1211}, but they may arise exclusively in the supraglottis, subglottis, hypopharynx {2348}, or trachea {4224}.

Clinical features

The most common symptoms are hoarseness (90%) and dyspnoea (10%) {1211,2893,3326}. Most patients present with

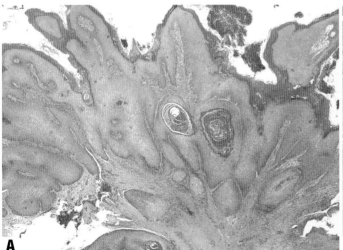
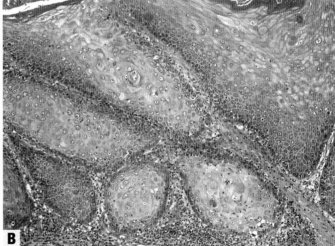

Fig. 3.17 Verrucous carcinoma. **A** Thickened, undulating projections and invaginations of well-differentiated squamous epithelium with marked surface keratinization. The invasive area has well-defined pushing borders extending below the level of the surrounding epithelium. **B** Invaginations and pushing projections of well-differentiated squamous epithelium with one layer of basal cells. The surrounding stroma is densely infiltrated by lymphocytes.

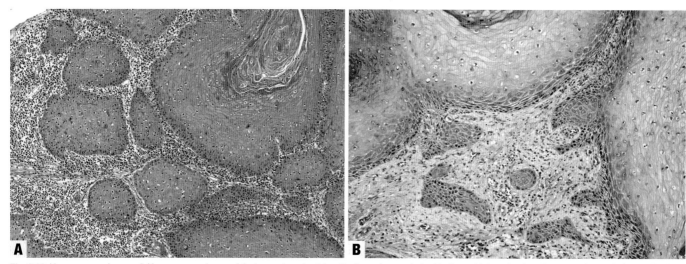

Fig. 3.18 Verrucous carcinoma. **A** Verrucous carcinoma of the larynx. Invasion takes the form of expanded epithelium, which pushes into the stroma in rounded nests that have abundant glassy cytoplasm, round nuclei with prominent nucleoli, and little mitotic activity. There is no stromal reaction. **B** Verrucous carcinoma with stromally invasive conventional squamous cell carcinoma (or hybrid verrucous carcinoma). The tumour shows a large, maturing verrucous component (above) and small, infiltrative, invasive nests (below).

stage I disease {2348}, and radiographic features are similar, stage for stage, to those of conventional SCC.

Epidemiology

VC is more common in men (M:F ratio: 12–14:1) and presents at about 60 years of age {1211}. Laryngeal VC accounts for < 1% of all head and neck carcinomas. As many as 90% of patients are White {2348}. Because VC has primarily been studied in the USA, it is difficult to identify global distribution and trends. Data suggest rates are decreasing over time {1189}.

Etiology

Studies show that VC is associated with smoking, similarly to conventional SCC {2893,2348}. Although early studies suggested an association with high-risk HPV, more recent studies using p16 plus HPV-specific testing and using HPV E6/E7 mRNA detection have shown conclusively that VC is not associated with transcriptionally active HPV {1079,3414,3262}.

Pathogenesis

VC has similar losses in microsatellite markers to well-differentiated, conventional SCC {854}.

Macroscopic appearance

VC presents as a fungating, exophytic, tan to white, broad-based tumour with a granular, shaggy surface. Cut surfaces are firm and tan to white, with clefts and very well defined margins {3326}.

Histopathology

Classic VC consists of thickened, undulating, crowded projections and invaginations of well-differentiated squamous epithelium. There are from one to several layers of basal cells and an extremely expanded spinous layer with cells with extremely prominent, densely eosinophilic cytoplasm, often described as "glassy" {1365}. There is marked surface keratinization and intraepithelial

microabscesses, and *Candida* superinfection may be present. Mitoses are rare and confined to the basal and parabasal cell layers {1211}. Invasion in VC is through a massive expansion in number and volume of cells in the existing squamous epithelium, with preservation of the basement membrane. Thus, the invasive areas of tumour have well-defined, pushing borders with no stromal desmoplasia, although a dense lymphoplasmacytic inflammatory infiltrate is usually present. By definition, VC extends below the level of the surrounding epithelium, and this may be difficult to assess on biopsy specimens. VC should have no more than mild/low-grade cytological pleomorphism. Although severe/high-grade dysplasia and limited carcinoma arising within VC may not necessarily result in worse outcomes {3414}, tumours with these latter features should still be termed invasive ("hybrid VC" or "invasive well-differentiated SCC with verrucous features"). Overtly invasive tumour arising in VC usually has morphological features identical to those of conventional SCC.

Differential diagnosis

The differential diagnosis includes verrucous hyperplasia, which is identical but lacks invasion below the level of the adjacent normal epithelium. Invasive well-differentiated SCC has more atypia, with frank nuclear hyperchromasia and pleomorphism; penicilliform, hyperchromatic basal nuclei; and irregular and infiltrative growth with stromal reaction. Florid pseudoepitheliomatous hyperplasia can be in the differential diagnosis, but this will lack the dense, glassy eosinophilic cytoplasm and bulbous rete, and will have more inflammation – either acute or giant cell / granulomatous, depending on the etiology.

Cytology

Not clinically relevant

Diagnostic molecular pathology

Not relevant

Essential and desirable diagnostic criteria

Essential: acanthotic, hyperkeratotic, and undulating bland squamous epithelium; smooth interface with the stroma; keratotic crypts; mitoses limited to basal/parabasal layers; pushing invasion below the level of the surrounding normal epithelium.

Desirable: dense lymphoplasmacytic submucosal chronic inflammation; glassy, eosinophilic cytoplasm.

Staging

Staging follows the eighth edition of the Union for International Cancer Control (UICC) / American Joint Committee on Cancer (AJCC) TNM staging system and is the same as for conventional laryngeal SCC.

Prognosis and prediction

VC is locally destructive through pushing invasion and expansive growth. It does not metastasize and has better prognosis than does conventional SCC, with reported 5-year survival rates of 85–95% {1211,4708}. Patients are best treated with primary surgery {1370}, although primary radiotherapy may also be effective {2711}. VC with dysplasia appears to have a similar clinical course to that of classic VC, but conventional SCC arising in VC has the potential for metastasis and should be treated as conventional SCC.

Basaloid squamous cell carcinoma

Bishop JA
Wenig BM

Definition
Basaloid squamous cell carcinoma (BSCC) is a distinctive form of squamous cell carcinoma (SCC) characterized by prominent basaloid morphology, squamous differentiation, and aggressive behaviour.

ICD-O coding
8083/3 Basaloid squamous cell carcinoma

ICD-11 coding
2B6C.0 & XH3GS1 Squamous cell carcinoma of piriform sinus & Basaloid squamous cell carcinoma

2B6D.0 & XH3GS1 Squamous cell carcinoma of hypopharynx and variants & Basaloid squamous cell carcinoma

2C23.10 & XH3GS1 Squamous cell carcinoma of larynx, glottis & Basaloid squamous cell carcinoma

2C23.20 & XH3GS1 Squamous cell carcinoma of larynx, supraglottis & Basaloid squamous cell carcinoma

2C23.30 & XH3GS1 Squamous cell carcinoma of larynx, subglottis & Basaloid squamous cell carcinoma

2C24.1 & XH3GS1 Squamous cell carcinoma of trachea & Basaloid squamous cell carcinoma

Related terminology
None

Subtype(s)
None

Localization
Most cases arise in the larynx, particularly the supraglottis; the hypopharynx (piriform sinus) and trachea are less commonly involved {4669,1271,1481,2672}.

Clinical features
Signs and symptoms vary by site and include haemoptysis, dysphagia, neck mass, cough, hoarseness, and otalgia. Patients often present at high stage, with frequent lymph node metastases and occasional distant metastases {1271,1481,2672}.

Epidemiology
BSCC is rare. It tends to affect older patients (27–88 years, median: 63 years), with a striking predilection for White men (80%) {1271,1481,2672}.

Etiology
Laryngeal and hypopharyngeal BSCC is strongly linked to smoking and alcohol consumption {4669,1271,1481,2672}. Typically, high-risk HPV is not found in laryngeal and hypopharyngeal BSCC cases {396,815}.

Pathogenesis
Unknown

Macroscopic appearance
BSCC has a nonspecific gross appearance of a tan-white, firm, poorly defined, endophytic, frequently ulcerated, and/or necrotic mass {1271}.

Histopathology
BSCC is characterized by a prominent basaloid component consisting of primitive-appearing cells with high N:C ratios growing as solid nests and lobules with frequent peripheral palisading. Myxoid to hyaline stromal matrix is often deposited in and between tumour nests, resulting in duct-like formations and a jigsaw puzzle–like or pseudocribriform appearance. Foci of clear cell change are common. The mitotic rate is high, with frequent apoptotic cells and comedonecrosis. Some cases show marked pleomorphism, whereas others appear more monotonous. Most BSCCs also exhibit overt squamous differentiation, in the form of either a component of conventional SCC (often intimately and abruptly associated with the basaloid areas) or dysplasia / carcinoma in situ of the overlying epithelium.

Immunohistochemistry
BSCC is diffusely positive for squamous markers like p40, p63, and CK5/6, and negative for neuroendocrine markers (synaptophysin, chromogranin, INSM1), SMA, S100, and thyroid transcription factor 1 (TTF1) {3981,2593}. It is also frequently positive for SOX10, KIT (CD117), and MYB, which are often unexpected and can result in diagnostic pitfalls {3020,590,3749}.

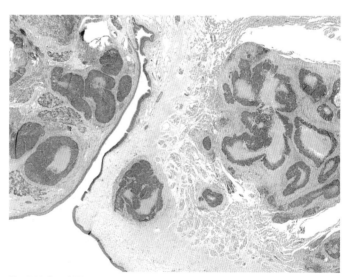

Fig. 3.19 Basaloid squamous cell carcinoma. This classic example consists primarily of infiltrative basaloid nests with comedonecrosis. There is a frequent jigsaw puzzle–like arrangement, with compact basaloid nests separated by thin strands of hyaline material.

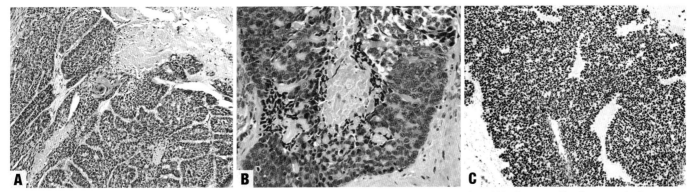

Fig. 3.20 Basaloid squamous cell carcinoma. **A** The tumour is characterized by compact solid nests and trabeculae of basaloid cells arranged in a jigsaw puzzle–like arrangement, separated by myxoid stroma. Abrupt keratinization (centre) and comedonecrosis (upper-right corner) are observed. **B** Within one of the basaloid nests are numerous deposits of hyaline basement membrane–like material, resulting in a pseudocribriform appearance. The tumour cells are pleomorphic, with vesicular chromatin and prominent nucleoli. **C** The tumour is characteristically positive for p40 in a strong, diffuse pattern, which helps to distinguish it from mimics like adenoid cystic carcinoma and small cell carcinoma.

Differential diagnosis

BSCC is distinguished from high-grade neuroendocrine carcinoma (NEC) by its diffuse squamous marker expression (e.g. p40, CK5/6) and lack of neuroendocrine marker (synaptophysin, chromogranin, INSM1) and TTF1 staining. Adenoid cystic carcinoma lacks overt squamous differentiation, exhibits some degree of true ducts and myoepithelial differentiation by immunohistochemistry (e.g. SMA, calponin, S100), is less diffusely positive for p40, and usually harbours a fusion in *MYB*, *MYBL1*, and/or *NFIB*. SOX10, KIT (CD117), and MYB immunostains are not helpful in this differential diagnosis. NUT carcinoma may look similar but is positive for NUT immunohistochemistry. Some HPV-associated oropharyngeal SCCs demonstrate prominent basaloid features but behave much more indolently and should be separated from BSCC {396}. Accordingly, direct detection assays for high-risk HPV must be performed on a laryngeal/hypopharyngeal BSCC that also involves the oropharynx.

Cytology

Smears show variably sized, tightly cohesive tissue fragments made up of basaloid cells with high N:C ratios, small to medium-sized round to oval hyperchromatic nuclei with granular chromatin, and single small nucleoli. The cytoplasm is scant, with moulding and apoptotic debris tending to be present. Single cells in variable numbers can be seen. Chromatinic smearing is not seen. Numerous mitotic figures are present, and the background is frequently necrotic. Single keratinized cells are a helpful clue, but keratinization is often scarce or absent {333,895, 2845}. Fragments of irregular magenta (Giemsa stain) basement membrane material can be present, and the differential

diagnosis includes adenoid cystic carcinoma, with its lesser degree of nuclear atypia and more rounded, sharply demarcated basement membrane material {895}.

Diagnostic molecular pathology

High-risk HPV is not typically found in laryngeal/hypopharyngeal BSCC {4669,815}.

Essential and desirable diagnostic criteria

Essential: a tumour with prominent basaloid morphology; presence of squamous differentiation and absence of neuroendocrine or myoepithelial differentiation by histology and/or immunohistochemistry.

Desirable: high-grade histological features, myxoid to hyaline stromal alterations.

Staging

Staging follows the eighth edition of the Union for International Cancer Control (UICC) / American Joint Committee on Cancer (AJCC) TNM staging system.

Prognosis and prediction

BSCC is traditionally regarded as an aggressive type of hypopharyngeal and laryngeal SCC, with most studies finding higher rates of nodal metastasis and distant metastasis, and worse overall and disease-free survival, than for conventional SCC. Some recent studies, however, have disputed the notion that BSCC behaves differently when matched stage for stage {1271, 1481,2672}. Studies that include more indolent HPV-associated oropharyngeal cases in their cohorts confound interpretation.

Papillary squamous cell carcinoma

Stelow EB
Wenig BM

Definition

Papillary squamous cell carcinoma (PSCC) grows exophytically, with papillary fronds covered by a malignant stratified squamous epithelium or with immature basaloid cells with minimal or no maturation.

ICD-O coding

8052/3 Papillary squamous cell carcinoma

ICD-11 coding

2B6C.0 & XH6S97 Squamous cell carcinoma of piriform sinus & Papillary squamous cell carcinoma

2B6D.0 & XH6S97 Squamous cell carcinoma of hypopharynx and variants & Papillary squamous cell carcinoma

2C23.10 & XH0UU4 Squamous cell carcinoma of larynx, glottis & Papillary squamous cell carcinoma

2C23.20 & XH0UU4 Squamous cell carcinoma of larynx, supraglottis & Papillary squamous cell carcinoma

2C23.30 & XH0UU4 Squamous cell carcinoma of larynx, subglottis & Papillary squamous cell carcinoma

2C24.1 & XH6S97 Squamous cell carcinoma of trachea & Papillary squamous cell carcinoma

Related terminology

None

Subtype(s)

None

Localization

Tumours can occur throughout the larynx and hypopharynx. The majority are glottic, supraglottic, and transglottic {4423}.

Clinical features

Patients most often present with hoarseness {4423}. Other symptoms can include dysphagia, sore throat, cough, and haemoptysis.

Imaging

This should be performed as per conventional laryngeal squamous cell carcinoma (SCC) and may demonstrate an exophytic soft tissue lesion.

Epidemiology

Tumours are much more common in men and are usually identified in or after the sixth decade of life {4423}.

Etiology

Tumours are related to tobacco and alcohol consumption and high-risk HPV infection at similar ratios to other non-keratinizing squamous cell carcinomas from the head and neck at the various subsites {4423,908,2107}.

Pathogenesis

The tumours are believed to arise through multistep squamous metaplasia and dysplasia {854,3992}.

Macroscopic appearance

Tumours have a grossly papillary appearance and lack grossly evident keratinization {4268}. They are typically friable and soft, and they vary in size.

Histopathology

Tumours are composed of numerous complex papillary and filiform structures extending in all planes, which often renders the assessment of definitive tissue invasion difficult {4215}. The papillary fronds are covered with a stratified squamous epithelium, which has overt features of malignancy, replete with lack

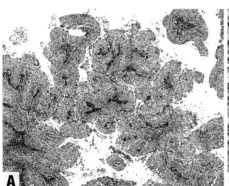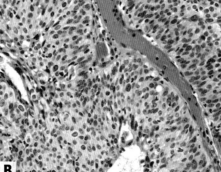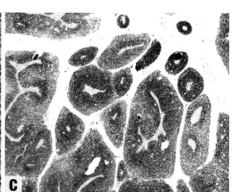

Fig. 3.21 Papillary squamous cell carcinoma. **A** This low-power image highlights the numerous delicate papillae seen with papillary squamous cell carcinoma. **B** At higher magnification, the papillae are covered by a malignant stratified squamous epithelium. **C** Diffuse, block-like p16 expression is seen with this hypopharyngeal papillary squamous cell carcinoma that was secondary to high-risk HPV infection.

of maturation, increased N:C ratios, nuclear irregularities, and numerous mitotic figures located throughout the entire thickness of the epithelium. These morphological features are related to the non-keratinizing type of PSCC. The keratinizing type shows papillae covered with high-grade keratinizing dysplasia {4782}. Koilocytic change is sometimes noted {4423}. Intracellular keratinization or dyskeratosis may be present; however, surface keratosis is most often not seen. The papillary fronds have fibrovascular cores that usually contain lymphocytes and plasma cells. The invasive component, when identified, will have infiltrating, irregular nests of squamous epithelium morphologically identical to most non-keratinizing SCCs.

Immunohistochemistry
Typical block-like p16 expression is seen with tumours secondary to high-risk HPV, especially in the non-keratinizing type, although testing by immunostaining is not currently recommended {2107}.

Differential diagnosis
Tumours must be distinguished from verrucous carcinoma, a tumour that typically has surface keratinization and lacks the atypia seen with PSCC. Laryngeal papillomas usually lack the cytological atypia of PSCC.

Cytology
Not clinically relevant

Diagnostic molecular pathology
Not relevant

Essential and desirable diagnostic criteria
Essential: exophytic growth composed predominantly of papillary fronds covered by a non-keratinizing malignant stratified squamous epithelium or, in the keratinizing type, by high-grade atypia.
Desirable: stromal infiltration.

Staging
Staging follows the eighth edition of the Union for International Cancer Control (UICC) / American Joint Committee on Cancer (AJCC) TNM staging system.

Prognosis and prediction
Tumours behave, stage for stage, similarly to or slightly better than conventional SCC at the site {908}. Because of their exophytic growth, they may be more likely to present at an early stage. Given the infrequency of high-risk HPV at many sites within the upper aerodigestive tract, it is unclear whether infection affects prognosis at sites outside of the oropharynx {2107}.

Spindle cell squamous cell carcinoma

Hernandez-Prera JC
Bishop JA
Zidar N

Definition
Spindle cell squamous cell carcinoma (SCSCC) is composed of spindle and/or epithelioid pleomorphic cells and is usually associated with intraepithelial dysplasia and/or invasive conventional squamous cell carcinoma (SCC).

ICD-O coding
8074/3 Squamous cell carcinoma, spindle cell

ICD-11 coding
2B6D.0 & XH6D80 Squamous cell carcinoma of piriform sinus & Squamous cell carcinoma, spindle cell
2B6D.0 & XH6D80 Squamous cell carcinoma of hypopharynx and variants & Squamous cell carcinoma, spindle cell
2C23.10 & XH6D80 Squamous cell carcinoma of larynx, glottis & Squamous cell carcinoma, spindle cell
2C23.20 & XH6D80 Squamous cell carcinoma of larynx, supraglottis & Squamous cell carcinoma, spindle cell
2C23.30 & XH6D80 Squamous cell carcinoma of larynx, subglottis & Squamous cell carcinoma, spindle cell
2C24.1 & XH6D80 Squamous cell carcinoma of trachea & Squamous cell carcinoma, spindle cell

Related terminology
Acceptable: spindle cell carcinoma; sarcomatoid carcinoma.
Not recommended: carcinosarcoma; pseudosarcoma.

Subtype(s)
None

Localization
The larynx is the most common site for SCSCC, followed by the oral cavity, sinonasal tract, oropharynx, nasopharynx, and

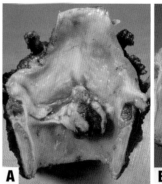
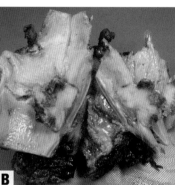

Fig. 3.22 Spindle cell squamous cell carcinoma. **A** Typical macroscopic appearance of laryngeal spindle cell squamous cell carcinoma showing a polypoid, bossed tumour of the glottis. **B** The cut surface of spindle cell squamous cell carcinoma is fleshy and haemorrhagic.

lastly the hypopharynx {1357,1135}. In the larynx, three quarters of cases involve the glottis {3296,4425}.

Clinical features
Hoarseness is a common symptom. An exophytic firm mass limited to the vocal cords is usually seen on a laryngoscopy examination {3296,4425}.

Imaging
Imaging is as per conventional SCC, most often with postcontrast CT.

Epidemiology
SCSCC represents < 1% of all laryngeal malignancies, occurs across a wide age range, has a peak incidence in the fifth and sixth decades of life, and shows a striking male predisposition {4425,1188,3692}.

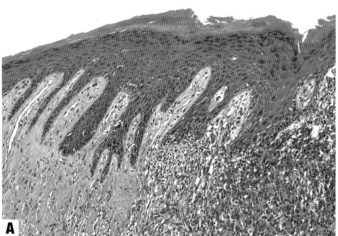
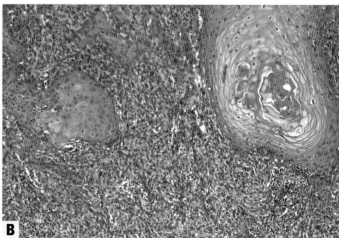

Fig. 3.23 Spindle cell squamous cell carcinoma. **A** Associated with high-grade keratinizing dysplasia. **B** Associated with a well-differentiated squamous cell carcinoma.

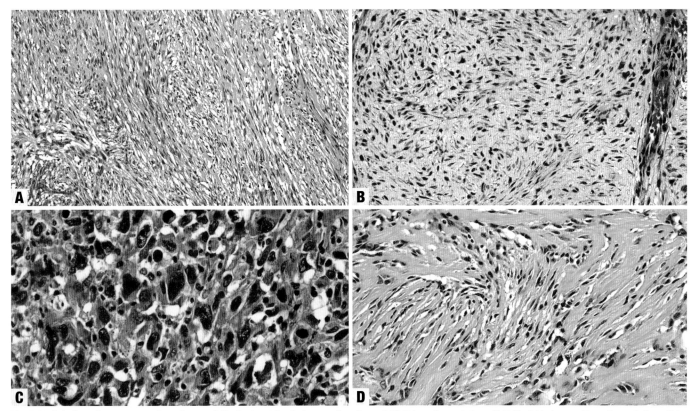

Fig. 3.24 Spindle cell squamous cell carcinoma. **A** Predominant fascicular growth pattern. **B** Stellate cell morphology. **C** Epithelioid pleomorphic cell morphology. **D** Increased stromal collagenization.

Etiology

Tobacco and alcohol abuse are strongly associated with SCSCC. Radiation history has been reported in a subset of patients {4425}. Regardless of location, the identification of high-risk HPV in SCSCC is rare {4744,476}.

Pathogenesis

SCSCC is an epithelial malignancy that has undergone epithelial–mesenchymal transition {1830,5050,2355,5048}.

Macroscopic appearance

SCSCC is usually a grossly polypoid tumour {4425}.

Histopathology

The histological hallmark of SCSCC is the presence of a spindle cell proliferation at a mucosa-based site. The spindle cells usually show overt pleomorphism, hyperchromasia, and increased mitotic activity. On rare occasions, SCSCC can exhibit bland cytomorphology, and tumour cells can have an epithelioid morphology. Most tumours are hypercellular and arranged in a diversity of patterns (fascicular, storiform, cartwheel). Hypocellular variants with increased stromal collagenization exist. Surface ulceration is common, and most tumours contain a certain degree of acute/chronic inflammation. The spindle cell component generally predominates; however, some tumours exhibit a biphasic morphology secondary to the presence of a differentiated SCC component. The latter can be in the form of intraepithelial dysplasia and/or invasive conventional SCC.

Heterologous differentiation occurs in up to 7% of cases and includes osseocartilaginous and rhabdomyoblastic elements {1633,4425,3776,3592}.

Immunohistochemistry

SCSCC shows variable reactivity for cytokeratin in 48–83% of cases {4988,1237,1830,2587,4425,207,476}. Immunoreactivity for p63 and p40 often mirrors the reactivity of cytokeratin; however, these are sometimes the only positive markers {2597,476}. SCSCC is consistently positive for vimentin and may express other mesenchymal markers, particularly SMA {4425,4641, 3592}. SCSCC exhibits a wide range of Ki-67 labelling, and a low proliferation index can be observed {3592}.

Differential diagnosis

Granulation tissue with reactive stromal changes, particularly after radiotherapy, can be distinguished from SCSCC by the lack of p40 reactivity {476}. Laryngeal sarcomas are extremely rare, and the most common one is chondrosarcoma {4617}. Therefore, in the absence of cytokeratin and/or p63/p40 reactivity, a mucosa-based malignant spindle cell neoplasm is SCSCC until proved otherwise. In such cases, careful evaluation of the overlying and adjacent mucosa is necessary and may identify intraepithelial dysplasia. Inflammatory myofibroblastic tumour can occur in the larynx and most commonly affects the glottis {4784}; it is characterized by various gene rearrangements involving *ALK*, *ROS1*, and *NTRK3*, not described in SCSCC {4904}.

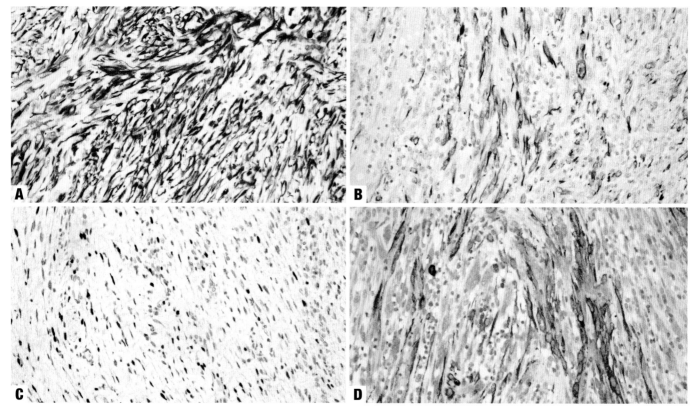

Fig. 3.25 Spindle cell squamous cell carcinoma. **A** Diffuse and strong pancytokeratin reactivity. **B** Focal pancytokeratin reactivity. **C** Focal p63 reactivity. **D** Weak SMA reactivity.

Cytology

Cellularity may be low and shows spindle cells with variable pleomorphism, sometimes admixed with epithelioid squamous cells showing varying degrees of keratinization with dense, well-defined cytoplasm and large hyperchromatic, pleomorphic nuclei {895}. The spindle cells can be seen singly, with poorly defined cytoplasm and hyperchromatic oval to (in some cases) large nuclei with large nucleoli. Multinucleation may be seen, and the differential diagnosis in the absence of the more characteristic keratinized squamous cells can include a sarcoma or melanoma.

Diagnostic molecular pathology

Not relevant

Essential and desirable diagnostic criteria

Essential: a mucosa-based carcinoma with a malignant spindle cell component.

Desirable: a polypoid tumour; intraepithelial dysplasia; invasive conventional SCC; immunoreactivity for cytokeratin and/or p63/p40 (in selected cases).

Staging

Staging follows the eighth edition of the Union for International Cancer Control (UICC) / American Joint Committee on Cancer (AJCC) TNM staging system.

Prognosis and prediction

The majority (62.1%) of laryngeal SCSCCs present as T1 tumours, compared with 10% of those in the hypopharynx {1188,1005}. In the larynx, the disease-specific survival rate at 10 years is 57.9%, comparable to that for conventional SCC. A glottic location confers a survival benefit due to early detection {4425,1571,1188}. The disease-specific overall survival rate for hypopharyngeal SCSCC at 10 years is 8%, significantly lower than that for conventional SCC {1005}. Tumours with a conventional SCC component appear to have a better prognosis {3592}. Radiotherapy-induced tumours have a worse prognosis than those arising de novo {4425}.

Adenosquamous carcinoma

Prasad ML
Wenig BM

Definition
Adenosquamous carcinoma (ASC) is a biphasic malignant tumour that arises from the surface epithelium and shows squamous and glandular differentiation.

ICD-O coding
8560/3 Adenosquamous carcinoma

ICD-11 coding
2B6D.Y & XH7873 Other specified malignant neoplasms of piriform sinus & Adenosquamous carcinoma

2B6D.Y & XH7873 Other specified malignant neoplasms of hypopharynx & Adenosquamous carcinoma

2C23.1Y & XH7873 Other specified malignant neoplasms of larynx, glottis & Adenosquamous carcinoma

2C23.2Y & XH7873 Other specified malignant neoplasms of larynx, supraglottis & Adenosquamous carcinoma

2C23.3Y & XH7873 Other specified malignant neoplasms of larynx, subglottis & Adenosquamous carcinoma

2C24.Y & XH7873 Other specified malignant neoplasms of trachea & Adenosquamous carcinoma

Related terminology
None

Subtype(s)
None

Localization
The larynx is the most frequently affected site in the head and neck {2205}, followed by the oral, pharyngeal, and sinonasal mucosa {2867,2534}.

Clinical features
Clinical symptoms are similar to those of squamous cell carcinoma (SCC) and include hoarseness, sore throat, dysphagia, haemoptysis, and/or a neck mass {2711}.

Epidemiology
ASC is rare and affects men 2–4 times as frequently as women, without any race predilection. The peak incidence is in the seventh and eighth decades of life (median: 66 years, range: 43–88 years) {2205,1191,2534}.

Etiology
As with SCC, smoking and alcohol consumption are likely predisposing factors {2240}. An association with HPV has been reported in ASC of the oropharynx and nasal cavity but not ASC of the larynx or hypopharynx {2867}.

Pathogenesis
Little is known about the etiopathogenesis of ASC, mainly because of its rarity and a lack of larger, controlled studies {2867}. However, cigarette smoking and alcohol consumption probably play an important role in the pathogenesis of ASC, similarly to other subtypes of SCC {135}.

Macroscopic appearance
Most ASCs present as glottic or supraglottic exophytic or polypoid masses (median size: 40 mm) or as mucosal induration or ulceration, similarly to SCC {1191}.

Histopathology
ASC has a biphasic morphology showing squamous and glandular differentiation. The squamous carcinoma is generally superficial and associated with dysplasia of the surface epithelium, and it may show keratinization including keratin pearls, whereas adenocarcinoma tends to be deeper and consists of

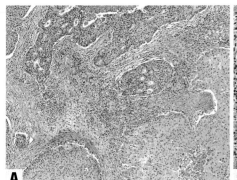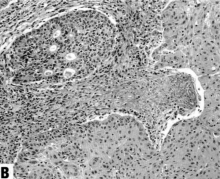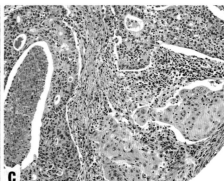

Fig. 3.26 Adenosquamous carcinoma. **A** Low-magnification view showing distinct areas of squamous carcinoma (right) and adenocarcinoma (left). The latter shows tubular structures and necrosis. **B** Higher-magnification view showing squamous carcinoma (right) and adenocarcinoma (left) adjacent to each other. **C** Higher-magnification view showing squamous carcinoma (lower-right corner) and adenocarcinoma (upper-right corner and left side) with necrosis.

Table 3.02 Differentiating adenosquamous carcinoma from mucoepidermoid carcinoma

Adenosquamous carcinoma	Mucoepidermoid carcinoma
Dysplastic changes in the overlying squamous epithelium	Dysplastic changes absent
Evidence of keratinization in the squamous component, including keratin pearls	Keratinization absent
Distinct squamous and glandular components adjacent to each other, with the former in the superficial part and the latter in the deeper infiltrative part of the tumour; mucin is often present but is not required for diagnosis	Columnar, mucinous, and squamous cells are closely intermixed within lobules of tumour; tumour cells with intracytoplasmic mucin are required for diagnosis
Secondary invasion of benign submucosal glands that maintain their bland cytomorphology	Originates in submucosal glands
Intermediate cells absent	Intermediate cells present
MAML2 translocation absent	*MAML2* translocation usually present {2205}

cribriform and tubuloglandular structures. Mucous cells may be present. The two components are distinct, separate or intermixed. Areas of transition and an undifferentiated basaloid or clear cell component may be seen {4409}. Necrosis, mitoses, and vascular and perineural invasion are frequent. Metastatic ASC may display one or both components.

Special stains
PAS, Alcian blue, and mucicarmine may demonstrate intraluminal (or, rarely, intracytoplasmic) mucin.

Immunohistochemistry
The tumour shows p63 expression in the squamous component, and CEA and low-molecular-weight cytokeratin (CAM5.2) in the adenocarcinomatous component. CK7 and high-molecular-weight cytokeratin may be seen in both components {2428}. CK20 is usually negative {2772}. Because CK7 may be focally expressed in head and neck SCC, the diagnosis requires the presence of distinct squamous and adenocarcinomatous components adjacent to each other on H&E.

Differential diagnosis
The differential diagnosis includes mucoepidermoid carcinoma (MEC) and adenoid, conventional, and basaloid SCC patterns invading submucous seromucinous glands. Distinction from MEC is important, because ASC has a worse prognosis (see Table 3.02). Demonstration of intracytoplasmic mucin and CEA helps to distinguish ASC from adenoid SCC. SCC invading or entrapping seromucinous glands is differentiated by a lobular architecture and the benign cytomorphology of the glandular cells. Basaloid SCC shows peripheral palisading and lacks glandular differentiation {4409}. Necrotizing sialometaplasia, rarely seen in the larynx, retains the lobular architecture of the seromucous glands (despite being replaced by squamous metaplasia) and may be associated with ischaemic necrosis of the acini, chronic inflammation, and pseudoepitheliomatous hyperplasia of the overlying squamous epithelium. Superficial

biopsies may be misdiagnosed as SCC because the glandular component tends to be deeper.

Cytology
Metastases may show features of predominantly keratinizing or non-keratinizing SCC with a lesser glandular component {895}.

Diagnostic molecular pathology
CRTC1::MAML2 translocation is important in distinguishing ASC from MEC. The *MAML2* translocation excludes the diagnosis of ASC, although negativity does not necessarily exclude MEC, especially high-grade MEC {2205}.

Essential and desirable diagnostic criteria
Essential: biphasic tumour with squamous and glandular components that are distinctly recognized adjacent to each other on H&E examination.
Desirable: evidence of origin from surface epithelium (e.g. squamous dysplasia); mucin production.

Staging
Staging follows the eighth edition of the Union for International Cancer Control (UICC) / American Joint Committee on Cancer (AJCC) TNM staging system.

Prognosis and prediction
ASC is more aggressive than conventional SCC, presenting at an advanced stage, with involvement of lymph nodes in 40% of cases and distant metastases in 10% of cases {1191}. Despite surgery and adjuvant chemotherapy and radiotherapy, tumours frequently recur and metastasize {1362,135}. The median survival is < 3 years, and 5-year survival rates range from 30% to 50% {2205,1191}. Advanced age and stage and large tumour size are associated with decreased survival {2534}. HPV-associated ASC in the oropharynx appears to have a better prognosis, like HPV-associated SCC {2867}.

Lymphoepithelial carcinoma of the larynx

Bishop JA
Nadal A
Wenig BM

Definition

Lymphoepithelial carcinoma (LEC) is a poorly differentiated form of squamous cell carcinoma characterized by its morphological similarity to the non-keratinizing, undifferentiated form of nasopharyngeal carcinoma.

ICD-O coding

8082/3 Lymphoepithelial carcinoma

ICD-11 coding

2B6C.0 & XH1E40 Squamous cell carcinoma of piriform sinus & Lymphoepithelial carcinoma

2B6D.0 & XH1E40 Squamous cell carcinoma of hypopharynx and variants & Lymphoepithelial carcinoma

2C23.10 & XH1E40 Squamous cell carcinoma of larynx, glottis & Lymphoepithelial carcinoma

2C23.20 & XH1E40 Squamous cell carcinoma of larynx, supraglottis & Lymphoepithelial carcinoma

2C23.30 & XH1E40 Squamous cell carcinoma of larynx, subglottis & Lymphoepithelial carcinoma

2C24.1 & XH1E40 Squamous cell carcinoma of trachea & Lymphoepithelial carcinoma

Related terminology

Not recommended: lymphoepithelial-like carcinoma; lymphoepithelioma; lymphoepithelioma-like carcinoma; undifferentiated carcinoma of the nasopharyngeal type; undifferentiated carcinoma with lymphoid stroma.

Subtype(s)

None

Localization

LEC occurs more frequently in the larynx (usually supraglottis) than the hypopharynx (piriform sinus), with only rare tracheal involvement {3311,4336,2523,1319}.

Clinical features

Patients present with hoarseness, neck mass, dysphonia, dysphagia, neck pain, and/or haemoptysis {2767,1174,4779,1319}.

Epidemiology

LEC of the larynx, hypopharynx, and trachea is rare, with < 50 reported cases. There is a marked male predominance, and it affects older patients (mean: 62 years). Unlike nasopharyngeal carcinoma, which most frequently affects people of Asian descent, laryngeal LEC usually occurs in White people {2987,3311,4204,2767,1174,4991,2523,4336,4779,2253,744}.

Etiology

Laryngeal/hypopharyngeal LEC is associated with smoking and alcohol consumption {2767,1174,4779}. Only rare cases are EBV-associated, but a subset harbour high-risk HPV {4991,4779,2253,25}.

Pathogenesis

LEC frequently harbours *TP53* mutations.

Macroscopic appearance

LEC appears as a nonspecific white, tan, or pink mass that may be endophytic or polypoid {2767}.

Histopathology

LEC is defined by its resemblance to undifferentiated nasopharyngeal carcinoma: sheet-like or nested architecture with syncytial growth, a prominent lymphoplasmacytic cell infiltrate, and tumour cells with vesicular chromatin and prominent

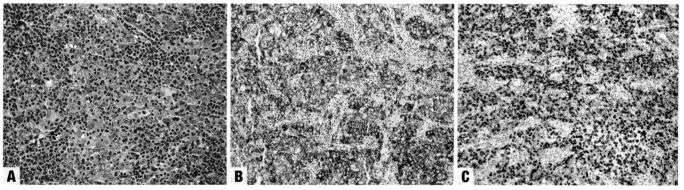

Fig. 3.27 Lymphoepithelial carcinoma. **A** The tumour is composed of large cells with indistinct cell borders and round nuclei with vesicular chromatin and prominent nucleoli, along with an intense infiltrate of chronic inflammatory cells. **B** The carcinoma expresses cytokeratins (AE1/AE3 immunocytochemistry). **C** The carcinoma shows strong nuclear expression of p40.

nucleoli. Mitotic figures and apoptotic cells are common. LEC can be pure or mixed with conventional squamous cell carcinoma either in the invasive tumour or in the surface epithelium (i.e. carcinoma in situ).

Immunohistochemistry
LEC is diffusely positive for pancytokeratin, and usually positive for squamous markers like CK5/6 and p40/p63.

Differential diagnosis
LEC is distinguished from large cell lymphoma and melanoma by its positivity for pancytokeratin and lack of staining for lymphoid markers (e.g. CD45, CD30, CD20) and melanoma markers (e.g. SOX10, S100, HMB45). Absence of EBV helps exclude spread from the nasopharynx.

Cytology
Not clinically relevant

Diagnostic molecular pathology
LECs are almost always negative for EBV, but a subset harbour high-risk HPV {2767,4991,4779,2253,25}.

Essential and desirable diagnostic criteria
Essential: a tumour with syncytial growth; inflammatory infiltrate; vesicular chromatin; prominent nucleoli.
Desirable: positivity for pankeratin and squamous markers (e.g. p40, CK5/6); exclusion of direct extension or metastasis.

Staging
Staging follows the eighth edition of the Union for International Cancer Control (UICC) / American Joint Committee on Cancer (AJCC) TNM staging system.

Prognosis and prediction
Laryngeal LEC has a 5-year disease-specific survival rate of approximately 65% {744,1319}. Regional lymph node metastasis occurs in 50–75%, with distant metastasis in 20–25% {2767, 1319}.

Laryngeal cartilaginous tumours

Thompson LDR
Hernandez-Prera JC
Magliocca K

Definition
Chondroma is a benign mesenchymal tumour of laryngeal hyaline cartilage. Chondrosarcoma is a malignant mesenchymal tumour of laryngeal hyaline cartilage.

ICD-O coding
9220/0 Chondroma
9220/3 Chondrosarcoma
9242/3 Clear cell chondrosarcoma
9243/3 Dedifferentiated chondrosarcoma

ICD-11 coding
2E90.6 & XH0NS4 Benign neoplasm of nasopharynx & Chondroma, NOS
2B6B.Y & XH8J23 Other specified malignant neoplasms of nasopharynx & Chondrosarcoma, NOS

Related terminology
None

Subtype(s)
Clear cell chondrosarcoma; dedifferentiated chondrosarcoma

Localization
Cricoid cartilage is the most common site (~70%) for laryngeal cartilaginous tumours, followed by the thyroid, arytenoid, and tracheal cartilages {2585,4415,296,3291,2514}; the epiglottis is rarely affected {4415,855}.

Clinical features
Both tumours grow slowly, producing an endolaryngeal mass, with symptoms depending on tumour site and size. Slowly progressive hoarseness, dyspnoea, dysphagia, and stridor are

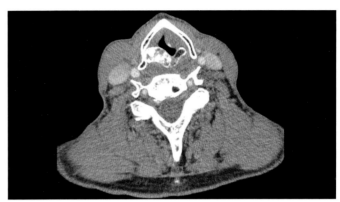

Fig. 3.28 Laryngeal chondrosarcoma. The posterior lamina of the cricoid cartilage is destroyed by a neoplasm with popcorn-type calcification (CT, axial plane).

usually present. Thyroid cartilage tumours may be a palpable mass {4415,296,3291}.

Imaging
High-resolution contrast-enhanced CT of laryngeal chondrosarcoma shows ring-like, arc, or popcorn calcifications within an expansile, bulky, destructive intracartilaginous mass below an intact mucosal surface. The tumour frequently expands outward into the perilaryngeal soft tissues. MRI shows a hyperintense mass on the T2 fat-suppressed short-tau inversion recovery (STIR) protocol {4834,4716,4415,296,389}. FDG PET may help with tumour grading, metastasis detection, and local recurrence assessment {3291}.

Epidemiology
Cartilaginous tumours account for 0.2–0.5% of all laryngeal tumours, with chondrosarcomas (the most common laryngeal

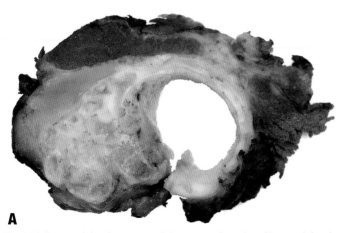

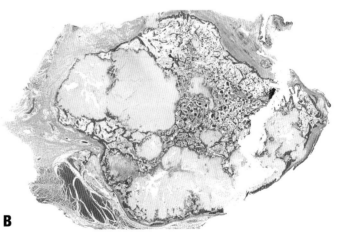

Fig. 3.29 Laryngeal chondrosarcoma. **A** A macroscopic section of laryngeal chondrosarcoma showing extension of the translucent cartilaginous tumour into the adjacent soft tissues. **B** A low-power image demonstrates islands of destructively invasive chondrocytes, expanding the bony trabeculae and extending into the perilaryngeal soft tissues.

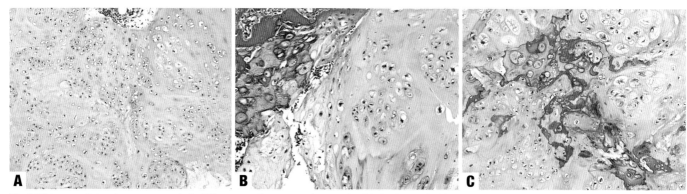

Fig. 3.30 Laryngeal chondrosarcoma, grade 1. **A** The tumour demonstrates increased cellularity, but no significant atypia. Cluster disarray is present. **B** Ischaemic change (granular blue cytoplasmic degeneration) is noted in the adjacent chondroma (left), and chondrosarcoma is noted on the right. **C** Calcification and residual bone from the endochondral ossification of the laryngeal cartilages may be seen within the background of the chondrosarcoma.

sarcomas) being significantly more common than chondromas {2585,697,1374,913,1190,3291,3873,4617}. Chondromas occur across a wide patient age range (24–79 years, median: 56 years), with an M:F ratio of 2.1 {2585}. Chondrosarcomas develop in slightly older patients, with a wide patient age range (25–91 years, median: 62 years), and the M:F ratio is 3.2:1 {2585,4415,1190,3291,842}. Chondrosarcomas are significantly more common in White people than in Black people (ratio: 7:1) {296}.

Etiology

The etiology is unknown, with several hypotheses, including the disordered ossification of hyaline cartilage in areas of muscle insertion {296}, and ischaemic changes in chondroma leading to malignant transformation {4415}. Other possible predisposing factors are radiotherapy, polytetrafluoroethylene (Teflon) injection, and repeated laryngeal trauma {1606,1736,3291}.

Pathogenesis

IDH1 and *IDH2* gene mutations are commonly seen in central-type chondrosarcomas, but they are detected in only 12% of laryngotracheal cases tested, suggesting an alternate tumorigenesis in laryngeal tumours {4348}.

Macroscopic appearance

Both tumours present as smooth, lobulated, submucosal masses with an intact mucosa. The cut surfaces are glassy, firm, white, or grey. Chondromas are ≤ 20 mm in greatest dimension, whereas chondrosarcomas are as large as 120 mm (median: 35 mm). Dedifferentiated chondrosarcomas have foci with a fleshy appearance {2585,4415,1540,697}.

Histopathology

Chondromas show mature hyaline cartilage histologically resembling normal cartilage and are hypocellular, with evenly distributed, bland-looking tumour cells in an abundant basophilic matrix. Chondrocytes have small, uniform, single nuclei surrounded by eosinophilic cytoplasm, with only one cell per lacuna. Cellular pleomorphism, mitoses, and binucleated chondrocytes are absent. Scattered foci of calcification and ossification may be seen.

Chondrosarcomas show a gradient of increased cellularity, pleomorphism, multinucleation, and mitoses, features used in tumour grading. Most laryngeal chondrosarcomas are low-grade (grade 1), showing a pattern of lobular disarray and destructive invasion of native cartilage and bone, with tumour lobules permeating and entrapping pre-existing bone trabeculae. The

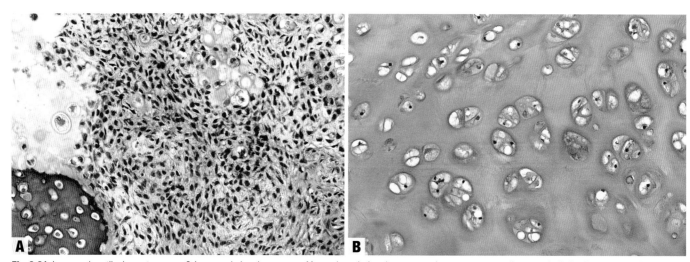

Fig. 3.31 Laryngeal cartilaginous tumours. **A** Laryngeal chondrosarcoma. Mesenchymal chondrosarcoma demonstrates a malignant spindled cell component immediately adjacent to islands of cartilaginous differentiation. **B** Laryngeal chondroma. There is a slightly increased cellularity within normally spaced chondrocytes that do not show cluster disarray. These tumours are < 20 mm by definition, without destructive growth by imaging.

cellularity is higher than in chondromas, with binucleation, slight nuclear pleomorphism, and nuclear hyperchromasia. Moderately differentiated (grade 2) tumours show a higher degree of cellularity and nuclear pleomorphism than do grade 1 tumours, and they may have scattered mitoses. The myxoid pattern {4415,297} shows a string-of-pearls pattern of neoplastic cells in a myxoid background. High-grade (grade 3) tumours have high cellularity; significant multinucleation, nuclear pleomorphism, and hyperchromasia; tumour necrosis; and increased mitoses. High-grade chondrosarcomas are rare, accounting for only about 5% of all laryngeal chondrosarcomas {4415}. Ossification and calcification can be seen in all tumour grades {2585,4415,296}.

Subtypes

These are rare in the larynx. Clear cell chondrosarcoma shows a sharp transition of conventional chondrosarcoma to a proliferation of tightly packed, large polygonal clear tumour cells with distinct cellular membranes but lacking the typical dense chondroid matrix {3808,2322,462,99,1839}. Dedifferentiated chondrosarcoma shows a biphasic appearance, with well-differentiated chondrosarcoma juxtaposed to a high-grade non-cartilaginous sarcoma {4415,1540,3700,3607,1388,2775,790}. Mesenchymal chondrosarcoma (separately discussed in *Mesenchymal chondrosarcoma*, p. 418) is an extremely rare malignancy of the larynx with a biphasic small blue round cell proliferation associated with islands of differentiated hyaline cartilage {1681,4411}.

Immunohistochemistry

Immunohistochemistry is rarely necessary, but the chondroid cells are immunoreactive for S100, SOX9, and D2-40, and negative for keratin and EMA {3758,1970,3858,2881}.

Differential diagnosis

The major differential is between chondroma and chondrosarcoma, and a size cut-off point of > 20 mm has been suggested to favour chondrosarcoma. However, in incisional biopsy or needle samples, distinction may be difficult. Some low-grade chondrosarcomas of the larynx may be better diagnosed as an atypical cartilaginous neoplasm, as is done at other sites {1216}, but without supporting evidence for laryngeal tumours specifically, this terminology is not advocated. Chondrometaplasia usually shows multiple elastic cartilage nodules affecting the vocal cord that blend into the adjacent stroma {87}. A spindle cell squamous cell carcinoma may have heterologous benign or malignant cartilage elements, but the cartilage is set within a malignant spindled epithelial cell population {4425}.

Cytology

Not clinically relevant

Diagnostic molecular pathology

Not clinically relevant

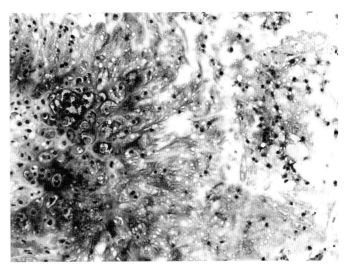

Fig. 3.32 Laryngeal chondrosarcoma. Myxoid pattern of chondrosarcoma, demonstrating myxoid change around the chondrocytes.

Essential and desirable diagnostic criteria

Chondroma

Essential: a lobular cartilaginous tumour without pleomorphism, binucleation, or destructive growth.
Desirable: tumour size ≤ 20 mm.

Chondrosarcoma

Essential: a malignant cartilaginous neoplasm with lobular cluster disarray, with destructive invasion of native cartilage and/or bone; increased cellularity with binucleation, nuclear pleomorphism, and nuclear hyperchromasia.
Desirable: imaging findings of an expansile, destructive intracartilaginous mass, usually with ring-like, arc, or popcorn calcifications.

Staging

Staging follows the eighth edition of the Union for International Cancer Control (UICC) / American Joint Committee on Cancer (AJCC) TNM staging system classification for head and neck sarcomas (chondrosarcoma).

Prognosis and prediction

The 1-year, 5-year, and 10-year disease-specific survival rates for laryngeal chondrosarcoma are 97%, 90%, and 85%, respectively, although the local recurrence rate is relatively high (18–50%), usually due to incomplete resection {4415,1190,842}. Tumour location, grade, subtype, and therapy do not seem to influence outcome (other than possibly for dedifferentiated tumours) {3700,842}, which encourages conservative, function-preserving surgery as the primary treatment {4415,697,3450}. Distant metastases are exceedingly rare {913}.

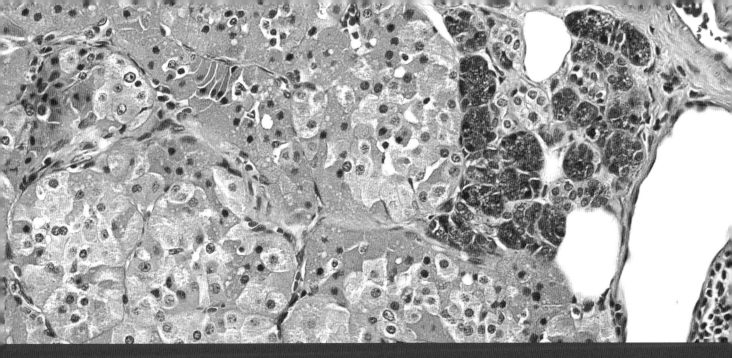

4

Salivary gland tumours

Edited by: Field AS, Hyrcza MD, Mehrotra R, Skalova A

Salivary gland tumours: Introduction

Skalova A
Bishop JA
Mehrotra R
Thompson LDR

The major and minor salivary glands are affected by a remark-able diversity of neoplasms. The reclassification of salivary gland tumours has seen unparalleled changes in recent years. Compared with tumours of other organs/systems, salivary gland neoplasms display some of the greatest morphological, pheno-typic, and genotypic diversity encountered in any single-organ system. Given the number of already existing entities that show considerable overlap of histological and immunohistochemi-cal features between different salivary gland neoplasms, only

very well documented new entities have been accepted in this edition. Reported tumours and different morphologies lacking consensus support and validation by independent investigators have not been included. This approach has resulted in the inclu-sion of microsecretory adenocarcinoma and sclerosing micro-cystic adenocarcinoma as the new malignant tumour entities; and keratocystoma, intercalated duct adenoma, and striated duct adenoma as new benign tumour entities. Furthermore, the neoplastic nature of sclerosing polycystic adenoma moved the

Table 4.01 Most common molecular changes in salivary tumours (adapted from {192}) (continued on next page)

Tumour type	Chromosomal region	Gene and mechanism	Prevalence	References
Pleomorphic adenoma	8q12	*PLAG1* fusions/amplification	> 50%	{184}
	12q13-15	*HMGA2* fusions/amplification	10–20%	{184}
Basal cell adenoma	3p22.1	*CTNNB1* mutations	37–80%	{4829,2108,3887}
	16q12.1	*CYLD* mutations	36%	{3705}
	16p13.3	*AXIN1* mutations	9%	{3887}
	5q22.2	*APC* mutations	3%	{3887}
Warthin tumour	Not reported			
Oncocytoma	Not reported			
Myoepithelioma, oncocytic subtype	8q12	*PLAG1* fusions	40%	{331}
Canalicular adenoma	Not reported			
Cystadenoma	Not reported			
Ductal papillomas	Not reported			
Sialadenoma papilliferum	7q34	*BRAF* p.V600E mutations	50–100%	{1931,3141}
Lymphadenoma	Not reported			
Sebaceous adenoma	Not reported			
Intercalated duct adenoma/hyperplasia	3p22.1	*CTNNB1* mutations	25%	{2907A}
	11p15.5	*HRAS* mutations	17%	{2907A}
Striated duct adenoma	15q26.1	*IDH2* mutations	100%	{3739A}
Sclerosing polycystic adenoma	3q26.32	*PIK3CA* mutation	45–50%	{4107,471}
	5q13.1	*PIK3R1* mutation	0–100%	{4107,471}
	10q23.31	*PTEN* loss	9–100%	{4107,471}
Keratocystoma	6p21.1	*RUNX2* fusions	100%	{476A}
Sialolipoma	Not reported			
Mucoepidermoid carcinoma	t(11;19)(q21;p13)	*CRTC1::MAML2*	40–90%	{405,469,2069}
	t(11;15)(q21;q26)	*CRTC3::MAML2*	6%	{3155}
	9p21.3	*CDKN2A* deletion	25%	{219}
Adenoid cystic carcinoma	6q22-23	*MYB* fusion/activation/amplification	~80%	{590,1176}
	8q13	*MYBL1* fusion/activation/amplification	~10%	{3028}
	9q34.3	*NOTCH* mutations	14%	{1376}
Acinic cell carcinoma	9q31	*NR4A3* fusion/activation	86%	{1740}
	19q31.1	*MSANTD3* fusion/amplification	4%	{196}

Table 4.01 Most common molecular changes in salivary tumours (adapted from {192}) (continued)

Tumour type	Chromosomal region	Gene and mechanism	Prevalence	References
	t(12;15)(p13;q25)	*ETV6::NTRK3* fusion	> 90%	{4126}
	t(12;10)(p13;q11)	*ETV6::RET* fusion	2–5%	{4125}
Secretory carcinoma	t(12;7)(p13;q31)	*ETV6::MET* fusion	< 1%	{3747}
	t(12;4)(p13;q31)	*ETV6::MAML3* fusion	< 1%	{1706}
	t(10;10)(p13;q11)	*VIM::RET* fusion	< 1%	{4108}
Microsecretory adenocarcinoma	t(5q14.3)(18q11.2)	*MEF2C::SS18* fusion	> 90%	{481}
Polymorphous adenocarcinoma				
Classic subtype	14q12	*PRKD1* mutations	73–81%	{4763}
	14q12	*PRKD1* fusions	38%	{4767,1733A}
Cribriform subtype	19q13.2	*PRKD2* fusions	14%	{4767,1733A}
	2p22.2	*PRKD3* fusions	5–19%	{4767,1733A}
Hyalinizing clear cell carcinoma	t(12;22)(q21;q12)	*EWSR1::ATF1* fusions	93%	{213}
		EWSR1::CREM fusions	< 5%	{761}
Basal cell adenocarcinoma	16q12.1	*CYLD* mutations	29%	{3705}
Intraductal carcinoma				
Intercalated duct subtype	10q11.21	*RET* fusions	47%	{4760}
Apocrine subtype	3q26.32	*PIK3CA* mutations	High	{4760}
	11p15.5	*HRAS* mutations	High	{4760}
	17q21.1	*ERBB2* (*HER2*) amplification	31%	{848}
	8p11.23	*FGFR1* amplification	10%	{848}
	17p13.1	*TP53* mutation	56%	{848}
	3q26.32	*PIK3CA* mutation	33%	{848}
	11p15.5	*HRAS* mutation	33%	{848}
Salivary duct carcinoma	Xq12	*AR* copy gain	35%	{3029}
	10q23.31	*PTEN* loss	38%	{848}
	9p21.3	*CDKN2A* loss	10%	{848}
	8q12	*PLAG1* rearrangements	27%	{847}
	12q13-15	*HMGA2* rearrangements	18%	{847}
Myoepithelial carcinoma	8q12	*PLAG1* fusions	38%	{1012}
	t(12;22)(q21;q12)	*EWSR1::ATF1* fusions	13%	{1012}
Epithelial-myoepithelial carcinoma	11p15.5	*HRAS* mutations	78%	{1224}
Mucinous adenocarcinoma	14q32.33	*AKT1* p.E17K mutations	100%	{3741}
	17p13.1	*TP53* mutations	88%	{3741}
Sclerosing microcystic adenocarcinoma	1p36.33	*CDK11B* mutation	1 case	{2086}
	8q12	*PLAG1* fusions/amplification	73%	{2207}
Carcinoma ex pleomorphic adenoma	12q13-15	*HMGA2* fusions/amplification	14%	{2207}
	17p13.1	*TP53* mutations	60%	{282}
Carcinosarcoma	Nonspecific			
Sebaceous adenocarcinoma	2p21	*MSH2* loss	10%	{4158}
Lymphoepithelial carcinoma	Not reported			
Squamous cell carcinoma	Not reported			
Sialoblastoma	Not reported			

lesion from a non-neoplastic epithelial lesion (WHO 2017 {1251}) into the "benign neoplasm" category.

Intraductal papillary mucinous neoplasm (IPMN) is an emerging entity comprising duct-centric tumours with low-grade mucinous morphology; it shares with mucinous adenocarcinoma frequent *AKT1* mutations. It is still not established whether IPMN should be classified separately or within the mucinous adenocarcinoma spectrum as a potential precursor {51,4920,3146}.

Molecular testing of salivary gland tumours for differential diagnostic accuracy and appropriate clinical management has become routine in many high-income countries {4123,3956}. Since the 2017 edition, molecular data have become widely reported, with many salivary gland neoplasms shown to harbour tumour-specific rearrangements (see Table 4.01, p. 160). The most common molecular alterations were included in the definition of the following entities: mucoepidermoid carcinoma, adenoid cystic carcinoma, secretory carcinoma, polymorphous adenocarcinoma, hyalinizing clear cell carcinoma, mucinous adenocarcinoma, and microsecretory adenocarcinoma.

Cytological findings have been included in most sections, in recognition of the importance of FNA as an initial diagnostic approach, with the Milan system recommended {1334}. Although FNA has emerged as the mainstay of the diagnostic workup of salivary gland–type tumours, core needle biopsies are still performed occasionally, especially after non-diagnostic aspirates. Although they offer more architectural information than FNAs, most core biopsies do not allow for the assessment of the interface between the tumour and the surrounding tissues and are therefore insufficient for distinguishing between neoplasms (i.e. myoepithelioma vs myoepithelial carcinoma). Only full resected specimens allow for diagnostic clarity in such cases.

The histological grading of salivary gland carcinomas has been shown to be an independent predictor of behaviour and plays a role in optimizing therapy. Still, most salivary gland carcinomas have an intrinsic biological behaviour, and attempted application of a universal grading scheme is not recommended {3951}. Carcinoma types for which validated grading systems exist include adenoid cystic carcinoma, mucoepidermoid carcinoma, and adenocarcinoma NOS {3953}. High-grade transformation has been shown to be an important concept of tumour progression in salivary gland carcinomas {4112}. The importance of this phenomenon is that tumours demonstrating high-grade transformation show an aggressive clinical course that deviates significantly from the usual behaviour for a given tumour type. High-grade transformation is included in the description of appropriate entities.

The following controversial issues remain:

1. Are IPMN and mucinous adenocarcinoma related? Are they part of a single spectrum? Is IPMN a precursor or preneoplastic condition? Is IPMN related to ductal papilloma? Further work and clarification are needed.

2. Clarification is needed regarding intraductal carcinoma and how to classify the tumour if invasion is noted, because recent data show that the myoepithelial layer is part of the tumour; therefore, these cases may be biphasic neoplasms rather than truly in situ neoplasms {480}.

3. There is no consensus about the existence of oncocytic carcinoma. Oncocytic appearance is a common change encountered in many different salivary gland tumours. In the past, carcinomas consisting entirely of oncocytes were frequently diagnosed as oncocytic carcinoma. Molecular studies have now shown many such tumours to be oncocytic variants of other salivary carcinomas. Therefore, it is unclear whether oncocytic carcinoma exists as an independent entity. For this reason, it has been included in the section on salivary gland carcinoma NOS.

4. It is not clear whether the sarcomatous component of salivary gland carcinosarcoma represents a true sarcoma or an epithelial–mesenchymal transition in the carcinomatous component. For this edition, it has remained as a separate entity.

Nodular oncocytic hyperplasia

Hellquist H
Gnepp DR
Rooper LM

Definition

Nodular oncocytic hyperplasia (NOH) is a non-neoplastic salivary gland lesion characterized by unencapsulated nodular proliferations of epithelial oncocytes and/or clear cells.

ICD-O coding

None

ICD-11 coding

DA04.1 Hypertrophy of salivary gland

Related terminology

Acceptable: multifocal nodular oncocytic hyperplasia; nodular oncocytosis; clear cell oncocytosis.

Subtype(s)

None

Localization

NOH is almost exclusively found in the parotid gland; it is rarely seen in the submandibular gland {3370,3750,3960}.

Clinical features

Patients with NOH present with a palpable painless mass, often present for years {3370,3750}.

Imaging

Imaging studies show a loss of normal architecture, usually with multiple nodules of various sizes, but this is not diagnostic {4017}.

Epidemiology

NOH constitutes < 1% of salivary tumours but accounts for approximately 7% of bilateral salivary lesions {1675,3888}. The peak incidence is in the fifth and sixth decades of life, and there is a slight female predilection {3960}.

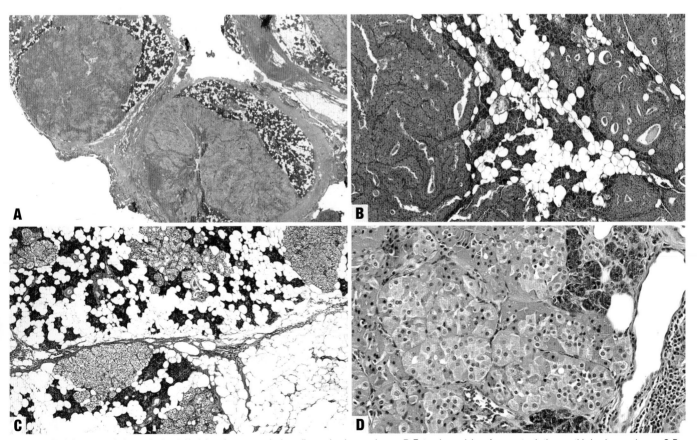

Fig. 4.01 Nodular oncocytic hyperplasia. **A** Nodules of oncocytes in the salivary gland parenchyma. **B** Extensive nodules of oncocytes in the parotid gland parenchyma. **C** Parotid gland showing multiple separate clear cell nodules. **D** High-power view of nodules in the parotid gland parenchyma demonstrating oncocytic cells with granular cytoplasm.

Etiology

Although the inciting factor is unknown, the oncocytic phenotype is associated with an accumulation of aberrant mitochondria and mitochondrial DNA mutations {1549,2421}.

Pathogenesis

Unknown

Macroscopic appearance

NOH displays multiple brown well-circumscribed but unencapsulated nodules. A partly encapsulated larger mass may indicate an oncocytoma arising in NOH {1983}.

Histopathology

NOH consists of irregularly shaped unencapsulated nodules of oncocytes in solid to tubulotrabecular patterns distributed throughout the salivary parenchyma {3370,1675,3888}. Lobular architecture is preserved. Clear cell change is frequent and can form small satellite foci that mimic invasive clear cell tumours. Unifocality and encapsulation can separate NOH from oncocytoma. Entrapped normal acini, ducts, and adipocytes within nodules and non-perivascular p63-positive basal cells distinguish NOH from acinic cell carcinoma or metastatic renal cell carcinoma {4756,2904}.

Differential diagnosis

Absence of *MAML2* rearrangement can rule out oncocytic mucoepidermoid carcinoma {4104}. Negativity for SOX10, S100, and *PLAG1* rearrangement helps distinguish NOH from pleomorphic adenoma and myoepithelioma with oncocytic metaplasia {331}.

Cytology

Smears are hypocellular, with small to medium-sized tissue fragments of oncocytic cells with well-defined cytoplasmic margins and coarsely granular dense cytoplasm, present in a clean background. These features overlap with those of oncocytoma (which cannot be distinguished from NOH) and those of the oncocytic cells seen in Warthin tumour, although that has lymphoid cells in a dense, proteinaceous, granular background {3750}.

Diagnostic molecular pathology

Not relevant

Essential and desirable diagnostic criteria

Essential: circumscribed but unencapsulated nodules of oncocytic and/or clear cells.
Desirable: multifocality.

Staging

Not relevant

Prognosis and prediction

NOH is a non-neoplastic lesion and recurrence is rare, although it is frequently multifocal and bilateral. Clear cell change may indicate an increased risk of recurrence {559}. Malignant transformation has not been reported.

Lymphoepithelial sialadenitis

Ihrler S
Laco J
Nagao T

Definition

Lymphoepithelial sialadenitis is a chronic, systemic, lymphocytic autoimmune inflammation of salivary glands causing acinar parenchymal atrophy and the formation of lymphoepithelial lesions.

ICD-O coding

None

ICD-11 coding

2E91.1 Benign lymphoepithelial lesion of salivary gland

Related terminology

Not recommended: benign lymphoepithelial lesion; myoepithelial sialadenitis; Mikulicz disease.

Subtype(s)

None

Localization

Typically, all salivary (and other mucosal) glands are affected. Minor glands are affected mostly microscopically, without enlargement, whereas the parotid glands often show bilateral enlargement.

Clinical features

Clinical symptoms of sicca syndrome (dry mouth, dry eye), frequently associated with bilateral parotid swelling.

Epidemiology

Patients are predominantly female (M:F ratio: 1:4) and in their sixth or seventh decade of life.

Etiology

Multiglandular lymphoepithelial sialadenitis is usually a histological correlate of the autoimmune condition Sjögren disease, characterized by progressive mucosal sicca syndrome, either as isolated disease or in combination with other autoimmune diseases, most frequently rheumatoid arthritis. The etiology is unclear {2007,1235}.

Pathogenesis

Not clinically relevant

Macroscopic appearance

Not clinically relevant

Histopathology

Early lesions show a minor to moderate degree of T cell–dominated periductal lymphocytic infiltration, rarely with reactive follicles and usually without lymphoepithelial lesions. They are typically encountered in minor labial glands and sampled for

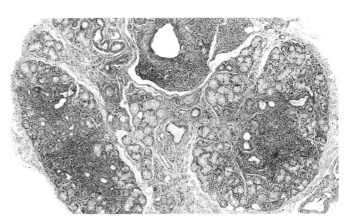

Fig. 4.02 Lymphoepithelial sialadenitis. Minor labial gland with four foci of dense periductal lymphocytic infiltration, representing a positive focus score in a female patient with clinical Sjögren syndrome.

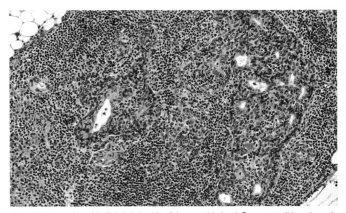

Fig. 4.03 Lymphoepithelial sialadenitis of the parotid gland. Dense small lymphocytic infiltration accompanied by lymphoepithelial lesions (islands).

diagnostic purposes in cases of suspected Sjögren disease {3538}. A positive focus is defined as ≥ 1 dense periductal aggregate of > 50 lymphocytes, representing a histological criterion within a diagnostic score {4642,4030}. Focus score is calculated as the number of lymphocytic foci per 4 mm^2.

Advanced lesions typically manifest as a tumorous enlargement of parotid (or, rarely, the submandibular or lacrimal) glands. They show intense, B cell–dominated, lymphoplasmacytic infiltrates with preserved lobular architecture; a variable (often massive) degree of parenchymal atrophy; multiple reactive follicles; and multiple, densely aggregated, partly cystic lymphoepithelial lesions. The pathognomonic lymphoepithelial lesions (islands) consist of a netlike proliferation of basaloid ductal cells and permeating (B-cell) lymphocytes {1781,2007,3538,1235}. Monocytoid B cells typically constitute narrow, bright haloes around lymphoepithelial lesions, whereas intensely expanded and confluent haloes might indicate progression to extranodal marginal zone lymphoma of mucosa-associated lymphoid tissue (see

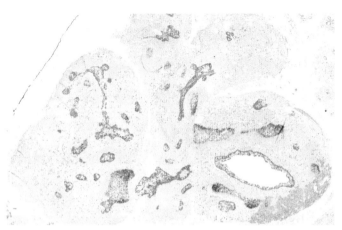

Fig. 4.04 Lymphoepithelial sialadenitis. Fully developed parotid lymphoepithelial sialadenitis with massive lymphocytic infiltration (haemalum, blue), total parenchymal atrophy, and preserved lobular architecture, with multiple lymphoepithelial lesions (CK14, brown), and reactive follicles (Ki-67, red), altogether representing an entirely reactive histological pattern (clinically Sjögren syndrome).

Extranodal marginal zone lymphoma of mucosa-associated lymphoid tissue, p. 553). Plasma cells may be frequent.

Immunohistochemistry
A keratin stain can be helpful for pattern analysis of preserved glandular architecture, including the frequency and distribution of lymphoepithelial lesions {2006,2007}. Immunohistological staining for kappa/lambda light chains or, alternatively, in situ hybridization detecting corresponding mRNA may demonstrate their polyclonal nature in lymphoepithelial sialadenitis, while molecular evidence of B-cell monoclonality may occur, but in the absence of further histological evidence it does not necessarily represent a malignant transformation. There is no association with EBV {1781,1235}.

Differential diagnosis
Cases with ductal dilatation, predominantly diffuse lymphocytic infiltration, and fibrosis represent nonspecific (e.g. traumatic or obstructive) sialadenitis of minor/labial glands. Sclerosis, obliterative phlebitis, and numerous IgG4-positive plasma cells,

as seen in IgG4-associated sialadenitis of the submandibular glands, are absent {2448}. HIV-associated cystic lymphoepithelial lesion is histologically similar but is usually bilateral, characterized by bizarre, enlarged follicles and massive cystically dilated lymphoepithelial lesions {994,2006}. Salivary lymphoepithelial carcinoma may show irregular lymphoepithelial lesions in a lobular arrangement but represents a bluntly infiltrating neoplasia with increased proliferation, cellular atypia, and the presence of EBV in a significant subset of cases {4802}. Clinical information is usually indispensable for correct differential diagnosis.

Cytology
Smears are cellular with a mixed lymphoid population including lymphocytes, larger lymphoid cells, dendritic cells and tingible-body macrophages from germinal centres, and plasma cells, along with a small number of cohesive ductal tissue fragments infiltrated by lymphocytes {3750}. The epithelial cells may show squamous metaplasia. Lymphoma (with its often more homogeneous lymphoid population) and metastatic squamous cell carcinoma (with its necrosis and more prominent nuclear pleomorphism) are in the differential diagnosis.

Diagnostic molecular pathology
None

Essential and desirable diagnostic criteria
Essential: a dense benign lymphocytic infiltrate, in salivary glands, with lymphoepithelial lesions.

Staging
None

Prognosis and prediction
The degree of lymphocytic infiltration, parenchymal atrophy, and corresponding clinical sicca syndrome is usually slowly progressive, lacking therapeutic options. Approximately 4% progress to extranodal marginal zone lymphoma of mucosa-associated lymphoid tissue (mostly unilateral in the parotid glands).

Pleomorphic adenoma

Hernandez-Prera JC Ihrler S
Altemani AM Katabi N
de Sousa SOM Wasserman JK
Faquin WC Weinreb I

Definition

Pleomorphic adenoma (PA) is a benign epithelial neoplasm characterized by cytomorphological and architectural diversity, with an admixture of ductal and myoepithelial cells usually embedded in a chondromyxoid or fibrous stromal component.

ICD-O coding

8940/0 Pleomorphic adenoma
8940/3 Metastasizing pleomorphic adenoma
8940/0 Oncocytic pleomorphic adenoma

ICD-11 coding

2E91 & XA5T23 & XH2KC1 Benign neoplasms of major salivary glands & Salivary gland apparatus & Pleomorphic adenoma

Related terminology

Acceptable: benign mixed tumour.

Subtype(s)

Benign metastasizing pleomorphic adenoma; oncocytic pleomorphic adenoma

Localization

Most PAs arise in the parotid gland (~70–80%), followed by the oral cavity and submandibular gland {4187,1306,2666,195, 4565,983}. In the oral cavity, the palate is the most common location {983}. Rare locations include the sinonasal tract, skull base, external auditory canal, and larynx {1192,3897,4420, 2399,3690}.

Clinical features

Generally, PA presents as a slowly growing, painless mass. Deep parotid lobe tumours present as parapharyngeal space masses; parotid tail tumours present as level II neck lesions; and minor salivary gland PAs may present with dysphagia, airway obstruction, or obstructive sleep apnoea {2666}. Recurrent PAs present as multinodular disease in the surgical bed or surrounding soft tissues {4835}. Malignant transformation can be suggested by rapid growth and facial nerve symptoms.

Benign metastasizing PA is a rare subtype that occurs after multiple recurrences and must be distinguished from malignancy. Biopsy-proven metastases are most commonly seen in bone, lung, and neck lymph nodes {4787,2339,4738}.

Imaging

MRI of PA demonstrates a number of typical features: a lobulated tumour with well-defined margins, extremely hyperintense on T2-weighted imaging, intermediate signal on T1-weighted imaging, and avidly enhancing after intravenous contrast. PAs have high apparent diffusion coefficient values (~1.6) on diffusion-weighted imaging. On ultrasound, PAs are hypoechoic with through-transmission; have lobulated, well-defined margins; and demonstrate internal vascularity. The use of Doppler imaging is mandatory to avoid mislabelling them as cysts. Although these features are characteristic of PA, they are also seen in other pathologies, and cytology/histology is required to confirm the diagnosis {955}.

Epidemiology

PA is the most common salivary gland neoplasm worldwide, accounting for 50–70% of all salivary gland tumours {4269, 4446,195,3853,4565,983}. With an estimated incidence of 4.2–4.9 cases per 100 000 person-years, PAs occur across a wide age range, with a peak incidence in the fifth and sixth decades of life and a slight female predilection {195,4565}.

The mean patient age at presentation of benign metastasizing PA is 49.5 years, and the mean interval between primary tumour diagnosis and metastatic disease is 14.9 years (range: 0–51 years) {4787,2339}. It often occurs after multiple recurrences {2339}.

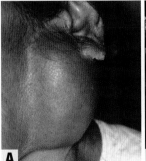 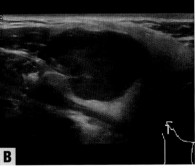 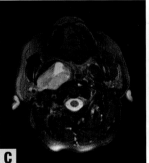 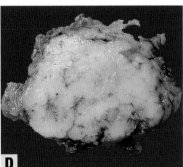

Fig. 4.05 Pleomorphic adenoma. **A** This slowly growing mass had been present for > 10 years. There is no ulceration or erythema of the skin. **B** This ultrasound shows a well-defined, solid mass that is hypoechoic compared with adjacent salivary tissue, with homogeneous internal echoes. **C** Classic marked hyperintensity (similar intensity to cerebrospinal fluid) on a T2-weighted fat-suppressed protocol. This right retropharyngeal mass shows connection to the deep lobe of the parotid gland. **D** The glistening, slightly bluish cut surface is a feature of the cartilaginous matrix seen in pleomorphic adenoma. There are multiple nodules and bosselations at the periphery, a finding common in pleomorphic adenoma.

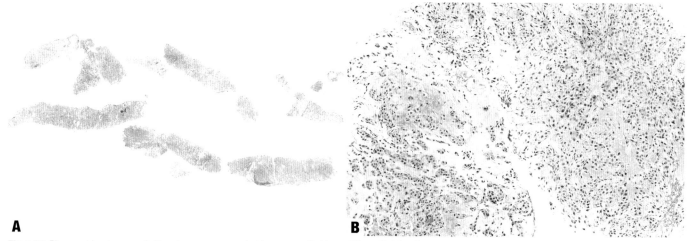

Fig. 4.06 Pleomorphic adenoma. **A** Many tumours are sampled by core needle biopsy. When all of the elements are present, a diagnosis can be made, while recognizing the sampling limitations. **B** High-power view of the core needle sample demonstrates the characteristic features of pleomorphic adenoma.

Etiology

The etiology is unknown, but radiation exposure and estrogen/progesterone have been suggested as risk factors {3923,4565, 4566}.

Pathogenesis

PAs harbour recurrent translocations or intrachromosomal rearrangements resulting in gene fusions involving *PLAG1* on 8q12 (> 50%) or *HMGA2* on 12q14.3 (10–15%) {4217}. Seven

recurrent fusion partner genes for *PLAG1* have been reported (*CTNNB1*, *FGFR1*, *LIFR*, *CHCHD7*, *TCEA1*, *NFIB*, and *BOC*), whereas *HMGA2* fuses with one of four recurrent fusion partners (*NFIB*, *WIF1*, *FHIT*, or *TMTC2*) {2201,4658,268,3490,4738, 32,3447}. Oncocytic PAs have been shown to contain *PLAG1* gene fusions with *GEM*, *CHCHD7*, *NTF3*, *FBXO32*, and *C1orf116* {331}. Concurrent or isolated *HMGA2* amplification has also been reported {3490,44}. Benign metastasizing PA is said to arise from embolism of benign tumour cells.

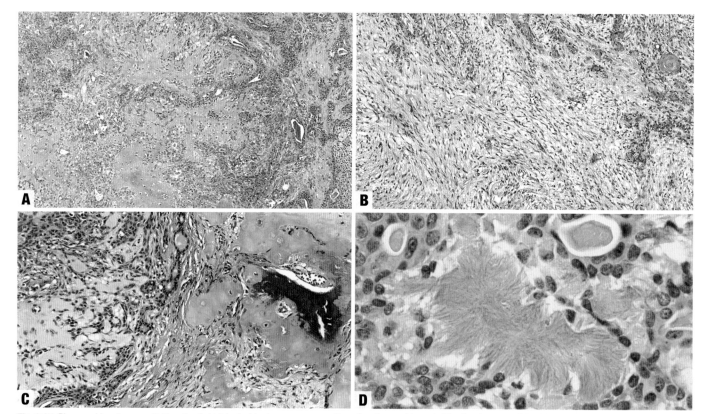

Fig. 4.07 Pleomorphic adenoma. **A** The classic histological features are seen, with a chondromyxoid matrix blending imperceptibly with the myoepithelial cells and showing small ducts in the background. **B** Tumours show remarkable variation in appearance, with a prominent spindled cell myoepithelial component illustrated. Focal squamous metaplasia is present. **C** Calcification and even bone formation may be seen in pleomorphic adenoma, often in those present for a long clinical duration. **D** Radially arranged collagen fibres, sometimes called collagenous crystalloids, are frequently seen in pleomorphic adenoma.

Macroscopic appearance

Tumours are well circumscribed, with smooth, lobular, or bosselated borders. The cut surface may be tan, chondroid white, or gelatinous. Cystic changes, haemorrhage, and infarction can occur.

Histopathology

The histological hallmark of PA is its morphological diversity derived from an admixture of bilayered ducts, myoepithelial cells, and stroma. PAs are well delineated and/or encapsulated. The capsule may be absent in minor salivary gland and chondromyxoid-predominant PAs.

The ductal and myoepithelial cells are commonly arranged in bilayered tubular structures, with the myoepithelial cells melding with the stroma. The cellular phenotype, particularly of the myoepithelial cells, is broad and includes epithelioid, basaloid, stellate, spindled, clear, oncocytic, and plasmacytoid morphology. The stroma can be mucoid, myxoid, hyalinized, chondroid, osseous, or lipomatous. The proportions of the three components vary in each tumour, and one element may predominate. Chondromyxoid-predominant stroma-rich lesions with few cellular structures can mimic true cartilaginous neoplasms. In cellular PAs, the ductal and/or myoepithelial cells are dominant over the stromal elements. Despite the increased cellularity, invasion is absent and immunohistochemical markers can highlight the biphasic nature of the tumour {1849}. Non-neoplastic acini merging at the periphery, capsular bosselation, pseudopodia, satellite nodules, and multinodular growth are not indicators of malignancy {4221,4992,3320,1849}. Intravascular tumour cells, possibly artefactually displaced during biopsy, should not be interpreted as angioinvasion {150,4106}. Bizarre tumour cells (ancient atypia) can be observed, and infarct-type necrosis can occur after biopsy {116,4344,2621}.

Most recurrent PAs exhibit multiple discrete round nodules of various sizes and chondromyxoid morphology contained within residual salivary gland or soft tissues {4993,4835}. The term "atypical PA" has been used to describe tumours with features that are suggestive of malignancy but insufficient for a diagnosis of carcinoma ex PA. Careful microscopic evaluation and extensive sampling is necessary in such cases {280}.

Benign metastasizing PA is histologically and molecularly indistinguishable from a benign tumour at a primary location

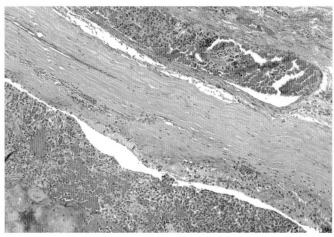

Fig. 4.08 Pleomorphic adenoma. Metastasizing pleomorphic adenoma. Neoplastic cells are noted within the vascular spaces in a salivary gland tumour that demonstrated pleomorphic adenoma in the lung parenchyma. The patient had had four previous surgeries.

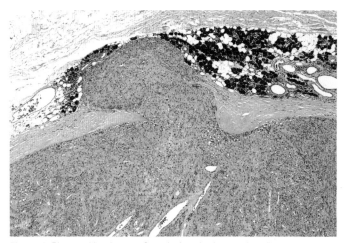

Fig. 4.09 Pleomorphic adenoma. Capsular invasion by pseudopodia.

{4787,4738}. No histological or molecular features can reliably predict metastasis {2339}.

The oncocytic subtype is mainly composed of cells with abundant eosinophilic granular cytoplasm {4114}.

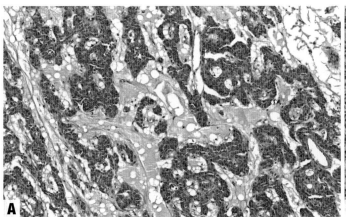

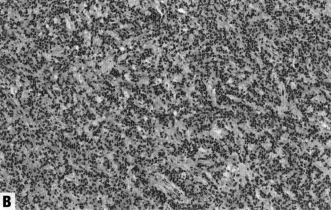

Fig. 4.10 Pleomorphic adenoma with canalicular adenoma–like growth pattern and *HMGA2::WIF1* fusion. **A** Anastomosing and branching cords, columns, and trabeculae are seen surrounded by myxoid stroma. **B** HMGA2 immunohistochemistry is homogeneously positive in all cells.

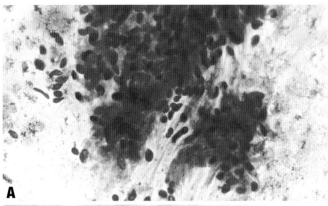

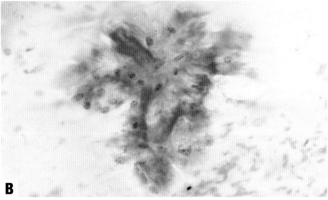

Fig. 4.11 Pleomorphic adenoma. **A** FNAC. Giemsa stain showing myoepithelial and ductal cells in a background of magenta fibrillary matrix. **B** FNAC (Pap) showing myoepithelial and ductal cells in a background of fibrillary matrix.

Immunohistochemistry
PLAG1 {2209}, and HMGA2 {3032}, respectively, are emerging as sensitive immunohistochemical markers for PA. There is usually strong and diffuse reactivity for pancytokeratin, AE1/AE3, CAM5.2, and CK7, which is often accentuated in the ductal or luminal cell areas, with various muscle, myoepithelial, and basal markers reactive, including calponin (most sensitive), SMA, S100, SOX10, p40 (better than p63), and CK5/6 {3280,2994, 2996A,3342A}. GFAP is usually more strongly expressed in myxoid and myoepithelial areas {3864B,985}.

The immunoexpression of S100 and SOX10 helps to differentiate oncocytic PA from other oncocytic tumours {331}.

Differential diagnosis
PAs can show squamous metaplasia and mucocytes, and mimic squamous cell carcinoma or mucoepidermoid carcinoma {2457}.

PA can be distinguished from squamous cell carcinoma by the absence of infiltrative growth, marked pleomorphism, and increased mitoses, and it can be separated from mucoepidermoid carcinoma by the identification of well-formed keratin pearls, the presence of myoepithelial differentiation, and the absence of *MAML2* rearrangements {4127}. PA can exhibit cribriform architecture mimicking adenoid cystic carcinoma, as well as areas of compact biphasic tubular structures reminiscent of epithelial-myoepithelial carcinoma {1849}. Myoepithelial carcinoma is often cytologically bland and may therefore be underrecognized as malignant and misclassified as a myoepithelial-rich PA {4887}.

Cytology
Usually, highly cellular smears show variable amounts of the characteristic fibrillary matrix, admixed with myoepithelial cells (which can be polygonal, plasmacytoid, spindled, clear, or round with bland round to oval nuclei) and ductal cells {2331}. The myoepithelial cells can be seen in the stroma and merge into the epithelial component. When the diagnostic fibrillary stroma is scant, the distinction from adenoid cystic carcinoma can be difficult, and squamous metaplasia can raise the possibility of high-grade mucoepidermoid carcinoma {1257,121}.

Diagnostic molecular pathology
Not applicable

Essential and desirable diagnostic criteria
Essential: an admixture of bilayered ducts, myoepithelial cells, and chondromyxoid/fibrous stroma; absence of invasion and malignant cytomorphological features.
Desirable: PLAG1 or HMGA2 alterations (in selected cases).

Staging
Not applicable

Prognosis and prediction
Complete surgical resection is curative and the treatment of choice. Recurrences occur in 2.9–6.7% of cases, mostly secondary to rupture and incomplete tumour excision {4993,195, 4565}. The overall rate of malignant transformation is difficult to assess because many carcinomas ex PA are diagnosed without a prior clinical history of a PA {1689}. In recurrent PAs, the rate of malignant transformation is about 3% {195,4565}. Out of 51 cases of benign metastasizing PA with reported survival data, 9 patients (17.6%) died secondary to the disease and 41 (80.4%) were alive at 1 year. Multiple metastases appear to confer a poor prognosis {2339}.

Basal cell adenoma

Seethala R
Fonseca I
Jo VY
Nagao T
Rossi ED
Yamamoto H

Definition

Basal cell adenoma (BCA) is a benign biphasic salivary gland neoplasm composed of basaloid and luminal cells, and often containing basement membrane material.

ICD-O coding

8147/0 Basal cell adenoma
8147/0 Membranous basal cell adenoma

ICD-11 coding

2E91.Z & XH60D1 Benign neoplasm of major salivary glands, unspecified & Basal cell adenoma

Related terminology

Not recommended: monomorphic adenoma; dermal analogue tumour.

Subtype(s)

Membranous basal cell adenoma

Localization

BCAs are largely restricted to major salivary glands, especially the parotid gland (> 80%) {1306,1285,4446,1532,989,3713}.

Clinical features

BCA usually presents as a well-defined, mobile, solitary mass {3713}, although syndromic cases may be multiple and associated with dermal cylindromas or trichoepitheliomas {3941}.

Epidemiology

BCAs account for about 1–4% of all salivary gland tumours {1306,1285,4446,1532,989,3713}. They present more frequently in the sixth and seventh decades of life, with a slight female predilection.

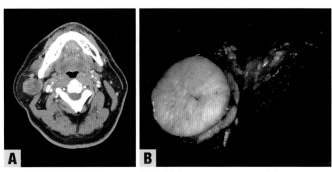

Fig. 4.12 Basal cell adenoma. **A** Axial CT demonstrates a smooth, homogeneous ovoid mass within the parotid gland. No destructive growth is noted. **B** Grossly, basal cell adenomas are well circumscribed and show a homogeneous grey-tan cut surface.

Etiology

Some BCAs occur in the setting of familial/multiple cylindromatosis syndromes {853,3713}.

Pathogenesis

CTNNB1 alterations are often present, usually in tubulotrabecular BCA {2108,2544,3887,3713}. *CYLD* (*CYLD1*) alterations are also common, more so with membranous BCA {3705,3713}.

Macroscopic appearance

BCAs are solitary and well circumscribed, and they range in size from 2 to 55 mm {4830}. The membranous type may be multifocal. They show a homogeneous solid grey texture, although cystic change is not uncommon {4445}.

Histopathology

BCAs are encapsulated or well circumscribed and show tubulotrabecular, cribriform, membranous, or solid growth. A subset show a distinct spindled S100-positive myoepithelial cell-derived stromal component {1028,3324}. The tumour shows

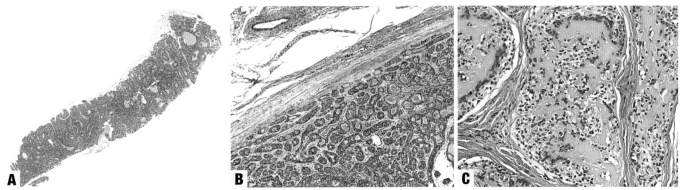

Fig. 4.13 Basal cell adenoma. **A** A basaloid salivary gland neoplasm is noted in this core needle sample. There is no plasmacytoid appearance and no chondromyxoid matrix. However, a definitive separation from basal cell adenocarcinoma cannot be reliably made from core needle or fine-needle samples. **B** Most tumours are encapsulated. **C** The basal and myoepithelial cells are intimately blended with the basement membrane material and separated into islands by collagenous tissue.

Chapter 4

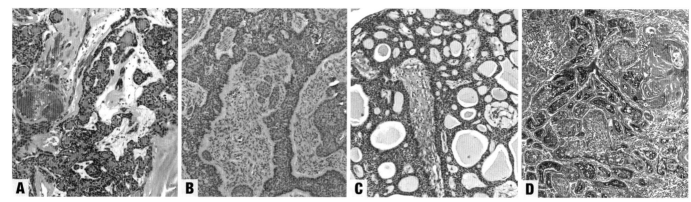

Fig. 4.14 Basal cell adenoma. Note the peripheral palisading in all patterns. **A** Tubulotrabecular pattern. **B** Trabecular pattern with a myoepithelial-derived stromal component. **C** Cribriform pattern. **D** Membranous pattern.

peripheral palisading of dark cells with luminal paler cells and ducts. Nuclei are vesicular {2234,4445,2605,4830,2729}. Tumours demonstrate stroma of variable amount and collagenous density, sometimes in drop-like hyaline material. A lipomatous subtype has been described {3506}.

Immunohistochemistry
Epithelial and myoepithelial markers highlight the dual cell composition {3128,3053}. Coexpression of nuclear β-catenin and LEF1 is detected in BCAs {2225,452,2108,2544}.

Differential diagnosis
BCAs are distinguished from cellular pleomorphic adenoma by their basaloid appearance, peripheral palisading, and lack of blending with associated myoepithelial-type stroma {3949}. BCAs are differentiated from basal cell adenocarcinoma by the absence of invasion.

Cytology
Smears are usually markedly cellular with small sheets and round, trabecular, or solid tissue fragments consisting of monomorphic small basaloid cells, with scant cytoplasm and frequent naked nuclei in a clean background. Stripped round nuclei show uniform fine hyperchromasia {4509}. A dense, thin layer of hyaline stroma most typically surrounds the basaloid tissue fragments and interdigitates the cells peripherally, and small rounded droplets of stroma may be seen, but no myxofibrillary stroma is seen. Squamoid and sebaceous features may be seen focally {4203}. Separating BCA from basal cell adenocarcinoma is difficult on FNAB, and the differential diagnosis from adenoid cystic carcinoma is not always possible; the term "basaloid neoplasm" is often appropriate.

Diagnostic molecular pathology
None

Essential and desirable diagnostic criteria
Essential: non-invasive; biphasic basaloid morphology; peripheral palisading; variable amount of collagenous stroma.
Desirable: dual population immunophenotype; nuclear β-catenin reactivity.

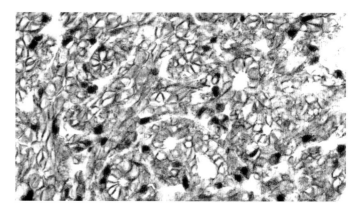

Fig. 4.15 Basal cell adenoma. These tumours often show nuclear localization of β-catenin, typically in the peripheral cell layer.

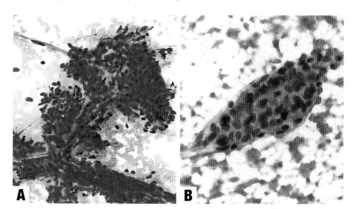

Fig. 4.16 Basal cell adenoma. **A** Tumour cells are monomorphic with scant cytoplasm. Here, they are arranged in arborizing fragments with scant, interdigitating hyaline stroma. Scattered naked nuclei are noted. (FNAC, Giemsa.) **B** Nuclei are vesicular and are accentuated at the periphery of cell fragments. (FNAC, Pap.)

Staging
Not applicable

Prognosis and prediction
Recurrence rates are low (< 2%), except for the membranous subtype (~25%). Malignant transformation can occur {3131}, more frequently with the membranous subtype {368}.

Warthin tumour

Simpson RHW
Di Palma S
Faquin WC
Pasricha S

Definition

Warthin tumour is a benign salivary gland tumour composed of oncocytic epithelial cells lining ductal, papillary, and cystic structures in a lymphoid stroma.

ICD-O coding

8561/0 Warthin tumour
8561/0 Infarcted/metaplastic Warthin tumour

ICD-11 coding

2E91.Z & XA5T23 & XH9ZB2 Benign neoplasm of major salivary glands, unspecified & Salivary gland apparatus & Adenolymphoma

Related terminology

Not recommended: adenolymphoma; papillary cystadenoma lymphomatosum; cystadenolymphoma.

Subtype(s)

Infarcted/metaplastic Warthin tumour

Localization

Tumours are almost exclusively restricted to parotid glands, especially the inferior pole, and periparotid lymph nodes {1231, 4591}; < 1% are found in the deep lobe {3805}. Tumours are multifocal in 12–20% of patients, either synchronously or metachronously, and are bilateral in 5–17% {2795,3500}. They may be associated with other salivary tumour types {1618,2148}.

Clinical features

Patients present with painless, slow-growing, and fluctuant swellings. Pain or facial nerve palsy may occur in metaplastic/infarcted variants {1305,1307}.

Imaging

Characteristic imaging findings include multifocality, parotid tail location, cystic change, and avidity on PET-CT {3657}.

Epidemiology

Warthin tumour accounts for 5–20% of all salivary tumours, except in Black Africans, in whom it is rare {2489}. The mean age at diagnosis is 62 years (range: 12–92 years) {763}. The M:F ratio has shifted in Europe and North America, from 10:1 in 1953 {763} to almost equal nowadays {1307}; however, a 2018 study found that the 10:1 ratio remains true in China {4893}.

Etiology

Warthin tumours, especially when bilateral, have been linked strongly to cigarette smoking {3549,3500,3799}. Other suggested risk factors include radiation exposure in atomic bomb survivors {3819}, and autoimmune diseases {1524,3314},

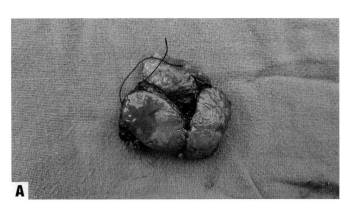

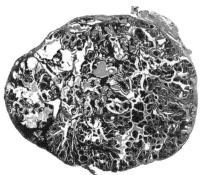

Fig. 4.17 Warthin tumour. **A** Gross image. A well-defined circumscribed tumour with a brown glistening homogeneous cut surface. **B** Numerous papillary structures are noted, lined by a double layer of oncocytically altered cells, all set within a very well developed lymphoid stroma.

especially thyroiditis. Some studies have suggested a role for IgG4 {33} and various viruses, but this is still unproven {777}.

Pathogenesis

Warthin tumour probably arises from salivary ductal inclusions in parotid lymph nodes {942,2908}. Clonality studies have suggested a non-neoplastic nature {1906,238}; however, a subset of metaplastic Warthin tumours have been found to harbour *KRAS* codon 12 mutations {48A}, which may suggest the existence of a different subtype with a neoplastic nature.

Macroscopic appearance

Most are well-circumscribed spherical-oval masses, 20–50 mm in diameter, although one example measured 200 mm {3825}. Solid areas and multiple cysts with papillary projections are apparent on cut surface.

Histopathology

Warthin tumour is composed of varying proportions of papillary-cystic structures lined by bilayered oncocytic epithelial cells, surrounded by a lymphoid stroma including germinal centres.

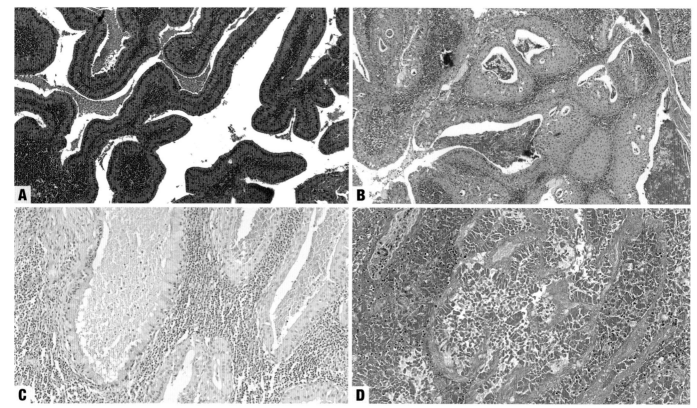

Fig. 4.18 Warthin tumour. **A** The double-layered (tram-tracking) appearance of the oncocytically altered cells is quite characteristic, whether they line the cystic spaces or are arranged in papillae. Note the lymphoid stroma. **B** Metaplastic Warthin tumour. The tumour is characterized by the replacement of the double layer of oncocytic cells by metaplastic epithelium. **C** Warthin tumour with mucinous metaplasia. Extensive mucinous metaplasia replacing bilayered papillary oncocytic epithelium. **D** Oncocytically altered tumours frequently undergo infarction or degeneration, especially after manipulation (FNA or core needle biopsy). However, papillary ghost cell outlines are noted, with degenerated lymphoid stroma adjacent.

The epithelial component comprises inner columnar and outer cuboidal cells. Limited foci of squamous, mucous, ciliated, and sebaceous cells can be present.

Subtype

In the infarcted/metaplastic subtype of Warthin tumour, the bilayered epithelium is replaced by squamous metaplastic epithelium without atypia. Mucinous metaplasia may also be present {4127,1120}. The infarcted/metaplastic subtype, which may follow FNA or trauma, shows areas of necrosis, in which a ghost papillary architecture may be discerned (highlighted with reticulin staining). There is usually marked squamous (less often, mucinous) metaplasia and a stromal reaction, including granuloma formation {1305,1120,3791}.

Differential diagnosis

The main differential diagnosis of the metaplastic Warthin tumour subtype is Warthin-like mucoepidermoid carcinoma; however, Warthin tumours lack *MAML2* gene rearrangement {4127,448}.

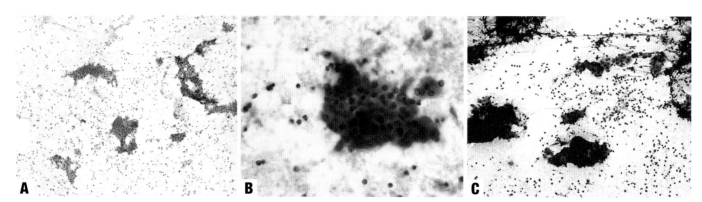

Fig. 4.19 Warthin tumour. **A** Smears show small cohesive sheets of oncocytes, numerous lymphocytes, and granular background debris (FNAB, Pap). **B** A smear showing a group of epithelial cells in a lymphoid background (FNAB, Pap). **C** Smears show numerous small cohesive sheets of oncocytes with lymphocytes in the background granular debris (FNAB, Giemsa).

Cytology

Smears show a characteristic triad of small cohesive sheets of oncocytes (with abundant granular cytoplasm, well-defined cytoplasmic margins, and central rounded nuclei with a prominent single nucleolus), numerous lymphocytes, and a smaller number of larger lymphoid cells, with granular background debris {2332}. The proportion of the three components can vary. Diagnostic challenges occur when there are metaplastic changes, including squamous and mucinous metaplasia raising a differential diagnosis with mucoepidermoid carcinoma, which lacks tissue fragments of bland oncocytic cells but may have a cystic background and a lymphoid component {323,121}.

Diagnostic molecular pathology

Diagnostic molecular pathology is not directly relevant, but an absence of *MAML2* alteration can exclude mucoepidermoid carcinoma {4127}.

Essential and desirable diagnostic criteria

Essential: a circumscribed mass with spaces lined by papillary bilayered oncocytic cells; lymphoid stroma.

Staging

Not applicable

Prognosis and prediction

Complete surgical excision with an adequate margin is usually curative {1280}. Uncommon local recurrences are probably due to multifocal tumours or inadequate excision {1284}. Malignant transformation in Warthin tumour is rare; a few examples have been reported of both epithelial {4113,4827,1439,1440,2291, 4893} and lymphoid neoplasms {3499,890,1118}.

Oncocytoma

Hellquist H
Baněčková M
Fonseca I

Definition
Oncocytoma is a benign encapsulated neoplasm composed of large epithelial cells with abundant eosinophilic granular cytoplasm due to the accumulation of mitochondria.

ICD-O coding
8290/0 Oncocytoma
8290/0 Clear cell oncocytoma

ICD-11 coding
2E91.1 & XH9Z86 Benign neoplasm of other specified major salivary glands & Oxyphilic adenoma

Related terminology
Acceptable: oncocytic adenoma, oxyphilic adenoma.

Subtype(s)
Clear cell oncocytoma

Localization
More than 80% of cases occur in the parotid, approximately 10% occur in the submandibular gland, and the rest occur in minor salivary glands and the sublingual gland {559,3370,4422, 665}.

Clinical features
Symptoms depend on anatomical location. Oncocytoma usually presents as a unilateral painless swelling.

Epidemiology
Oncocytomas represent < 1.5% of salivary gland tumours. The incidence peak is in the seventh decade of life, with no sex predilection {559,3370}. Tumours may be multifocal and bilateral {1618,1983,4556}.

Etiology
A history of radiotherapy or long-term radiation exposure has been reported {559}. The oncocytic phenotype is associated with mitochondrial DNA mutations {665,1549}.

Pathogenesis
Oncocytoma may arise in the background of multinodular oncocytic hyperplasia.

Macroscopic appearance
Oncocytomas are usually small, single, lobulated, well-circumscribed, brownish tumours with or without a cystic component and/or central fibrosis.

Histopathology
Oncocytomas are well-circumscribed tumours consisting of oncocytes with abundant eosinophilic granular cytoplasm, arranged in nests and sheets, separated by a thin fibrovascular stroma. The nuclei are uniform, vesicular, and centrally placed, with prominent single nucleoli. Dark cells with pyknotic nuclei, probably representing degenerated oncocytes, are present. Tumours lack entrapped normal parenchyma.

Subtype
In clear cell oncocytoma, the presence of glycogen and fixation artefacts causes the clear cell change {1234}.

Immunohistochemistry and differential diagnosis
The presence of p63-positive basal cells excludes metastatic renal cell carcinoma and acinic cell carcinoma {2904,4756}. An absence of PAX2 and/or PAX8 expression favours oncocytoma over metastatic renal carcinoma {638}. *MAML2* rearrangement helps distinguish oncocytic mucoepidermoid carcinoma {4104}. SOX10 and S100 immunopositivity and *PLAG1* gene rearrangement distinguishes pleomorphic adenoma and myoepithelioma with extensive oncocytic metaplasia {331}.

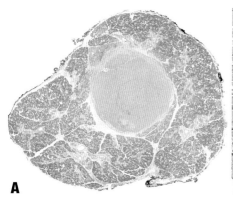 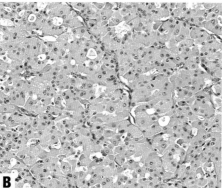 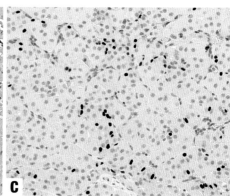

Fig. 4.20 Oncocytoma. **A** Oncocytoma of the parotid gland. The tumour is composed predominantly of sheets of oncocytes, large bland cells with eosinophilic granular cytoplasm. **B** Sheets of monomorphic cells with oncocytic cytoplasm. **C** Several p63+ basal cells.

Cytology

Smears of oncocytoma are indistinguishable from those of nodular oncocytic hyperplasia {3919}. The nuclei tend to be round, with prominent nucleoli. Acinic cell carcinoma can be distinguished by the finely vacuolated cytoplasm that is often lost in smears. A DOG1, p63, and S100 panel on FNA cell blocks is useful in differential diagnosis {3919}.

Diagnostic molecular pathology

Not relevant

Essential and desirable diagnostic criteria

Essential: a circumscribed mass composed of large oncocytic epithelial cells; lack of entrapped normal parenchyma.
Desirable: basal cells positive for p63; absence of SOX10 and S100 (in selected cases).

Staging

Not relevant

Prognosis and prediction

Oncocytomas do not recur if completely resected. Malignant transformation is exceedingly rare {1831}.

Salivary gland myoepithelioma

Katabi N
Agaimy A
Fonseca I
Gnepp DR
Simpson RHW

Definition

Myoepithelioma (ME) is a benign salivary gland neoplasm that is composed almost exclusively of myoepithelial cells and the stroma they produce.

ICD-O coding

8982/0 Myoepithelioma

ICD-11 coding

2E91.1 & XH3CQ8 Benign neoplasm of other specified major salivary glands & Myoepithelioma

Related terminology

Not recommended: myoepithelial cell tumour; myoepithelial adenoma.

Subtype(s)

None

Localization

Most MEs occur in the parotid gland, followed by the palate; less commonly, they occur in submandibular gland {4953}.

Clinical features

The tumour usually presents as a painless slow-growing mass.

Epidemiology

ME accounts for 1.5% of all salivary gland tumours. It constitutes 2.2% and 5.7% of major and minor salivary gland tumours, respectively. The patient age range is 9–85 years (mean: 44 years), and it affects both sexes equally {1029,2671,347, 3940,4078,133,4518}.

Etiology

Unknown

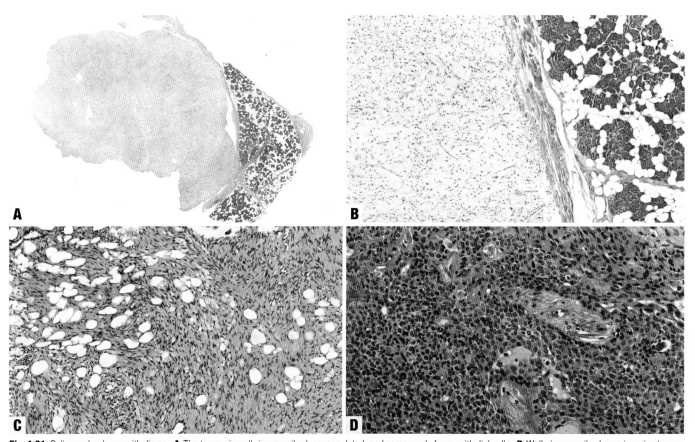

Fig. 4.21 Salivary gland myoepithelioma. **A** The tumour is well circumscribed, encapsulated, and composed of myoepithelial cells. **B** Well-circumscribed, non-invasive tumour surrounded by a capsule composed of spindle-shaped cells with myoepithelial differentiation. **C** Spindle cell with adipose metaplasia. The tumour is composed of spindled myoepithelial cells with adipose metaplasia. **D** Epithelioid and plasmacytoid myoepithelial cells.

Pathogenesis

A few cases show *EWSR1* rearrangements, with no correlation with histological patterns {3208}. *NTF3::PLAG1*, *FBXO32::PLAG1*, and *GEM::PLAG1* fusions have been detected in oncocytic ME {331}.

Macroscopic appearance

Tumours are solid and well-circumscribed, and they exhibit tan to yellow glistening cut surfaces.

Histopathology

ME shows well-circumscribed and often encapsulated borders. The myoepithelial cells can be spindled, epithelioid, plasmacytoid, or clear, or in variable combinations thereof {2368,3872}, and they may be arranged in nested, cord-like, trabeculated, or reticular patterns. The stroma can be myxoid, collagenous, or vascular. Abundant intracellular mucin is a rare reported finding {1612,1614,4110}, and oncocytic changes may be found. Encapsulation is uncommon in the minor salivary gland tumours.

Immunohistochemistry

ME is positive for keratins, S100, SOX10, and myoepithelial markers such as p63, calponin, and SMA.

Differential diagnosis

The well-defined borders of the tumour and the lack of invasive growth distinguish ME from myoepithelial carcinoma {2368,4887}. The characteristic basaloid biphasic pattern, peripheral palisading, and minimal to absent myxoid stroma of basal cell adenoma help to separate it from ME. Monomorphic histology and rare or absent ductal structures in ME separate it from pleomorphic adenoma {2666,4953}. Distinguishing from soft tissue ME may be difficult, given the overlapping histological features and the presence of *PLAG1* gene rearrangements in both {216}.

Cytology

Smears show variable cellularity, with bland myoepithelial cells (spindled, epithelioid, clear, or plasmacytoid) as a single cell type or mixed, in loosely cohesive tissue fragments with strands of hyaline stroma or as single cells. There is no myxofibrillary stroma. Necrosis and nuclear atypia suggest myoepithelial carcinoma, but because tumour invasion cannot be assessed, it is impossible to differentiate ME from myoepithelial carcinoma on cytopathology {2368}.

Diagnostic molecular pathology

Detection of *PLAG1* rearrangement by cytogenetics or other methods can be helpful {3208,331}.

Essential and desirable diagnostic criteria

Essential: almost exclusive myoepithelial differentiation and absence of invasion.
Desirable: tumour encapsulation (except in minor salivary glands).

Staging

Not applicable

Prognosis and prediction

ME is a benign tumour that shows a low recurrence rate. The tumour is treated by complete surgical resection. Malignant transformation to myoepithelial carcinoma has been reported but seems to be extremely rare {516,3895}.

Canalicular adenoma

Thompson LDR
Agaimy A
Bloemcna E

Definition
Canalicular adenoma is a benign salivary gland neoplasm of monomorphic epithelial cells arranged in anastomosing cords within a loose, vascularized stroma.

ICD-O coding
8149/0 Canalicular adenoma

ICD-11 coding
2E91.Z & XH1TD7 Benign neoplasm of major salivary glands, unspecified & Canalicular adenoma

Related terminology
Not recommended: canalicular tumour; canalicular mixed tumour; monomorphic adenoma, canalicular type; cystic adenoma; adenomatosis of accessory salivary glands.

Subtype(s)
None

Localization
Canalicular adenomas occur in the upper lip (80%), followed by the buccal mucosa, lower lip, hard palate, and soft palate {4413}.

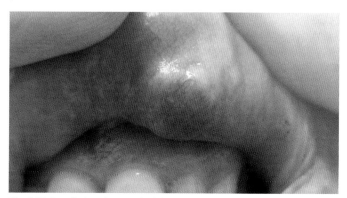

Fig. 4.22 Canalicular adenoma. A clinical image showing an upper-lip subepithelial nodule, characteristic of canalicular adenoma.

Clinical features
Patients present with a slowly growing, mobile, painless, non-ulcerated mass {4413}. Multifocal tumours are seen in 9% of cases {3021,3188,3772,4931}.

Epidemiology
Canalicular adenoma accounts for < 1% of all salivary gland tumours {2035,2122} and 4–6% of all benign minor salivary gland

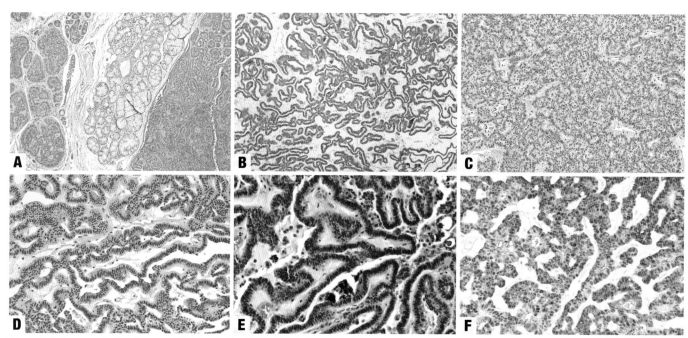

Fig. 4.23 Salivary canalicular adenoma. **A** Multifocality identified by identical tumour foci that are separate from the main tumour mass. **B** Low-power view demonstrates the interlacing canals and ribbons of neoplastic cuboidal-columnar cells separated by a loose, oedematous stroma. **C** This cellular tumour demonstrates a tight, glandular, ribbon-like architecture composed of a syncytium of short columnar epithelial cells. **D** Adjacent ribbons of cells come together and form a knot (beading), a feature quite characteristic of canalicular adenoma. **E** The canals contain squamoid morules, histiocytes, and calcifications. **F** All of the neoplastic cells show a strong and diffuse nuclear and cytoplasmic reaction for S100.

neoplasms {4674,2727,3021,3686,2120,2706,1448,3550,4413, 1428}. There is an M:F ratio of 1:1.7 {1008,4413}, with a wide age range (33–91 years) but a peak in the seventh decade of life.

Etiology
Unknown

Pathogenesis
Canalicular adenomas consistently lack the *IDH2* mutations of striated duct adenoma {3739A}.

Macroscopic appearance
Tumours range in size from 2 to 30 mm. They are well circumscribed, often cystic, showing light-yellow to tan to brown translucent nodules {4413}.

Histopathology
Tumours have a bosselated or lobulated surface and are occasionally multifocal. The tumour cells are relatively monotonous, high cuboidal to columnar, and arranged in one or two cell layers. These layers anastomose to create a lattice of cords, canaliculi, tubules, and/or strands. Papillary projections into cystic spaces are common. The cell ribbons frequently abut one another (termed "beading") with knots of cells joining parallel rows {1008,4413}. The nuclei appear pseudostratified. Intraluminal squamoid morules may be seen in the canals. The nuclei are round to oval with coarse chromatin. There is a syncytial appearance to the cells. There is no basal or myoepithelial layer. The stroma is sparse, loose, fibrillary, and oedematous, and it sometimes contains histiocytes. Laminated microliths are frequently present {4494,4413}. Mitoses are limited. Rare hybrid or collision tumours have been reported {3964}.

Immunohistochemistry
The cells are immunoreactive for pancytokeratin, CK7, S100, SOX10, and KIT (CD117), but non-reactive for DOG1, desmin, and actins {1377,3577,2759,4748,1215,1214,4413}. There is a characteristic linear peripheral GFAP immunoreactivity {985,4413}.

Differential diagnosis
The entities in the differential diagnosis include basal cell adenoma, polymorphous adenocarcinoma, adenoid cystic

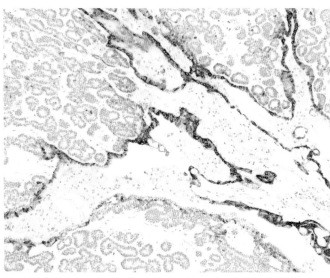

Fig. 4.24 Salivary canalicular adenoma. There is a curious peripheral GFAP immunoreactivity, while the central tumour cells are non-reactive.

carcinoma, reticulated myoepithelioma, selected odontogenic tumours, and skin basal cell carcinoma.

Cytology
Not clinically relevant

Diagnostic molecular pathology
None

Essential and desirable diagnostic criteria
Essential: minor salivary gland location; monotonous, isomorphic syncytium of cuboidal to columnar cells anastomosing in a lattice of cords and canaliculi; no basal/myoepithelial layer.

Staging
Not applicable

Prognosis and prediction
Complete conservative removal is best, although multifocality may suggest recurrence {4413}.

Cystadenoma of the salivary glands

Agaimy A
Nakaguro M
Seethala R
Simpson RHW

Definition
Cystadenoma is a rare, predominantly multicystic, benign epithelial salivary gland neoplasm that is lined by proliferative epithelium with variable papillary architecture and frequent oncocytic cytology.

ICD-O coding
8440/0 Cystadenoma
8450/0 Papillary cystadenoma
8440/0 Oncocytic cystadenoma
8470/0 Mucinous cystadenoma

ICD-11 coding
2E91.Z & XH5RJ2 Benign neoplasm of major salivary glands, unspecified & Cystadenoma, NOS

Related terminology
Not recommended: cystic duct adenoma; intraductal papillary hyperplasia.

Subtype(s)
Papillary cystadenoma; oncocytic cystadenoma; mucinous cystadenoma

Localization
Cystadenomas seem equally distributed between major and minor salivary glands. Almost half of all cases originate in the parotid, followed by minor glands of the lip and buccal mucosa {4463}.

Clinical features
Cystadenomas present as slowly growing, painless nodules or masses. Minor salivary gland tumours are covered by smooth mucosa, frequently mimicking mucocoele. Major salivary gland tumours are clinically not distinguishable from other indolent cystic salivary gland lesions {4463}.

Epidemiology
Cystadenomas represent 1–4% of all salivary gland neoplasms. Women are more frequently affected than men, with a mean age in the fifth to seventh decade of life {4463}.

Etiology
None

Pathogenesis
The pathogenesis of cystadenoma is not well understood. Three tumours (two oncocytic) with genetic data lacked mutations in *BRAF, AKT1, PIK3CA, HRAS, KRAS,* and *GNAS* {3146}.

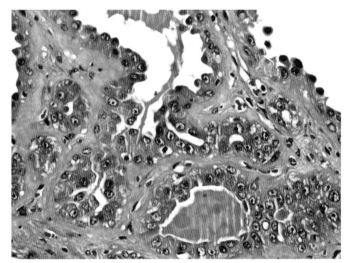

Fig. 4.25 Cystadenoma of the salivary gland. The cysts in this tumour are lined predominantly by apocrine cells.

Macroscopic appearance
Tumours vary from unilocular to multilocular with variably sized cystic spaces. Their lining varies from flat and smooth to a granular-papillary lining. The cyst contents vary depending on the predominant epithelial type and range from watery to thick mucoid {4463,1598}.

Histopathology
Cystadenomas are well circumscribed but unencapsulated, with entrapment of salivary tissue at the periphery. As many as 20% of cases are unicystic. The cysts are variably sized and lined by epithelial cells of different types with a variable papillary configuration. The lining epithelium shows an admixture of columnar, cuboidal, and oncocytic cells in variable combinations. Mucinous, squamous, apocrine, and ciliated epithelia are uncommon. Cystadenomas lack cytological atypia, mitotic activity, and invasive growth. They also lack the complex arborizing and hierarchical papillary tufting of intercalated-type intraductal carcinoma and other entities {4117}.

Subtypes
The papillary oncocytic subtype closely mimics lymphocyte-poor Warthin tumour. Purely or predominantly mucinous and squamous subtypes are rare.

Immunohistochemistry
The lining cells show a simple luminal phenotype (CK8/18+), supported by a p63+ basal cell layer {1430}. S100 and SOX10 are usually absent or only focally expressed.

Differential diagnosis

Cystadenoma should be distinguished from other papillary ductal proliferations by established criteria {35}. Immunohistochemistry may help to exclude macrocystic secretory carcinoma (S100+, SOX10+, mammaglobin+, MUC4+) and intercalated-type intraductal carcinoma (S100+, SOX10+, mammaglobin+) {1846, 4378}. The mucinous subtype has organoid epithelium lacking the irregularly distributed intermediate and epidermoid cells and distorted mucous cell component seen in purely cystic mucoepidermoid carcinoma {1598,2467}.

Cytology

Not described

Diagnostic molecular pathology

Diagnostic molecular pathology is not directly relevant. However, testing can exclude other cystic tumour entities (i.e. *ETV6* for secretory carcinoma, *NR4A3* for acinic cell carcinoma, and *MAML2* for mucoepidermoid carcinoma).

Essential and desirable diagnostic criteria

Essential: a unicystic or multicystic non-invasive bland neoplasm with an oncocytic or mixed epithelial lining; no lymphoid stroma; exclusion of other cystic salivary gland tumours.
Desirable: oncocytic cells and other variable cell types; a variable papillary component; a demonstrable basal cell layer.

Staging

Not applicable

Prognosis and prediction

Cystadenoma is cured by simple excision. Recurrence is rare. Rare cases of invasive carcinoma originating from cystadenoma have been reported {4073,2982}.

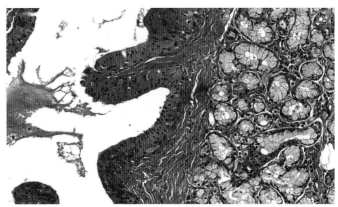

Fig. 4.26 Cystadenoma of the salivary gland, oncocytic–papillary subtype. A unicystic lesion lined by oncocytic epithelium with a variable papillary configuration.

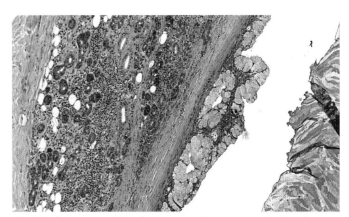

Fig. 4.27 Cystadenoma of the salivary gland, mucinous subtype. A multicystic tumour composed of large cysts lined by well-oriented mucinous cells with basal nuclei and focal papillae supported by a basal cell layer. No *MAML2* fusion was detected

Ductal papillomas

Foschini MP
Katabi N
Nakaguro M

Definition

Ductal papillomas (DPs) are benign epithelial neoplasms arising from the main excretory salivary ducts.

ICD-O coding

8503/0 Intraductal papilloma

ICD-11 coding

2E91.Z & XA5T23 & XH4LZ4 Benign neoplasm of major salivary glands, unspecified & Salivary gland apparatus & Intraductal papilloma

Related terminology

Acceptable: intraductal papilloma; inverted ductal papilloma.

Subtype(s)

None

Localization

Preferential sites are intraoral minor salivary glands, with the lower lip, buccal mucosa, and palate being the most frequent {569,35,1831}. Rare DPs affect the parotid or unusual sites {1768,4286}.

Clinical features

DPs present as slowly growing, painless submucosal lesions or as polypoid intraoral lesions. The duration of symptoms ranges from a few weeks to several years {569,1789}.

Epidemiology

DPs constitute about 0.3% of oral salivary gland tumours {35}. They usually affect adults, with no sex predilection {852,2391, 3248}. Rare paediatric cases have been reported {569,35,1831}.

Etiology

A relationship with trauma has been reported {3824}.

Pathogenesis

HPV DNA was detected in only 1 case {2016,1142}. No genetic changes were identified {3146}.

Macroscopic appearance

DPs appear as cystic nodules measuring < 15 mm {569}.

Histopathology

DP may be described as intraductal papilloma or inverted ductal papilloma, according to the growth pattern {569,1831, 35}. Intraductal papillomas are usually located at the ostia of the salivary excretory ducts, presenting as a unicystic lesion with well-defined borders and filled with papillary projections. Papillae are lined by columnar cells intermingled with rare mucoid cells. Inverted ductal papilloma is an unencapsulated, endophytic epithelial tumour with well-defined borders and a central opening that is frequently in contact with the surface mucosa. It is composed of mucinous and non-keratinizing squamous cells. No atypia is seen, and mitoses are rare {852, 2391,3248}.

Immunohistochemistry

Immunohistochemistry is of little help in the diagnosis.

Differential diagnosis

The entities include other salivary gland papillary lesions {35} such as mucinous adenocarcinoma {51} and mucoepidermoid carcinoma. The presence of branching papillae lined by numerous pale, gastric-like cells favours mucinous adenocarcinoma. Atypia, invasive borders, and the presence

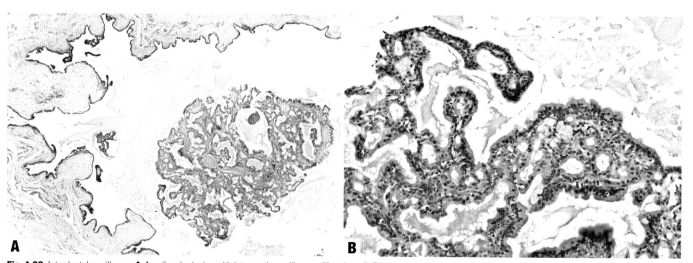

Fig. 4.28 Intraductal papilloma. **A** A unilocular lesion with intracystic papillary proliferation. **B** Bland cuboidal to columnar tumour cells are admixed with some mucoid cells.

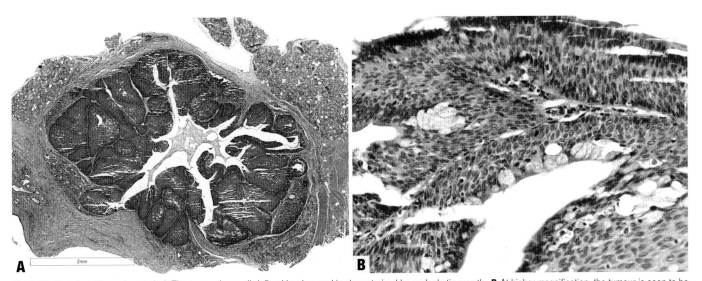

Fig. 4.29 Ductal papilloma, inverted. **A** The tumour has well-defined borders and is characterized by endophytic growth. **B** At higher magnification, the tumour is seen to be composed of squamoid cells and some mucous cells, with no atypia.

of *MAML2* fusion favour the diagnosis of mucoepidermoid carcinoma.

Cytology

Rarely reported cases show smears with papillary tissue fragments and sheets of ductal or oncocytic columnar cells with bland nuclei, and histiocytes in the background {1767,4172}.

Diagnostic molecular pathology

Not relevant

Essential and desirable diagnostic criteria

Intraductal papilloma

Essential: a unicystic lesion with internal papillae, lined by columnar cells lacking atypia.

Inverted ductal papilloma

Essential: well-delineated borders and endophytic growth, composed of squamous and mucoid cells devoid of atypia.

Staging

Not relevant

Prognosis and prediction

DPs are benign, cured by complete surgical excision {569}.

Sialadenoma papilliferum

Hsieh MS
Foschini MP
Katabi N
Nakaguro M

Definition

Sialadenoma papilliferum (SP) is a polypoid neoplasm with both exophytic and inward papillary proliferation of mucosal and salivary ductal epithelium.

ICD-O coding

8406/0 Sialadenoma papilliferum

ICD-11 coding

2E91.Z & XH65F9 Benign neoplasm of unspecified major salivary glands & Sialadenoma papilliferum

Related terminology

None

Subtype(s)

None

Localization

Most SPs occur in the hard palate, followed by the buccal mucosa. Other sites include the soft palate, tongue, mouth floor, parotid gland, bronchus, and oesophagus {3141,794}.

Clinical features

SP usually presents as a raised sessile or pedunculated mucosal lesion {794}.

Epidemiology

SP is rare and tends to occur in older adults. The age range is 2–91 years (median: 62 years) {19,1446,1931}. There is a male predominance {794}.

Etiology

Unknown

Pathogenesis

BRAF p.V600E mutation is consistently reported in SP {1931, 3141}.

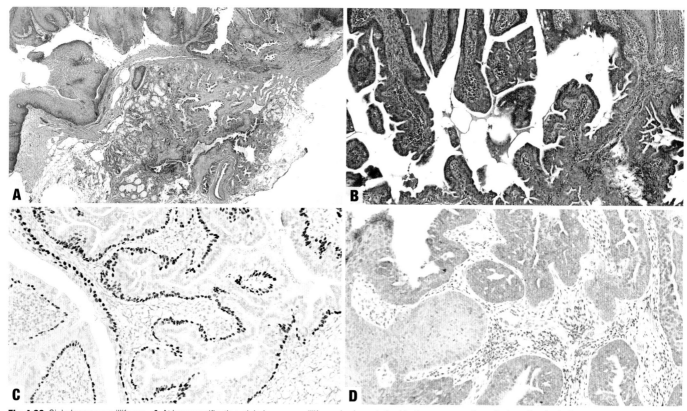

Fig. 4.30 Sialadenoma papilliferum. **A** At low magnification, sialadenoma papilliferum is characterized by the presence of exophytic and endophytic components. **B** The upper exophytic part shows a papillary proliferation of squamous cells mixed with ductal cells. The lower part shows the ductal component with a cystic-papillary pattern. **C** The ductal component has p63-positive basal cells. **D** Both the squamous and ductal components are positive for BRAF p.V600E by immunohistochemistry.

Macroscopic appearance

SP is typically polypoid with a papillary surface and well-circumscribed margins. The size is usually < 10 mm, and cystic spaces might be grossly visible on cut section {19,1446,1931, 794}.

Histopathology

SP is characterized by the presence of both exophytic surface squamous and endophytic ductal papillary proliferation. The exophytic squamous proliferation is directly contiguous with submucosal salivary gland ductal epithelium that shows endophytic papillary infoldings and cystic-like spaces {19,1446, 3146}. The ductal epithelium has a biphasic pattern, with luminal cuboidal or columnar cells and basally located basal cells {1446}. A lymphoplasmacytic stromal infiltrate is common. The ductal luminal cells may show oncocytic metaplasia {1931,794}. Cases with endophytic ductal proliferation with *BRAF* mutation but no exophytic component are called "SP-like intraductal papillary tumours" {3146}.

Immunohistochemistry

The ductal cells are positive for CK7 and SOX10; the basal cells are positive for p63. The exophytic squamous cells are positive for p63 and CK13, and may be focally positive for CK7 {2793, 1931,794}. Positive immunohistochemistry for BRAF p.V600E staining can be seen in both squamous and ductal components of SP {3146,794}.

Differential diagnosis

The presence of a typical exophytic and endophytic growth pattern can distinguish SP from other salivary duct papillary tumours including squamous cell papilloma, ductal papilloma, or cystadenoma. A lack of invasion and overt atypia distinguishes SP from adenosquamous carcinoma.

Cytology

Not reported

Diagnostic molecular pathology

Demonstration of *BRAF* p.V600E mutation by PCR or other methods may be helpful.

Essential and desirable diagnostic criteria

Essential: surface exophytic mucosal squamous proliferation and submucosal ductal cystic-like spaces.
Desirable: evidence of *BRAF* p.V600E mutation (in selected cases).

Staging

Not applicable

Prognosis and prediction

Surgical removal is curative for SP. Recurrence and malignant transformation are very rare {794}.

Lymphadenoma

Gnepp DR
Chiosea S
Layfield LJ
Prasad ML
Vazmitsel M

Definition
Lymphadenoma is a benign salivary gland tumour consisting of a proliferation of ductal or sebaceous epithelial cells forming nests within a reactive lymphoid background.

ICD-O coding
8563/0 Lymphadenoma
8563/0 Sebaceous lymphadenoma
8563/0 Non-sebaceous lymphadenoma

ICD-11 coding
2E91.Z & XH7J33 Benign neoplasm of major salivary glands, unspecified & Lymphadenoma

Related terminology
None

Subtype(s)
Sebaceous lymphadenoma; non-sebaceous lymphadenoma

Localization
Most sebaceous lymphadenomas occur in the parotid/periparotid area or submandibular gland {4989,3429,1547}; lacrimal and minor salivary gland tumours have been reported {2864, 3431}. Non-sebaceous lymphadenomas frequently occur in parotid gland or periparotid tissue {2678,3431,4639}.

Clinical features
Patients present with a slowly growing, painless mass of a few months' to several years' duration {2678}.

Epidemiology
Lymphadenomas represent 0.1% of salivary gland neoplasms and < 0.5% of salivary gland adenomas {3961}. The sebaceous type is more common. The patient age range is 10–78 years (median: 59 years) {3961}. Non-sebaceous lymphadenomas tend to affect younger patients, including children {2749, 1030,4281,3665,3071}. Sebaceous lymphadenomas have an M:F ratio of 4:3, and non-sebaceous lymphadenomas may show a slight female preference {3961}.

Etiology
Unknown

Pathogenesis
Unknown

Macroscopic appearance
Sebaceous lymphadenomas are slightly larger than non-sebaceous lymphadenomas: 29 mm (range: 10–60 mm) and 15 mm (range: 6–50 mm), respectively. They are typically well

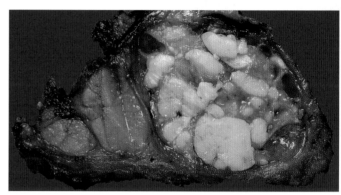

Fig. 4.31 Sebaceous lymphadenoma. The cut surface of this parotid gland tumour shows numerous cysts filled with yellow, greasy sebaceous material.

circumscribed to encapsulated, with a grey-white / tan-yellow solid or multicystic cut surface {3431}.

Histopathology
Sebaceous lymphadenomas are well circumscribed and variably macrocystic or microcystic. They are composed of variably sized ducts, with foci of sebaceous differentiation in a benign lymphoid background containing reactive lymphoid follicles with germinal centres {2749,3961,4015,5006}. Pleomorphism and cytological atypia are minimal; necrosis and mitoses are uncommon. Squamous differentiation and oncocytic metaplasia may be seen {1065,4989}. Histiocytes and/or foreign body giant cells, from sebum leakage, are common {2749,3961, 5006}. Non-sebaceous lymphadenomas are similar but without sebaceous cells {2749,3961,5006}.

Immunohistochemistry
Sebocytes stain for p63, EMA, adipophilin, and perilipin. Basal cells are positive for CK5/6 and p63; luminal epithelial cells are positive for CK7, CK18, and CK19 {4919,3961}. Lymphocytes are polytypic. The Ki-67 index is < 10%. p16 is positive in sebaceous lymphadenoma; HPV, EBV, and KSHV/HHV8 are negative {3961}.

Differential diagnosis
Absence of invasion, extensive epidermoid islands, and *MAML2* gene rearrangement help to distinguish lymphadenomas from the Warthin-like variant of mucoepidermoid carcinoma {5006}.

Cytology
Smears are cellular, showing 3D tissue fragments that may be glandular or solid, composed of bland basaloid or columnar cells, with lymphocytes and histiocytes in a proteinaceous background {699,4610,4639}. Sebaceous differentiation with abundant finely vacuolated microvesicular cytoplasm and central nuclei is not prominent.

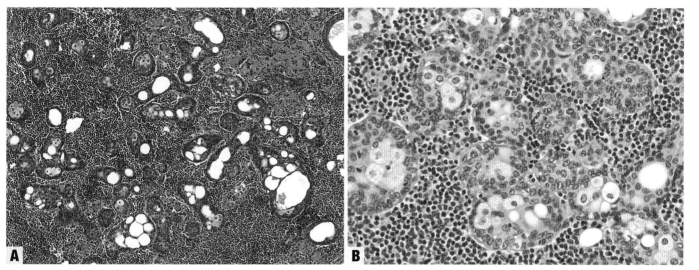

Fig. 4.32 Lymphadenoma. **A** Numerous cystic spaces and small ducts are noted, many showing microvesicular cytoplasm as would be expected in sebaceous differentiation. **B** Sebaceous lymphadenoma. Small glands are lined by cuboidal cells, and numerous sebocytes are noted throughout, a finding seen in sebaceous lymphadenoma. Note the lymphoid stroma in the background.

Diagnostic molecular pathology
Not applicable

Essential and desirable diagnostic criteria
Essential: for lymphadenoma, sebaceous subtype: epithelial nests/ducts, sebaceous cells/nests, and a benign lymphoid background; for lymphadenoma, non-sebaceous subtype: epithelial nests/ducts in a benign lymphoid background.
Desirable: a well-defined capsule.

Staging
Not applicable

Prognosis and prediction
These are benign tumours, which do not recur if completely excised. Malignant transformation is extremely rare and has been reported in the sebaceous, basaloid, and lymphoid components {974,1616,3961,4610}.

Sebaceous adenoma

Gnepp DR
Di Palma S
Thompson LDR
Weinreb I
Williams MD

Definition

Sebaceous adenoma is a benign, well-circumscribed tumour composed of irregularly sized and shaped nests of sebaceous cells without cytological atypia, frequently with areas of cystic change and squamous differentiation.

ICD-O coding

8410/0 Sebaceous adenoma

ICD-11 coding

2E91.Z & XH1NC5 Benign neoplasm of major salivary glands, unspecified & Sebaceous adenoma

Related terminology

None

Subtype(s)

None

Localization

Approximately 60% arise in the major salivary glands (typically the parotid gland) and 40% arise in the oral cavity (frequently the buccal mucosa) {1613}.

Clinical features

Patients usually present with a painless mass.

Epidemiology

Sebaceous adenoma is rare, accounting for 0.1% of all salivary gland neoplasms and slightly less than 0.5% of all adenomas {1831}. The mean age at initial clinical presentation is in the sixth decade of life (range: 22–90 years), with an M:F ratio of 4:3 {1613,1831}.

Etiology

Unknown

Pathogenesis

Unknown

Macroscopic appearance

These tumours range in size from 4 to 60 mm in greatest dimension. They are commonly encapsulated or sharply circumscribed, varying in colour from greyish-white to pinkish-white to yellow or yellowish-grey {1616}.

Histopathology

Tumours are composed of closely associated dilated or microcystic salivary ducts with foci of prominent sebaceous differentiation, often with areas of squamous change. Atypia and pleomorphism are minimal; invasion of surrounding tissues is not found. Sebaceous glands vary markedly in tortuosity and

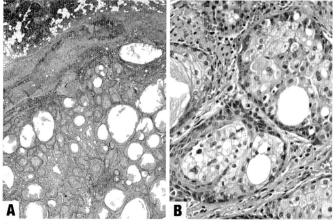

Fig. 4.33 Sebaceous adenoma. **A** The tumour is encapsulated and is composed of numerous closely associated nests with prominent sebaceous differentiation. The cystic spaces previously contained sebum. **B** Nests of cells exhibiting prominent sebaceous differentiation.

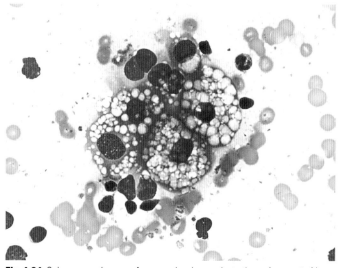

Fig. 4.34 Sebaceous adenoma. A smear showing a minute tissue fragment of large vacuolated epithelial cells with centrally located scalloped nuclei (FNAB, Giemsa).

size; they are frequently embedded in fibrous stroma. Marked oncocytic metaplasia may be found, and histiocytes and/or foreign body giant cells due to extravasated sebum can be seen focally. Lymphoid infiltrates and follicles, cytological atypia, necrosis, and mitoses are not compatible with a diagnosis of sebaceous adenoma {1616,1613}.

Cytology

Smears are moderately cellular, with tissue fragments consisting of large epithelial cells with abundant foamy, finely granular or finely vacuolated sebaceous cytoplasm and centrally located bland round nuclei with slightly irregular nuclear contours and inconspicuous nucleoli {699,4610,4639}. Basaloid cells, squamous cells, and lymphocytes can be present, as well as histiocytes. Oncocytes are not seen. Necrosis, nuclear atypia, and mitotic figures are absent {1096,223}.

Diagnostic molecular pathology
Not clinically relevant

Essential and desirable diagnostic criteria
Essential: numerous closely packed sebaceous glands with minimal or no atypia, arising in salivary gland tissue.

Staging
Not relevant

Prognosis and prediction
The tumours do not recur after complete excision.

Intercalated duct adenoma and hyperplasia

Chiosea S
Di Palma S
Thompson LDR
Weinreb I
Williams MD

Definition

Intercalated duct adenoma and hyperplasia are benign salivary ductal proliferations resembling bilayered (epithelial and myoepithelial) intercalated ducts.

ICD-O coding

None

ICD-11 coding

2E91.Z Benign neoplasm of unspecified major salivary glands

Related terminology

Not recommended: adenomatous ductal proliferation.

Subtype(s)

None

Localization

The majority (85%) of cases arise in the parotid gland, followed by the submandibular gland (11%) and the oral cavity (4%) {1139,818,4958,2735,4764,3167,806,452}.

Clinical features

Most cases are incidental, identified concurrently with other salivary gland lesions (e.g. basal cell adenoma, epithelial-myoepithelial carcinoma) {818,4764,3053,452}.

Epidemiology

Intercalated duct adenoma and hyperplasia are rarely reported {1139,818,4958,2735,4764,3167,806,3053,452}. There is an M:F ratio of 2:3, occurring in middle age (mean age: 52 years).

Etiology

Unknown

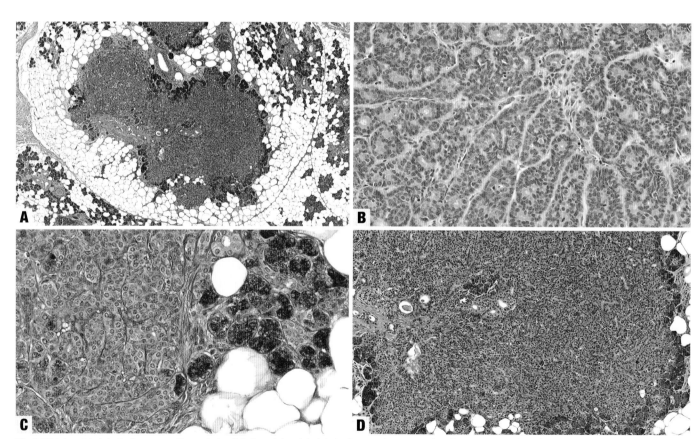

Fig. 4.35 Intercalated duct adenoma and hyperplasia. **A** Salivary intercalated duct adenoma. Low-power view demonstrates an irregular periphery, with multinodularity. The proliferation is a monotonous single-cell population, with acinar cells at the periphery. **B** Salivary intercalated duct adenoma. A monotonous proliferation of cuboidal cells arranged in an acinar configuration. Note the delicate eosinophilic cytoplasmic granules. **C** Intercalated duct hyperplasia. Proliferation of small eosinophilic tubules with transition from acini. **D** Salivary intercalated duct lesion. The separation of adenoma from hyperplasia is challenging, because sometimes there is a blending at the periphery with acinar cells (dark blue cytoplasmic granules), whereas the proliferation contains eosinophilic cytoplasmic granules.

Pathogenesis

Adenomas have been shown to harbour hotspot *HRAS* pathogenic variants, while hyperplasia often has *CTNNB1* mutations {2907A}.

Macroscopic appearance

Intercalated duct adenoma and hyperplasia are rarely detected macroscopically. Most lesions are < 5 mm {4764}.

Histopathology

Intercalated duct lesions manifest as a nodular, occasionally multinodular, proliferation of cuboidal ductal cells with attenuated myoepithelial cells, sometimes containing acinic cells. Intercalated duct lesions are subdivided into adenoma when well circumscribed or encapsulated, and hyperplasia when blending with adjacent acini {4764,2907A}.

Differential diagnosis

If well circumscribed, it should be distinguished from striated duct adenoma (which lacks myoepithelial cells) {4764,4766}.

Cytology

Smears show cohesive large tissue fragments of epithelial cells with high N:C ratios and bland oval nuclei, with admixed thin stromal strands {3043}.

Diagnostic molecular pathology

Not clinically relevant

Essential and desirable diagnostic criteria

Essential: a monotonous proliferation of cuboidal ductal cells surrounded by myoepithelial cells, sometimes with acinic cells.

Staging

Not applicable

Prognosis and prediction

Most are incidental lesions, with an excellent prognosis.

Chapter 4

Striated duct adenoma

Weinreb I
Hellquist H
Perez-Ordonez B
Wasserman JK

Definition
Striated duct adenoma (SDA) is a benign salivary gland tumour composed of ducts resembling normal striated ducts lined by a single layer of luminal cells with minimal intervening stroma.

ICD-O coding
8503/0 Striated duct adenoma

ICD-11 coding
2E91.Z Benign neoplasm of unspecified major salivary glands

Related terminology
Not recommended: ductal adenoma.

Subtype(s)
None

Localization
SDA can involve both the major and minor salivary glands, with a predominance in the parotid {4766,2037}.

Clinical features
SDA presents as a painless mass {4766,2037}.

Epidemiology
SDAs are rare tumours. Those described have been in adults (age range: 47–78 years), with a slight female predominance {4766,2037}.

Etiology
Unknown

Pathogenesis
In one study, *IDH2* p.R172 pathogenic variants were found in all tested cases {3739A}.

Macroscopic appearance
SDAs present as solid masses with a yellow cut surface.

Histopathology
SDAs are well circumscribed and encapsulated. They are composed of small, closely spaced ducts with minimal intervening

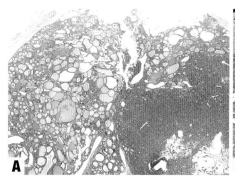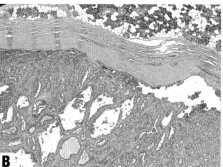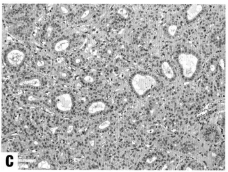

Fig. 4.36 Striated duct adenoma. **A** Low-power image of a striated duct adenoma with variable small-calibre ducts and microcysts. **B** The tumours are made of a pure population of eosinophilic ducts with minimal intervening stroma. Some lumina contain numerous red blood cells. **C** The majority of the ductal spaces are similarly sized to normal striated ducts and have bland nuclei. Luminal secretions may resemble colloid.

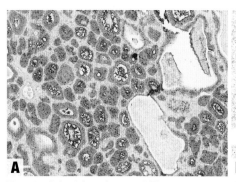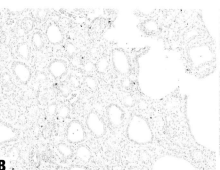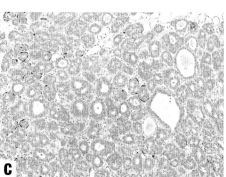

Fig. 4.37 Striated duct adenoma. **A** These tumours are diffusely positive for S100, unlike their closest mimics, namely oncocytomas. **B** Striated duct adenomas are unilayered, with minimal contribution from basal or myoepithelial cells. Therefore, p63 immunohistochemistry stains only focal abluminal cells, if any. **C** Calponin (shown here) or actins show only focal abluminal staining, if any, in striated duct adenoma.

stroma. Small cysts can also be seen. The tumour may be highly vascular, and some contain staghorn blood vessels. The ducts are lined by a single layer of columnar cells with eosinophilic cytoplasm, unlike intercalated duct lesions {4764}. Occasionally, the luminal spaces may contain eosinophilic material reminiscent of colloid, as well as red blood cells. Some cases show hyalinization and may mimic oncocytoma with oncocytosis. Occasional cases will show striated duct hyperplasia of the background parotid. The duct calibre is comparable to that of normal striated ducts. Fat cells may be focally or diffusely present {4928,4766}.

Immunohistochemistry
SDAs are strongly positive for keratins, including CK7 and CK5/6. Most tumours show strong nuclear and cytoplasmic staining for S100 (unlike oncocytoma). In contrast, calponin, SMA, SMMHC, and p63 highlight isolated abluminal cells only, which should not be interpreted as a true basal or myoepithelial layer. Markers of thyroid differentiation, such as thyroid transcription factor 1 (TTF1) and thyroglobulin, are negative {4766}.

Differential diagnosis
SDAs do not show chondromyxoid stroma or any other matrix. They do not show morphologically visible bilayering {4766}. They do not have the deeply eosinophilic cytoplasm characteristic of oncocytoma.

Cytology
Not reported

Diagnostic molecular pathology
IDH2 mutations may help to confirm the diagnosis in selected cases {3739A}.

Essential and desirable diagnostic criteria
Essential: closely spaced ducts with minimal intervening stroma lined by a single layer of eosinophilic luminal cells.
Desirable: absence of myoepithelial cells by immunohistochemistry (in selected cases).

Staging
Not applicable

Prognosis and prediction
SDAs do not recur, according to the limited case reports to date, and they do not metastasize {4766,2037}.

Sclerosing polycystic adenoma

Bishop JA
Losito NS
Petersson BF
Prasad ML
Thompson LDR

Definition

Sclerosing polycystic adenoma (SPA) is a circumscribed salivary gland neoplasm composed of large acinar cells with brightly eosinophilic intracytoplasmic granules, and variable ductal and cystic components, including foamy, vacuolated, and apocrine cells.

ICD-O coding

8140/0 Sclerosing polycystic adenoma

ICD-11 coding

2E91.Z Benign neoplasm of unspecified major salivary glands

Related terminology

Not recommended: sclerosing polycystic adenosis.

Subtype(s)

None

Localization

The majority (80%) arise in the parotid gland, with occasional sinonasal, submandibular, and lacrimal gland involvement {1619,3237,1723,2916,4259,3519,4107}.

Clinical features

SPA is a slow-growing, painless mass. It is rarely multifocal {1619,3510,2817}.

Epidemiology

SPA is rare {1619}. The mean age at presentation is 40 years (range: 7–84 years), and there is a slight female predominance {4110}.

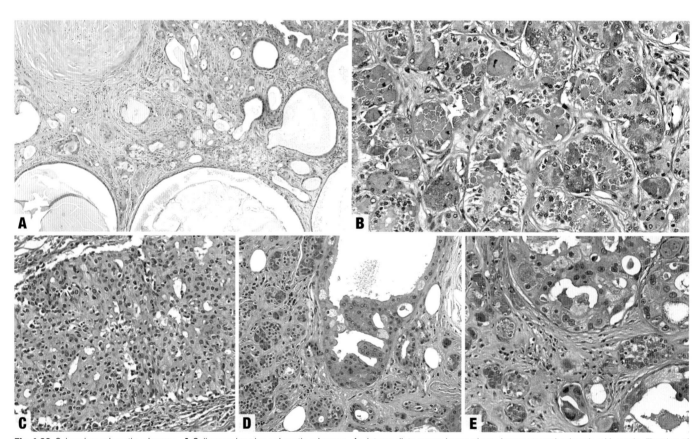

Fig. 4.38 Sclerosing polycystic adenoma. **A** Salivary sclerosing polycystic adenoma. An intermediate-power image shows heavy stromal sclerosis with cystic dilatation of hyperplastic-appearing epithelium showing ducts and acinar cells. Apocrine change is present, and foamy cytoplasm is seen in degenerating cells. **B** Salivary sclerosing polycystic adenoma. Eosinophilic, spherical laminated hyaline globules are noted in association with epithelial nests, which also have cells with prominent eosinophilic cytoplasmic granules. **C** Foci of homogeneous solid, micropapillary, and cribriform intraductal epithelial proliferations reminiscent of the intercalated duct cell variant of intraductal carcinoma. The intraductal proliferations are composed of intercalated duct cell–like epithelium and show solid and cribriform patterns. **D** Salivary sclerosing polycystic adenoma. This case shows a mixed population of acinar cells and ducts in a fibrous stroma. The cystic duct in the centre shows apocrine hyperplasia that, by itself, is indistinguishable from apocrine intraductal carcinoma. **E** Salivary sclerosing polycystic adenoma. Closely attached solid, tubular, and cribriform epithelial proliferations are composed of apocrine cells with nuclear atypia and finely granular cytoplasm. These cells are positive for AR and negative for SOX10.

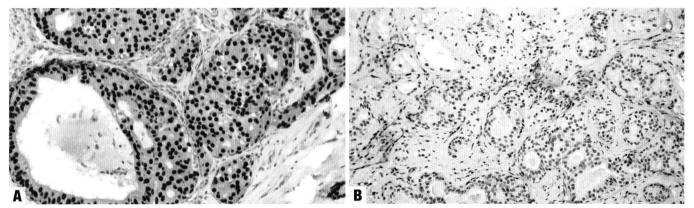

Fig. 4.39 Sclerosing polycystic adenoma. **A** The intraductal proliferations show rigid bridging and cribriform patterns and are composed of intercalated duct cell–like epithelium positive for SOX10. **B** Salivary sclerosing polycystic adenoma. PTEN immunohistochemistry shows an abnormal loss of expression in the ductal and apocrine elements but retained staining in the stromal and myoepithelial cells.

Etiology

Rare cases are associated with polycystic/dysgenetic disease {2143} and Cowden syndrome {1848}.

Pathogenesis

SPA was originally regarded as pseudoneoplastic {4144, 4116}, until monoclonality was demonstrated by polymorphism of human androgen receptor assay {4111}. Consistent mutations in PI3K pathway genes, most frequently *PTEN*, confirm its neoplastic nature and suggest links with apocrine intraductal carcinoma and salivary duct carcinoma {471,472, 483,1848,4107}.

Macroscopic appearance

SPA is a well-circumscribed, often encapsulated nodule measuring 10–120 mm (mean: 30 mm). The cut section is partially solid and cystic.

Histopathology

SPA is characterized by a cystic and multilobular pattern, composed of variably sized and shaped ducts lined by flattened, cylindrical, or apocrine foamy or vacuolated epithelium, embedded in a sclerotic collagenous stroma with focal lymphoid aggregates {4115,4110,483}. The hallmark of SPA is the presence of acini containing large, brightly eosinophilic cytoplasmic granules/globules. SPA often display solid, cribriform, and micropapillary proliferations with variable degrees of cytological atypia, surrounded by myoepithelial cells, resembling intraductal carcinoma {3505}. SPA is rarely associated with invasive carcinoma {652,1848,4107}.

Immunohistochemistry

Each cellular component demonstrates its expected immunophenotype: SOX10 in ductules, myoepithelial cells, and acini; SMA, p40, and calponin in myoepithelial cells; and AR and GCDFP-15 in apocrine cells. There is frequent loss of PTEN in ductal and acinar cells, but not in myoepithelial cells {471,1848}.

Cytology

Smears show a mix of flat, cohesive sheets of epithelial cells with variably granular oncocytic cytoplasm and round nuclei; sheets of apocrine-type epithelium; and histiocytic cells in a proteinaceous background. The coexistence of different cell types in a single sheet is helpful {1286,1503,4115}.

Diagnostic molecular pathology

None

Essential and desirable diagnostic criteria

Essential: mixtures of ductal and myoepithelial cells, with acinar cells containing large hypereosinophilic cytoplasmic granules.
Desirable: apocrine metaplasia and intraductal proliferation creating a resemblance to low-grade ductal carcinoma in situ; cystic appearance; PTEN loss by immunohistochemistry (in selected cases).

Staging

Not applicable

Prognosis and prediction

There is local recurrence in 10% of incompletely excised or multifocal cases {4144,4116,3505,1614,483}. Rare invasive carcinomas ex SPA have been reported {652,4107}.

Keratocystoma

Nagao T
Gnepp DR
Nibu K

Definition

Keratocystoma is a benign salivary gland tumour characterized by multicystic spaces, lined by stratified squamous epithelium, containing keratotic lamellae and focal solid epithelial nests.

ICD-O coding

8052/0 Keratocystoma

ICD-11 coding

2E91.Z Benign neoplasm of unspecified major salivary glands

Related terminology

None

Subtype(s)

None

Localization

All reported tumours arose in the parotid gland.

Clinical features

The tumour manifests as a painless, slowly growing parotid gland mass.

Epidemiology

The patient age range is 8–49 years {3965,3129,5016,1953, 4720,2365}.

Etiology

Unknown

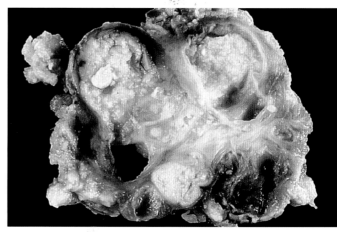

Fig. 4.40 Keratocystoma. Cut surface of the parotid tumour, showing multiple cystic formations filled with keratin-like material.

Pathogenesis

Keratocystoma is characterized by *RUNX2* rearrangements, mostly with *IRF2BP2::RUNX2* fusion {476A}.

Macroscopic appearance

Tumours range in size from 13 to 40 mm. The cut surface shows a multilocular cystic lesion filled with a keratin-like substance.

Histopathology

The tumour consists mainly of multiple cysts containing keratotic lamellae. Stratified squamous epithelium lines the cystic spaces and shows a parakeratotic or orthokeratotic surface, usually without a granular cell layer. The stratification

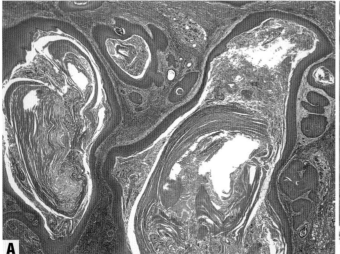
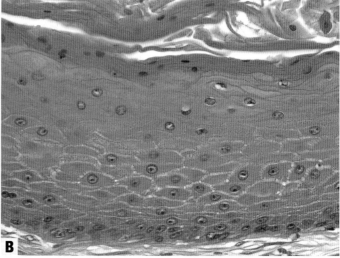

Fig. 4.41 Keratocystoma. **A** Multiple cysts with focal bud-like epithelial outer protrusions and a few solid epithelial cell nests. The cystic spaces contain lamellar keratin material. **B** The cyst wall is lined by bland stratified squamous epithelium with keratinization through parakeratotic cells. Note the lack of a granular cell layer.

of the epithelium is oriented regularly from the outer basal to the inner keratotic cell layers. Focally, the outer layer demonstrates bud-like protrusions, but no skin appendages are seen. In some areas, solid squamous cell islands with sharply defined margins are surrounded by collagenous stroma. The solid areas of squamous cell nests are localized partly within the parenchyma of the parotid gland adjacent to an excretory duct and should not be interpreted as invasive growth. Transformation from parotid ductal epithelium to neoplastic cells, through a squamous metaplasia–like process, may be present.

Cells of the neoplastic squamous epithelium have uniform, bland nuclei and abundant eosinophilic cytoplasm. There is no oncocytic or mucous cell differentiation and no myxochondroid component. Foci of foreign body reaction against keratin and a dense lymphoid infiltration may be evident.

Immunohistochemistry
Immunostaining for S100, SMA, and calponin is negative.

Differential diagnosis
The differential diagnoses include primary and metastatic squamous cell carcinoma, mucoepidermoid carcinoma, metaplastic Warthin tumour, and necrotizing sialometaplasia. The absence of necrosis, invasion, and cytological atypia in keratocystoma weighs against malignancy.

Cytology
Not reported

Diagnostic molecular pathology
Not clinically relevant

Essential and desirable diagnostic criteria
Essential: multicystic structures containing keratinized lamellae; bland stratified squamous epithelial lining without a granular layer.
Desirable: the presence of sharply defined solid squamous cell islands.

Staging
Not applicable

Prognosis and prediction
The tumours behave in a benign manner, with no recurrence after excision or subtotal parotidectomy.

Mucoepidermoid carcinoma

Leivo I
Bishop JA
Cipriani NA
Costes-Martineau V
Inagaki H
Vielh P

Definition

Mucoepidermoid carcinoma (MEC) is a malignant salivary gland neoplasm characterized by mucous, intermediate, and epidermoid (squamoid) tumour cells forming cystic and solid growth patterns, usually associated with *MAML2* rearrangement.

ICD-O coding

8430/3 Mucoepidermoid carcinoma
9270/3 Central intraosseous mucoepidermoid carcinoma

ICD-11 coding

2B67.Y & XH1J36 Other specified malignant neoplasms of parotid gland & Mucoepidermoid carcinoma
2B68.2 & XH1J36 Other specified malignant neoplasms of submandibular or sublingual gland & Mucoepidermoid carcinoma
2B65.Z & XH1J36 Malignant neoplasms of palate, unspecified & Mucoepidermoid carcinoma
2B66 & XH1J36 Malignant neoplasms of other or unspecified parts of mouth & Mucoepidermoid carcinoma

Related terminology

Not recommended: mucoepidermoid tumour.

Subtype(s)

Central intraosseous mucoepidermoid tumour

Localization

Approximately half of all MECs occur in major salivary glands, predominantly in the parotid gland, followed by the submandibular and sublingual glands. Intraorally, the most frequent site is the palate, followed by the buccal mucosa and other sites {996}. Rare central intraosseous MECs occur in the mandible or maxilla {1061}.

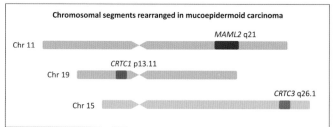

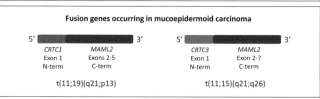

Fig. 4.42 Mucoepidermoid carcinoma. Chromosomal segments rearranged in mucoepidermoid carcinoma (upper panel) and fusion genes occurring in mucoepidermoid carcinoma (lower panel). Chr, chromosome; term, terminus.

Clinical features

MEC usually presents as a firm and fixed tumour, but occasional tumours may be largely cystic with only minor solid areas. Tumours situated below an intact oral surface epithelium may have a bluish appearance and mimic vascular lesions or mucocoele. Largely cystic tumours may present diagnostic problems on imaging and FNA.

Epidemiology

MEC is reported as the most frequent salivary malignancy in North America, many European countries, and Brazil. The reported annual incidence of MEC in the United Kingdom and Japan is 0.2–0.4 cases per 100 000 population {541,555, 3976,1804}. Patients with MEC have a wide age range, from childhood to old age (mean age: 45 years), and there is a female predominance (M:F ratio: 1:1.1–1.5) {1155}.

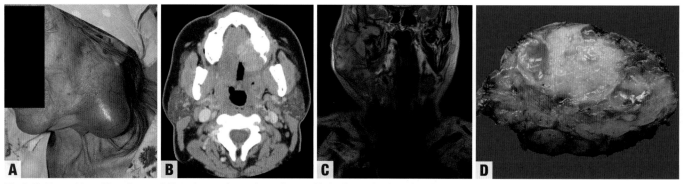

Fig. 4.43 Mucoepidermoid carcinoma. **A** There is a very large, destructive parotid gland mass that has thinned the overlying skin. **B** Axial CT shows a mass within the palate, with areas of cystic change. **C** T2-weighted coronal MRI shows a hyperintense, large, destructive right parotid gland mass, with significant soft tissue extension. **D** Multiple cysts are noted in this parotid gland tumour, showing an irregular periphery to the tumour.

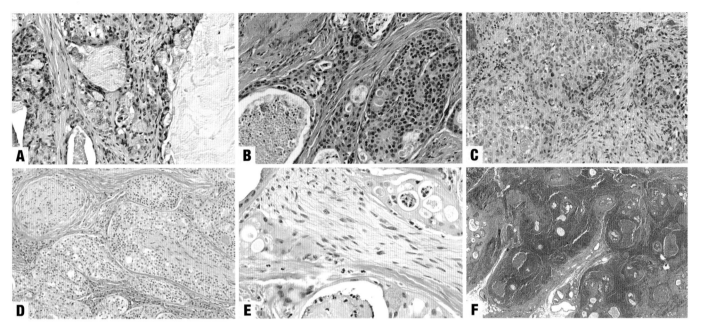

Fig. 4.44 Mucoepidermoid carcinoma. **A** Low-grade tumour. Cystic spaces are partly lined by mucous cells. Other cell types include intermediate, squamoid, and partly clear cells. **B** Intermediate-grade tumour. Largely solid nests of tumour cells with some ductal, mucinous, and oncocytoid features, and tumour necrosis. There is nerve invasion in the adjacent field (not shown). **C** High-grade tumour. Poorly differentiated high-grade carcinoma with minor amounts of mucinous cells. **D** Perineural invasion is frequently identified and is used as part of the grading of tumours. **E** Perineural invasion is seen, with the transitional epithelium and mucocytes intimately admixed with the nerve fibres. **F** It is not uncommon to have a very well developed tumour-associated lymphoid proliferation associated with mucoepidermoid carcinoma, which can sometimes simulate a lymph node.

Etiology

An increased occurrence of childhood MEC has been reported after nuclear disasters and chemotherapy {1155}.

Pathogenesis

Most MECs harbour a tumour type–specific translocation at t(11;19)(q21;p13), expressing the *CRTC1::MAML2* fusion gene {3955,2069,3285}. Rare cases display a t(11;15)(q21;q26) translocation with *CRTC3::MAML2* fusion {3155}, or a highly unusual t(6;22)(p21;q12) translocation with *EWSR1::POU5F1* fusion {3046}. The *CRTC1::MAML2* fusion is seen in most low- and intermediate-grade tumours and some high-grade tumours. Low-grade MECs show negligible copy-number variation {2069} and few somatic mutations, such as *TP53* and *POU6F2* {2163}.

Macroscopic appearance

MECs are usually firm or soft, partly cystic to solid masses with circumscribed or infiltrative borders. Occasionally a large cyst predominates.

Histopathology

MEC is characterized by mucous (mucin-producing), intermediate, and squamoid cells. Architectural configurations include cystic and solid areas where proportions of tumour cell types vary widely. Cystic spaces are partly lined by mucous cells with abundant mucinous cytoplasm and peripherally situated nuclei, and they display intracytoplasmic mucicarmine or PAS staining with diastase resistance. Intermediate cells are often the most frequent cell type in tumours. Extracellular mucin may be present. Significant keratinization is exceptional. Cell populations with clear, columnar, or oncocytic cells may be present, and occasionally they predominate. Sclerosing {4894}, clear cell {4330}, oncocytic {4104}, Warthin-like {2030,469}, ciliated {469}, spindle cell {1623}, and mucoacinar {625} patterns of MEC have been described.

Subtype

Central mucoepidermoid carcinoma is a location-specific jaw intraosseous subtype {1061}.

Grading

MECs are graded into three grades using a variety of grading systems {281,1653,560,2206} (see Table 4.02, p. 202). Low-grade MECs are usually circumscribed, partly cystic, and contain groups of mucous cells. Intermediate-grade MECs generally have more solid areas, whereas high-grade neoplasms are solid with fewer mucous cells and may display nuclear pleomorphism, mitotic figures, and necrosis, as well as perineural, lymphovascular, or bony invasion. Clinicopathological studies show that patients with low- and intermediate-grade MECs have similar clinical outcomes {2206,898,3990,4383}, favouring the use of two histological grades instead of three. US Armed Forces Institute of Pathology (AFIP) grading evaluates five histological features, which may enhance grading reproducibility, but some tumours graded as low-grade may behave more aggressively {281,1653}. Brandwein grading evaluates many histological features and tends to upgrade MECs compared with AFIP {560}. Memorial Sloan Kettering Cancer Center (MSK) grading evaluates tumours qualitatively based on the predominance of their features, but many criteria are not well defined {2206}.

Immunohistochemistry

Immunohistochemical p63 or p40 expression in the absence of S100/SOX10 staining may help to differentiate MEC from other salivary tumours {3846}; however, a subset of solid/trabecular MECs may be entirely negative for p63 and p40 {483A,73A}.

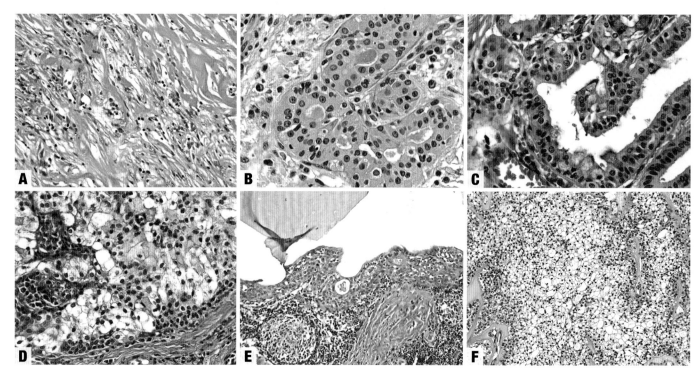

Fig. 4.45 Mucoepidermoid carcinoma. **A** Sclerotic pattern. Tumour cells are embedded in a sclerotic collagenous matrix. **B** Oncocytic pattern. Prominent oncocytoid features and very few hardly visible mucous cells. *CRTC1::MAML2* fusion was detected. **C** Ciliated pattern. Tumour cells lining cystic spaces display luminal cilia. **D** Clear cell pattern. Tumour cells have largely clear cytoplasm. **E** Warthin-like pattern. Tumour cells have oncocytoid and mucous features, and form cystic spaces. Tumour areas are surrounded by lymphatic tissue reminiscent of the architecture of Warthin tumour. **F** This tumour demonstrates a predominantly clear cell morphology, although more classic areas of mucoepidermoid carcinoma were noted in other areas of the same tumour.

Table 4.02 Comparison of mucoepidermoid carcinoma grading systems

Feature	AFIP[a] system (Auclair et al., 1992 {281}; Goode et al., 1998 {1653})	Brandwein[a] system (Brandwein et al., 2001 {560})	MSK system (Katabi et al., 2014 {2206})
Cysts/architecture	2 (< 20% cystic)	2 (< 25% cystic)	LG: predominantly cystic IG/HG: predominantly solid
Perineural invasion	2	3	n/a
Necrosis	3	3	LG/IG: absent HG: present
Mitoses[b]	3 (4 per 10 HPF)	3 (5 per 10 HPF)	LG: 0–1 per 10 HPF IG: 2–3 per 10 HPF HG: ≥ 4 per 10 HPF
Nuclear anaplasia/pleomorphism	4	2	LG/IG: not significant
Border / invasive front	n/a	2 (small nests and islands)	LG: circumscribed IG/HG: infiltrative
Lymphovascular invasion	n/a	3	n/a
Bony invasion	n/a	3	n/a
Stroma	n/a	n/a	n/a
Low grade	0–4	0	Qualitative assessment
Intermediate grade	5–6	2–3	Qualitative assessment
High grade	7–14	≥ 4	Qualitative assessment

AFIP, US Armed Forces Institute of Pathology; HG, high grade; IG, intermediate grade; LG, low grade; MSK, Memorial Sloan Kettering Cancer Center; n/a, not applicable.
[a]Points are assigned in the AFIP and Brandwein systems. If a pathological feature is present, relevant points are assigned as listed in the table. Final grade is determined by the sum of the points.
[b]For this table, the traditional denominator of 10 HPF could not be further defined as a precise area expressed in mm².

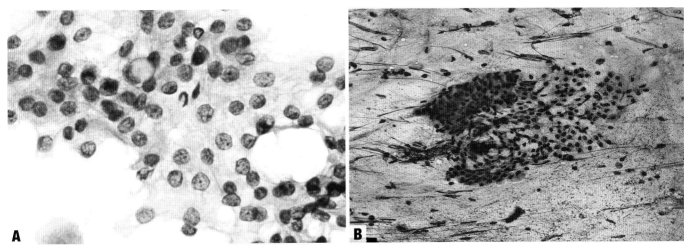

Fig. 4.46 Mucoepidermoid carcinoma. **A** There is a sheet-like appearance to this smear, where a mucocyte is noted within the field. **B** Smears from the tumour contain malignant cells, indicative of low-grade mucoepidermoid carcinoma (FNAC, parotid gland; Pap).

Differential diagnosis

The entities in the differential diagnosis of low-grade MEC include mucocoele, necrotizing sialometaplasia, sclerosing sialadenitis with mucous metaplasia, pleomorphic adenoma and Warthin tumour with oncocytic or squamous metaplasia, sclerosing polycystic adenoma, and secretory carcinoma. High-grade MEC must be distinguished from carcinoma ex pleomorphic adenoma, poorly differentiated squamous cell carcinoma, adenosquamous carcinoma, salivary duct carcinoma, and metastatic carcinomas.

Cytology

MEC produces variably cellular smears showing varying numbers of mucinous cells admixed with intermediate cells having relatively dense cytoplasm and arranged in sheets and tissue fragments, together with polygonal, epidermoid (squamoid) cells that are large and have moderate to copious dense cytoplasm {2334}. The mucinous cells can resemble goblet cells with bland round nuclei and abundant granular to finely vacuolated eccentric cytoplasm, or glandular cells with single vacuoles in which mucin droplets can be seen. Well-differentiated MEC with mucinous cells in intermediate cell sheets can be diagnosed confidently, but these tumours often show cystic degeneration, and smears may show only a mucinous or granular proteinaceous background with a variable number of histiocyte-like mucinous cells, raising a differential diagnosis with mucocoele-like lesions: any salivary gland FNAB yielding mucin must be considered atypical. In intermediate and high-grade MEC, there are fewer mucinous cells and a greater number of intermediate and squamoid cells, and nuclear enlargement, hyperchromasia, pleomorphism, and larger nucleoli become more prominent. Necrosis can be associated with high-grade lesions. FNAB cytopathology attempts to grade MEC as only low- and high-grade. Lymphocytes may be prominent. Very occasional focal partial keratinization may be present in some cases, but extensive keratinization is not seen and its presence in a high-grade lesion is in keeping with squamous cell carcinoma.

Diagnostic molecular pathology

Among salivary tumours, the *CRTC1::MAML2* fusion gene is specific for MEC and useful in diagnostic workups. A FISH result positive for *MAML2* rearrangement should be validated by *MAML2* PCR or next-generation sequencing.

Essential and desirable diagnostic criteria

Essential: salivary gland carcinoma with mucous, intermediate, and squamoid cells.
Desirable: *MAML2* rearrangement (in selected cases).

Staging

Staging follows the eighth edition of the Union for International Cancer Control (UICC) / American Joint Committee on Cancer (AJCC) TNM staging system.

Prognosis and prediction

Decreased overall and disease-free survival in MEC is associated with advanced stage, advanced age, male sex, a high histological grade, and a positive resection margin {996,4383}. A lack of *CRTC1::MAML2* fusion is associated with worse survival; however, fusion-negative tumours may actually represent other high-grade non-mucoepidermoid carcinomas {2069,898, 3285,1350}. The 5-year overall survival rates of low-, intermediate-, and high-grade MEC are reported as 90%, 86%, and 55%, respectively {996,4383}.

Adenoid cystic carcinoma

Inagaki H
Faquin WC
Stenman G
Urano M

Definition

Adenoid cystic carcinoma (AdCC) is an invasive carcinoma composed of epithelial and myoepithelial neoplastic cells arranged in tubular, cribriform, and solid patterns associated with basophilic matrix and reduplicated basement membrane material, often associated with *MYB*, *MYBL1*, or *NFIB* rearrangement.

ICD-O coding

8200/3 Adenoid cystic carcinoma

ICD-11 coding

2B68.0 & XH4302 Malignant neoplasms of major salivary glands, NOS & Adenoid cystic carcinoma
2B65.Y & XH4302 Other specified malignant neoplasm of palate & Adenoid cystic carcinoma
2B68.2 & XH4302 Other specified malignant neoplasms of submandibular or sublingual glands & Adenoid cystic carcinoma

Related terminology

None

Subtype(s)

None

Localization

Approximately 60% of AdCCs occur in the major salivary glands and 30% occur in the minor salivary glands {495}. The parotid, submandibular, and minor glands of the palate are the predominant sites {1531,495}.

Clinical features

Patients usually present with a swelling or a slow-growing mass. Neural symptoms like pain, numbness, and paraesthesia are commonly reported {911}. Lymph node involvement is uncommon, but in AdCC with high-grade transformation, the clinical course tends to be accelerated, with a high propensity for lymph node metastasis {1833}. Distant metastases are frequent, most commonly to the lungs, followed by bone, liver, and brain {2229, 718}.

Imaging

AdCC usually presents as a poorly defined mass {2263}.

Epidemiology

The incidence of AdCC is 1–2 cases per 100 000 person-years {1232,4796}. It is one of the most common salivary malignancies, accounting for 25% of all primary salivary carcinomas {4796}. The median patient age at diagnosis is approximately 60 years. AdCC has a slight female predilection {1232,541}.

Etiology

Germline mutations in *BRCA1/2* {4022} and DNA double-strand repair genes {1887} may increase the risk of salivary gland AdCC.

Pathogenesis

The genomic hallmark of AdCC is t(6;9) or t(8;9) translocation, resulting in *MYB::NFIB* and *MYBL1::NFIB* fusions, respectively {4218,3491,577,3028}. The former alteration is found in > 50% of cases and the latter in approximately 5% of cases {1491}. *MYB::NFIB* activation due to gene fusion or other mechanisms is a key event in AdCC pathogenesis {1176,182,1471,183}. Losses of 1p, 6q, and 15q are associated with high-grade tumours,

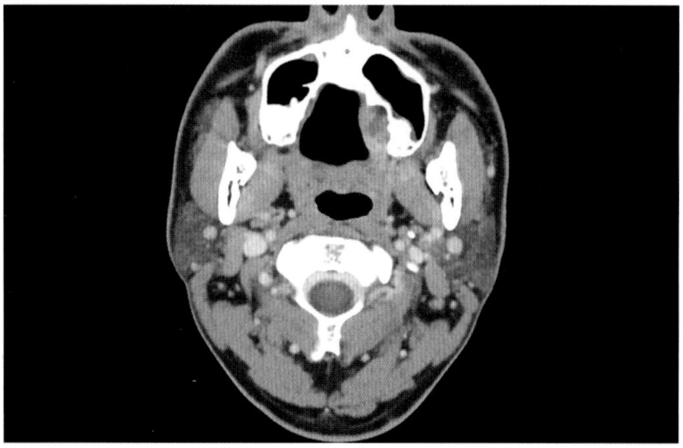

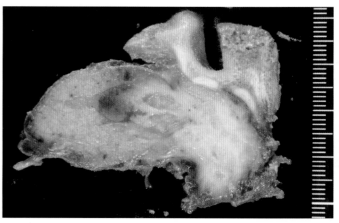

Fig. 4.47 Adenoid cystic carcinoma. Axial CT demonstrates a destructive mass involving the left palate, with bone remodelling. Although not diagnostic of adenoid cystic carcinoma, it is supportive of a malignant salivary gland neoplasm.

Fig. 4.48 Adenoid cystic carcinoma. Gross photograph showing a firm, unencapsulated, and infiltrative mass with a greyish-white, homogeneous cut surface in the left parotid gland.

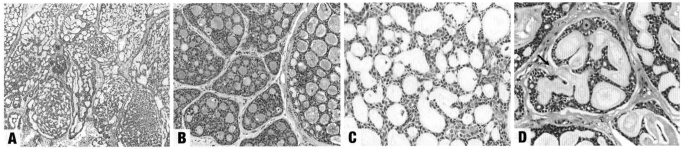

Fig. 4.49 Adenoid cystic carcinoma. **A** Low-power view of adenoid cystic carcinoma showing a prevailing cribriform growth pattern. **B** The cribriform pattern of adenoid cystic carcinoma is one of the most helpful features in the diagnosis. This image shows glycosaminoglycan material creating the Swiss-cheese or telephone-dial appearance. Note the stromal-epithelial clefting. **C** Cribriform growth pattern. **D** Cribriform pattern (*MYB::NFIB*-positive case). Myoepithelial tumour cells with clear cytoplasm and angular nuclei surround multiple cyst-like areas (pseudocysts) that are contiguous with the stroma of the neoplasm (arrow). A small lumen surrounded by eosinophilic, cuboidal cells (asterisk) indicates a focus of true ductal differentiation.

and loss of 14q is exclusively seen in low-grade tumours {3492,4212}. Next-generation sequencing identified mutations in genes in the FGF/IGF/PI3K, chromatin-remodelling, and NOTCH signalling pathways {1885,4223,1887}.

Macroscopic appearance

AdCC typically presents as a poorly circumscribed, tan, grey or white, firm, solid mass. Necrosis and/or haemorrhage are rare; their presence may indicate a high-grade tumour.

Histopathology

AdCC consists of two main cell types: ductal cells and myoepithelial cells. Ductal cells have eosinophilic cytoplasm and uniform round nuclei, and myoepithelial cells have clear cytoplasm and hyperchromatic angular nuclei. Mitotic figures are infrequent. Perineural invasion is a hallmark of AdCC, sampling dependent.

AdCC shows three growth patterns: tubular, cribriform, and solid {3948}. The tubular pattern consists of well-formed ducts and tubules lined with luminal ductal and abluminal myoepithelial cells. The cribriform pattern, which is most frequent, is characterized by nests of tumour cells with microcystic-like spaces filled with hyaline or basophilic mucoid material. The spaces are pseudocysts contiguous with the tumour stroma. The solid pattern is characterized by tumour sheets composed of basaloid cells lacking tubular or cribriform formations. Combinations of these growth patterns are common. Identification of both pseudocysts and true glandular lumina is usually required to make the diagnosis.

AdCC with high-grade transformation shows a pleomorphic, mitotically active high-grade carcinoma component, typically a poorly differentiated adenocarcinoma or anaplastic carcinoma {1833,1832,4112}. The high-grade component is negative for myoepithelial markers {3957,4112}.

Generally, AdCCs with > 30% solid component pursue a more aggressive clinical course {3948,4584,3074}. In recent studies, the presence of any solid tumour component has been emphasized as an objective high-grade tumour marker {4584, 3074}.

Immunohistochemistry

Pancytokeratin is strongly positive in ductal cells and weakly positive in myoepithelial cells. CK7 and KIT (CD117) are typically positive in ductal cells {188}, whereas p63, p40, calponin,

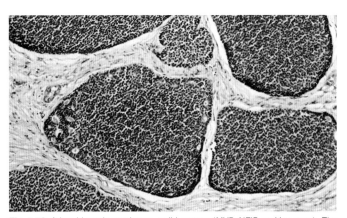

Fig. 4.50 Adenoid cystic carcinoma, solid pattern (*MYB::NFIB*-positive case). The solid pattern is characterized by dense cellular tumour nests lacking the pseudocystic spaces observed in the cribriform and tubular patterns.

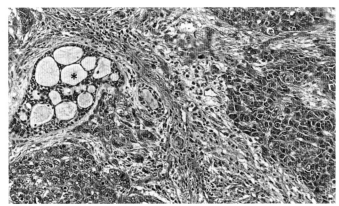

Fig. 4.51 Adenoid cystic carcinoma, high-grade transformation (*MYB::NFIB*-positive case). A typical cribriform tumour nest (asterisk) is surrounded by tumour nests best characterized as poorly differentiated adenocarcinoma.

and α-SMA are positive in myoepithelial cells. MYB protein overexpression is common in AdCC, but its diagnostic value is limited by its suboptimal specificity {590,3061,3738,3993, 4287}.

Differential diagnosis

The main salivary gland tumours to be distinguished from AdCC include pleomorphic adenoma, polymorphous adenocarcinoma, epithelial-myoepithelial carcinoma, and basal cell adenoma/adenocarcinoma. Because AdCC often shows mild cytological atypia

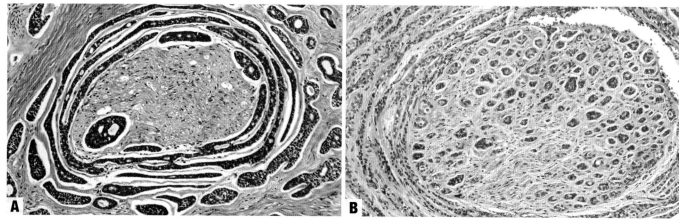

Fig. 4.52 Adenoid cystic carcinoma. **A** A *MYB::NFIB*-positive case. The tumour shows prominent perineural and intraneural invasion. **B** Adenoid cystic carcinoma of the tongue with perineural and intraneural invasion.

and a cribriform pattern, its distinction from benign tumours with a cribriform pattern, especially the cribriform subtype of basal cell adenoma, is critical {4528}.

Cytology

AdCCs usually show highly cellular smears with cohesive tissue fragments that form sheets, or they show tubular, complex, or cribriform architecture containing hard-edged balls of stroma. These tissue fragments consist of uniform basaloid cells with high N:C ratios and oval to angulated and hyperchromatic nuclei. Atypia is generally mild, and the distinction from other basaloid salivary gland neoplasms can be difficult in the absence of the typical cribriform pattern and stromal matrix, particularly the stromal balls, and the predominance of sheets of basaloid cells in the solid subtype. These cases raise differential diagnoses with pleomorphic adenoma and basal cell adenoma and should be regarded as atypical or suspicious for malignancy. High nuclear grade can occur and be associated with mitoses and necrosis. Romanowsky–Giemsa-type stains highlight the characteristic discrete spheres and branching tubules of the acellular magenta matrix {2333}.

Diagnostic molecular pathology

Demonstration of *MYB/MYBL1* rearrangements or gene fusions by FISH or other methods can help establish a diagnosis of AdCC.

Essential and desirable diagnostic criteria

Essential: hyperchromatic, angulated nuclei; a mixture of tubular, cribriform, and solid patterns associated with a basophilic matrix and reduplicated basement membrane material.
Desirable: perineural invasion; demonstration of *MYB* or *MYBL1* rearrangements (in selected cases).

Staging

Staging follows the eighth edition of the Union for International Cancer Control (UICC) / American Joint Committee on Cancer (AJCC) TNM staging system.

Prognosis and prediction

AdCC is characterized by a prolonged clinical course, with frequent local recurrences, late onset of metastases, and a fatal

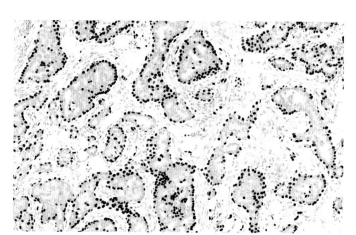

Fig. 4.53 Adenoid cystic carcinoma. Immunostaining for p40 decorates the basal cell layer.

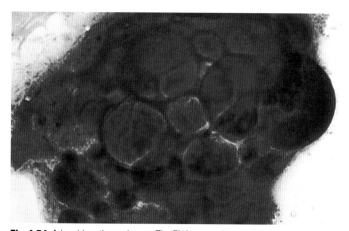

Fig. 4.54 Adenoid cystic carcinoma. The FNA smear demonstrates the characteristic discrete spheres and branching tubules of the acellular magenta matrix (Romanowsky–Giemsa stain).

outcome. Overall survival and recurrence-free survival rates at 10 years are approximately 50% and 60%, respectively {495, 4796}. Factors influencing survival include patient age, tumour site, tumour grade, TNM stage, surgical margins, and *NOTCH1* mutation status {171,4878,2229}. The median overall survival time after diagnosis of distant metastasis is 36 months {1531}.

Acinic cell carcinoma

Stevens TM
Agaimy A
Faquin WC
Hellquist H
Hsieh MS
Kiss K
Simpson RHW

Definition

Acinic cell carcinoma is a salivary gland carcinoma exhibiting serous acinar differentiation and lacking mucinous differentiation.

ICD-O coding

8550/3 Acinic cell carcinoma

ICD-11 coding

2B68.2 & XH3PG9 Other specified malignant neoplasms of submandibular or sublingual glands & Acinic cell adenocarcinoma

Related terminology

Acceptable: acinic cell adenocarcinoma.

Subtype(s)

None

Localization

About 90–95% of cases arise in the parotid gland. The remainder involve intraoral sites, the submandibular gland, and (exceptionally) the sinonasal tract {492,4589}.

Clinical features

Patients typically present with slow-growing, painless masses. High-grade tumours may be rapidly growing and fixed to adjacent structures, with facial nerve paralysis.

Epidemiology

Acinic cell carcinoma represents 10% of all salivary gland malignancies and as many as 18.7% of parotid carcinomas. It is the second most common salivary gland malignancy in children {4589,4797}. The M:F ratio is 1:1.5 {4121,3416,4412,4589}. It occurs over a wide age range (average age: 47.7–52 years) {845,4589}. Acinic cell carcinoma with high-grade transformation occurs on average two decades later than conventional examples.

Etiology

Unknown

Pathogenesis

The majority of cases harbour a t(4;9)(q13;q31) rearrangement that places the active enhancer regions of the secretory calcium-binding phosphoprotein (SCPP) gene cluster upstream of

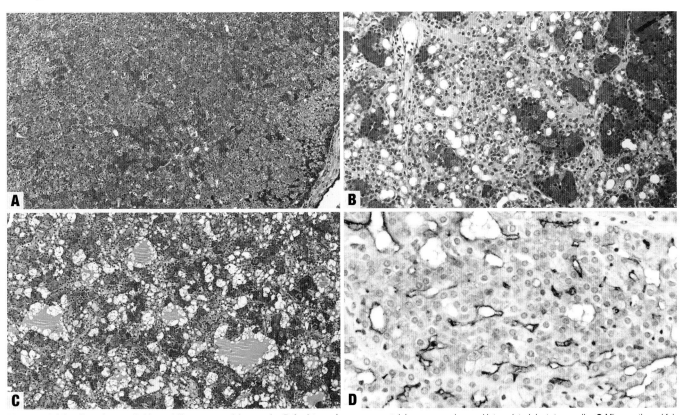

Fig. 4.55 Acinic cell carcinoma. **A** A basophilic, zymogen-rich example. **B** A mixture of zymogen-containing serous acinar and intercalated duct–type cells. **C** Microcystic and follicular growth patterns. **D** DOG1 immunohistochemistry shows a membranous, canalicular or apical-luminal, and cytoplasmic reaction in the neoplastic cells of acinic cell carcinoma.

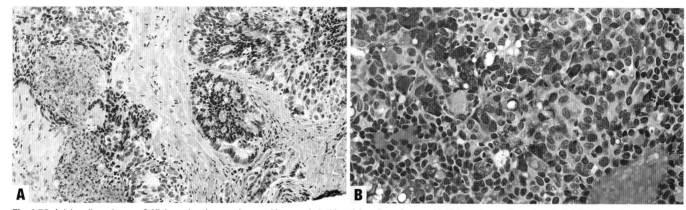

Fig. 4.56 Acinic cell carcinoma. **A** High-grade adenocarcinoma with necrosis in this acinic cell carcinoma with high-grade transformation. **B** Acinic cell carcinoma with high-grade transformation. High-grade tumour cells that feature nuclear enlargement and pleomorphism (upper right) can be seen admixed with conventional, low-grade tumour cells (lower left) in this high-grade example.

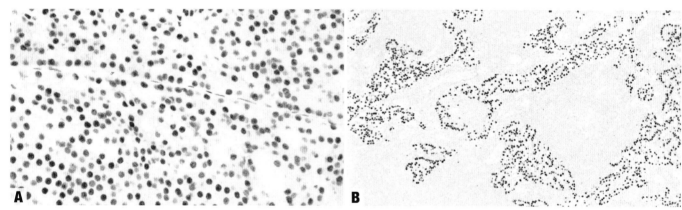

Fig. 4.57 Acinic cell carcinoma. **A** All of the neoplastic nuclei show strong and diffuse immunoreactivity for NR4A3 (endothelial cells are a negative internal control). **B** Nuclear expression of NR4A3 in the neoplastic acinar cells of acinic cell carcinoma with a lymphoid-rich stroma.

the *NR4A3* (*NOR1*) gene, resulting in the upregulation of NR4A3 via enhancer hijacking {1740,1744,1743}.

Macroscopic appearance

Well circumscribed to variably lobulated, unencapsulated or variably pseudoencapsulated, solid to variably cystic. Infiltrative growth is more common in high-grade tumours.

Histopathology

The tumour exhibits solid, microcystic, follicular, to less commonly papillary-cystic architectures, often with a prominent lymphoid stroma. Neoplastic cells are heterogeneous with the most common cell type being the serous acinar cell which features PAS-positive, diastase-resistant basophilic cytoplasmic zymogen granules, with variable intercalated duct–type, nonspecific glandular, vacuolated, oncocytic, and (rarely) clear cells. Cytoplasmic borders are poorly defined and nuclei are small and peripherally placed {1236,4589,4972}. High-grade (HG) tumours exhibit, in addition to conventional areas, a component of high-grade adenocarcinoma (with variable cribriform, solid, trabecular growth patterns) or poorly differentiated/undifferentiated carcinoma. Acinic cell carcinomas with high-grade transformation show nuclear enlargement and pleomorphism, coarse chromatin, necrosis, increased mitotic activity and Ki-67 index, and more frequent perineural and lymphovascular invasion. Increased expression of cyclin-D1

and membranous β-catenin have been described {4121,4412, 4972}.

Immunohistochemistry

Acinic cell carcinoma cells express SOX10 and DOG1, and are negative for p40/p63, mammaglobin and S100, however S100 may label intercalated cells {806,3280}. Nuclear staining for NR4A3 (NOR1) or NR4A2 (NURR1) have been identified in 98% and 2% of cases, respectively {1744,1743}. The sensitivity and

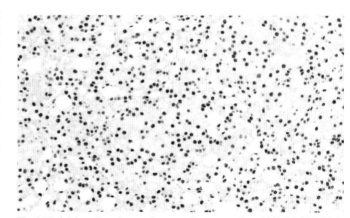

Fig. 4.58 Acinic cell carcinoma. Strong nuclear expression of NR4A2 (NURR1) in neoplastic cells in an acinic cell carcinoma.

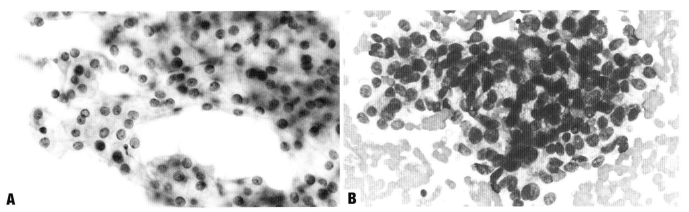

Fig. 4.59 Acinic cell carcinoma. **A** The smear shows round to oval nuclei with delicate, vacuolated cytoplasm (FNAB, Pap). Characteristic coarse cytoplasmic zymogen granules that stain basophilic in Pap preparations may be seen (not shown). **B** Round to oval nuclei with delicate, vacuolated cytoplasm (FNAB, Pap).

specificity of immunohistochemistry for NR4A3 are 94.4% and 99%, respectively {1744,4600,1743,3205,4133,4842,808,3342}.

Cytology

The usually highly cellular smears show irregular, loosely cohesive sheets and tissue fragments with a variable microacinar architecture and occasional association with thin branching capillaries, in a granular background with plentiful stripped round nuclei. The cells are polygonal with round to oval nuclei; usually small but occasionally larger nucleoli; and abundant eccentric, delicate, finely vacuolated cytoplasm, best seen in Romanowsky–Giemsa-type stains. The Pap may show coarse basophilic cytoplasmic zymogen granules {2330}. Cystic degeneration can occur, but mitoses and necrosis are usually absent. There is no association with normal grape-like acinar architecture or ducts. Lymphoid cells can be prominent, raising a differential diagnosis with Warthin tumour and also with metastatic carcinoma in a lymph node.

Diagnostic molecular pathology

Molecular pathology is typically not needed for diagnosis. However, demonstrating NR4A subfamily rearrangements or positive immunohistochemistry for NR4A3 or NR4A2 may be confirmatory in challenging cases.

Essential and desirable diagnostic criteria

Essential: a salivary gland carcinoma with serous acinar differentiation.

Desirable: nuclear staining for NR4A3 (NOR1) or NR4A2 (NURR1), or molecular demonstration of *NR4A3* rearrangement (in selected cases).

Staging

Staging follows the eighth edition of the Union for International Cancer Control (UICC) / American Joint Committee on Cancer (AJCC) TNM staging system.

Prognosis and prediction

Acinic cell carcinomas with a complete fibrous pseudocapsule, diffuse dense lymphoid stroma, and microcystic growth pattern have superior outcomes {2985}. The mean 5- and 10-year survival rates are approximately 95–97.2% and 83–93.8%, respectively {2588,3416,4589}. Distant metastasis drops the survival rate to about 22% and occurs in about 20% of cases {4589}; 72.7% of 25 patients with acinic cell carcinoma with high-grade transformation had died at a mean time of 2.9 years {4412}. Local recurrence rates are approximately 35% and 80% and lymph node metastases occur in about 10% and 50% of conventional and high-grade tumours, respectively {4121,845,492,4412,632}.

Secretory carcinoma

Skalova A
Bishop JA
Kholova I
Urano M

Definition

Secretory carcinoma (SC) is a monophasic salivary gland carcinoma composed of cells with abundant eosinophilic or bubbly secretions, arranged in microcystic, tubular, and solid structures. It is usually characterized by a specific rearrangement of the *ETV6* or *RET* gene, and it harbours *ETV6::NTRK3* or *ETV6::RET* fusion in most cases.

ICD-O coding

8502/3 Secretory carcinoma

ICD-11 coding

2B67.Y & XH44J4 Other specified malignant neoplasms of parotid gland & Secretory carcinoma

2B68.2 & XH44J4 Other specified malignant neoplasms of submandibular or sublingual glands & Secretory carcinoma

2B65.Y & XH44J4 Other specified malignant neoplasm of palate & Secretory carcinoma

2B60 & XH44J4 Malignant neoplasms of the lip & Secretory carcinoma

2B66.Y & XH44J4 Other specified malignant neoplasms of other or unspecified parts of mouth & Secretory carcinoma

Related terminology

Acceptable: mammary analogue secretory carcinoma.

Subtype(s)

None

Localization

The most common site of occurrence is the parotid gland, followed by the oral cavity and submandibular gland {4126,939,

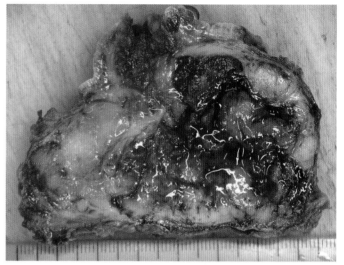

Fig. 4.60 Secretory carcinoma of the parotid gland with high-grade transformation (*ETV6::NTRK3* fusion was confirmed). Gross photograph showing an unencapsulated, haemorrhagic, infiltrative mass with a focally cystic cut surface.

4103,3994}. In the oral cavity, the lip, soft palate, and buccal mucosa are the most commonly affected subsites {465,492}. Rare cases originating from the minor salivary glands of the sinonasal mucosa have been reported {2738,4883,329}.

Clinical features

SC most commonly presents as a painless, slowly growing mass {4126,310,291}. SC with high-grade transformation is associated with an aggressive clinical behaviour, a high propensity for cervical lymph node metastasis, a risk of distant metastasis, and a poor prognosis {4124,2799,4227,310,330A}.

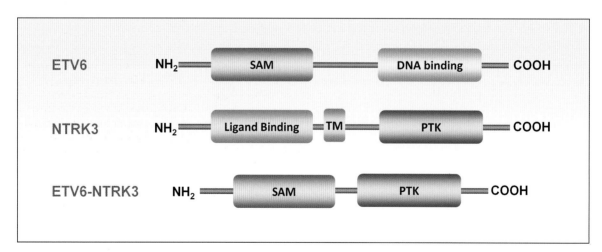

Fig. 4.61 The ETV6::NTRK3 chimeric tyrosine kinase of secretory carcinoma. This fusion combines the sterile alpha motif dimerization domain (SAM) of the ETV6 DNA-binding domain with the protein tyrosine kinase domain (PTK) of the transmembrane (TM) NTRK3 tyrosine kinase, generating a ligand-independent constitutively active chimeric tyrosine kinase.

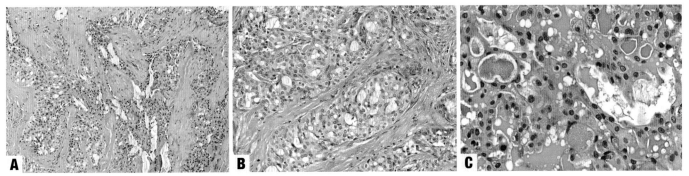

Fig. 4.62 Secretory carcinoma. **A** Perineural invasion is seen in the upper right corner. **B** Microcystic architecture, pale mucinous secretions, and typical nuclear morphology. **C** Secretory carcinoma of the buccal mucosa. The tumour cells of secretory carcinoma have low-grade vesicular nuclei with finely granular chromatin and distinctive centrally located nucleoli, surrounded by pale-pink granular or vacuolated cytoplasm.

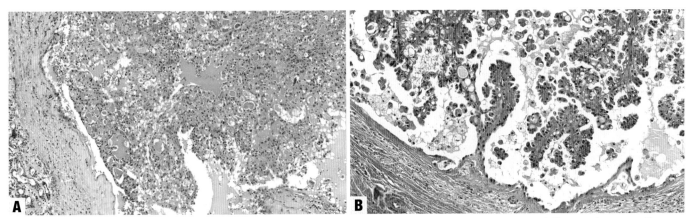

Fig. 4.63 Secretory carcinoma. **A** Histology of a secretory carcinoma with the classic *ETV6::NTRK3* fusion demonstrates a microcystic/cribriform growth pattern and homogeneous and bubbly eosinophilic secretory material. **B** Secretory carcinoma of the parotid gland with *ETV6::NTRK3* fusion. The papillary-cystic architectural pattern shows some degree of cyst formation with micropapillary features and hobnailing of the cells.

Imaging

Imaging of SC typically shows a well-defined, predominantly cystic lesion with solid papillary projections, and a low incidence of associated pathological lymph nodes. Cystic areas are usually T1-hyperintense or have a fluid-fluid level including a T1-hyperintense area. It has also been suggested that haemosiderin deposition on MRI may help differentiate SC from acinic cell carcinoma {2203,2439,1834}.

Epidemiology

SC usually occurs in adults, with a mean patient age of 46.5 years (range: 10–86 years) and an equal sex distribution {4126,939,465,4103,3994,330A}.

Etiology

Unknown

Pathogenesis

Most cases of SC harbour a characteristic chromosomal translocation, t(12;15)(p13;q25), resulting in an *ETV6::NTRK3* fusion {4126}. A small subset of cases demonstrate divergent molecular findings, with alternate *ETV6::RET* {2038,4128,4125}, *ETV6::MET* {3747}, *ETV6::MAML3* {1706}, and *VIM::RET* {4108} fusions.

Macroscopic appearance

Grossly, SC has a rubbery, tan cut surface. The tumours are generally well circumscribed and may have a prominent cystic component {465,2799,1846}.

Histopathology

SC is usually well circumscribed but not encapsulated. The tumours have a lobulated growth pattern separated by fibrous septa and are composed of microcystic/solid, tubular, follicular, and papillary-cystic structures with distinctive luminal secretions. It may have an infiltrative pattern with occasional perineural invasion and may show abundant fibrosclerotic stroma with prominent, thick, hyalinized septa. Some SCs show a macrocystic morphology. The tumour cells have low-grade vesicular round to oval nuclei with finely granular chromatin and distinctive, centrally located nucleoli. The pale pink cytoplasm is granular to vacuolated. Cellular atypia is usually mild, and mitoses are rare. High-grade transformation is uncommon.

Histochemistry

Abundant eosinophilic to bubbly secretions are positive for PAS (before and after diastase digestion) and Alcian blue. Unlike acinic cell carcinoma, SC does not show true PAS-positive secretory zymogen cytoplasmic granules.

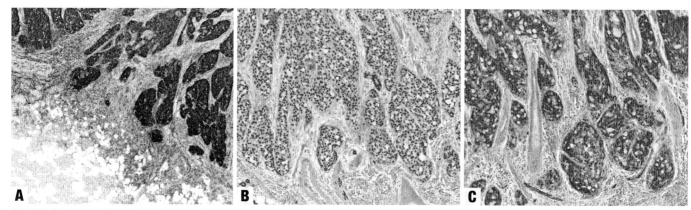

Fig. 4.64 Secretory carcinoma. **A** Mammaglobin immunohistochemistry shows diffuse cytoplasmic positivity in the tumour cells. **B** SOX10 immunohistochemistry shows diffuse nuclear staining in the tumour cells. **C** S100 immunohistochemistry shows diffuse cytoplasmic staining in the tumour cells.

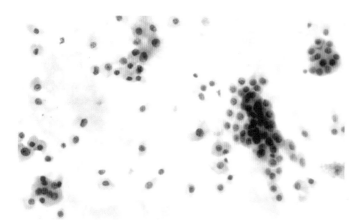

Fig. 4.65 Secretory carcinoma with *ETV6::NTRK3* fusion. Papillary-like structures and clusters of epithelial cells with rich, finely granulated cytoplasm and round to oval mildly polymorphic nuclei with discernible nucleoli in a mucinous background (FNAC, Pap).

Immunohistochemistry

SCs are positive for CK7, S100, SOX10, vimentin, and mammaglobin, and negative for p63, p40, NR4A3, and DOG1 {4126, 3994,4547}.

Differential diagnosis

In contrast to SC, acinic cell carcinomas demonstrate intense apical membranous staining for DOG1 around lumina and variable cytoplasmic positivity in most cases {806}.

Cytology

The moderately cellular smears show loosely cohesive sheets and papillary or cribriform tissue fragments and dispersed cells in a usually mucinous background, although in some cases haemosiderophages and blood may be seen. The cells show low to moderate N:C ratios; abundant finely granular or vacuolated cytoplasm (with some cells resembling signet-ring cells with large vacuoles indenting the nuclei); and uniform round to oval nuclei with fine chromatin, distinct single nucleoli, and mild atypia {494,1688,1864,2144,2306,2990}.

Diagnostic molecular pathology

Approximately 90% of SCs harbour a characteristic chromosomal rearrangement, t(12;15)(p13;q25), resulting in an *ETV6::NTRK3* fusion {4126}. A small subset of cases demonstrate divergent molecular findings, with alternate *ETV6::RET* {2038,4128,4125}, *ETV6::MET* {3747}, *ETV6::MAML3* {1706}, and *VIM::RET* {4108} gene fusions.

Essential and desirable diagnostic criteria

Essential: a malignant salivary gland neoplasm of a single cell type with vacuolated, colloid-like secretory material; no zymogen cytoplasmic granules; immunohistochemical positivity for S100, SOX10, and mammaglobin; lack of immunohistochemical staining for p40 and/or p63.
Desirable: *ETV6* or *RET* rearrangement demonstrated by FISH, RNA sequencing, or PCR (in selected cases).

Staging

Staging follows the eighth edition of the Union for International Cancer Control (UICC) / American Joint Committee on Cancer (AJCC) TNM staging system.

Prognosis and prediction

SC is usually an indolent salivary gland malignancy. Lymph node metastases are reported in as many as 25% of cases {3985,3994,4547,291}, but distant metastases are uncommon {844,4547,3994,2799,532,330A}. Clinical stage and high-grade transformation are the main adverse prognostic factors {4124, 2799,4227,310,330A}. There are no current predictive biomarkers in SC, but translocation status itself may be a predictive marker with the ongoing development of selective TRK inhibitors {1178,1177}.

Microsecretory adenocarcinoma

Bishop JA
Mikami Y
Weinreb I

Definition
Microsecretory adenocarcinoma (MSA) is a low-grade malignancy with an intercalated duct-like phenotype and *MEF2C::SS18* fusion.

ICD-O coding
8502/3 Microsecretory adenocarcinoma

ICD-11 coding
2B66.Y Other specified malignant neoplasms of other and unspecified parts of mouth
2B65.Y Other specified malignant neoplasm of palate

Related terminology
None

Subtype(s)
None

Localization
Almost all MSAs have arisen in the oral cavity, with palate and buccal mucosa being the most frequently affected subsites. A single case involved the parotid gland {484,2228,481}. Cases have been reported affecting the skin {490}.

Clinical features
Patients present with a painless, slow-growing mass.

Epidemiology
Fewer than 30 cases have been reported. The mean patient age is 49.5 years (range: 17–83 years), and there is a slight female predominance {484,2228,481}.

Etiology
Unknown

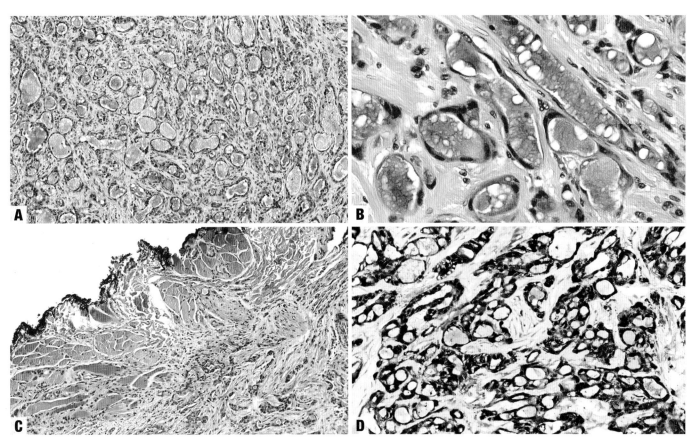

Fig. 4.66 Microsecretory adenocarcinoma. **A** The prototypical appearance of microsecretory adenocarcinoma is microcysts filled with pale, bluish secretions, set in a cellular fibromyxoid stroma. **B** The tumour cells are flattened, with modest amounts of eosinophilic to clear cytoplasm and monotonous, hyperchromatic oval nuclei. **C** The tumour often initially appears circumscribed, but close inspection reveals subtle infiltration into nearby tissues such as skeletal muscle. **D** The tumour has a consistent immunoprofile, with strong and diffuse immunoexpression of S100.

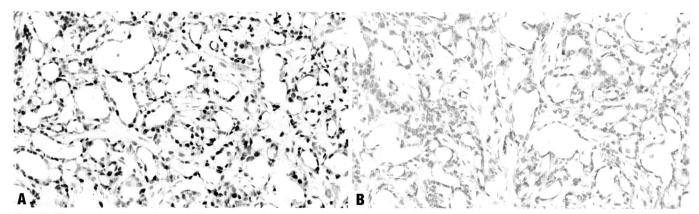

Fig. 4.67 Microsecretory adenocarcinoma. **A** Microsecretory adenocarcinoma has a consistent immunoprofile, with strong and diffuse immunoexpression of p63. **B** The lack of nuclear reactivity for p40, coupled with the strong p63, helps in reaching a diagnosis for this tumour category.

Pathogenesis

MSA is characterized by chromosomal rearrangement and fusion of the *MEF2C* gene (5q14.3) with *SS18* (18q11.2). Rare reported cases with an alternate fusion *SS18::ZBTB7A* may represent a different tumour type {4761A,481}.

Macroscopic appearance

MSA grossly appears to be a non-ulcerated, well-circumscribed mass. The masses average 11 mm (range: 6–30 mm).

Histopathology

MSA has very consistent morphological features: (1) a microcystic-predominant growth pattern with occasional cribriform structures or cords; (2) uniform intercalated duct-like tumour cells with attenuated eosinophilic to clear cytoplasm; (3) monotonous oval hyperchromatic nuclei with indistinct nucleoli; (4) abundant basophilic luminal secretions; (5) a variably cellular fibromyxoid stroma; and (6) rounded borders with subtle infiltrative growth into nearby skeletal muscle, fat, or minor salivary glands. Occasionally, MSA is accompanied by pseudoepitheliomatous hyperplasia, tumour-associated lymphoid proliferation, or metaplastic bone formation. Perineural invasion is rare, necrosis is absent, and mitotic rates are low.

Immunohistochemistry

MSA has a consistent immunophenotype. It is positive for S100, SOX10, and p63, and negative for p40, mammaglobin, and calponin. Occasional cases are focally positive for SMA.

Differential diagnosis

Secretory carcinoma has more abundant cytoplasm, pink secretions, mammaglobin positivity, and harbours different fusions (usually *ETV6::NTRK3*). Polymorphous adenocarcinoma shows more architectural diversity and different genetic alterations (mutations or rearrangements of *PRKD1*, *PRKD2*, or *PRKD3*). Adenoid cystic carcinoma has two cell populations, is far more infiltrative, and harbours rearrangements of *MYB*, *MYBL1*, and/or *NFIB*. Sclerosing microcystic adenocarcinoma is less cellular, with more stroma, more cord-like growth, and a subtly biphasic tumour population.

Cytology

Not reported

Diagnostic molecular pathology

MEF2C::SS18 fusion can be demonstrated by RNA sequencing, RT-PCR, or *SS18* break-apart FISH {484,2228,475,481}.

Essential and desirable diagnostic criteria

Essential: a salivary gland malignancy with a microcystic-predominant growth pattern; bluish secretions; fibromyxoid stroma; monotonous tumour cells; positivity for S100 and p63 but not p40 or mammaglobin.

Desirable: *SS18* rearrangement demonstrated by FISH, RNA sequencing, or PCR (in selected cases).

Staging

Staging follows the eighth edition of the Union for International Cancer Control (UICC) / American Joint Committee on Cancer (AJCC) TNM staging system.

Prognosis and prediction

MSA usually behaves in an indolent manner, with only rare reported cases of distant or regional metastasis {2132A,1702A}.

Polymorphous adenocarcinoma

Weinreb I
Leivo I
Michal M
Simpson RHW

Vander Poorten VLM
Wasserman JK
Xu B

Definition

Conventional polymorphous adenocarcinoma (PmA) is a malignant epithelial tumour characterized by cytological uniformity, morphological diversity, and an infiltrative growth pattern, and it is usually associated with alterations in the PRKD gene family.

Cribriform polymorphous adenocarcinoma (cribriform adenocarcinoma of the salivary glands; CASG) is characterized by a predominant papillary and glomeruloid growth pattern, clear nuclei, and common *PRKD1*, *PRKD2*, or *PRKD3* fusions.

ICD-O coding

8525/3 Polymorphous adenocarcinoma
8525/3 Polymorphous adenocarcinoma, conventional subtype
8525/3 Polymorphous adenocarcinoma, cribriform subtype (cribriform adenocarcinoma of the salivary glands)

ICD-11 coding

2B61 & XH5SD5 Malignant neoplasm of base of tongue & Polymorphous adenocarcinoma
2B65.Y & XH5SD5 Other specified malignant neoplasm of palate & Polymorphous adenocarcinoma
2B67.Y & XH5SD5 Other specified malignant neoplasms of parotid gland & Polymorphous adenocarcinoma
2B6A.Y & XH5SD5 Other specified malignant neoplasms of oropharynx & Polymorphous adenocarcinoma
2B6B.Y & XH5SD5 Other specified malignant neoplasms of nasopharynx & Polymorphous adenocarcinoma
2B6D.Y & XH5SD5 Other specified malignant neoplasms of hypopharynx & Polymorphous adenocarcinoma

Related terminology

Acceptable: polymorphous low-grade adenocarcinoma; cribriform adenocarcinoma of tongue / salivary gland.

Subtype(s)

Polymorphous adenocarcinoma, conventional subtype; polymorphous adenocarcinoma, cribriform subtype (cribriform adenocarcinoma of the salivary glands)

Localization

More than 95% of PmAs involve minor salivary glands or seromucous glands of the upper aerodigestive tract. The palate is the most common site {705,1299,3958,3423,1228,4881}. Other sites include the buccal mucosa, retromolar trigone, floor of the mouth, and sinonasal tract / nasopharynx {705,1299, 3958,3423,1228,4881}. CASGs are localized mostly in the tongue; other sites include the soft palate, retromolar buccal mucosa, tonsils, and upper lip {4110}. Fewer than 5% of cases affect major salivary glands {4767,4881,3946}.

Clinical features

PmA typically presents as a slowly growing, painless mass of variable duration {705}. Very few patients with PmA present with lymph node metastasis {4884}, but cervical lymph node metastases are common in CASG {4120,2978,4110,4884}.

Imaging

PmA has nonspecific imaging features, including occasional invasion/erosion of adjacent bone, but otherwise smooth borders with a T2-hypointense fibrous capsule and progressive enhancement pattern. Imaging is used to assess local tumour extent and identify potential metastatic lymph nodes {3318}.

Epidemiology

PmA is the second most common intraoral salivary gland carcinoma {4674}, with an incidence rate of 0.051 cases per 100 000 person-years {3367}. The M:F ratio is about 1:2 {705,

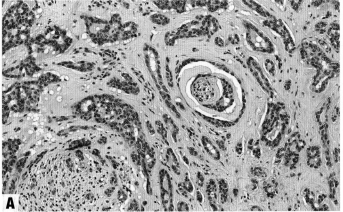
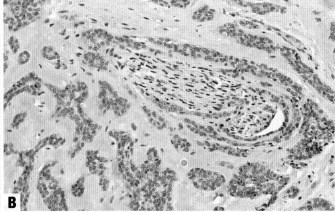

Fig. 4.68 Polymorphous adenocarcinoma, classic subtype. **A** Various patterns, including tubules, trabeculae, microcysts, and cribriform architecture, are seen in a mucoid/myxoid background. The tumour is often arranged in a targetoid or streaming fashion in the periphery or around nerves. **B** The tumour cells have uniform small oval nuclei, scant cytoplasm, open chromatin, and inconspicuous nucleoli. Neurotropism is seen.

1299,3423,4881}. The patient age range is 16–94 years, with a mean in the seventh decade of life {705,1299,3423,4881}.

Etiology
Unknown

Pathogenesis
Pathogenic alterations of the PRKD gene family are highly prevalent. Approximately 70–89% of PmAs and 0–20% of CASGs harbour *PRKD1* p.E710D activating hotspot mutations, whereas 70–94% of CASGs and 6–11% of PmAs contain a rearrangement of *PRKD1*, *PRKD2*, or *PRKD3* {4767,4763,3946,4884}.

Macroscopic appearance
PmAs often present as firm, solid, unencapsulated, yellow/tan, ovoid submucosal masses {705}. Papillary-cystic tumours, particularly in CASG, may have gross cystic change and haemorrhage.

Histopathology
The conventional subtype of PmA is typically an unencapsulated submucosal mass. The tumours are characterized by cytological uniformity, histological diversity, and an infiltrative growth pattern. Neoplastic cells are uniform in shape, with scant cytoplasm, bland oval nuclei, open chromatin, occasional small nucleoli, and nuclear grooves. A prominent feature is the wide variation in architectural patterns, including single file, fascicular, trabecular, tubular, microcystic, solid, and (rarely) papillary-cystic. Streaming or eddy-like formations can be present at the peripheral boundary of the tumour. Foci of oncocytic, clear, squamous, apocrine, or mucous cells and microcalcifications can be observed. Tumour stroma can be myxoid, mucinous, or hyalinized. Perineural involvement is frequent, being seen in approximately two thirds of cases, often in a targetoid pattern. This pattern is also observed around vessels. High-grade transformation characterized by marked nuclear atypia, mitotic activity, and prominent necrosis, has been reported in PmA {4079, 2281}.

CASG was initially reported at the base of the tongue {2984} and later in other minor salivary gland sites {4120} and the parotid gland {4884}. CASG is considered to be a separate entity by some authors {2984,4120,2978} and a subtype within the PmA morphological spectrum by others {4884}. CASG is characterized by a multinodular growth pattern separated by fibrous septa; a relatively uniform solid, cribriform, and microcystic architecture; and optically clear nuclei. Glomeruloid and papillary structures, peripheral palisading, and clefting are typically observed. CASG is associated with a higher risk of lymph node metastasis, and a higher frequency of PRKD gene rearrangement {4120,4767,3946}.

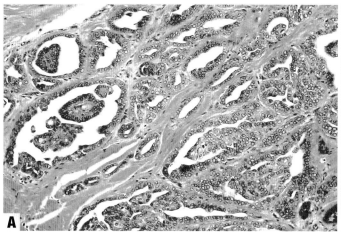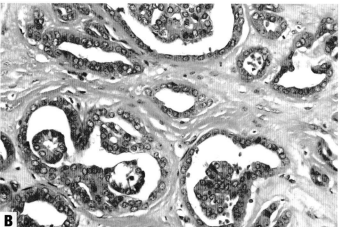

Fig. 4.69 Polymorphous adenocarcinoma, cribriform subtype. **A,B** Glomeruloid structures.

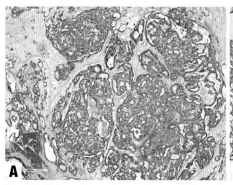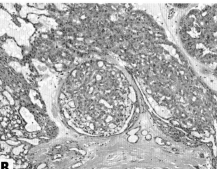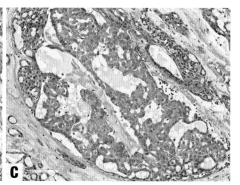

Fig. 4.70 Polymorphous adenocarcinoma, cribriform subtype. **A** The low-power photomicrograph demonstrates numerous patterns, with easily identified papillary structures and glomeruloid bodies. Fibrous connective tissue stroma is present. The nuclei show open chromatin, even at this magnification. **B** Islands of neoplastic cells are separated by a fibrous connective tissue stroma. The cells show glomeruloid projections into the lumen with clefting artefacts. The nuclei are monotonous. **C** Numerous patterns, with easily identified papillary structures and glomeruloid bodies. The nuclei show open chromatin. Fibrous connective tissue stroma is present.

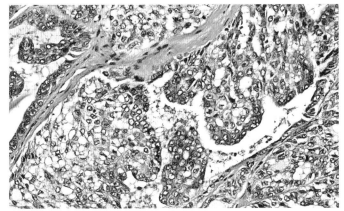

Fig. 4.71 Polymorphous adenocarcinoma, cribriform subtype. Optical nuclear chromatin clearing is a characteristic finding in this tumour. Note the papillary and glomeruloid architecture.

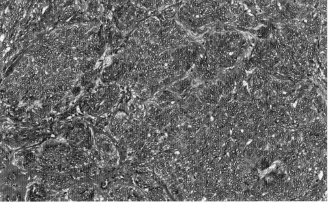

Fig. 4.72 Polymorphous adenocarcinoma, cribriform subtype. Solid growth pattern and optically clear nuclei reminiscent of papillary thyroid cancer nuclei.

Immunohistochemistry

PmA is immunoreactive as a single population for cytokeratins (e.g. CK7, in 100% of cases) {2915} and S100 (97–100%) {3474,4881}. Staining for p63 is reported in 78–100% of cases, whereas p40 is typically negative; this pattern is helpful in the differential diagnosis {4881}. Other positive immunomarkers include mammaglobin (67–100%), KIT (CD117) (60%), CEA (54%), GFAP (15%), MSA (13%), and EMA (12%) {3474,3460, 3579,493,3596}.

Cytology

Because of their intraoral location, PmAs are rarely sampled by FNAB and are rarely seen in metastases to neck lymph nodes. In accessible cases, smears show uniform polygonal, moderately sized tumour cells with relatively dense cytoplasm and round to oval nuclei, forming pseudopapillary, tubular, and irregular solid tissue fragments. Small acini and some dense hyalinized stroma may also be seen {2089}. Occasional nuclear grooves and small metachromatic globules may be seen, and misinterpretation as papillary thyroid carcinoma is a rare pitfall. The differential diagnosis is with pleomorphic adenomas, which have fibrillary stroma, and adenoid cystic carcinoma with its usual cribriform architecture.

Diagnostic molecular pathology

Detection of a *PRKD1* p.E710D hotspot mutation or translocation of *PRKD1*, *PRKD2*, or *PRKD3* is highly specific for the diagnosis of PmA {193}.

Essential and desirable diagnostic criteria

Essential: a salivary gland malignancy with cytological uniformity; architectural diversity; infiltrative border.
Desirable: immunopositivity for S100; *PRKD1* hotspot mutation (for PmA) or translocation of *PRKD1*, *PRKD2*, or *PRKD3* (for CASG) in selected cases.

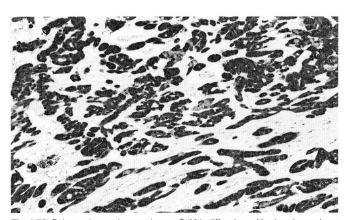

Fig. 4.73 Polymorphous adenocarcinoma. S100 is diffusely positive in polymorphous adenocarcinoma, regardless of morphological subtype.

Staging

Staging follows the eighth edition of the Union for International Cancer Control (UICC) / American Joint Committee on Cancer (AJCC) TNM staging system.

Prognosis and prediction

The overall prognosis of PmA is excellent, with a 10-year disease-specific survival rate of 94–99% {705,3958,2311,3423,1228}. The rates of local recurrence and regional metastasis are 5–33% and 9–15%, respectively {705,2311,3423,4881}. Rare cases of distant metastases have been reported {3958,3423,4881}.

Factors that are associated with a high risk of regional metastasis and/or an unfavourable prognosis include high-grade transformation {3958}, cribriform/CASG histology {4120}, PRKD gene fusion {3946}, various proportions cribriform and papillary architecture {4881}, necrosis, extrapalatal and hard palate location, angiolymphatic and bone invasion, and/or perineural infiltration around large nerves {4588}.

Hyalinizing clear cell carcinoma

Weinreb I
Simpson RHW
Wasserman JK
Wenig BM

Definition

Hyalinizing clear cell carcinoma (HCCC) is a carcinoma composed of clear and eosinophilic cells in a variably hyalinized stroma, usually associated with *EWSR1* rearrangement.

ICD-O coding

8310/3 Hyalinizing clear cell carcinoma

ICD-11 coding

2B61 & XH6L02 Malignant neoplasm of base of tongue & Clear cell carcinoma, NOS

2B65.Y & XH6L02 Other specified malignant neoplasm of palate & Clear cell carcinoma, NOS

2B67.Y & XH6L02 Other specified malignant neoplasms of parotid gland & Clear cell carcinoma, NOS

2B6A.Y & XH6L02 Other specified malignant neoplasms of oropharynx & Clear cell carcinoma, NOS

2B6B.Y & XH6L02 Other specified malignant neoplasms of nasopharynx & Clear cell carcinoma, NOS

2B6D.Y & XH6L02 Other specified malignant neoplasms of hypopharynx & Clear cell carcinoma, NOS

Related terminology

Acceptable: clear cell carcinoma.

Subtype(s)

None

Localization

Most HCCCs arise from oral minor salivary glands in locations including the soft palate, tongue, floor of the mouth, lips, buccal mucosa, retromolar trigone, and gingival sites {3001,213,1847}. A minority develop in other sites including the oropharynx, nasopharynx, parotid, sinonasal tract, larynx, and hypopharynx {3001, 213,1847}. Clear cell odontogenic carcinoma is morphologically and genetically similar and arises within the gnathic bones {456}.

Clinical features

Most HCCCs present with localized swelling. The overlying mucosa may be ulcerated. Pain and symptoms associated with cranial nerve involvement are rare {4758}.

Imaging

Typical findings are a well-defined lesion, usually in the oral cavity or tongue base, which has smooth margins and is hypoechoic to isoechoic on ultrasound. It is homogeneous, T2-hyperintense, and enhances uniformly on CT and MRI. Cervical lymph node and distant metastases are uncommon {4555,4906}.

Epidemiology

HCCC has a slight female predominance {213}. The tumour develops in adults, with a median age at diagnosis of 56 years (range: 23–87 years) {3001,213,1847}.

Etiology

Unknown

Pathogenesis

Most HCCCs harbour a translocation involving *EWSR1* and *ATF1*, which typically results in a fusion between *EWSR1* exon 11 and *ATF1* exon 3 {213}. Other fusions (*EWSR1* exon 15 and *ATF1* exon 5; *EWSR1::CREM*) have been described {761,1875}.

Macroscopic appearance

Tumours range in size from 4 to 50 mm. The cut surface is white-tan and solid. The tumour is well circumscribed but unencapsulated. Gross invasion into surrounding structures may be seen {213,4758,1847}.

Histopathology

HCCC is composed of clear or eosinophilic cells. Despite its name, tumours composed entirely of clear cells are rare, and some completely lack clear cells. The tumour is arranged in

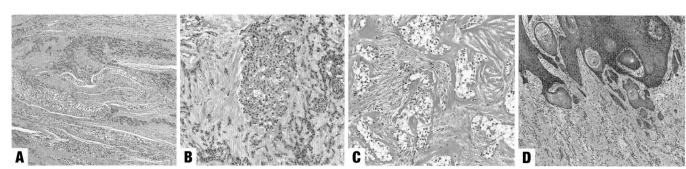

Fig. 4.74 Hyalinizing clear cell carcinoma. **A** The tumour shows a combination of clear and eosinophilic cords of cells with perineural invasion. **B** Some hyalinizing clear cell carcinomas have minimal clear cell change. This tumour is mostly eosinophilic, with only a small focus of clear cells. **C** The tumour shows bland clear cells in cords and small nests in a sclerotic stroma. **D** The tumour may connect to the surface in the oral cavity and may show pagetoid spread, or pseudoepitheliomatous hyperplasia of the squamous mucosa (shown here).

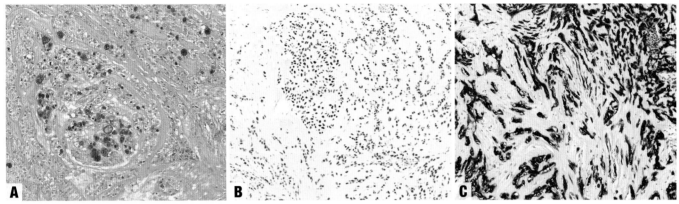

Fig. 4.75 Hyalinizing clear cell carcinoma. **A** About half of all cases show focal mucin, and occasional cases have conspicuous goblet-type mucinous cells (mucicarmine). **B** The majority of cases stain diffusely with p63. **C** Most hyalinizing clear cell carcinomas stain diffusely with high-molecular-weight keratins. This staining pattern reflects a squamous phenotype and is a pitfall in the differential diagnosis with mucoepidermoid carcinoma.

nests, cords, and trabeculae. Ducts and small cysts may be seen. Squamous differentiation and mucocytes are common {4081,3001,4162,3335,213,4758}. Increased mitoses, marked atypia, and necrosis are rare; when seen, they represent high-grade transformation {2091,4112}.

HCCCs are unencapsulated, with cells infiltrating the surrounding tissues, particularly skeletal muscle. Tumours arising in the oral cavity may connect with the overlying epithelium and show a pagetoid pattern of spread. Perineural invasion is seen in about half of all cases. The stroma ranges from densely hyalinized basement membrane–like to desmoplastic or fibrocellular, and the juxtaposition of these two stroma types is largely pathognomonic of HCCC.

Histochemistry
The clear cells are PAS-positive and diastase-sensitive. Mucicarmine highlights intracellular mucin {4758}.

Immunohistochemistry
The tumour cells express epithelial markers including CK7, CK19, CK14, CAM5.2, and EMA. They also usually express p63, p40, and CK5/6, supporting squamous differentiation. Myoepithelial markers including S100, MSA, SMA, and calponin are negative {4081,3001,4162,3335,213,4758}. Some tumours express p16, which can be a diagnostic dilemma when the tumour arises in the oropharynx; however they lack transcriptionally active HPV {479}.

Differential diagnosis
The entities include clear cell mucoepidermoid carcinoma, epithelial-myoepithelial carcinoma, myoepithelial carcinoma, oncocytoma, myoepithelioma, and metastatic clear cell carcinoma, with distinction sometimes requiring molecular studies.

Cytology
HCCCs have been sampled rarely by FNAB, and have shown large cells with clear to eosinophilic cytoplasm, distinct cell borders, round nuclei lacking prominent nucleoli, and (in some cases) metachromatic stroma {4968}.

Diagnostic molecular pathology
Demonstration of an *EWSR1* fusion gene is helpful in selected cases.

Essential and desirable diagnostic criteria
Essential: a salivary gland malignancy with nests, cords, and trabeculae of clear and/or eosinophilic cells in a hyalinized stroma.
Desirable: EWSR1 fusion (in selected cases).

Staging
Staging follows the eighth edition of the Union for International Cancer Control (UICC) / American Joint Committee on Cancer (AJCC) TNM staging system.

Prognosis and prediction
HCCCs are slow-growing, with a good prognosis. The 5-year rates of local recurrence, lymph node metastasis, and distant metastasis are 19%, 3%, and 2%, respectively {1847}. Locoregional recurrence may be associated with incomplete resection and/or perineural invasion. Cases with high-grade transformation have been described, with distant metastases identified {2091,4112}. Death from disease is rare {3317}.

Basal cell adenocarcinoma

Seethala R
Fonseca I
Jo VY
Nagao T
Rossi ED
Yamamoto H

Definition
Basal cell adenocarcinoma (BCAC) is a malignant infiltrative basaloid salivary gland tumour composed of a mixture of basal and ductal cells.

ICD-O coding
8147/3 Basal cell adenocarcinoma

ICD-11 coding
2B67.Z & XH9SA7 Malignant neoplasms of parotid gland, unspecified & Basal cell adenocarcinoma

Related terminology
Not recommended: carcinoma ex monomorphic adenoma; malignant dermal analogue tumour.

Subtype(s)
None

Localization
Most BCACs occur in the parotid gland (> 90%) {1238,1433, 3395,987}.

Clinical features
BCAC usually presents as a slow-growing nodule in the parotid gland. Patients with syndromic BCAC may also have multiple skin adnexal tumours {1238,1984,4959,3941}.

Epidemiology
BCAC accounts for < 3% of malignant salivary tumours {1433, 3395,987}. Most affected patients are in their sixth or seventh decade of life {1433,3713,3395,987}. There is no sex predilection.

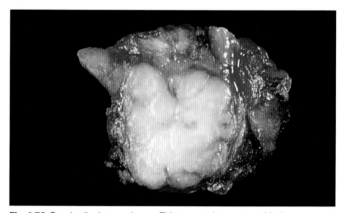

Fig. 4.76 Basal cell adenocarcinoma. This tumour shows a tan-white homogeneous cut surface and a multinodular pushing border that may be deceptively innocuous.

Etiology
Some BCACs (~15%) occur in the setting of Brooke–Spiegler syndrome {3941}. Most BCACs arise de novo, but a few develop from pre-existing basal cell adenoma (BCA) {2736,786,3131, 1932}.

Pathogenesis
BCAC may show a complex genetic profile {2108,4829}. A subset of cases show CYLD or CTNNB1 alterations {853,3887, 3705,3347}.

Macroscopic appearance
BCACs typically range in size from 20 to 40 mm {5004,3713} and present as a firm, unencapsulated, tan mass.

Histopathology
BCACs show tubulotrabecular, membranous, or solid growth, with the latter two patterns predominating. Tumour nests show

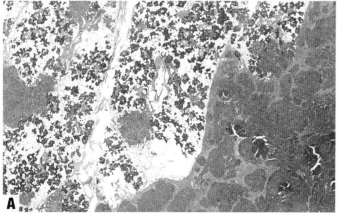
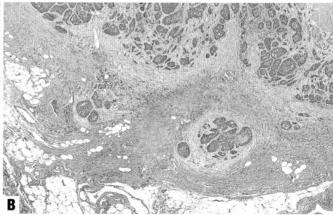

Fig. 4.77 Basal cell adenocarcinoma. **A** Syndromic setting. The carcinoma (right) is arising in a background of multiple precursor lesions (left). Compared with the precursor lesions, tumour nests are larger and bounded by more profound sclerosis. **B** The tumour shows infiltration into soft tissue.

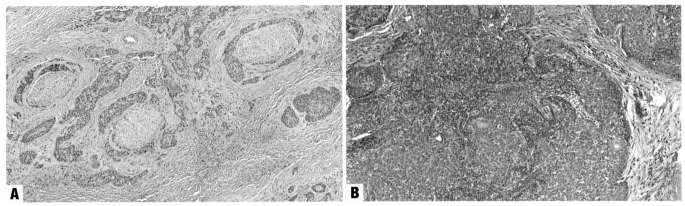

Fig. 4.78 Basal cell adenocarcinoma. **A** Perineural invasion can be noted. **B** Most tumours show a solid and/or membranous pattern, although any pattern can be seen.

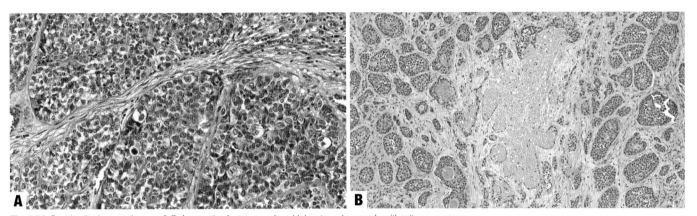

Fig. 4.79 Basal cell adenocarcinoma. **A,B** Aggressive features such as high cytonuclear grade with mitoses are rare.

peripheral palisading of dark cells with paler cells and centrally located ducts. Squamous and sebaceous elements may be seen. Nuclei are vesicular. About 25% show perineural and vascular invasion; anaplasia is rare.

Immunohistochemistry
Epithelial and myoepithelial markers highlight the dual cell composition of BCAC. Nuclear β-catenin immunoexpression is present in a subset of BCACs {2131,2108,2544,3887,3347}.

Differential diagnosis
The presence of peripheral palisading and focal squamous metaplasia can help to separate BCAC from adenoid cystic carcinoma. BCAC is distinguished from BCA by infiltration, necrosis, and mitoses (especially when > 4 mitoses/2 mm²) {3130}.

Cytology
BCAC shows very similar cytopathological features to those of BCA (see *Basal cell adenoma*, p. 171). Squamoid and sebaceous features may be seen focally, helping to distinguish BCAC from adenoid cystic carcinoma {4203}; however, differentiating BCA from BCAC and from adenoid cystic carcinoma is

not always possible, and the term "basaloid neoplasm" is often appropriate.

Diagnostic molecular pathology
None

Essential and desirable diagnostic criteria
Essential: a salivary gland malignancy with invasive growth; basaloid morphology; peripheral palisading with paler inner cells and ducts; dual population immunophenotype.

Staging
Staging follows the eighth edition of the Union for International Cancer Control (UICC) / American Joint Committee on Cancer (AJCC) TNM staging system.

Prognosis and prediction
Local recurrence rates are about 37% {3112}, but complete surgical excision with clear margins is curative in > 90% of cases. Regional lymph node and distant metastasis and disease-related death are rare (< 10%). Age and T categorization are key prognosticators {5004}.

Intraductal carcinoma

Bishop JA
Agaimy A
Nagao T
Thompson LDR
Weinreb I

Definition
Intraductal carcinoma (IDC) is a salivary gland malignancy characterized by papillary, cribriform, and solid proliferations that are entirely or predominantly intraductal.

ICD-O coding
8500/2 Intraductal carcinoma
8500/2 Intercalated duct intraductal carcinoma
8500/2 Apocrine intraductal carcinoma
8500/2 Oncocytic intraductal carcinoma
8500/2 Mixed intraductal carcinoma

ICD-11 coding
B67.Z & XH4V32 Malignant neoplasms of parotid gland, unspecified & Ductal carcinoma in situ, NOS
2E60.0 Carcinoma in situ of lip, oral cavity, or pharynx

Related terminology
Acceptable: intercalated duct carcinoma.
Not recommended: low-grade cribriform cystadenocarcinoma; low-grade salivary duct carcinoma; ductal carcinoma.

Subtype(s)
Intercalated duct IDC; apocrine IDC; oncocytic IDC; mixed IDC

Localization
IDC arises predominantly in the parotid gland {787,561,4760, 3147,4129,4117}, with uncommon involvement of the intraparotid lymph nodes {561,4759,3751}, submandibular gland {561}, and oral cavity {787,824}.

Clinical features
Patients present with longstanding painless swellings. IDCs are indolent neoplasms, but rare cases of invasive carcinoma ex IDC have been reported {4760,4117}.

Epidemiology
IDC is rare. It affects adults, with a wide age range (25–93 years) and an even sex distribution {787,561,4759,4760,3147,4117, 3751,4467}.

Etiology
Unknown

Pathogenesis
Intercalated duct IDC usually has *NCOA4::RET* and rarely has *STRN::ALK*, *TUT1::ETV5*, or *KIAA1217::RET*; some cases are fusion-negative {4760,4117,3751}. The oncocytic type may harbour *TRIM33::RET*, *NCOA4::RET*, or *BRAF* p.V600E pathogenic variants; some cases have no alterations {3147, 477}. Mixed intercalated duct–apocrine IDC usually harbours *TRIM27::RET* and occasionally harbours *NCOA4::RET* {4129,

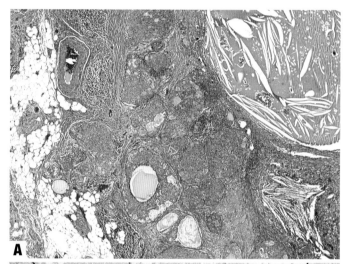

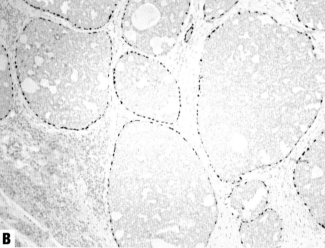

Fig. 4.80 Intraductal carcinoma. **A** Intercalated duct cell subtype. This intraductal carcinoma has a typical low-power appearance of large cysts and rounded lobules with solid, cribriform, and micropapillary growth. Although cell morphology cannot be seen at this magnification, the blue appearance is in keeping with intercalated duct–type intraductal carcinoma. Haemorrhage and cholesterol clefts are evident. This case harboured *NCOA4::RET*. **B** Intercalated duct type. All forms of intraductal carcinoma are characterized by a rim of myoepithelial cells completely surrounding the tumour lobules. Here, the myoepithelial cells are highlighted by p40 immunostaining.

4117}. Purely apocrine IDC harbours multiple pathogenic variants (e.g. *HRAS*, *PIK3CA*, *TP53*); some cases are fusion-negative {4760,480} or harbour *TRIM27::RET* fusion {4129}. One study reported that myoepithelial and ductal cells of IDC harbour the same fusion {480}.

Macroscopic appearance
IDC is well circumscribed and variably solid and cystic, measuring as large as 46 mm (mean: 14 mm).

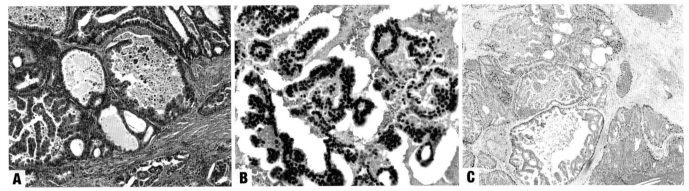

Fig. 4.81 Intraductal carcinoma, apocrine subtype. **A** Intraductal papillary proliferations with widespread apocrine differentiation. **B** The tumour cells are positive for AR. **C** Almost intact abluminal myoepithelial layer decorated by p63 immunostaining.

Table 4.03 Subtypes of intraductal carcinoma

Subtype	Grade	S100 and SOX10	AR	Genetics	Associated invasion
Intercalated duct	Low	++	−	Usually *NCOA4::RET* Rarely *STRN::ALK, TUT1::ETV5, KIAA1217::RET* Occasionally fusion-negative	Rare
Apocrine	Low or high	−	++	Complex, with multiple mutations (*HRAS, PIK3CA*, others) No fusions	Common
Oncocytic	Low	++	−	*TRIM33::RET* *BRAF* p.V600E mutation Occasionally *NCOA4::RET* or fusion/mutation-negative	Unknown
Mixed	Low or high	++ in intercalated duct and oncocytic areas	++ in apocrine areas	Usually *TRIM27::RET* Occasionally *NCOA4::RET*	Rare

Histopathology

All subtypes of IDC display rounded cysts and lobules, with variable solid, cribriform, micropapillary, and Roman bridge–type ductal proliferations, surrounded by a continuous, flattened layer of myoepithelial cells. The ductal cells vary with each subtype (see Table 4.03).

Subtypes

Intercalated duct IDC has small amphophilic to eosinophilic cells with oval nuclei. Apocrine IDC has large cells with bubbly eosinophilic cytoplasm with snouting and decapitation secretions. Oncocytic IDC has cells with abundant granular eosinophilic cytoplasm and round nuclei with prominent nucleoli, whereas mixed IDC shows hybrid features.

Intercalated duct and oncocytic IDCs exhibit low-grade features and low mitotic rates, whereas IDCs with apocrine components can be low- or high-grade. The background often shows degenerative changes (fibrosis, inflammation, cholesterol clefts, haemorrhage). Frank invasive growth with loss of myoepithelial cells can occasionally be seen in all subtypes of IDC {4760, 4117}.

Immunohistochemistry

Intercalated duct and oncocytic IDCs are positive for S100, SOX10, and mammaglobin, but negative for AR and GCDFP-15, whereas apocrine IDC has the opposite staining pattern. Mixed IDC shows mixed immunoprofiles of the components present.

Myoepithelial cells of IDC are consistently positive for p40/p63, CK14, SMA, and calponin.

Differential diagnosis

Intraductal proliferations seen in carcinoma ex pleomorphic adenoma and sclerosing polycystic adenoma are distinguished

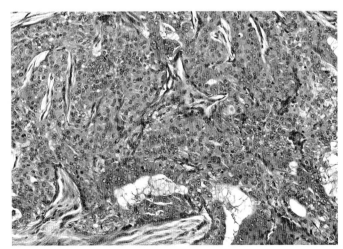

Fig. 4.82 Intraductal carcinoma, oncocytic subtype. This case consists of tightly packed, solid nests of oncocytic cells with abundant granular eosinophilic cytoplasm and round nuclei with small, distinct nucleoli. This tumour was positive for S100 and negative for AR (not shown), and it harboured *BRAF* p.V600E.

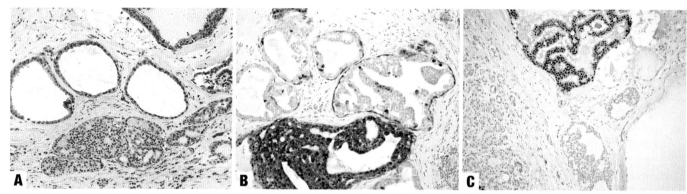

Fig. 4.83 Intraductal carcinoma, mixed intercalated duct–apocrine subtype. **A** Two different morphologies can be seen in this mixed intraductal carcinoma. Apocrine cells (top) have eosinophilic cytoplasm, apical snouting, and large nucleoli. Intercalated duct cells (bottom) have less cytoplasm, which is more amphophilic; smaller nuclei; and indistinct nucleoli. The nests of both components are rimmed by a subtle layer of flattened myoepithelial cells. This case harboured *TRIM27::RET*. **B** S100 is diffusely positive in the intercalated duct component (bottom), whereas in the apocrine component (top) only the surrounding myoepithelial cells stain. **C** Only the apocrine tumour component (top) of this mixed intraductal carcinoma was positive for AR.

by their background elements (chondromyxoid stroma and acinar cells, respectively). Cystadenoma lacks a fenestrated or cribriform appearance and the complete layer of myoepithelial cells. Mucoepidermoid carcinoma, secretory carcinoma, and salivary duct carcinoma do not have a complete circumferential layer of myoepithelial cells, and in epithelial-myoepithelial carcinoma the myoepithelial cells are larger and much more prominent.

Cytology
Low-grade IDCs exhibit populations of both mildly atypical ductal cells and smaller myoepithelial cells with a clean background, whereas high-grade apocrine IDC has large pleomorphic ductal cells and necrosis {3368,4640}.

Diagnostic molecular pathology
Demonstration of molecular alteration can assist in diagnosis. Routine break-apart FISH is often falsely negative in IDC with *NCOA4::RET*, which is a tight inversion due to an intrachromosomal rearrangement {4760,4129,480}.

Essential and desirable diagnostic criteria
Essential: a salivary gland malignancy with rounded lobules of ductal neoplastic cells; a surrounding rim of myoepithelial cells; ductal cells positive for S100, SOX10, and mammaglobin and/or AR.

Desirable: a cystic component; identification of *RET* fusion (for intercalated duct, oncocytic, or mixed IDC), *BRAF* p.V600E mutations (for oncocytic IDC), or PI3K pathway mutations (for apocrine IDC) in selected cases.

Staging
IDC is currently regarded as an in situ disease according to the eighth edition of the Union for International Cancer Control (UICC) / American Joint Committee on Cancer (AJCC) TNM staging system. Staging of invasive carcinoma ex IDC follows the TNM classification.

Prognosis and prediction
Pure IDCs of all types behave indolently after complete excision. Frankly invasive carcinomas ex IDC can behave aggressively {4760,4117}.

Salivary duct carcinoma

Chiosea S
Agaimy A
Hellquist H
Nagao T
Simpson RHW
van Herpen CML

Definition

Salivary duct carcinoma (SDC) is an aggressive carcinoma resembling mammary ductal carcinoma, most typically with an apocrine phenotype.

ICD-O coding

8500/3 Salivary duct carcinoma
8033/3 Sarcomatoid salivary duct carcinoma
8481/3 Mucin-rich salivary duct carcinoma
8265/3 Micropapillary salivary duct carcinoma
8500/3 Basal-like salivary duct carcinoma
8290/3 Oncocytic salivary duct carcinoma

ICD-11 coding

XH7KH3 & XA5CM1 Infiltrating duct carcinoma, NOS & Salivary duct

Related terminology

None

Subtype(s)

Sarcomatoid SDC; mucin-rich SDC; micropapillary SDC; basal-like SDC; oncocytic SDC

Localization

Most tumours involve major salivary glands {4575,2045,2065}.

Clinical features

SDC presents as a rapidly growing tumour, with facial nerve palsy, pain, and cervical lymphadenopathy. If arising from pleomorphic adenoma, a rapid increase in size of a longstanding pre-existing mass is common.

Imaging

On cross-sectional imaging, SDC most commonly presents as a poorly defined, infiltrative salivary gland mass with frequent calcification and necrosis. Foci of marked hypointensity on T2-weighted MRI may be a useful radiological feature to suggest the diagnosis {4794}.

Epidemiology

SDC has a distinct male predilection and a peak incidence in the fifth to seventh decades of life {4821,3143}.

Etiology

None

Pathogenesis

AR copy-number gain and splice variants have been reported {3029}. The most frequent genetic alterations are mutations in *TP53* (55%), *HRAS* (23%), and *PIK3CA* (23%); amplification of *ERBB2* (35%) {1011}; *PTEN* deletion; and *BRAF* pathogenic

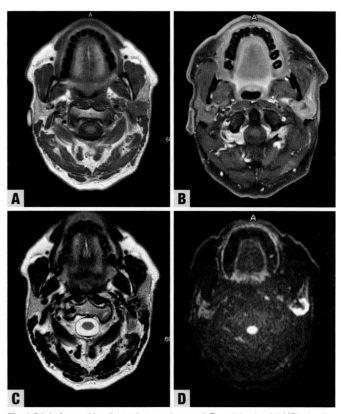

Fig. 4.84 Left parotid salivary duct carcinoma. **A** T1-weighted axial MRI showing intermediate signal lesion spanning superficial and deep lobes. **B** Postcontrast fat-suppressed T1-weighted axial MRI showing heterogeneous enhancement. **C** T2-weighted axial MRI showing intermediate to low signal intensity (compare with hyperintense pleomorphic adenoma). **D** Axial b1000 diffusion-weighted imaging showing restricted diffusion in enhancing areas.

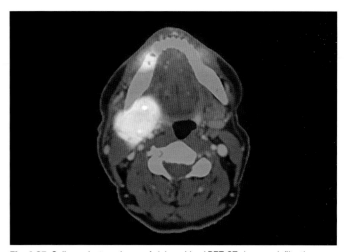

Fig. 4.85 Salivary duct carcinoma. Axial combined PET-CT shows an infiltrative mass with avid FDG uptake arising from the submandibular gland.

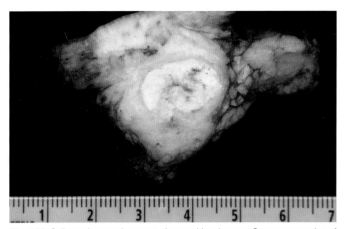

Fig. 4.86 Salivary duct carcinoma ex pleomorphic adenoma. Gross presentation of salivary duct carcinoma ex pleomorphic adenoma. Irregular tan-white mass involves the parotid gland (right) and extends to the skin. In the centre of the mass, there is a rounded focus of pre-existing hyalinized pleomorphic adenoma.

variants {848,4038,3144}. *PLAG1* or *HMGA2* rearrangements, markers of pre-existing pleomorphic adenoma, are identified in about half of all SDCs {313,2207,847}. A small subset of SDCs harbour *ALK* {1147,36} and *ETV6::NTRK3* fusions {4465}.

Macroscopic appearance

SDCs are infiltrative, firm, tan-white masses, frequently involving adjacent structures, and they may contain well-defined nodules of pre-existing pleomorphic adenoma.

Histopathology

SDCs display complex solid, cribriform, and papillary-cystic architecture with frequent comedonecrosis {2321}. The cells have large pleomorphic nuclei with coarse chromatin and prominent nucleoli, and abundant eosinophilic, typically apocrine, cytoplasm {848,4821}. Lymphovascular and perineural invasion are common {3143}. A hyalinized nodule of a pre-existing pleomorphic adenoma may be present. Rarely, SDC may be purely in situ {4077}.

Subtypes

The sarcomatoid subtype of SDC contains areas of highly atypical spindle cells, occasionally with foci of heterologous differentiation (e.g. osteoid production) {1841,3357}. In mucin-rich SDC there are significant pools of extracellular mucin {4080,2427}. Micropapillary SDC includes small tumour nests, without fibrovascular cores, with prominent retraction from adjacent stroma, and an inside-out pattern of EMA immunostaining {4076}. Basal-like SDC is characterized by a less abundant and more amphophilic, rather than apocrine, cytoplasm {1119,4076}. Oncocytic SDC is defined by abundant granular eosinophilic cytoplasm {4076}. SDC with rhabdoid-like features contains usually dyscohesive ovoid cells with eccentric nuclei; immunohistochemically, the rhabdoid cells are positive for cytokeratin and negative for myoepithelial markers {2429}. The current definition of SDC subtypes does not include a universally agreed-on minimal threshold for variant morphology. All subtypes are commonly accompanied by areas of conventional SDC.

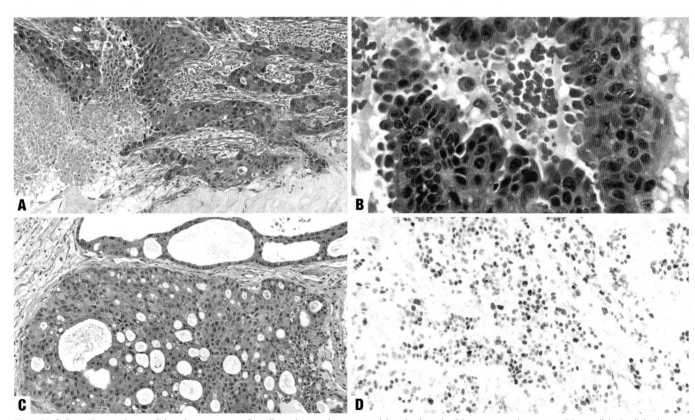

Fig. 4.87 Salivary duct carcinoma. **A** Invasive component of a salivary duct carcinoma comprising glands and solid nests, necrotic areas, and hypocellular hyalinized stroma of probably pre-existing pleomorphic adenoma (lower part of the image). **B** Salivary duct carcinoma cells (oncocytic subtype) characterized by abundant eosinophilic cytoplasm with apocrine-type secretions and enlarged pleomorphic nuclei with prominent nucleoli. **C** Complex architecture with cribriforming glands and a Roman-bridge pattern. **D** Moderate to strong immunopositivity for AR.

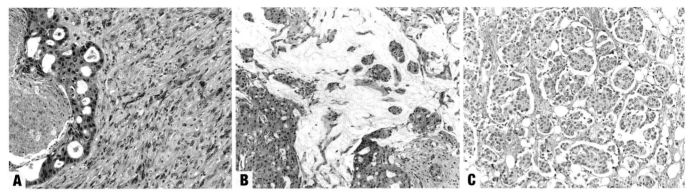

Fig. 4.88 Salivary duct carcinoma. **A** Sarcomatoid subtype. Conventional salivary duct carcinoma (left) is adjacent to sarcomatoid atypical spindle cells (right). **B** Mucin-rich subtype. Mucin lakes and cells of conventional salivary duct carcinoma. **C** Micropapillary subtype. Small clusters of tumour cells, devoid of fibrovascular cores, surrounded by clear spaces.

Immunohistochemistry

AR is expressed in about 90% of SDCs, indicative of an apocrine immunophenotype {2170,1119,2873,4821,4343,531}. Diffuse and strong immunoreactivity for ERBB2 is identified in about one third of SDCs {4343,531,3144,3634}. CK7 is consistently positive, whereas S100 and SOX10 are negative. Staining for p63 may help to identify the intraductal component by highlighting basal/myoepithelial cells surrounding neoplastic cells.

Differential diagnosis

The differential diagnosis includes other salivary carcinomas with high-grade transformation {3126,4821,4112}.

Cytology

Markedly cellular smears show irregular crowded tissue fragments (which may show a cribriform architecture), with large polygonal cells showing well-defined cytoplasm, pleomorphic nuclei, prominent nucleoli, and plentiful mitoses, in a necrotic background, resembling poorly differentiated carcinoma, no special type, of breast {2329,2226,3144}.

Diagnostic molecular pathology

Because systemic therapies targeting AR, *ERRB2* amplification, the PI3K pathway (including *PIK3CA* mutations and *PTEN* loss), and *BRAF* p.V600E are being investigated, molecular analysis may be warranted {3863,4535,3634}.

Essential and desirable diagnostic criteria

Essential: a high-grade carcinoma, most typically with apocrine features.
Desirable: AR expression.

Staging

Staging follows the eighth edition of the Union for International Cancer Control (UICC) / American Joint Committee on Cancer (AJCC) TNM staging system.

Prognosis and prediction

SDC is the most aggressive salivary gland malignancy, with most patients presenting with regional lymph node or distant metastases {2065,4821,531} and disease progression within 3–5 years {2045,2065,2117,3143}.

Myoepithelial carcinoma

Katabi N
Di Palma S
Nagao T
Stenman G

Definition

Myoepithelial carcinoma (MECA) is an invasive malignant salivary gland neoplasm that is almost exclusively composed of myoepithelial cells.

ICD-O coding

8982/3 Myoepithelial carcinoma

ICD-11 coding

2B67.Y & XH43E6 Other specified malignant neoplasms of parotid gland & Myoepithelial carcinoma
2B65.Y & XH43E6 Other specified malignant neoplasms of palate & Myoepithelial carcinoma
2B68.2 & XH43E6 Other specified malignant neoplasms of submandibular or sublingual glands & Myoepithelial carcinoma

Related terminology

Not recommended: malignant myoepithelioma.

Subtype(s)

None

Localization

Most tumours occur in the parotid gland, followed by the palate and the submandibular gland {2368,4105}.

Clinical features

Patients often present with a painless mass, sometimes with recent rapid growth {2368,4882}.

Imaging

Cross-sectional imaging shows an irregular, lobulated, poorly defined, heterogeneously enhancing salivary gland mass, with avid FDG uptake on PET-CT. Lesions are often T1- and T2-hypointense on MRI, and some demonstrate punctate calcification on CT. Imaging is used to assess the primary tumour

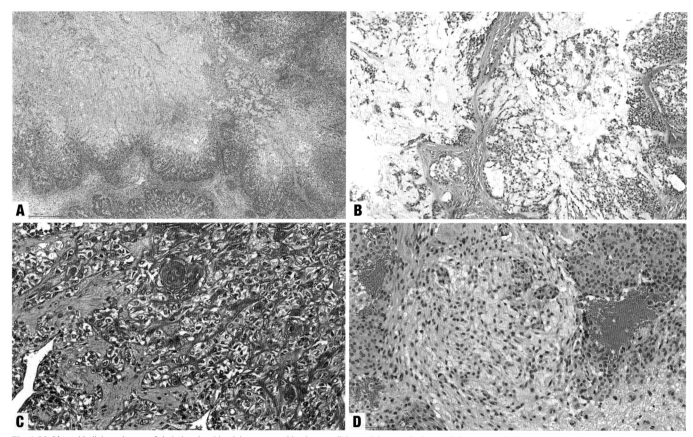

Fig. 4.89 Myoepithelial carcinoma. **A** Lobulated multinodular pattern with a hypercellular periphery and a hypocellular centre. **B** Myoepithelial carcinoma of the parotid gland. The tumour has a multinodular architecture divided by fibrous bands. A characteristic feature is a zonal arrangement with a hypercellular peripheral rim surrounding a hypocellular and often myxoid centre. **C** Myoepithelial carcinoma of the parotid gland. Clear cells represent a prominent component of a subset of myoepithelial carcinomas. Squamous pearls or overt squamous differentiation are present. **D** Spindle and epithelioid/plasmacytoid myoepithelial cells with a myxoid stroma.

and the presence of lymph node and distant metastases (including to the lungs, skin, liver, bone and brain) {4970,2607}.

Epidemiology
MECA is underrecognized. It may present at any age and has no sex predilection {2368,4882}.

Etiology
Unknown

Pathogenesis
PLAG1 fusions are identified in > 50% of cases of both de novo MECA and MECA ex pleomorphic adenoma (PA), with different fusion partner genes, including *FGFR1*, *TGFBR3*, and others {1012,4105}. *HMGA2* and *EWSR1* fusions are detected in small subsets of tumours {1012,4886}. *EWSR1* rearrangement without fusion may be present in clear cell MECA {4130,4105}.

Macroscopic appearance
The tumour is typically unencapsulated and has a grey to tan-white cut surface. Haemorrhage, necrosis, and cystic change may occur.

Histopathology
MECA may arise de novo or within a pre-existing PA and is the second most common histological subtype of carcinoma ex PA {2208,2368}. It exhibits diverse morphologies with different cell types (spindle, epithelioid, plasmacytoid, vacuolated, oncocytic, and clear) and architectures (solid, trabecular, and reticular) {2983,3133,363}. The stroma can be myxoid, myxochondroid, or hyalinized. The uniform cellular myoepithelial proliferation with the multinodular pattern and the transition from peripheral hypercellular zones to central hypocellular areas are characteristic and help to differentiate MECA from PA {4887}. Focal duct-like or squamous differentiation may occur {4130}. The presence of PA and tumour necrosis correlates with a worse outcome {2368}.

MECA expresses cytokeratins, SOX10, S100, and myoepithelial markers such as SMA, calponin, and p63/p40 {3133,2208, 2368,4887}.

Differential diagnosis
MECA is often cytologically bland and may therefore be underrecognized as malignant and misclassified as a myoepithelial-rich PA {4887}.

Cytology
In cytological specimens, MECA shows a mixture of spindle, plasmacytoid, and epithelioid cells. MECA cannot be distinguished from cellular PA on cytology {834,4887}.

Diagnostic molecular pathology
Not clinically relevant

Essential and desirable diagnostic criteria
Essential: a salivary gland malignancy showing nearly exclusively myoepithelial differentiation; invasive growth.
Desirable: a zonal pattern with a hypercellular periphery and a hypocellular centre.

Staging
Staging follows the eighth edition of the Union for International Cancer Control (UICC) / American Joint Committee on Cancer (AJCC) TNM staging system.

Prognosis and prediction
MECA has a varied clinical behaviour but is relatively aggressive, even when it is intracapsular or minimally invasive MECA ex PA {2208,2368,4887}. The risks of local recurrence and distant metastasis are 35% and 22%, respectively {4887}. MECA seems to have a propensity to distant rather than lymph node metastasis {4266,4688,2368,4887}.

Epithelial-myoepithelial carcinoma

Nagao T
Inagaki H
Nakaguro M
Seethala R

Definition

Epithelial-myoepithelial carcinoma (EMC) is a salivary gland malignancy characterized by biphasic tubular structures, usually composed of tightly coupled inner ductal and prominent outer myoepithelial cells.

ICD-O coding

8562/3 Epithelial-myoepithelial carcinoma

ICD-11 coding

2B67.Y & XH9JP2 Other specified malignant neoplasms of parotid gland & Epithelial-myoepithelial carcinoma
2B68.2 & XH9JP2 Other specified malignant neoplasms of submandibular or sublingual glands & Epithelial-myoepithelial carcinoma

Related terminology

None

Subtype(s)

None

Localization

The majority of EMCs develop in the parotid gland; the remainder affect the other major or minor salivary glands, sinonasal tract, and bronchus {1434,3954}.

Clinical features

EMC usually presents as a slow-growing, painless mass. Lymphadenopathy is rare.

Imaging

Features are nonspecific, but lesions are frequently slow-growing and fairly well defined on CT and MRI, with intermediate signal on T1- and T2-weighted MRI and with heterogeneous enhancement. Biopsy is required to differentiate them from other low-grade salivary gland masses {3554}.

Epidemiology

EMC is an uncommon neoplasm, accounting for 1% of all salivary gland tumours {3954}. It mostly occurs in the sixth and seventh decades of life, with a slight female predilection.

Etiology

A small subset arise in association with intercalated duct hyperplasia {4764,2907A}. EMC may also arise in a pre-existing pleomorphic adenoma {3954,1224,4548}.

Pathogenesis

A significant number of EMCs harbour *HRAS* mutations, most commonly at codon 61 {846,1696,1224,4548}.

Macroscopic appearance

The mean tumour size is 30 mm {3142}. The cut surface shows a white-tan, nodular, firm mass. Cystic changes may be noted {3954,3142}.

Histopathology

EMC generally exhibits multinodular invasive growth. The histological hallmark is a biphasic arrangement of inner (luminal) eosinophilic ductal epithelial cells and outer (abluminal), often clear myoepithelial cells {1156,945}. The myoepithelial component varies from single-layered to multilayered or even

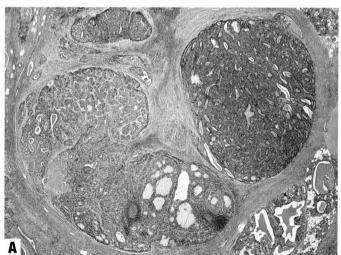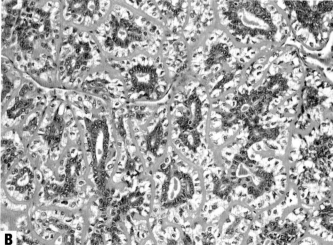

Fig. 4.90 Epithelial-myoepithelial carcinoma. **A** Low-power view shows a multinodular growth pattern. **B** Bilayered tubular structures, consisting of inner eosinophilic ductal cells and outer polygonal clear myoepithelial cells.

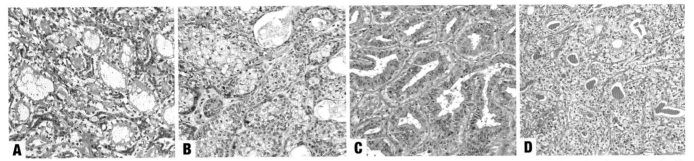

Fig. 4.91 Epithelial-myoepithelial carcinoma, histological variations. **A** A cribriform pattern with multiple pseudocysts. **B** Sebaceous differentiation featuring tumour cells with bubbly cytoplasm. **C** Apocrine differentiation of ductal cells. **D** A double-clear tubular pattern. Both inner ductal cells and outer myoepithelial cells exhibit clear cytoplasm.

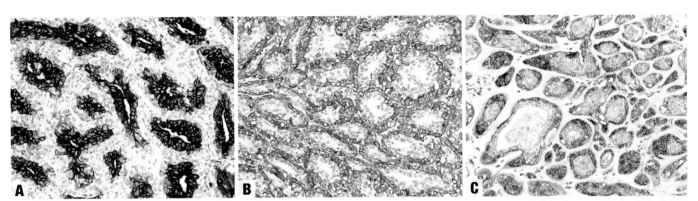

Fig. 4.92 Epithelial-myoepithelial carcinoma. **A** Immunostaining for CK7 highlights the luminal ductal cells. **B** The abluminal myoepithelial cells are positive for SMA. **C** RAS p.Q61R is expressed in the abluminal myoepithelial cells.

solid. Nuclear atypia is mild to moderate. There are several histological patterns and morphologies, including cribriform, basaloid, sebaceous, apocrine/oncocytic, and double-clear appearances, as well as squamous differentiation {3954,4045, 3959,1971,3952,488}. High-grade transformation rarely occurs {134,3775,3126,4112}.

Immunohistochemistry
The luminal cells are positive for CK7, whereas abluminal cells are usually positive for SMA, calponin, and p63/p40 {3954, 3142}. Diffuse and membranous/cytoplasmic RAS p.Q61R expression is observed in 65% of EMCs {3145}.

Differential diagnosis
The differential diagnosis includes other salivary gland tumours with biphasic and/or clear cell morphology, such as adenoid cystic carcinoma, basal cell adenocarcinoma, pleomorphic adenoma, myoepithelial carcinoma, and clear cell carcinoma {3142}.

Cytology
Aspirates classically show 3D clusters with a dual epithelial and myoepithelial cell population {2335,3003}.

Diagnostic molecular pathology
Assessment of *HRAS* mutations is useful for discriminating EMC from mimics {4548,3142}.

Essential and desirable diagnostic criteria
Essential: a salivary gland malignancy, usually with multinodular invasive growth; at least partly with a dual arrangement of inner ductal cells and outer prominent, usually clear, myoepithelial cells.

Staging
Staging follows the eighth edition of the Union for International Cancer Control (UICC) / American Joint Committee on Cancer (AJCC) TNM staging system.

Prognosis and prediction
EMC has a favourable prognosis {4612,1659,3142} but occasionally recurs locally; lymph node and distant metastases are rare. High-grade transformation is clearly a poor prognosticator {134,3775,3126,4112}. Other adverse features include size, necrosis, angiolymphatic invasion, and margin status {1434,3954,3775}.

Mucinous adenocarcinoma

Rooper LM
Agaimy A
Bishop JA
Gnepp DR
Leivo I

Definition

Mucinous adenocarcinoma (MA) is a primary salivary carcinoma that displays prominent intracellular and/or extracellular mucin, lacks diagnostic features of other tumour types, and is usually associated with *AKT1* alterations.

ICD-O coding

8480/3 Mucinous adenocarcinoma

ICD-11 coding

2B66.Y & XH1S75 Other specified malignant neoplasms of other or unspecified parts of mouth & Mucinous adenocarcinoma

Related terminology

Not recommended: papillary cystadenocarcinoma; mucinous cystadenocarcinoma; mucin-producing adenopapillary carcinoma; colloid carcinoma; signet ring carcinoma.

Subtype(s)

None

Localization

MA is most common in intraoral minor salivary glands {1441, 4896,3741}.

Clinical features

Most patients have painless masses or swellings. Nodal metastases are occasionally seen at presentation {2000,1337}.

Epidemiology

MA has a peak incidence in the eighth decade of life and a relatively equal sex distribution {4896,3741,1441}.

Etiology

Unknown

Pathogenesis

MA has a recurrent *AKT1* p.E17K mutation, usually accompanied by *TP53* mutations {3741}.

Macroscopic appearance

Tumours are solid or cystic, with a gelatinous cut surface.

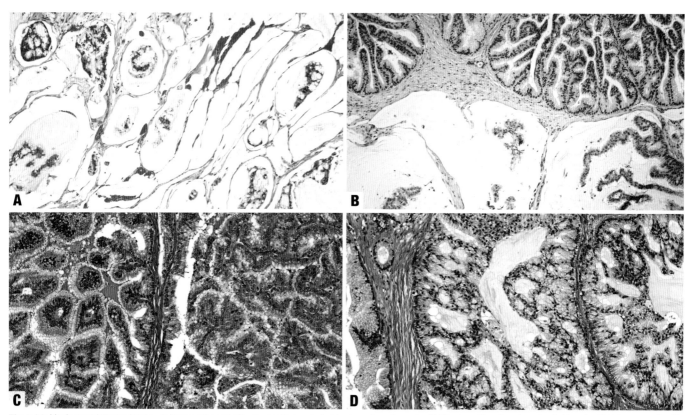

Fig. 4.93 Mucinous adenocarcinoma. **A** Nests and cords of tumour cells suspended in stromal mucin pools. **B** Mixed papillary fronds and colloid pools. **C** Columnar cells with apical mucin caps forming complex papillary fronds. **D** Complex mucin-producing papillary fronds projecting into cystic spaces.

Histopathology

MA is defined by abundant intracellular and/or extracellular mucin production in multiple forms, including goblet cell–like vacuoles, apical caps, foveolar-type cytoplasmic droplets, or stromal pools. Tumours show variable papillary, colloid, or signet-ring architecture, with 40% displaying mixed patterns {1042, 1534,4896,3741}. Most tumours display complex or simple papillary fronds projecting into cystic spaces. The colloid pattern is the second most common, with tumour nests suspended in mucin pools. Discohesive signet-ring cells are rarely seen. Cytological atypia varies widely.

Immunohistochemistry

MA is positive for CK7 and negative for CK20, CDX2, p63, p40, thyroid transcription factor 1 (TTF1), S100, calponin, SMA, and AR {1534,3741}.

Differential diagnosis

To diagnose MA, other mucin-producing salivary gland carcinomas must be excluded, including mucin-rich mucoepidermoid carcinoma (epidermoid/intermediate cells; p63/p40+), mucinous and rhabdoid variants of salivary duct carcinoma (apocrine cytology; AR+), and the mucinous/secretory pattern of myoepithelial carcinoma (nested/corded pattern; S100, calponin, or SMA+). Metastasis from gastrointestinal, pancreaticobiliary, or lung adenocarcinomas should be ruled out clinically.

Cytology

Not reported

Diagnostic molecular pathology

The identification of *AKT1* p.E17K mutation can support the diagnosis.

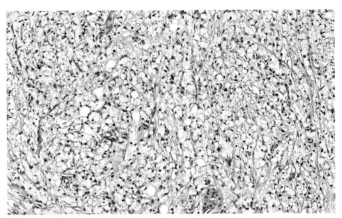

Fig. 4.94 Mucinous adenocarcinoma. Dyscohesive signet-ring cells with prominent intracytoplasmic mucin vacuoles.

Essential and desirable diagnostic criteria

Essential: a salivary gland malignancy with abundant intracellular or extracellular mucin; CK7+, CK20−; no features of other mucin-producing salivary gland neoplasms.
Desirable: *AKT1* p.E17K mutation (in selected cases).

Staging

Staging follows the eighth edition of the Union for International Cancer Control (UICC) / American Joint Committee on Cancer (AJCC) TNM staging system.

Prognosis and prediction

Although papillary-predominant tumours are generally indolent, dominant colloid or signet-ring patterns are associated with recurrence and metastases {1441,2000,1337}.

Sclerosing microcystic adenocarcinoma

Wenig BM

Definition

Sclerosing microcystic adenocarcinoma (SMA) is an indolent infiltrative salivary gland carcinoma composed of a biphasic population of ductal and myoepithelial cells embedded in a dense collagenous stroma.

ICD-O coding

8407/3 Sclerosing microcystic adenocarcinoma

ICD-11 coding

2B66.Z & XH17P2 Malignant neoplasms of other or unspecified parts of mouth, unspecified & Microcystic adnexal carcinoma

Related terminology

Acceptable: microcystic adnexal carcinoma of the tongue; sclerosing sweat duct–like carcinoma; syringomatous adenocarcinoma.

Subtype(s)

None

Localization

SMA arises from intraoral minor salivary glands in sites including the tongue, lip mucosa, floor of the mouth, and buccal mucosa {3007,3739}. A single case was reported in the nasopharynx {3007}.

Clinical features

Patients most commonly present with a painless mass or swelling; less common symptoms include dysphagia {3916}, numbness {5018}, and diplopia {3007}.

Epidemiology

SMA is more common in women than men and occurs from the fifth to the eighth decades of life (mean age: 56 years) {522, 3916,5018,2086}.

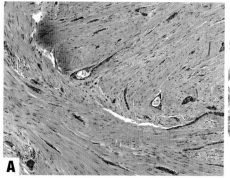 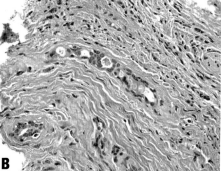 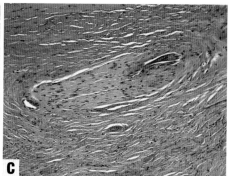

Fig. 4.95 A,B Sclerosing microcystic carcinoma. **A** The cords of neoplastic cells are usually compressed by the heavy stromal sclerosis. **B** The neoplasm is composed of ducts and tubules, along with strands and cords within a sclerosing stroma. **C** Sclerosing microcystic adenocarcinoma. A finding that assists in confirming a diagnosis of malignancy (i.e. adenocarcinoma) is the presence of perineural invasion, which is commonly present.

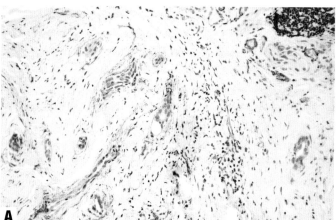 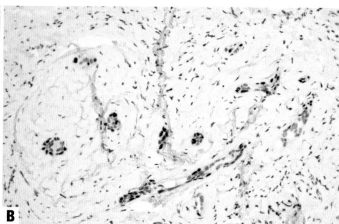

Fig. 4.96 Sclerosing microcystic adenocarcinoma. **A** The myoepithelial cells are highlighted by SMA. **B** The myoepithelial cells can also be highlighted with p40 immunohistochemistry.

Etiology

Unknown

Pathogenesis

Whole-exome sequencing revealed a moderate mutation burden and putative loss-of-function mutations in *CDK11B*, but an absence of mutations in genes including *CDKN2A*, *CDKN2B* {2086}, *TP53*, and *JAK1* {748}.

Macroscopic appearance

Gross examination of the surgical resection specimen revealed a poorly defined white-tan submucosal mass in a single case report {5018}.

Histopathology

SMA is characterized by deeply infiltrative ducts/tubules, strands/cords, nests, and (rarely) single cells embedded in a densely collagenous stroma. The tumour is composed of a biphasic cell population including luminal-lining bland-appearing ductal cells with round to oval monotonous nuclei, evenly dispersed chromatin, occasional nucleoli, and eosinophilic to clear cytoplasm. Ductal lining cells are peripherally surrounded by flattened myoepithelial cells. Mitotic figures are not conspicuous. Perineural invasion is commonly seen, and apposition to and/or invasion of minor salivary glands can be seen.

Histochemistry

Mucicarmine-positive luminal eosinophilic globular secretory material is seen.

Immunohistochemistry

Duct lining cells are positive for pancytokeratin and CK7, and the peripheral myoepithelial cell population expresses p40/p63, S100, SMA (smooth muscle actin), and calponin {4849,5018, 3739}. KIT (CD117) is negative {3007,5018}. Low proliferation indexes are seen with Ki-67 (MIB1) staining.

Differential diagnosis

The biphasic cell population, bland cytology, immunoreactive staining pattern, and lack of keratinization are helpful features in the differentiation from squamous cell carcinoma, polymorphous adenocarcinoma, adenoid cystic carcinoma, mucoepidermoid carcinoma, and hyalinizing clear cell carcinoma.

Cytology

Not reported

Diagnostic molecular pathology

Not clinically relevant

Essential and desirable diagnostic criteria

Essential: an infiltrative low-grade adenocarcinoma embedded in a dense sclerotic stroma; a biphasic cell population with an attenuated myoepithelial cell layer.
Desirable: perineural invasion.

Staging

Staging follows the eighth edition of the Union for International Cancer Control (UICC) / American Joint Committee on Cancer (AJCC) TNM staging system.

Prognosis and prediction

Surgical excision is the treatment of choice. Adjunctive radiotherapy may be used in margin-positive excision {5018}. SMA has a uniformly good outcome, without locoregional recurrence or distant metastases {5018,3739}.

Carcinoma ex pleomorphic adenoma

Katabi N
Altemani AM
Chiosea S
Fonseca I
Ihrler S
Klijanienko J

Definition
Carcinoma ex pleomorphic adenoma (CXPA) is an epithelial and/or myoepithelial malignancy that arises in association with a primary or recurrent pleomorphic adenoma (PA).

ICD-O coding
8941/3 Carcinoma ex pleomorphic adenoma

ICD-11 coding
2B67 & XH42V2 Malignant neoplasms of parotid gland & Carcinoma ex pleomorphic adenoma

Related terminology
Acceptable: carcinoma ex benign mixed tumour.

Subtype(s)
None

Localization
Most CXPAs arise in the parotid gland, but they may originate from the submandibular gland or minor salivary glands {4483, 2208,217,2296,4757,4468}.

Clinical features
The typical clinical presentation is that of a longstanding painless mass with recent rapid progression, or of a previous diagnosis of a PA. Occasionally, the tumour may be asymptomatic {217}. Facial nerve palsy, pain, or skin ulceration may occur {2208}.

Imaging
The majority of CXPAs present as an irregular, lobular, and heterogeneously enhancing mass with uneven margins on CT and MRI. Internal calcification is regarded as a specific sign for this tumour. Cervical lymph node and distant metastases are commonly found {4687}.

Epidemiology
CXPA accounts for 3.6% of all salivary gland tumours and 12% of all salivary gland malignancies {1689}. It occurs in the setting of a recurrent PA in about 12% of cases. Patients present in their sixth or seventh decade of life. The tumour is slightly more common in women {4757,1689,2207}.

Etiology
Unknown

Pathogenesis
About two thirds of CXPAs display *PLAG1* or *HMGA2* rearrangements and/or amplification, markers of a pre-existing PA. Additionally, tumours may exhibit the following markers of progression to carcinoma: mutations of *TP53*, *HRAS*, *PIK3CA*;

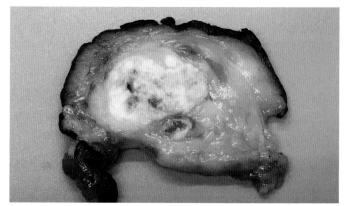

Fig. 4.97 Carcinoma ex pleomorphic adenoma. Macroscopic view showing the invasive carcinoma at the top and a residual well-circumscribed sclerotic pleomorphic adenoma component at the bottom.

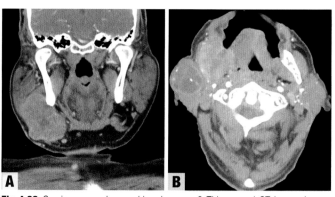

Fig. 4.98 Carcinoma ex pleomorphic adenoma. **A** This coronal CT image demonstrates a large destructive soft tissue–density mass in the right parotid gland. **B** This axial CT image shows small calcifications within a large destructive right parotid gland tumour.

amplification of *MYC*; and/or amplification of *EGFR* {3732,2860, 3490,4649,847}.

Macroscopic appearance
Tumour sizes range from 10 to 250 mm {4483,2586}. Grossly, the tumour is often poorly demarcated and may show a gross residual PA component that occasionally exhibits a well-circumscribed encapsulated sclerotic nodule {2586,2208}.

Histopathology
In most cases, the carcinoma component constitutes > 50% of the tumour volume {2586}. The PA component, which may have variable cellularity, can be intermixed with the carcinoma or appear as a discrete nodule (often hyalinized or rarely entirely sclerotic). CXPA can be subclassified according to the extent of invasion beyond the PA borders as follows: (1) intracapsular, when the carcinoma is confined within the PA capsule; in situ

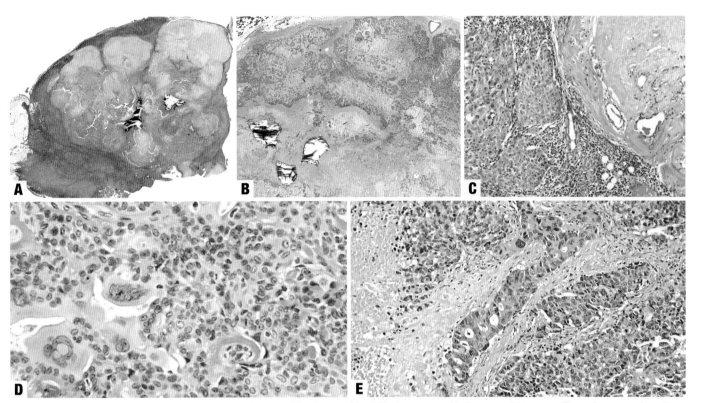

Fig. 4.99 Carcinoma ex pleomorphic adenoma. **A** Nodules of pleomorphic adenoma with calcifications are noted in the centre of this tumour. The malignant transformation to carcinoma is seen surrounding the tumour. **B** The lower half demonstrates the heavy stromal hyalinization within the pleomorphic adenoma with associated calcifications, while the area of myoepithelial carcinoma expands into the adjacent tissues. **C** A heavily hyalinized residuum of pleomorphic adenoma is noted. The carcinoma is seen immediately adjacent. **D** In many instances, the initial alterations are identified as profoundly pleomorphic epithelial cells within the lumen of ducts in the pleomorphic adenoma. This degree of atypia is beyond that of a benign tumour. **E** High-power view of the invasive carcinoma showing the histology of salivary duct carcinoma.

intracapsular, when the malignant tumour cells replace the ductal cells while retaining an intact myoepithelial layer; (2) minimally invasive, when the carcinoma invades < 4–6 mm beyond the PA borders; and (3) invasive, when the invasion beyond the PA capsule measures ≥ 6 mm.

Additionally, the histological type of the malignant component should be reported. The carcinoma component can be of any type, but the most common is salivary duct carcinoma, followed by myoepithelial carcinoma and adenocarcinoma NOS {289, 1224,2430}. Carcinosarcoma is a rare, aggressive tumour that is composed of malignant epithelial and sarcomatous components and can arise in association with a PA {1715,2213}.

Immunohistochemistry
Expression of PLAG1 and HMGA2 may help to identify the PA component {3767,1048,2209}. Staining for AR may be indicative of salivary duct CXPA {4703,4476}.

Differential diagnosis
Myoepithelial carcinoma and epithelial-myoepithelial carcinoma ex PA can mimic cellular PA especially when intracapsular or minimally invasive. The invasive multinodular pattern helps to differentiate these tumours from PA.

Cytology
FNAB smears can show poorly differentiated adenocarcinoma or salivary duct carcinoma, or other salivary gland carcinomas including mucoepidermoid carcinoma, adenoid cystic carcinoma, and carcinosarcoma, or the FNAB may show PA, depending on sampling. It is uncommon that both components are identified, and necrosis in an otherwise pleomorphic adenoma may be the only clue apart from a previous history of a longstanding mass or previous biopsy {2326,2327,3283,2830}.

Diagnostic molecular pathology
PLAG1 or *HMGA2* rearrangements detected by FISH serve as a marker of pre-existing PA and can assist in the diagnosis of CXPA.

Essential and desirable diagnostic criteria
Essential: evidence of a pre-existing PA, clinically or histologically, with a carcinoma (epithelial and/or myoepithelial).

Staging
Staging follows the eighth edition of the Union for International Cancer Control (UICC) / American Joint Committee on Cancer (AJCC) TNM staging system.

Prognosis and prediction
Most CXPAs are aggressive, with local and distant recurrences occurring in as many as 70% of cases. The 5-year survival rate ranges from 25% to 75% {2586,2208,4757,1689,1714}. Invasive CXPA has worse outcomes than intracapsular and minimally invasive CXPA {2586,2208,4757,1689,2004}. A large size (> 40 mm), multiple positive lymph nodes, and distant metastasis have been reported to increase the mortality risk {1714}.

Carcinosarcoma of the salivary glands

Ihrler S
Katabi N

Definition

Salivary carcinosarcoma is characterized by a variable combination of malignant epithelial and sarcomatous tumour components, which may develop from a pre-existent pleomorphic adenoma or de novo.

ICD-O coding

8980/3 Carcinosarcoma

ICD-11 coding

2B67.Y & XH2W45 Other specified malignant neoplasms of parotid gland & Carcinosarcoma, NOS

2B68.2 & XH2W45 Other specified malignant neoplasms of submandibular or sublingual glands & Carcinosarcoma, NOS

Related terminology

Not recommended: (true) malignant mixed tumour.

Subtype(s)

None

Localization

Most cases of carcinosarcoma manifest in major salivary glands (parotid, 70%; submandibular, 19%); minor gland occurrences are rare {1611}.

Clinical features

Carcinosarcomas are typically rapidly growing, large, and infiltrative tumours.

Epidemiology

The mean age at presentation is 58 years (range: 14–87 years), with no sex predilection {1611}.

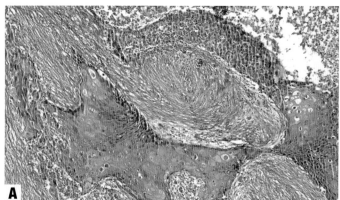
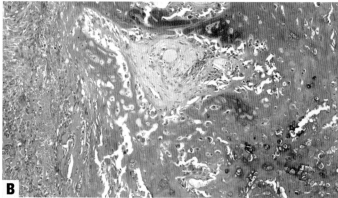

Fig. 4.100 Carcinosarcoma ex pleomorphic adenoma of the parotid gland. **A** Undifferentiated and squamous carcinomatous components. **B** Osteoid and chondroid sarcomatous components.

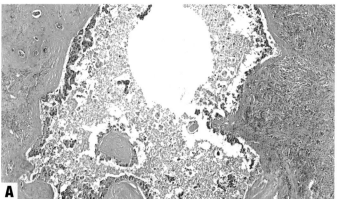
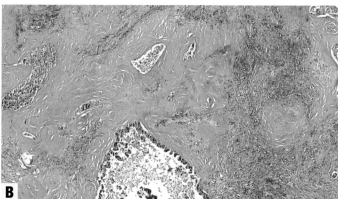

Fig. 4.101 Carcinosarcoma ex pleomorphic adenoma of the parotid gland. **A** The tumour is composed of high-grade adenocarcinomatous and high-grade sarcomatous components. **B** The tumour is composed of spindle-shaped sarcomatous and high-grade adenocarcinomatous structures. There is a hyalinized focus of pre-existing pleomorphic adenoma in the upper-left part of the picture.

Etiology

Approximately half of all cases develop from a pre-existent pleomorphic adenoma {4222,1769}. However, it has been shown that some carcinosarcomas arise de novo {1829,1611}. A few cases occurred after radiotherapy {4192}.

Pathogenesis

A subset of carcinosarcomas harbour *PLAG1* or *HMGA2* fusions {2005A}; however, molecular alterations are heterogeneous.

Macroscopic appearance

They are predominantly large, infiltrating tumours (as large as 50–100 mm, mean: 39 mm), frequently with necrosis and haemorrhage. A smaller, often sclerotic nodule may represent a pre-existent pleomorphic adenoma.

Histopathology

The carcinomatous component is most commonly a squamous cell carcinoma or adenocarcinoma, whereas the most common sarcomatous component is a chondrosarcoma {1611}. The sarcomatous components frequently dominate. Approximately half of the tumours show a pre-existing, often sclerotic pleomorphic adenoma, usually with a carcinomatous (rarely sarcomatous) intracapsular component. Pure intracapsular carcinosarcoma ex pleomorphic adenoma is very rare {1829}.

Immunohistochemistry

Immunohistochemistry is recommended for characterizing the usually heterologous sarcomatous component, and especially for distinguishing carcinosarcoma from other malignancies with high-grade transformation {1829,1611,3508}.

Cytology

Scattered irregular tissue fragments of large epithelial cells with abundant cytoplasm, large pleomorphic hyperchromatic nuclei, and prominent nucleoli are present, along with occasional giant cells and spindle cells showing atypical nuclei in a background of necrosis. The epithelial component can show squamoid features {173}.

Diagnostic molecular pathology

Not relevant

Essential and desirable diagnostic criteria

Essential: a combined salivary gland tumour with malignant epithelial and mesenchymal components; exclusion of sarcomatoid subtypes of other salivary gland malignancies.

Staging

Staging follows the eighth edition of the Union for International Cancer Control (UICC) / American Joint Committee on Cancer (AJCC) TNM staging system.

Prognosis and prediction

The prognosis is poor, with a high frequency of local recurrence and lymphatic and haematogenous spread. The largest series showed a mortality rate of 50% and a mean survival time of 3.6 years {4222,1611}. Most cases have been reported as case reports with insufficient clinical follow-up {1769,4198,3508}.

Sebaceous adenocarcinoma

Gnepp DR
Altemani AM
Layfield LJ
Vazmitsel M

Definition

Sebaceous adenocarcinoma is a malignant tumour arising in salivary gland composed mainly of neoplastic sebaceous cells.

ICD-O coding

8410/3 Sebaceous adenocarcinoma

ICD-11 coding

2B67.Y & XH4VR2 Other specified malignant neoplasms of parotid gland & Sebaceous carcinoma

2B68.2 & XH4VR2 Malignant neoplasms of submandibular or sublingual gland & Sebaceous carcinoma

2B66.Y & XH4VR2 Other specified malignant neoplasms of other or unspecified parts of mouth & Sebaceous carcinoma

Related terminology

Acceptable: sebaceous carcinoma.

Subtype(s)

None

Localization

Most (~70%) arise in the parotid gland, but they may occur in the sublingual, submandibular {1613,4158}, or minor glands {2064}.

Clinical features

Patients present with painful masses, varying degrees of facial nerve paralysis, and occasional skin fixation. Rare patients present with tumour metastasis (head/neck or lung) or a non-tender mass {1613}.

Epidemiology

Sebaceous adenocarcinoma is rare and shows two peak incidences, in the third and seventh/eighth decades of life (age range: 6–93 years) {1613,4332}. There is a slight female predominance {4158}. Rare cases are associated with Muir–Torre syndrome {3174,4158}.

Etiology

Sebaceous adenocarcinoma associated with Muir–Torre syndrome (MIM number: 158320) shows microsatellite instability and loss of expression of the DNA mismatch repair genes *MLH1*, *MSH2*, and *MSH6*; these findings are not usually seen in sporadic sebaceous adenocarcinoma {3174,4199,2337,4158,3874}.

Pathogenesis

Unknown

Macroscopic appearance

Tumours range in size from 6 to 95 mm and are frequently well circumscribed or partially encapsulated, with pushing or locally infiltrating margins. Cut surfaces are yellow, tan-white, grey-white, white, or pale pink {1613}.

Histopathology

The tumours are composed of multiple invasive, variably sized nests and/or sheets of cells with hyperchromatic nuclei, abundant clear vacuolated to eosinophilic cytoplasm (sebocytes), and mild to marked cellular pleomorphism. Necrosis is frequent. Perineural invasion is noted in about 20% of cases; vascular

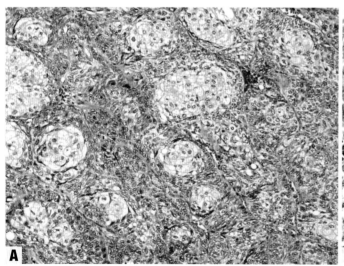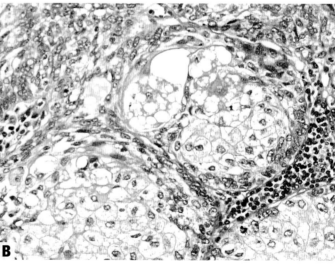

Fig. 4.102 Sebaceous adenocarcinoma. **A** Locally infiltrating, closely packed tumour nests with prominent sebaceous differentiation, surrounded by peripheral basal cells with mild to moderate cytological atypia. **B** Several tumour nests with prominent central sebaceous differentiation, composed of large, moderately pleomorphic, vacuolated cells with an area of holocrine secretion (centre); nuclei are pleomorphic. These cells are surrounded by atypical basal cells. A few infiltrating lymphocytes are noted.

invasion is rare. Oncocytes and foreign body giant cells are rare {1613}. A lymphocytic infiltrate is commonly present.

Immunohistochemistry
Sebaceous/basal epithelial cells are positive for CK5/6, CK7, CK14, and EMA {206}; sebocytes are positive for CD15, lactoferrin, GCDFP-2, and adipophilin {4158}.

Differential diagnosis
The differential diagnosis includes other salivary carcinomas with dense lymphoid reaction and sebaceous differentiation {279}.

Cytology
In a background of plentiful mature lymphocytes, small epithelial tissue fragments are present, consisting of large cells resembling sebaceous cells, with abundant finely to coarsely vacuolated cytoplasm and (usually) bland round nuclei with single conspicuous nucleoli. There is a second population of basaloid cells. There are some reports of sebaceous cells showing malignant nuclei {974}, but others report that the adenocarcinoma shows similar features to sebaceous adenoma {974,4610}.

Diagnostic molecular pathology
Loss of MSH2 expression is uncommon and may characterize tumours in Muir–Torre syndrome {3174,4158}.

Essential and desirable diagnostic criteria
Essential: an invasive salivary gland malignancy; neoplastic sebaceous cells of varying maturity.
Desirable: tumour necrosis.

Staging
Staging follows the eighth edition of the Union for International Cancer Control (UICC) / American Joint Committee on Cancer (AJCC) TNM staging system.

Prognosis and prediction
Tumours may recur and (rarely) metastasize. The 5-year overall survival rate is 62%, lower than that of sebaceous adenocarcinoma of the skin or orbit (84.5%) {1613}. Oral tumours may have a better prognosis with short-term follow-up {88}.

Lymphoepithelial carcinoma

Seethala R
Nagao T
Thompson LDR
Wenig BM
Whaley RD

Definition

Lymphoepithelial carcinoma (LEC) is a morphologically undifferentiated carcinoma with an associated prominent, non-neoplastic lymphoplasmacytic cell infiltrate.

ICD-O coding

8082/3 Lymphoepithelial carcinoma

ICD-11 coding

2B67.Y & XH1E40 Other specified malignant neoplasms of parotid gland & Lymphoepithelial carcinoma
2B68.2 & XH1E40 Other specified malignant neoplasms of submandibular or sublingual glands & Lymphoepithelial carcinoma

Related terminology

None

Subtype(s)

None

Localization

The majority (> 90%) of LECs arise in the major salivary glands, with the parotid gland predominating (> 75%) {5005,4802,4702, 4439}, as well in the larynx (see *Lymphoepithelial carcinoma of the larynx*, p. 153) and sinonasal cavities (see *Sinonasal lymphoepithelial carcinoma*, p. 71).

Clinical features

Patients present with a mass of varying duration; pain (occurring in ~5% of cases) and nerve findings (~2.5%) are rare {4014, 2416,4689}. Cervical lymphadenopathy is noted in about 17% of cases. Most patients show evidence of EBV infection (i.e. IgA antibodies to VCA), which occasionally precedes actual tumour presentation {2466,3896}.

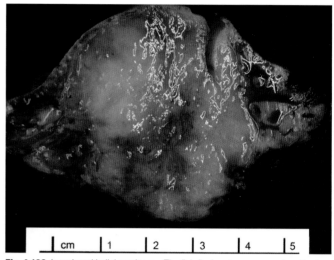

Fig. 4.103 Lymphoepithelial carcinoma. The fish-flesh cut appearance is quite characteristic of lymphoepithelial carcinoma in the salivary glands.

Imaging

CT and MRI may show a homogeneous, enhancing soft tissue lesion with a lobulated shape and relatively well defined margins. However, as many as 50% may be heterogeneous, particularly those that have metastasized to intraglandular or extraglandular lymph nodes {4710}.

Epidemiology

In some ethnic groups (in particular, in Inuit, southern Chinese, Japanese, northern African, and Mongolian populations) {90,1750, 2574,4503,3127,4014}, LEC accounts for 3.6–92% of malignant tumours, but in non-endemic regions it represents only 0.3–0.7% of malignancies {2122,5005}. It affects a wide age range (median: 46 years; patients in non-endemic regions tend to be a decade older). No sex predilection is noted {1525,3869,2812,4013,5005}.

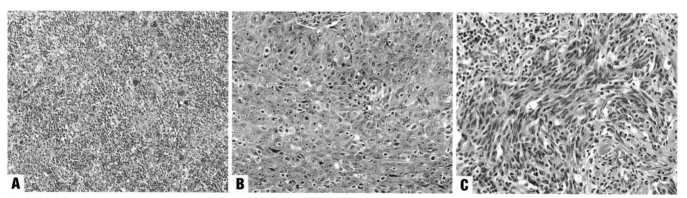

Fig. 4.104 Salivary lymphoepithelial carcinoma. **A** The almost-1:1 ratio of neoplastic epithelial cells to lymphoid cells may make identification of the neoplastic elements challenging. Isolated multinucleated tumour giant cells are seen. **B** The neoplastic cells are arranged in a syncytium, showing large round nuclei with prominent nucleoli and nuclear chromatin clearing. **C** Tumour cell spindling may occasionally be the dominant finding in lymphoepithelial carcinomas.

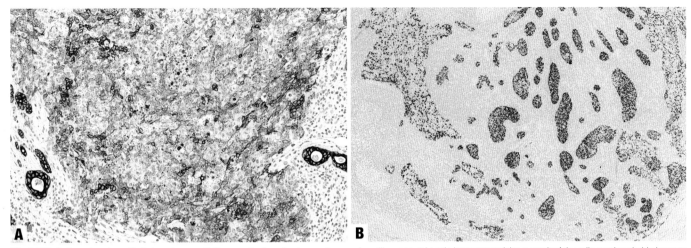

Fig. 4.105 Salivary lymphoepithelial carcinoma. **A** The neoplastic cells show a sieve- or lace-like pancytokeratin immunoreactivity, a result of the adjacent lymphoid elements compressing the cytoplasm (AE1/AE3). **B** All of the neoplastic cell nuclei demonstrate a strong and diffuse reaction for EBER in situ hybridization, a characteristic finding of this neoplasm.

Etiology
EBV infection is the major etiological factor and is more frequent in endemic populations.

Pathogenesis
EBV-related LEC pathogenesis in the salivary gland is presumed {90,2466,1750,2389,251,1525,743,1749,3127,2416,2812,2611}. HIV infection imparts an increased risk {4013}. Some cases arise in the setting of lymphoepithelial sialadenitis {785,3925}.

Macroscopic appearance
Tumours are unencapsulated, with a lobulated, firm, tan-white cut surface, and vary from well demarcated to infiltrative {3869, 4779,5005,4439}.

Histopathology
The histological features of LEC are essentially identical to those of non-keratinizing nasopharyngeal carcinoma; namely, nests of large anaplastic carcinoma cells within a lymphoid stroma. A basaloid morphology has been described, showing a sclerotic stroma, limited lymphoid tissue, and angulated cord or syringoma-like nests {1474}. The adjacent parenchyma often shows lymphoepithelial sialadenitis {2812,3925,4779}.

Differential diagnosis
LEC must be distinguished from large cell undifferentiated carcinoma and from metastasis from the nasopharynx {4779}.

Cytology
Cellular smears show syncytial tissue fragments comprising markedly atypical undifferentiated epithelial cells and spindle cells with high-grade vesicular nuclei and prominent nucleoli in a lymphoplasmacytic background, which may largely obscure the epithelial component, along with necrosis. The features raise a differential diagnosis of high-grade mucoepidermoid carcinoma, sinonasal LEC, or non-keratinizing nasopharyngeal carcinoma {3869,1870}.

Diagnostic molecular pathology
In situ hybridization for EBV-encoded small RNA (EBER) establishes EBV status.

Essential and desirable diagnostic criteria
Essential: a salivary gland malignancy of undifferentiated morphology with lymphoid stroma; exclusion of other tumours with associated lymphoid proliferation; exclusion of metastasis.
Desirable: EBER positivity.

Staging
Staging follows the eighth edition of the Union for International Cancer Control (UICC) / American Joint Committee on Cancer (AJCC) TNM staging system.

Prognosis and prediction
The 5-year survival rate is about 81% {11,4014,4689,2611,4779, 5005}. Nodal disease is present in about 17%; distant metastases are uncommon (~6%) {2466,536,367,4689,3869,2611, 5005} but are more frequent in endemic areas {5005}. This is a key prognosticator.

Squamous cell carcinoma

Wenig BM
Bishop JA
Chiosea S

Definition
Primary salivary gland squamous cell carcinoma (SCC) is a malignant epithelial neoplasm with exclusive squamous differentiation. The diagnosis can only be established after the exclusion of metastatic SCC.

ICD-O coding
8070/3 Squamous cell carcinoma, NOS

ICD-11 coding
2B67.1 Squamous cell carcinoma of parotid gland
2B68.1 Squamous cell carcinoma of submandibular or sublingual gland

Related terminology
None

Subtype(s)
None

Localization
Approximately 80% of cases occur in the parotid gland, with the remainder primarily in the submandibular gland {4018,2968}.

Clinical features
Patient presentations include a mass (with or without pain) and facial nerve palsy {1554}.

Epidemiology
Primary salivary SCC is very rare {2968}. The majority of reported cases of salivary SCC are cutaneous SCC with secondary invasion or metastasis to the salivary gland {4190, 1554,2844,1420,4937,792,2968}. SCC is more common in men than in women, and it occurs mostly in the seventh to eighth decades of life.

Etiology
Radiotherapy is associated with an increased risk of developing SCC {4191,4018}, with a median time to development of 15.5 years {4191} (range: 7–32 years {3922}). SCC may arise independently of prior radiotherapy {1554}.

Pathogenesis
Work done on mouse models has demonstrated that mice with increased WNT/β-catenin signalling developed rapidly growing, aggressive salivary gland SCC {4935}.

Macroscopic appearance
Most tumours are firm and infiltrative.

Histopathology
SCC is an infiltrating well- to moderately differentiated carcinoma with associated desmoplasia. Intracellular keratin, keratin pearl formation, and intercellular bridges are seen. Less often, the tumour is poorly differentiated and may include spindle-shaped (sarcomatoid) cells. Acantholytic (adenoid) features may uncommonly be present. Invasion includes infiltration of salivary gland parenchyma, infiltration of extraglandular fibroconnective tissues, neurotropism, lymphovascular invasion, and/or osseous invasion. Direct invasion and/or metastasis to intraparotid lymph nodes may be present. Salivary duct changes may include squamous metaplasia and/or dysplasia, and transition from

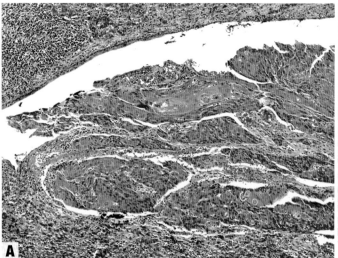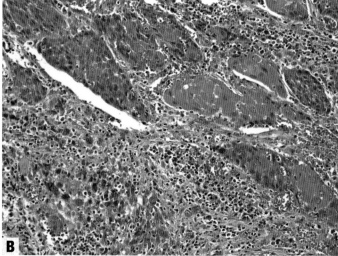

Fig. 4.106 Squamous cell carcinoma, primary in parotid gland. **A** Invasive keratinizing squamous cell carcinoma protruding into a salivary duct. Residual intact attenuated epithelial cells line the duct superior to the carcinoma. **B** Invasive squamous cell carcinoma comprising an admixture of well-, moderately, and poorly differentiated carcinoma.

normal to dysplastic duct epithelium (sialodochodysplasia) and to SCC may occasionally be identified.

Immunohistochemistry
SCCs are immunoreactive for cytokeratins and p63/p40 and are negative for AR, S100, mammaglobin, and DOG1. SCCs may overexpress p16 but are negative for high-risk HPV RNA.

Differential diagnosis
Primary SCC must be distinguished from metastases (cutaneous or mucosal), as well as from high-grade transformation of adenoid cystic carcinoma with squamoid pattern {3957}. A lack of mucous and intermediate cells and the presence of keratinization are most helpful in differentiating SCC from a mucoepidermoid carcinoma {805}.

Cytology
Smears vary depending on the degree of keratinization. Keratinized SCCs show cohesive tissue fragments and dispersed spindle, polygonal, and tadpole cells showing varying degrees of keratinization with dense light-blue (Giemsa stain) or orangeophilic (Pap) well-defined cytoplasm. Nuclei can show pyknosis in the keratinized cells, or larger central nuclei with coarse chromatin and prominent nucleoli. Keratinous debris can be prominent in the background. Poorly keratinizing carcinomas show predominantly large sheets and tissue fragments consisting of cells with well-defined dense but non-keratinized cytoplasm, large central pleomorphic nuclei with coarse chromatin, and one or more large and pleomorphic nucleoli. Necrosis may be present in the background. Primary SCC in the salivary gland cannot be distinguished on FNAB, core needle biopsy, or even excision from a metastatic tumour. The clinical history is crucially important, and the presence of prominent lymphoid material intermingled with the carcinoma may suggest a metastasis.

Diagnostic molecular pathology
Not clinically relevant

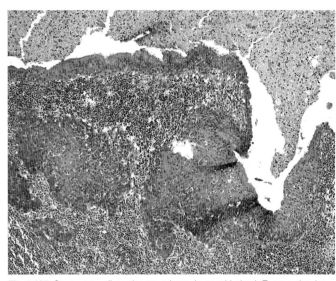

Fig. 4.107 Squamous cell carcinoma, primary in parotid gland. Tumour showing a salivary duct lined in part by (normal) respiratory epithelial cells transitioning to squamous cell carcinoma, the latter infiltrative (centre left). Note the area of squamous metaplasia of the duct epithelium (lower right).

Essential and desirable diagnostic criteria
Essential: a primary salivary gland malignancy with exclusively squamous differentiation; no history of another primary SCC.
Desirable: presence of salivary duct dysplasia.

Staging
Staging follows the eighth edition of the Union for International Cancer Control (UICC) / American Joint Committee on Cancer (AJCC) TNM staging system.

Prognosis and prediction
The prognosis and predictive factors are unknown due to rarity. An overall survival rate of 50% at 5 years {1554} and a median disease-free survival time of 13 months were reported {2968}.

Sialoblastoma

Katabi N
Cohen MC
Perez-Atayde AR

Definition
Sialoblastoma is a low-grade malignant primitive salivary gland anlage neoplasm.

ICD-O coding
8974/1 Sialoblastoma

ICD-11 coding
2B67.Z Malignant neoplasms of parotid gland, unspecified
2B68.Z Malignant neoplasms of submandibular or sublingual glands, unspecified
2B67.Y & XH0G00 Other specified malignant neoplasms of parotid gland & Sialoblastoma

Related terminology
Not recommended: embryoma; basaloid adenocarcinoma; congenital basal cell adenoma; congenital hybrid basal cell adenoma; adenoid cystic carcinoma.

Subtype(s)
None

Localization
The majority (two thirds) of tumours arise in the parotid gland, followed by the submandibular gland; there are only rare reports of tumours in the minor salivary glands {3395,4028,865,4098, 1117}.

Clinical features
Patients present with painless facial swelling; rare cases show nerve involvement or skin ulceration {29,558,1947,4375,865}. Other tumours (naevi and hepatoblastoma) may be coexistent {4167,1685,3349,3942}. Elevated serum AFP has been reported {3349}.

Imaging
This lesion is usually diagnosed in the neonatal period but is occasionally seen on antenatal imaging. MRI may show a mass, hypointense to brain on T1-weighted images and mildly hyperintense on T2-weighted images, containing foci of haemorrhage and necrosis. Heterogeneous, weak postcontrast enhancement is described, as is invasion of adjacent structures including bone and muscle {4930,3388}.

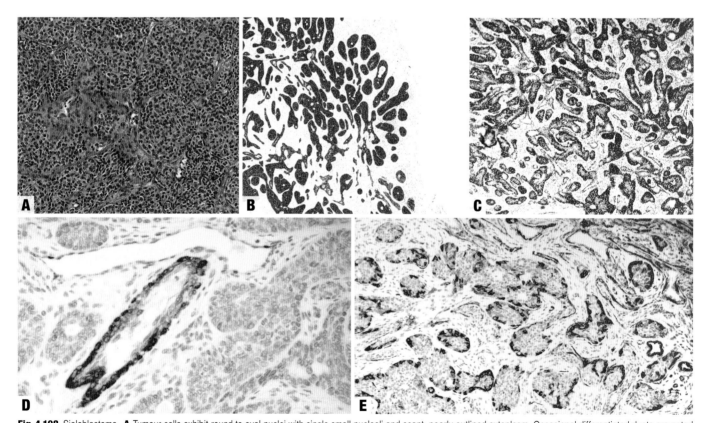

Fig. 4.108 Sialoblastoma. **A** Tumour cells exhibit round to oval nuclei with single small nucleoli and scant, poorly outlined cytoplasm. Occasional differentiated ducts are noted within the tumour nests. **B** CK7 shows strong immunoreactivity in the basaloid nests and ducts. The myoepithelial differentiation is highlighted by p63 (**C**), calponin (**D**), and SMA (**E**).

Epidemiology

The vast majority of tumours are identified at birth or within the first few months of life, with only rare reports in adults. There is no sex predilection {865,4712}.

Etiology

None

Pathogenesis

The tumour may originate from retained blastema cells rather than basal reserve cells {4098}.

Macroscopic appearance

Tumours are lobulated, well defined, and encapsulated, or they may show infiltration to the surrounding tissue. The cut surface is usually grey or yellow and solid. Tumours range from 15 mm to 150 mm in size. Focal haemorrhage or necrosis may be present {4075,4381,3769}.

Histopathology

Sialoblastoma typically exhibits solid organoid nests composed of primitive basaloid epithelial cells, separated by dense fibrous stroma. Tumour cells have indistinct cell borders, scant cytoplasm, a high N:C ratio, and round to oval vesicular nuclei with occasional nucleoli. In addition, differentiated budding ducts lined by cuboidal to columnar epithelium with intraluminal basophilic secretions or a cribriform pattern may be present. Peripheral nuclear palisading is occasionally present. Tumour cells may exhibit apoptosis, necrosis, and nuclear pleomorphism, with increased mitoses. Sialoblastoma is not graded.

Immunohistochemistry

Tumours are reactive for SOX10, p63, and β-catenin, and variably reactive with cytokeratins (including CK5/6, CK7, and CK19), S100, SMA, KIT (CD117), and calponin {2604}.

Differential diagnosis

The primitive histological features and the patients' young age help to differentiate sialoblastoma from other basaloid salivary gland tumours such as basal cell adenoma/adenocarcinoma, adenoid cystic carcinoma, and adamantinoma-like Ewing sarcoma {3323,4631,1932,4712,3746,2604}.

Cytology

Highly cellular smears show cohesive tissue fragments of basaloid cells with scant cytoplasm, round to oval vesicular nuclei, and occasional inconspicuous nucleoli, and they may contain ductal cells and dense, metachromatic, magenta hyaline globular material with smooth, rounded outlines. The features raise a differential diagnosis with basal cell adenoma, adenoid cystic carcinoma, and cellular pleomorphic adenoma {1947,2210}. FNAB in paediatric patients requires careful planning.

Diagnostic molecular pathology

Not relevant

Essential and desirable diagnostic criteria

Essential: a salivary gland malignancy showing primitive solid organoid nests; basaloid epithelial cells with vesicular chromatin; cuboidal to columnar ductal cells.
Desirable: dividing fibrous stroma and peripheral palisading.

Staging

Staging follows the eighth edition of the Union for International Cancer Control (UICC) / American Joint Committee on Cancer (AJCC) TNM staging system.

Prognosis and prediction

Local recurrence is seen in about one third of patients, whereas regional and distant metastases are seen in about 15% {2027}. Death from disease is rare {1546,4375,865,2027,4712,1117}. A less aggressive behaviour is suggested for tumours in the submandibular gland than for those at other anatomical sites. Histological features associated with a worse prognosis include tumour necrosis and an increased mitotic count and/or a high Ki-67 proliferation index.

Salivary gland carcinoma NOS

Ihrler S
Bishop JA

Definition
Salivary gland carcinoma NOS represents a heterogeneous spectrum of carcinomas forming epithelial, ductal, and/ or glandular structures, and it is a diagnosis of exclusion, specifically of otherwise-defined salivary gland carcinoma entities.

ICD-O coding
8140/3 Adenocarcinoma, NOS
8290/3 Oncocytic adenocarcinoma
8144/3 Intestinal-type adenocarcinoma

ICD-11 coding
2B67.Z Malignant neoplasms of parotid gland, unspecified
2B68.Z Malignant neoplasms of submandibular or sublingual glands, unspecified
2B60.Z Malignant neoplasms of lip, unspecified
2B65.Z Malignant neoplasms of palate, unspecified
2B66.Z Malignant neoplasms of other or unspecified parts of mouth, unspecified

Related terminology
Not recommended: unclassified adenocarcinoma; ductal adenocarcinoma; (papillary) cystadenocarcinoma.

Subtype(s)
Oncocytic adenocarcinoma; intestinal-type adenocarcinoma

Localization
More than 50% of cases arise in the parotid gland {4188,1441, 496}, and 40% arise in minor glands, most often in the hard palate, buccal mucosa, and lips {1441,4691}.

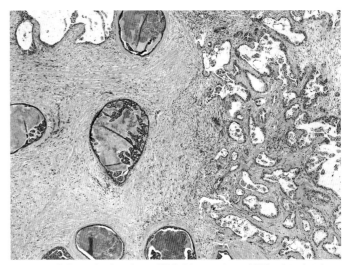

Fig. 4.109 Salivary gland carcinoma NOS. Adenocarcinoma NOS ex intraductal carcinoma. Adjacent to an intercalated duct–type intraductal carcinoma (left), there is a frankly infiltrative tumour (right) comprising irregular glands and micropapillae. Both components harboured *NCOA4::RET*.

Clinical features
Patients with tumours of major glands usually present with asymptomatic, solitary, firm or cystic masses. Occasionally, they may be painful. Tumours in the palate often ulcerate and may erode bony structures {4188}.

Epidemiology
Because of morphogenetic identification of new types of salivary gland adenocarcinoma {3007,484}, the entity adenocarcinoma NOS now accounts for only 5–10% of salivary gland carcinomas

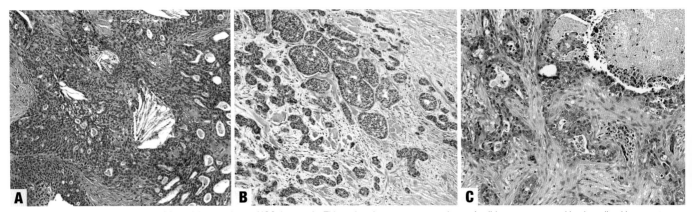

Fig. 4.110 Salivary gland carcinoma NOS. **A** Adenocarcinoma NOS, low-grade. This oral cavity tumour was made up of solid nests punctuated by ducts lined by monotonous round nuclei. It does not conform to any known tumour type and was negative for fusions by RNA sequencing. **B** Adenocarcinoma NOS, intermediate-grade. This submandibular gland tumour consisted of one cell type with monotonous dark nuclei, arranged as infiltrative solid and cribriform nests, cords, and ducts in a myxoid stroma. The tumour was negative for fusions by RNA sequencing. **C** Adenocarcinoma NOS, high-grade. This submandibular gland tumour has irregular ducts lined by pleomorphic cells with necrosis and a high mitotic rate. There are no overtly apocrine features, and AR (not shown) was negative.

{4188,496}. The average patient age is 58 years, with a wide age range {4668,496}. They are extremely rare in children.

Etiology
Unknown

Pathogenesis
Unknown

Macroscopic appearance
Tumours may be partly circumscribed but usually have an irregular and infiltrative appearance. The cut surface is commonly tan or yellow, sometimes with areas of necrosis and haemorrhage.

Histopathology
Tumours display a wide range of ductal or glandular proliferation patterns, with or without a cystic component or necrosis. There is a variety of architectural growth patterns, including small confluent nests or cords, large islands, and (often) associated densely cellular stroma. Tumour cells can be cuboidal, columnar, polygonal, clear, mucinous, oncocytoid, or plasmacytoid. Ductal and glandular structures are predominant in low- and intermediate-grade tumours, but less frequent in high-grade tumours {2614,2005}.

Proof of an intraductal component supports a salivary gland origin {2005}.

Subtypes
These include oncocytic adenocarcinoma {1441,4896} and intestinal-type {409,4139,1589} adenocarcinoma, the latter of which is often positive for CK20 and CDX2.

Immunohistochemistry
Immunohistochemistry is helpful in distinguishing adenocarcinoma NOS from acinic cell carcinoma (NR4A3, DOG1) {2003}, tumours with myoepithelial/basal cell composition (calponin, CK5/6, p63), and metastatic adenocarcinoma (site-specific markers) {3221}.

Differential diagnosis
For the diagnosis of adenocarcinoma NOS to be rendered, other primary carcinoma types must be excluded, including salivary duct carcinoma, mucoepidermoid carcinoma, polymorphous adenocarcinoma, and high-grade transformation of other types of salivary carcinoma {3221}. Tumours with significant mucinous differentiation may be better regarded as mucinous adenocarcinoma.

Cytology
Smears show adenocarcinoma with (usually) high-grade nuclei in a necrotic background, and they lack the features of other salivary gland carcinomas, resulting in a differential diagnosis of metastases from colon and lung. Oncocytic and intestinal types are recognized {4188}.

Diagnostic molecular pathology
Molecular alterations are heterogeneous and not diagnostic {4703}.

Essential and desirable diagnostic criteria
Essential: a salivary gland carcinoma lacking the morphological, immunohistochemical, and molecular features of other salivary carcinomas; exclusion of metastasis is mandatory.

Staging
Staging follows the eighth edition of the Union for International Cancer Control (UICC) / American Joint Committee on Cancer (AJCC) TNM staging system.

Prognosis and prediction
Prognosis is influenced by location, histological grade, and clinical stage {4188,5003}. High-grade adenocarcinoma NOS is an aggressive malignancy. A study showed 15-year survival rates of 54%, 31%, and 3% for low-, intermediate-, and high-grade tumours, respectively {4188}. The survival rate for adenocarcinoma with a significant cystic component is more favourable {1441}. The reports of intestinal-type adenocarcinoma suggest an aggressive behaviour {409,1589}.

Sialolipoma

Ihrler S
Bullerdiek J
Flucke U
Wenig BM

Definition
Sialolipoma is a neoplastic lipomatous proliferation within salivary glands, with an oncocytic (oncocytic lipoadenoma) or non-oncocytic (sialolipoma) epithelial component.

ICD-O coding
8850/0 Sialolipoma
8850/0 Oncocytic lipoadenoma

ICD-11 coding
2E91.0 & XH8P28 Benign neoplasm of parotid gland & Lipoadenoma
2E90.3 & XH8P28 Benign neoplasm of other or unspecified parts of mouth & Lipoadenoma

Related terminology
Acceptable: lipoadenoma.
Not recommended: adenolipoma; oncocytic sialolipoma.

Subtype(s)
Oncocytic lipoadenoma

Localization
Conventional lipomas (see *Lipomas*, p. 461) predominate in parotid glands (≥ 80%), whereas sialolipoma and oncocytic lipoadenoma manifest in minor glands (50%) and in parotid glands (40%) {3134,3234,4206,982}. In the oral cavity, the lower lip and tongue are the most common locations {982}.

Clinical features
Patients typically present with a slow-growing swelling. The salivary gland location is verified by radiological or intraoperative localization and/or by histological demonstration of a rim of salivary parenchyma {3134,45,4206}.

Epidemiology
The mean age at presentation regardless of site is 51.5 years, with an equal sex distribution {2054}. In minor salivary gland cases, the mean age of 10 patients was 46.1 years (range: 11–71 years) and the M:F ratio was 1:2.3 {982}.

Etiology
Unknown

Pathogenesis
Unknown

Macroscopic appearance
Sialolipomas are well-circumscribed tumours measuring 30–40 mm on average.

Histopathology
Combined lipoepithelial salivary gland lesions comprise a spectrum of morphological subtypes from sialolipoma to oncocytic lipoadenoma. Sialolipoma combines lobules of salivary parenchyma with dominating and evenly interspersed adipose tissue. The salivary parenchyma rarely shows focal sebaceous differentiation and is usually devoid of oncocytic epithelium. The term "sialolipoma" indicates that the adipocytic component is regarded as neoplastic {3134,3234,45,982}.

Subtype
The rare oncocytic lipoadenoma subtype typically demonstrates a predominance of epithelial elements with a varying oncocytic component, reminiscent of oncocytoma. A minor sebaceous component may occur. The term "oncocytic lipoadenoma" indicates that the oncocytic/epithelial component is regarded as neoplastic {45}.

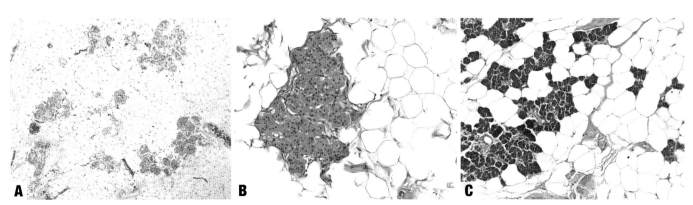

Fig. 4.111 Sialolipoma. **A** Isolated salivary gland elements are seen within a predominantly adipocytic proliferation. **B** Oncocytic lipoadenoma. The tumour consists of salivary gland lobules with oncocytic features and mature adipose tissue. **C** Sialolipoma of the parotid gland. Isolated salivary gland elements are seen within a predominantly adipocytic proliferation. In all three tumours, a well-developed capsule was seen around the periphery.

Differential diagnosis

The entities include extrasalivary lipomatous tumours (see Chapter 9: *Soft tissue tumours*) and epithelial salivary tumours with lipomatous metaplasia, especially pleomorphic adenoma / myoepithelioma {4122}, and a fatty replacement (lipomatosis) in atrophic salivary parenchyma secondary to chronic inflammation or old age {3134,45}.

Cytology

Cytological preparations may show mature adipocytic and salivary epithelial elements in varying proportions.

Diagnostic molecular pathology

Not relevant

Essential and desirable diagnostic criteria

Essential: a lipoma with benign salivary epithelial components.

Staging

None

Prognosis and prediction

There are no reported recurrences. All types are cured by excision.

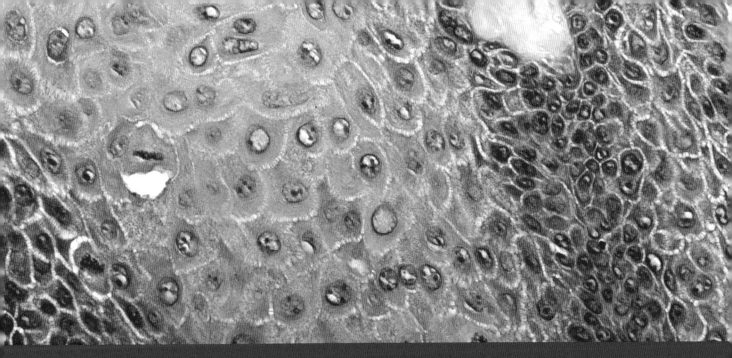

5

Oral cavity and mobile tongue tumours

Edited by: Muller S, Odell EW, Tilakaratne WM

Oral cavity and mobile tongue tumours: Introduction

Muller S
Tilakaratne WM

The classification of oral cavity and mobile tongue tumours in this fifth edition volume shares similarities with that in the previous edition, but the classification of oral mucosal diseases continues to be refined as molecular discoveries and immunohistochemical advances evolve.

This chapter now includes a dedicated group of sections on non-neoplastic lesions. Necrotizing sialometaplasia is included, chiefly to highlight the clinical and histological features of this reactive, self-limiting entity, because it may mimic squamous cell and salivary gland carcinomas {675}. The condition forms an ulcerative mass lesion almost exclusively in the oral cavity, so it is covered here rather than with salivary gland tumours. Multifocal epithelial hyperplasia has been moved to this section in view of its clinical behaviour of spontaneous regression {3986}. Melanoacanthoma is another new entity in this edition because the clinical and histological presentation needs to be distinguished from oral mucosal melanoma {659}.

The sections on epithelial tumours are organized by tumour behaviour, with squamous cell carcinoma discussed last. Oral potentially malignant disorders (OPMDs) and oral epithelial dysplasia (OED) have been expanded to reflect advances in clinical, histological, and molecular findings. Dysplasia grading of OED continues to be contentious, with different grading applied in different regions of the world. The criteria for grading OED have been updated and include additional architectural features that alone may confer a diagnosis of dysplasia {3109,4847,3265}. A three-tiered grading system of OED is maintained, with the acknowledgement that defining dysplasia in this manner oversimplifies the inherent difficulties of grading.

The clinical and histological features of proliferative verrucous leukoplakia (PVL) have been better defined and updated since the last edition {4427}. The subtle histological features of early PVL (which may easily be overlooked) are presented, along with the panoply of histological findings at all stages of PVL. A section on oral submucous fibrosis has been added, with a description of histology and clinical significance, because it is such an important OPMD in some parts of the world. Three conditions have been removed from the table of OPMDs. *Candida* infection is frequent in dysplastic epithelium, and infection

is more frequent with higher grade, but no good evidence has emerged that *Candida* is an independent risk factor for malignant transformation. Syphilis remains endemic in many regions of the world {2360}, but syphilitic leukoplakia in tertiary syphilis appears extremely rare. A risk of oral carcinoma in syphilis has remained {2986}, but syphilitic leukoplakia appears to have all but disappeared. Its status as an OPMD was considered to be largely of historical interest in the 2005 edition and so it has been removed from the list of OPMDs. Actinic keratosis is the key condition predisposing patients to lip vermilion squamous carcinoma. It was included in previous editions primarily because ICD coding groups the lip and oral cavity together. However, its etiology is distinct, and anatomically the condition is extraoral. It has therefore been removed from the list of OPMDs, although its significance in cutaneous lip cancer is not in dispute.

Because of improvements in characterization, and for consistency with classification at other body sites, HPV-associated OED has been classified as a separate entity from conventional OED {2273}. Despite strong p16 immunoexpression in HPV-associated OED, there are insufficient data to recommend this as a surrogate marker for HPV infection in the oral cavity {1051}.

Both carcinoma cuniculatum and verrucous carcinoma are described separately from conventional oral squamous cell carcinoma on the basis of their distinctive presentation, histopathological appearance, and behaviour. The oral cavity is the most common location in the head and neck for both these entities {2348,1335}.

Under tumours of uncertain histogenesis, ectomesenchymal chondromyxoid tumour has been updated since the previous edition to reflect the molecular findings of a *RREB1::MRTFB* fusion in 90% of cases {1128}. The anterior dorsal tongue is still the most prevalent site, but additional cases have been identified in the palate and mandible.

The previous edition included various soft tissue neoplasms in this chapter that are now included in the chapter on soft tissue tumours. Oral melanoma now appears in the chapter on melanocytic tumours, and intraoral salivary gland lesions are included in the chapter on salivary gland tumours.

Necrotizing sialometaplasia

Slootweg PJ
Aguirre A

Definition
Necrotizing sialometaplasia is a reactive, self-limiting, inflammatory condition of the salivary glands, usually resulting in necrosis or degeneration of salivary acini, and ductal squamous metaplasia.

ICD-O coding
None

ICD-11 coding
DA04 Diseases of salivary glands

Related terminology
Not recommended: adenometaplasia.

Subtype(s)
None

Localization
The most common location is the posterolateral hard palate, but it can occur in other minor salivary sites, including the tongue, oral floor, lacrimal glands, upper airway, proximal oesophagus, trachea, and bronchi {568,18,4780,3360,1110,574,1644}. Major salivary gland involvement is rare.

Clinical features
The classic palatal presentation is a single lateral ulcer near the junction of the hard and soft palate. Bilateral or metachronous lesions may rarely occur. Swelling is typical and may precede the development of a crater-like ulcer ranging in size from 10 to 15 mm, which clinically can mimic a malignancy {5046}. Most cases are asymptomatic; a burning sensation, mild pain, or numbness is occasionally identified {568}.

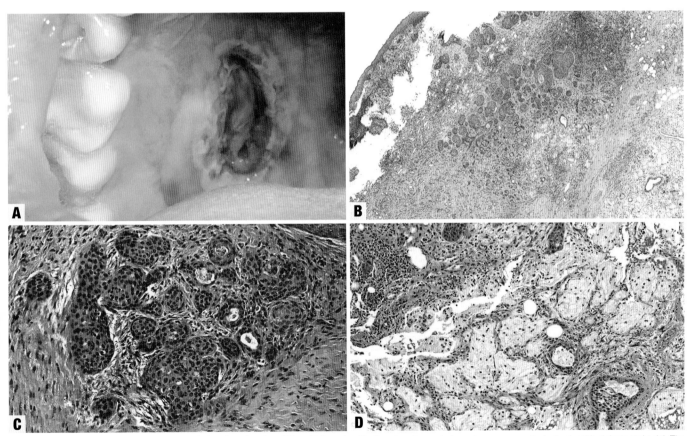

Fig. 5.01 Necrotizing sialometaplasia. **A** Palatal ulcer lateral to the midline. **B** Pseudoepitheliomatous hyperplasia and squamous metaplasia of residual ducts and acini. The lobular architecture of the glands is preserved, with the outlines of the necrosed residual acini. Inflammation is also present. **C** The lobular architecture of the minor salivary glands is preserved and also involves ducts. Smooth contours and regenerative atypia of the lobules is evident among a reactive myxocollagenous stroma. **D** Necrosis of acini (with loss of nuclei and cell borders) with squamous metaplasia. Lobular configuration is maintained.

Epidemiology

Necrotizing sialometaplasia typically presents in the fourth decade of life, with a male predilection {568}.

Etiology

The etiology of necrotizing sialometaplasia is uncertain, but it is probably associated with trauma, vascular compromise, and/or hypoxia {124}.

Pathogenesis

The pathogenesis involves vascular compromise leading to ischaemic infarction of seromucous glands and subsequent regeneration {290}.

Macroscopic appearance

Necrotizing sialometaplasia appears as an ulcer 10–15 mm in diameter {568}.

Histopathology

Pre-existing salivary lobular architecture is usually preserved {675}. Early lesions display acinar infarction/necrosis accompanied by mucus spillage. Ulceration varies. As lesions mature, involved ducts and acini undergo squamous metaplasia. Generally, cytological features remain bland, but keratinocytic regenerative atypia with mitotic activity may be present. Remnants of ductal cells, interspersed mucocytes, granulation reaction, and stromal subacute inflammation may comingle.

Recognition is most challenging when lobular preservation is poor, or when pseudoepitheliomatous hyperplasia of the intact overlying mucosa merges with ductal squamous metaplasia, simulating squamous carcinoma {20,675}. Differential diagnosis should include subacute necrotizing sialadenitis {1444,4299}.

Cytology

Not relevant

Diagnostic molecular pathology

Not relevant

Essential and desirable diagnostic criteria

Essential: preservation of a lobular architecture with squamous metaplasia of ducts and acini.
Desirable: infarction/necrosis of acini; pseudoepitheliomatous hyperplasia.

Staging

Not relevant

Prognosis and prediction

Necrotizing sialometaplasia heals spontaneously in 6–10 weeks, but healing may take as long as 6 months. Close follow-up is needed to ensure proper healing. If healing does not occur, or if the lesion recurs, repeat biopsy is indicated to rule out neoplasia or vasculopathy {20,2178}.

Multifocal epithelial hyperplasia

Carlos R
Mainville GN
Mosqueda-Taylor AA

Definition

Multifocal epithelial hyperplasia (MEH) is a benign squamous epithelial proliferation caused by HPV.

ICD-O coding

None

ICD-11 coding

1E82.0 Focal epithelial hyperplasia of the oral mucous membranes

Related terminology

Acceptable: Heck disease.
Not recommended: focal epithelial hyperplasia.

Subtype(s)

None

Localization

The lesions predominantly affect the borders and tip of the tongue, the buccal mucosa along the occlusal plane, and the lips. The lower labial mucosa is more frequently affected than the upper labial mucosa. When lesions involve the mucosal lip vermilion, they do not extend to perioral skin. The keratinized hard palate and gingiva, floor of the mouth, and the soft palate are rarely affected {3807}.

Clinical features

Patients with MEH usually present with multiple painless, sessile, smooth-surfaced papules that are similar in colour to adjacent mucosa (papulonodular presentation). Early lesions can grow to 10 mm in diameter. They can coalesce to form cobblestone plaques with increased keratinization. In the uncommon papillomatous presentation, the papules have a rough, pebbly surface {3807}. Individual lesions are well demarcated and tend to flatten when the mucosa is extended, a helpful distinguishing feature.

Epidemiology

MEH is not limited to specific ethnic groups or geographical regions. It occurs in children and adolescents, but it has not been reported in patients aged < 2 years. Adults are infrequently affected. An M:F ratio of 3:4 is reported. Household transmission is common {3986}.

Etiology

MEH is caused predominantly by HPV subtypes 13 and 32, although other genotypes have also been detected {3986}. PCR and DNA or RNA in situ hybridization for HPV13 and HPV32 is positive {3807,3936}.

Risk factors

Low socioeconomic status, malnutrition, and overcrowded living conditions are significant contributing factors {3986} that could explain the striking epidemiological differences between high-income and low- and middle-income countries. Household spread of HPV13 through saliva and through the sharing of contaminated objects has been reported {2716}. Medical conditions that lead to immunosuppression are also associated with MEH. The condition is not considered to be transmitted during vaginal birth or sexually, because HPV13 and HPV32 have not been reported in the genital mucosa to date {3807}.

Genetic factors

HLA-DR4 (DRB1*0404) has been associated with genetic susceptibility to the disease {1541,3257}.

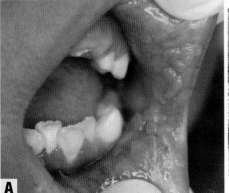 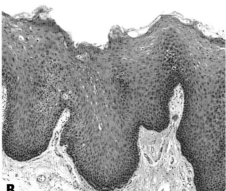 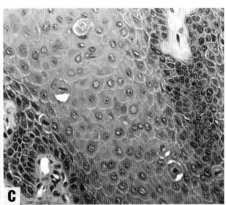

Fig. 5.02 Multifocal epithelial hyperplasia. **A** Multiple coalescing papules on the retrocommissural mucosa in an 8-year-old boy. **B** Acanthotic epithelium with minimal superficial keratosis. Rete pegs show elongation and widening, with a tendency to coalesce. Cell maturation is well preserved. **C** Characteristic mitosoid bodies representing cytopathic viral nuclear damage.

Pathogenesis

Social conditions play an important role and are probably related to poor nutrition, which in turn leads to cellular immunodeficiency during childhood growth. Infection with HPV13 or HPV32, depending on tissue-site specificity and combination with local trauma, causes multiple papillomas {3257,3807}. Trauma is exacerbated by poor dental status and sharp edges on teeth, explaining the clinical distribution of oral lesions.

Macroscopic appearance

MEH appears macroscopically as thickened epithelium with a cobblestone appearance.

Histopathology

MEH shows prominent exophytic acanthosis, broad and confluent rete ridges, and normal epithelial maturation. A papillary surface architecture is infrequently present. Occasional keratinocytes with fragmented nuclei that may mimic a mitotic figure (mitosoid bodies) are present in the upper epithelium, a viral cytopathic nuclear effect. Occasional koilocytes can be present within the superficial epithelial layers {3807,3986}.

HPV subtypes 13 and 32 do not cause functional inactivation of *RB1*, therefore p16 immunohistochemistry has no diagnostic value.

Cytology

Not clinically relevant {3807,3986}

Diagnostic molecular pathology

Routine detection of HPV in MEH is rarely required {3807}.

Essential and desirable diagnostic criteria

Essential: a sessile or occasionally papilloma-like lesion; cobblestone surface appearance; acanthotic epithelium, with mitosoid bodies in the upper epithelium.

Staging

Not relevant

Prognosis and prediction

Most patients experience spontaneous regression when reaching puberty or with improved living conditions {3986}.

Oral melanoacanthoma

Fitzpatrick SG
Freedman PD

Definition

Oral melanoacanthoma is a non-neoplastic process that is distinct from the neoplastic cutaneous melanoacanthoma. It is characterized by a dual proliferation of epithelial and melanocytic cells with a characteristic clinical profile of rapid initial growth but indolent behaviour.

ICD-O coding

None

ICD-11 coding

2E90.3 Benign neoplasm of other or unspecified parts of mouth

Related terminology

Acceptable: melanoacanthosis.

Subtype(s)

None

Localization

The buccal mucosa is affected in approximately half of all cases, although it may occur on any oral mucosal surface, including the palate, gingiva / alveolar mucosa, labial mucosa, or tongue {594,659}.

Clinical features

Patients with melanoacanthoma present with a rapidly growing, pigmented lesion that is usually smooth but can be slightly raised in appearance {594,1438}. It is most frequently asymptomatic, but mild symptoms such as pain, itching, or burning have been described {1438}. Unifocal lesions are most common, with multifocal lesions occurring in a minority of cases {594,659}.

Epidemiology

Melanoacanthoma occurs most frequently in people with higher natural levels of skin pigmentation. There is a female predominance. It affects patients of all ages, from children to the elderly, with an average age at presentation in the third to fifth decades of life {1438,594,659}.

Etiology

Although the etiology is unknown, multiple reactive factors have been proposed, including chronic trauma and reactions to oral care products such as toothpaste or mouthwash {659}. Oral melanoacanthoma has been rarely reported in association with Laugier–Hunziker syndrome and Addison disease {4982,1026}.

Pathogenesis

Although the pathogenesis is not proven, it is thought that chronic or acute trauma may stimulate melanocyte proliferation in oral melanoacanthoma in as many as 75% of cases {659}.

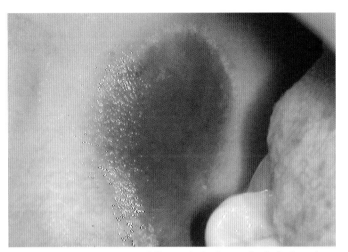

Fig. 5.03 Oral melanoacanthoma. Diffuse melanin pigmentation in the buccal mucosa of rapid onset but otherwise asymptomatic.

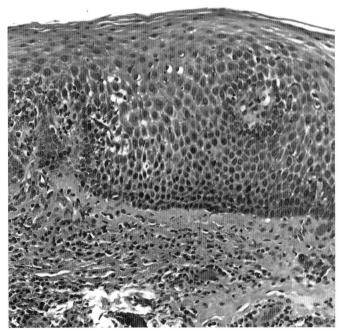

Fig. 5.04 Oral melanoacanthoma of the buccal mucosa. Acanthosis of the epithelium is apparent, along with melanin deposition in the basal layer and dendritic melanocytes within the epithelium.

Macroscopic appearance

Pigmented mucosal tissue

Histopathology

Epithelial and melanocytic proliferation with acanthosis and dendritic melanocytes are present throughout the epithelium.

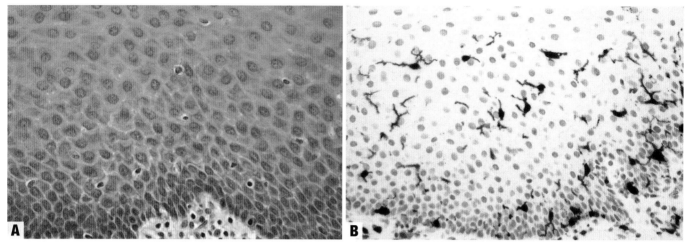

Fig. 5.05 Melanoacanthoma. **A** Dendritic melanocytes within the intercellular spaces of the acanthotic epithelium may be seen, but S100 immunohistochemisty is helpful when they are scarce or lightly pigmented. **B** The dendritic melanocytes are highlighted by S100 immunohistochemisty.

Spongiosis and submucosal chronic inflammatory infiltrate are noted, and exocytosis of lymphocytes may also be seen {1438}. Melanin deposition in the basal layer is frequent. Langerhans cells may also be prominent. Nuclear pleomorphism, hyperchromatism, and nesting of melanocytes are not present {594}. Immunohistochemistry for S100, HMB45, or melan-A highlights dendritic melanocytes {594,1032}. Mucosal melanoma is the most important differential diagnosis {659}.

Cytology
Not clinically relevant

Diagnostic molecular pathology
Not clinically relevant

Essential and desirable diagnostic criteria
Essential: dendritic melanocyte proliferation high in the epithelium; spongiosis; absence of atypia and invasion of melanocytic nests.
Desirable: epithelial acanthosis; melanin deposition in the basal layer.

Staging
Not relevant

Prognosis and prediction
Oral melanoacanthoma frequently regresses after biopsy, even with incomplete removal {94,1438,1032}. Malignant transformation has not been described.

Squamous papilloma

Bradley G
O'Regan EM

Definition
Squamous papilloma is a benign, well-demarcated, exophytic-papillary epithelial neoplasm with finger-like surface projections or a cauliflower-like morphology, usually associated with low-risk or non-oncogenic HPV.

ICD-O coding
8052/0 Squamous papilloma

ICD-11 coding
2E90.3 & XH50T2 Benign neoplasm of other or unspecified parts of mouth & Squamous cell papilloma, NOS

Related terminology
Acceptable: squamous cell papilloma.

Subtype(s)
Condyloma acuminatum; verruca vulgaris

Localization
Any site in the oral cavity may be involved, but the soft and hard palate, tongue, lips, and gingiva are most commonly affected {5,1478}.

Clinical features
Most lesions are < 10 mm in diameter, pedunculated, and white, with a rough, cauliflower-like or finger-like surface. Larger lesions (as large as 20 mm) are rarely seen, but these are still well defined and regular in shape. Sessile lesions are less common and may be pink in colour {5,1478}. Squamous papilloma is usually a solitary, well-defined lesion, and the occurrence of two or more lesions simultaneously is rare {1478}. The clinical differential diagnosis includes verruca vulgaris, condyloma acuminatum, verruciform xanthoma, and giant cell fibroma {437}. Immunocompromised individuals, particularly those with HIV/AIDS, frequently present with multiple or florid lesions that may be difficult to distinguish from condyloma acuminatum and multifocal epithelial hyperplasia. In such cases, lesions with overlapping clinical appearances may be referred to as "benign HPV-associated oral lesions" {648}. Patients on long-term highly active antiretroviral therapy (HAART) also have an increased number of HPV-associated oral lesions {179}.

Epidemiology
Squamous papillomas are common and can occur at any age, from childhood to old age, although they are found most frequently in adults, with a mean age in the fourth to fifth decades of life, and with no sex predilection {5,3595,1478}.

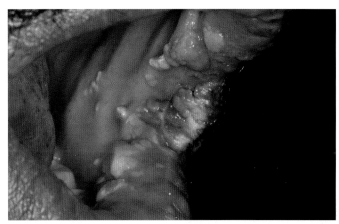

Fig. 5.06 Condyloma acuminatum. Multiple coalescing condylomas in a male patient with HIV.

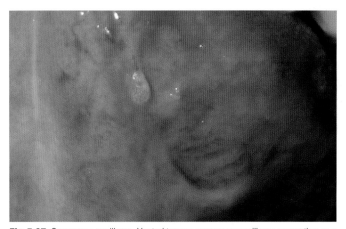

Fig. 5.07 Squamous papilloma. Ventral tongue squamous papilloma presenting as a solitary, white, somewhat sessile lesion with finger-like fronds.

Etiology
HPV is the most important etiological factor, and studies have shown an association with HPV6 and HPV11 {1994}. There is no association with high-risk, carcinogenic HPV types {4153, 4502}. The reported prevalence of low-risk HPV DNA in oral squamous cell papillomas varies considerably, with some of this variability attributed to technical differences, the characteristics of the HPV life cycle, and the presence of non-pathogenic or passenger HPV in the normal oral mucosa in a small percentage of individuals {1478,4350,437}. Studies that used DNA in situ hybridization have identified the presence of HPV DNA in 13–62% of squamous papillomas {5000,4957}. Studies that used the more sensitive technique of PCR showed prevalence rates between 21% and 68% {4731,4502}.

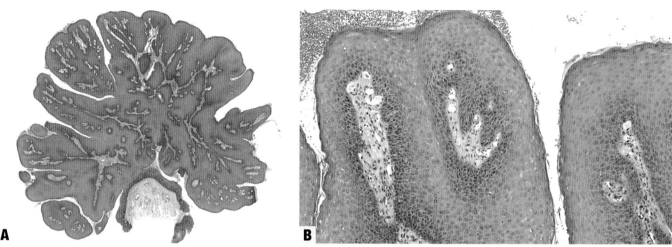

Fig. 5.08 Squamous papilloma. **A** Exophytic, pedunculated, papillary lesion consisting of a thin, branching core of fibrovascular connective tissue covered by hyperplastic stratified squamous parakeratinized epithelium. **B** Papillary projections covered by stratified squamous parakeratinized epithelium with basal cell hyperplasia and orderly maturation.

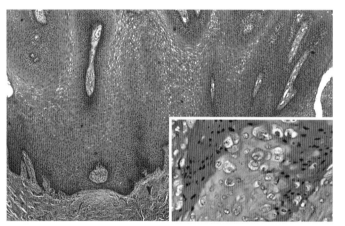

Fig. 5.09 Condyloma acuminatum. Exophytic broad-based proliferation with blunted papillae supported by fibrovascular cores. **Inset:** Koilocytes are characterized by vacuolated keratinocytes with shrunken nuclei.

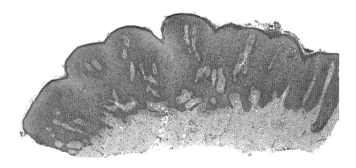

Fig. 5.10 Squamous papilloma. Lacking exophytic papillary projections, sessile papillomas have blunted, rounded papillae. Koilocytes generally are absent. The architecture may be a reflection of frictional forces in the oral cavity.

Pathogenesis

The pathogenesis of squamous papilloma involves HPV-induced proliferation of basal squamous epithelial cells. Immunohistochemistry for low-risk HPV types has yielded variable findings, where 4–41% of cases showed intranuclear staining in the upper epithelial layers {2252}. HPV-negative cases may be

due to a low level of detectable viral antigen expression {1478}. HPV DNA in situ hybridization labels nuclei of both koilocytic and non-koilocytic cells in the upper epithelial layers {5000, 2899}.

Macroscopic appearance

Exophytic, pedunculated, or sessile papillary epithelial projections

Histopathology

Squamous papilloma is an exophytic papillary proliferation of hyperplastic stratified squamous epithelium with a narrow branching core of fibrovascular connective tissue with dilated capillaries {1478,437}. The papillary projections may be pointed or round {1302}. The majority of lesions show parakeratosis, but orthokeratotic or non-keratinized lesions may be seen {5}. The sessile type generally lacks the finger-like projections, imparting a blunted, cauliflower-like appearance. The stratified squamous epithelium shows an orderly maturation, with no signs of dysplasia {2899}. Koilocytes are infrequent in squamous papillomas compared with verruca vulgaris and condyloma acuminatum. Basal cell hyperplasia with mild nuclear atypia and increased mitotic activity may be present but can be attributed to HPV-induced hyperplasia, or trauma or inflammation {5,1478,4237}.

Condyloma acuminatum exhibits an exophytic broad-based growth of acanthotic stratified squamous epithelium with bulbous rete that may interconnect {437}. The papillary fronds are more blunted than squamous papillomas, with invagination of the parakeratin that fills the crypts between the papillae. Koilocytes are usually present in the upper spinous layer.

Verruca vulgaris is uncommon intraorally, and the histological features are identical to cutaneous verruca vulgaris, with a papillary architecture and extensive keratinization {4237,437}. At the periphery of the lesion, the rete ridges are inwardly facing. Coarse keratohyalin granules and koilocytic change in the upper spinous layer are present, but epithelial maturation is maintained.

There can be histological overlap between the benign papillomatous lesions of the oral cavity. Squamous papillomas that are sessile and show koilocytes in the upper spinous layers may be difficult to differentiate from verruca vulgaris and condyloma acuminatum {1301,437}. More importantly, squamous papilloma should be distinguished from dysplastic papillary epithelial proliferations and verrucous dysplastic lesions {2899,437}. Clinical information of an irregular-shaped lesion > 10 mm in size with the histological finding of dysplasia should raise the suspicion of atypical papillary, potentially malignant, lesions arising in the setting of proliferative verrucous leukoplakia.

Cytology
Not relevant

Diagnostic molecular pathology
Not relevant

Essential and desirable diagnostic criteria
Essential: exophytic, pedunculated or sessile, papillary architecture in a benign squamous cell proliferation; epithelial hyperplasia; parakeratosis/orthokeratosis; fibrovascular cores; no evidence of dysplasia.
Desirable: superficial koilocytes; low-risk or non-oncogenic HPV type (in selected cases).

Staging
Not relevant

Prognosis and prediction
Treatment is simple excision, and recurrence is rare {1478, 4470}. Immunocompromised patients may require multiple excisions, cryotherapy, and/or immunomodulatory agents.

Oral potentially malignant disorders

Muller S
Tilakaratne WM

Definition

Oral potentially malignant disorders (OPMDs) constitute a heterogeneous group of clinically defined conditions associated with a variable risk of progression to oral squamous carcinoma. Most produce clinically visible lesions.

ICD-O coding

None

ICD-11 coding

DA01.00 Disturbances of oral epithelium

Related terminology

Acceptable: epithelial precursor lesion.
Not recommended: precancerous lesion; precancerous condition.

Subtype(s)

See Box 5.01.

Localization

OPMDs can involve any intraoral site. Lesions presenting on the lateral/ventral tongue and the floor of the mouth are more closely associated with cancer progression {4847}.

Clinical features

Most high-risk OPMDs form red, white, or speckled lesions. "Leukoplakia" is a clinical term used to describe a white plaque of questionable risk after having excluded other known diseases {4733}. Leukoplakia varies in thickness, and its surface ranges from flat, thin, uniform, and homogeneous in colour, to granular, fissured, nodular, or verrucous, the latter types having a higher risk. Erythroplakia is defined as a red patch that cannot be characterized clinically or pathologically as another definable

Box 5.01 Oral potentially malignant disorders {4733}

Erythroplakia

Erythroleukoplakia

Leukoplakia

Proliferative verrucous leukoplakia

Submucous fibrosis

Palatal lesions associated with reverse smoking

Oral lichenoid lesions[a]

Oral lichen planus

Smokeless tobacco keratosis[b]

Oral graft-versus-host disease

Lupus erythematosus

Familial cancer syndromes including Fanconi anaemia, dyskeratosis congenita, xeroderma pigmentosum, Li–Fraumeni syndrome, Bloom syndrome, ataxia–telangiectasia, and Cowden syndrome

[a]Oral lesions resembling lichen planus but lacking typical clinical or histopathological appearances. [b]Risk varies with tobacco type.

lesion. Erythroplakia is a thin, or slightly depressed, red patch of the oral mucosa and is less common than leukoplakia. Erythroleukoplakia or speckled leukoplakia has both an erythroplakia component and a leukoplakia component. Erythroplakia is much less common than leukoplakia but is much more likely to be associated with high-grade dysplasia or carcinoma (> 90%) {4847,4733}. Diagnosis of the common OPMDs is partly by exclusion and therefore usually requires biopsy.

Epidemiology

Oral leukoplakia is considered to be the most common OPMD, and the mean global prevalence of leukoplakia ranges from 1% to 4%; however a much higher prevalence is reported in south-eastern Asia {2934}. In contrast, erythroplakia is rare, with

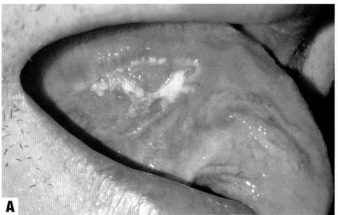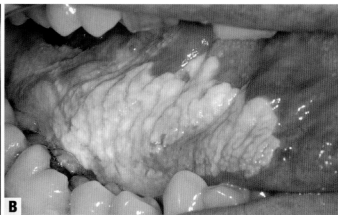

Fig. 5.11 Oral leukoplakia. **A** Depressed lesion on the lateral tongue with light keratosis around the periphery and zones of keratosis within it, together with mucosa with a lightly stippled surface. Biopsy showed moderate dysplasia. **B** Large leukoplakia on the lateral and ventral tongue. Some margins are well defined but fade to normal posteriorly.

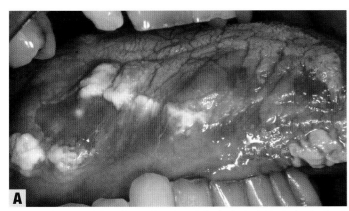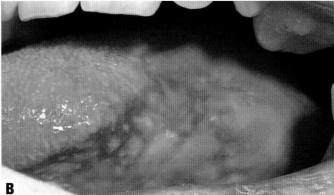

Fig. 5.12 Oral potentially malignant disorders. **A** Erythroleukoplakia. A mixed red and white patch on the lateral tongue. The leukoplakia component is non-homogeneous, with nodular keratotic areas. **B** Erythroplakia. An irregular, flat, fiery-red patch of the lateral tongue. Severe dysplasia was present on biopsy.

a prevalence of < 0.1% {1903}. Leukoplakia is more common in men, but women have a higher risk of malignant transformation {71}. Advanced age is also associated with an increased risk of cancer development. Features of oral submucous fibrosis, proliferative verrucous leukoplakia (PVL), and HPV-associated dysplasia are given in their separate sections. Prevalence data are given in Table 5.01.

Etiology
Tobacco (smoked and smokeless), and to a lesser degree alcohol abuse, are strongly associated with most OPMDs. The use of areca nut, with or without tobacco, causes submucous fibrosis. However, for PVL and many cases of OPMD, there is no tobacco association and the etiopathogenesis is unknown, although genetic, oral microbiome, immune, or other undiscovered factors may play a role {2023}. HPV-associated oral dysplasia is rare and covered separately.

Pathogenesis
The pathogenesis varies between OPMDs {4733}.

Macroscopic appearance
The appearance varies between OPMDs but most present as white or erythematous macules, papules, or verrucous plaques, which can coalesce.

Histopathology
The histopathological features vary between OPMDs. In most OPMDs the risk is considered to relate to the presence and degree of oral epithelial dysplasia, ranging from minimal to severe. However, some OPMDs, particularly PVL and leukoplakia with a verrucous architecture, have minimal dysplastic changes for their risk of malignant transformation.

Cytology
Not clinically relevant

Diagnostic molecular pathology
Not clinically relevant

Essential and desirable diagnostic criteria
Individual diagnostic criteria are presented in each section.

Table 5.01 Prevalence of oral premalignant disorders in adults by geographical area and clinical diagnosis {2934}

Geographical area	Prevalence % (95% CI)
Asia	10.5 (4.6–18.6)
Europe	3.1 (1.6–4.9)
Middle East	3.7 (2.9–4.7)
South America and the Caribbean	3.9 (2.4–5.8)
North America	0.1 (0.004–0.4)
Clinical presentation	**Overall prevalence % (95% CI)**
Leukoplakia	4.1 (2–7)
Homogeneous	2.0 (0.4–4.6)
Non-homogeneous	0.2 (0.1–0.3)
Erythroplakia	0.2 (0.1–0.3)
Oral submucous fibrosis	4.9 (2.3–8.6)

Staging
Not relevant

Prognosis and prediction
The transformation risk in most OPMDs is low. A meta-analysis of leukoplakia showed a mean global annual transformation rate of 1.56% {2023}. Both a large lesion size and erythroleukoplakia are associated with an increased risk of cancer {1904}. The status of lichen planus as potentially malignant is generally accepted, but the degree of risk remains a matter of controversy despite many studies. A lack of definitive clinical and histological diagnostic criteria and an overlap in histological features between lichen planus and dysplasia confound analysis. A wide variation in risk is reported, with a higher risk associated with disease lacking typical features (sometimes called lichenoid lesions) {4590,3645}. The early stages of PVL resemble lichen planus both clinically and histologically {2911}, and it may be impossible to differentiate oral lichen planus from mild dysplasia in some patients, although the distinction may become possible with time {809,3110}. Similar uncertainty surrounds lupus erythematosus within the oral cavity, as opposed to on the cutaneous lip vermilion border {4733}.

Proliferative verrucous leukoplakia

Eisenberg E
Fitzpatrick SG
Kallarakkal TG
Warnakulasuriya S

Definition

Proliferative verrucous leukoplakia (PVL) is a clinicopathological subtype of oral leukoplakia that is multifocal, persistent, and progressive, with a high rate of recurrence and a high risk of progression to squamous cell carcinoma.

ICD-O coding

None

ICD-11 coding

DA01.00 Leukoplakia

Related terminology

Acceptable: proliferative leukoplakia, proliferative multifocal leukoplakia.

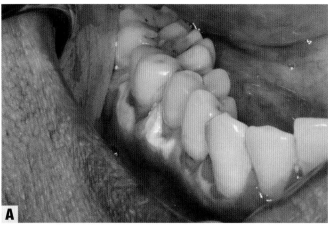

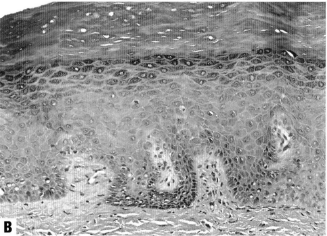

Fig. 5.13 Proliferative verrucous leukoplakia. **A** A well-demarcated leukoplakia with a prominent linear marginal pattern common to proliferative verrucous leukoplakia lesions involving the gingiva. **B** Early lesion exhibiting subtle histology with orthokeratosis, epithelial atrophy, no cytological atypia, and variable or no inflammation.

Not recommended: atypical verrucoid epithelial proliferation; atypical verrucous hyperplasia; papillary or verrucous hyperkeratosis with dysplasia.

Subtype(s)

None

Localization

The gingiva and alveolar ridge are the most frequently involved sites, followed by the buccal mucosa, tongue {664,4480,2911}, and hard palate {3461,82}.

Clinical features

Initial lesions in patients with PVL are often indistinguishable from oral lichen planus and homogeneous oral leukoplakias, forming smooth to fissured/verruciform or verrucous white or mixed white-and-red patches, usually without ulceration {82,4427}. Multiple non-contiguous lesions or a single lesion > 40 mm involving one site, or a single lesion > 30 mm involving contiguous sites, are characteristic {4632}. Thick, verrucoid marginal gingival leukoplakias that encircle the tooth, especially when multifocal, are characteristic of PVL {4544}.

Epidemiology

PVL occurs predominantly in elderly women, with no racial predilection and a mean age of 66.8 years {664,4632}.

Etiology

The etiology is unknown. PVL does not seem to be correlated with the major risk factors for oral carcinoma, including tobacco (smoked and smokeless), alcohol abuse, and areca nut / betel quid chewing {3461}. There is no apparent etiological association between PVL and HPV, EBV, or *Candida albicans* {1590, 4543,3284}.

Pathogenesis

The pathogenesis is unknown. Like tissue in other dysplastic lesions, tissue in PVL lesions shows a loss of heterozygosity and DNA ploidy anomalies {3284}.

Macroscopic appearance

PVL appears macroscopically as white mucosa, ranging from flat to thickened, sometimes with a corrugated surface or exophytic nodules.

Histopathology

Early lesions of PVL are unremarkable flat keratoses with architectural features that may be atypical, possibly premature keratinization, sharp lateral margins, increased keratin, and no cytological atypia. They are readily misdiagnosed as hyperkeratosis without dysplasia or lichen planus but gradually develop the typical verrucous morphology.

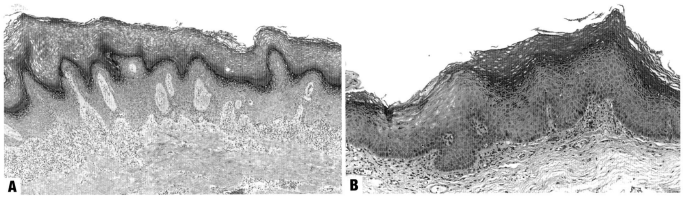

Fig. 5.14 Early lesions of proliferative verrucous leukoplakia. **A** Abrupt transition to marked hyperorthokeratosis and epithelial corrugation with lichenoid inflammation. **B** Sharp transitions and skip zones of corrugated orthokeratosis.

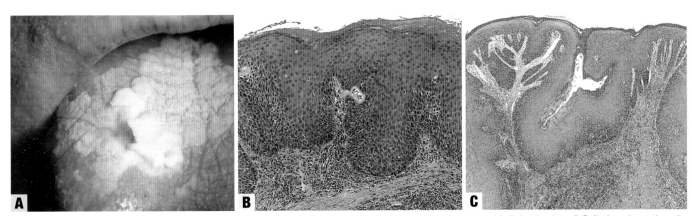

Fig. 5.15 Proliferative verrucous leukoplakia. **A** Diffuse, rough, variably thickened leukoplakia with prominent fissuring and indistinct borders. **B** Bulky hyperkeratotic endophytic proliferation with lichenoid inflammation. Bulky endophytic proliferative epithelium showing bland cells with broad, blunted rete pegs that appear to merge towards one another as they attain a uniform depth. **C** Bulky hyperkeratotic proliferation with lichenoid inflammation. An exophytic and endophytic growth pattern covered by parakeratin, with an undulating surface and surface crypts filled with parakeratin.

Corrugated hyperkeratotic lesions exhibit verrucopapillary or disproportionate flat hyperorthokeratosis/hyperparakeratosis with minimal or no dysplasia. Skip areas of normal to abnormal to normal tissue are a common finding. A sharp, abrupt transition from adjacent unaffected normal epithelium is usually seen.

Proliferative bulky epithelial lesions demonstrate atypical, hyperkeratotic epithelial architecture with/without dysplasia. Both an exophytic and an endophytic growth pattern can be present, and the epithelium shows bulbous rete pegs that sometimes coalesce.

At all stages of PVL, lymphocytic infiltration in the epithelial–stromal interface can be mistaken for lichen planus; intact basal cells and/or dysplasia preclude(s) that diagnosis {3109,4847}. A strict, stepwise histopathological continuum from the corrugated hyperkeratotic stage to the proliferative epithelial stage and progression to malignancy does not always occur (see Box 5.02) {3109,4427}.

Cytology
Not relevant

Diagnostic molecular pathology
Not relevant

Box 5.02 Spectrum of histopathological features in proliferative verrucous leukoplakia {4427}

Early (initial) phase: Solitary or multifocal corrugated hyperkeratotic lesion
- Corrugated, undulating, or flat, dense surface hyperorthokeratosis (usually) or hyperparakeratosis
- Surface keratin excessive relative to the width of the underlying epithelial compartment
- +/− Sharp keratin crests
- +/− Skip areas of surface orthokeratinization or parakeratinization
- Sharp, abrupt transitions from adjacent unaffected normal epithelium
- +/− Stratum granulosum
- +/− Epithelial atrophy, flattened rete ridges
- Minimal to no cytological dysplasia
- +/− Lichenoid interface inflammation

Progressive phase: Bulky epithelial proliferation
- Undulating surface with keratin-filled crypts
- Voluminous epithelial cellular compartment
- +/− Exophytic papillary surface projections
- Rete ridges
  - Elongated
  - Endophytic down to uniform depth
  - Bulky, broad, bulbous configuration
- Cytological atypia – minimal
- Significant architectural disturbances
- +/− Lichenoid lymphoplasmacytic infiltrate

Essential and desirable diagnostic criteria

Essential: a clinical presentation consistent with PVL; for early lesions: premature keratinization and minimal cytological atypia; for later lesions: verrucous, nodular, or bulky architecture and variable dysplasia.

Desirable: lichenoid host response.

Staging

Not relevant

Prognosis and prediction

PVL is best managed by active patient surveillance, with biopsy when clinically indicated {3,3109,308}. Laser ablation, surgical excision, and radiotherapy are associated with a high recurrence rate and are often ineffective {3,664}. Disease progression is unpredictable. A systematic review of 17 studies reported progression to malignancy in 43.87% (95% CI: 31.93–56.13%) of PVL cases {3644}.

Submucous fibrosis

Warnakulasuriya S
Ranganathan K

Definition
Oral submucous fibrosis (OSF) is a chronic, insidious disease characterized by the progressive fibrosis of submucosal tissues of the oral cavity and the oropharynx with a risk of transformation to squamous cell carcinoma.

ICD-O coding
None

ICD-11 coding
DA02.2 Oral submucous fibrosis

Related terminology
Not recommended: atrophia idiopathica (trophica) mucosae oris; idiopathic scleroderma of the mouth; idiopathic palatal fibrosis; sclerosing stomatitis.

Subtype(s)
None

Localization
OSF involves the oral cavity and oropharynx, and it may extend to the upper third of the oesophagus {4451}.

Clinical features
Fibrous banding in the buccal mucosa, lip, or palate leads to a progressive limitation of mouth opening. Associated features include burning mouth, depapillation of the tongue, blanching, and leathery mucosa {3652}. Clinical grades are described with increasing severity (see Table 5.02, p. 270).

Epidemiology
OSF is described almost exclusively in populations in India; Pakistan; Sri Lanka; Nepal; and Taiwan, China; as well as among Pacific Islanders. However, there have been case reports from the southern Chinese provinces of Hunan and Hainan, southern Viet Nam, and Thailand, as well as among migrants from the Indian subcontinent to Europe, the USA, and southern and eastern Africa {4736}. A systematic review found OSF to be a prevalent oral potentially malignant disorder worldwide (prevalence in adults: 4.96%; 95% CI: 2.28–8.62%), with significant differences between populations {2934}.

Etiology
The International Agency for Research on Cancer (IARC) has identified that areca nut chewing is the main etiological factor for OSF {1993}. The relative risk estimates for OSF reported

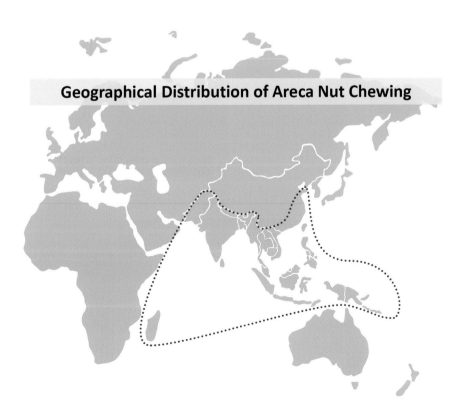

Geographical Distribution of Areca Nut Chewing

Fig. 5.16 Map showing countries reporting areca nut consumption.

Table 5.02 Clinical grading of oral submucous fibrosis (OSF) (modified from Kerr et al., 2011 {2255})

Grade	Features
Grade 1 (mild)	Interincisal opening > 35 mm
	With any of the following symptoms: burning mouth, depapillation of tongue, blanching or leathery mucosa
Grade 2 (moderate)	Limited interincisal opening, 20–35 mm
	With palpable fibrous bands and any of the above symptoms associated with OSF
Grade 3 (severe)	Limited interincisal opening, < 20 mm
	With palpable fibrous bands and any of the above symptoms associated with OSF
Grade 4 (advanced)	With broad fibrous bands and features of OSF + any other oral potentially malignant disorder (leukoplakia, erythroplakia, exophytic verrucous hyperplasia)
Grade 5 (advanced)	With broad fibrous bands and features of OSF + oral squamous cell or verrucous carcinoma

in case–control studies among areca nut chewers from India; Pakistan; Sri Lanka; and Taiwan, China, ranged from 1.8 to 172 {4448}. Arecoline, a principal alkaloid in the areca nut, has been shown to induce fibroblastic proliferation and increased collagen formation {3636,4451,1222,1991}.

Pathogenesis

The main pathological change in OSF is the increased accumulation of collagen I within the subepithelial tissues. Decreased levels of matrix metalloproteinases and increased amounts of tissue inhibitors of matrix metalloproteinases have been reported {3555}. Polyphenols of the areca nut such as flavonoids, catechin, and tannins cause collagen fibres to cross-link, and thereby make them resistant to degradation by collagenase. Lysyl oxidase, encoded by *LOX*, is upregulated {4496}. Cytokines such as TGF-β induce transdifferentiation of fibroblasts into myofibroblasts {2269}. αvβ6-dependent TGF-β1 activation is also implicated {2011,3097}.

Macroscopic appearance

The affected area shows a leathery mucosal texture and pale whitish mucosa, with loss of lingual papillae.

Histopathology

A spectrum of histopathological changes is evident from early to advanced disease {3650,3381,441,3458,4024}. Initially the epithelium is hyperplastic, and it subsequently progresses to marked atrophy with a loss of rete ridges. Epithelial dysplasia starts to appear unpredictably with progression of the disease. Budding rete morphology is a very early dysplastic feature. Changes in the submucosa in the early stage are minimal, with a slightly increased vascularity, inflammatory infiltrate, increased fibrillar collagen, and collagen fibre bundles with interspersed

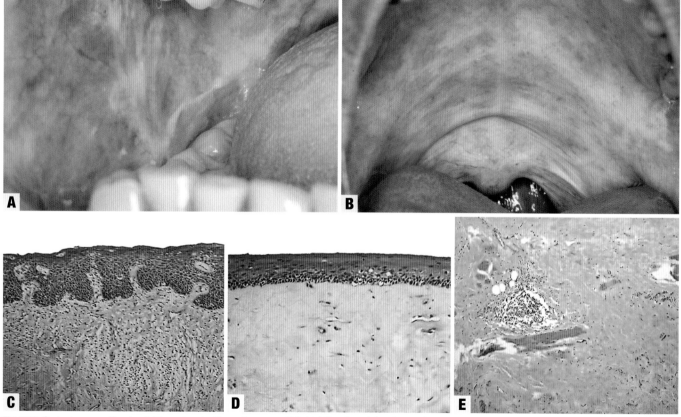

Fig. 5.17 Oral submucous fibrosis. **A** Fibrous bands of buccal mucosa. **B** Palatal fibrosis and shrunken uvula. **C** Epithelium showing dysplastic changes. The submucosa is fibrosed and contains a diffuse inflammatory cell infiltrate. **D** Marked epithelial atrophy, flattening of rete ridges, juxtaepithelial hyalinization, and homogeneous collagen. **E** An advanced case showing fibrosis involving muscles, muscle degeneration, and foci of chronic inflammatory cells.

fibroblasts. Later the collagen becomes homogeneous, starting superficially with juxtaepithelial hyalinization. Advanced cases show a loss of vascularity, hyalinization of collagen, and dense fibrosis extending to the underlying tissues, with muscle degeneration and the complete replacement of loose connective tissue (areolar and reticular tissue) by fibrous tissue. Attempts have been made to classify OSF into histopathological stages, but different parts of the oral mucosa can be affected to varying degrees, so histopathological grading may not be representative {3548,4551,3381,3652}.

Cytology
Not clinically relevant

Diagnostic molecular pathology
Unknown

Essential and desirable diagnostic criteria
Essential: palpable fibrous bands in the oral mucosa; subepithelial hyalinization and fibrosis.

Desirable: limitation of mouth opening; fibrosis extending to muscle; loss of tongue papillae; epithelial atrophy.

Staging
Staging is based on clinical features and histopathology. Clinical stages are based on mouth opening (> 35 mm, 20–35 mm, < 20 mm), the presence of an oral potentially malignant disorder (leukoplakia, erythroplakia, proliferative verrucous hyperplasia), and transformation to carcinoma {2255}.

Prognosis and prediction
OSF is a fertile background for squamous carcinoma, which develops in 4.2% (95% CI: 2.7–5.6%) of patients, and cases with oral epithelial dysplasia have a higher potential for malignant transformation than cases without dysplasia {2402}. There are no established molecular predictive markers. Loss of heterozygosity in genes within the 13q14-q33 region, hypoxia, and reactive oxygen species may have some predictive value for transformation {4449,1222}.

Oral epithelial dysplasia

Lingen MW
Kujan O
Kurago ZB
Poh CF
Ranganathan K
Vigneswaran N

Definition

Oral epithelial dysplasia (OED) is a spectrum of architectural and cytological epithelial changes resulting from an accumulation of genetic alterations, usually arising in a range of oral potentially malignant disorders (OPMDs), and indicating a risk of malignant transformation to squamous cell carcinoma.

ICD-O coding

8077/0 Low-grade squamous intraepithelial lesion
8077/2 High-grade squamous intraepithelial lesion

ICD-11 coding

None

Related terminology

Acceptable: epithelial precursor lesions.
Not recommended: intraepithelial neoplasia; squamous intraepithelial lesions; carcinoma in situ.

Subtype(s)

None

Localization

OED can involve any intraoral site, but its presence on the lateral/ventral tongue, retromolar area, and floor of the mouth is associated with a higher risk of malignant transformation than at other sites {4847}. The gingiva and buccal mucosa are other frequently affected sites. The hard palate is rarely affected.

Clinical features

OED itself has no clinical meaning or consistent presentation, and its clinical features vary widely depending on the OPMD. Erythroplakia and erythroleukoplakia are the presentations most likely to be associated with dysplasia or carcinoma (> 90%), on initial biopsy or subsequently {4847}.

Epidemiology

Most cases of OED arise in OPMDs, each of which have distinct epidemiological features. The prevalence of the various OPMDs is included separately {2934}.

Etiology

Most cases of OED are associated with the use of tobacco (smoked and smokeless) or areca nut, alone or in combination, or (to a lesser degree) with alcohol abuse, but for many cases of OED the etiopathogenesis remains unknown {3109,2023}.

Pathogenesis

OED is associated with the progressive accumulation of genetic and epigenetic changes, including loss of heterozygosity / copy-number alterations, hypermethylation, changes in RNA molecule expression (mRNA and microRNA), and somatic mutations. These lead to chromosomal and genomic instability at an early stage {3266}.

Macroscopic appearance

The macroscopic appearance varies depending on the OPMD.

Histopathology

OED comprises changes resulting from the abnormal proliferation, maturation, and differentiation of epithelial cells {4452,4450, 4907}. Box 5.03 lists the architectural and cytological disturbances that are used to diagnose OED. Individually these features are relatively nonspecific, but the number and combination of features, which vary between OPMDs, are used to determine the presence of epithelial dysplasia. OED can be diagnosed on

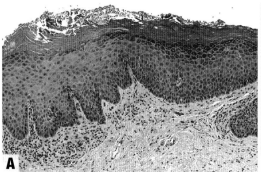 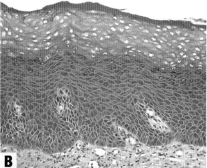 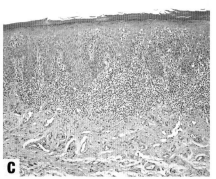

Fig. 5.18 Oral epithelial dysplasia, mild. **A** Architectural features of dysplasia include a sharp lateral demarcation of the epithelium with an abrupt change to orthokeratosis. Mild anisonucleosis and hyperchromatism, as well as a slightly disorganized basal cell layer with generalized premature keratinization, are seen. **B** Primarily an architectural or differentiated pattern of dysplasia with loss of basal cell polarization, budding of the rete, increased hyperchromasia, and mitotic figures confined to the basal and parabasal layers with generalized premature keratinization. **C** Band-like inflammatory infiltrate at the epithelial–stromal interface imparting a lichenoid appearance including apoptotic degeneration of keratinocytes but with general preservation of a slightly expanded and hyperchromatic basal cell layer.

the basis of architectural or cytological features alone. Traditionally, OED is divided into three grades, and determining the number of thirds of the epithelium affected is one factor in assigning grade. Architectural and cytological atypia usually increases in higher-grade lesions, with mild dysplasia characterized by cytological atypia limited to the basal third, moderate dysplasia by extension to the middle third, and severe dysplasia by extension to the upper third. However, defining dysplasia grade only in this manner oversimplifies the complexity of grading. Cytological atypia confined to the basal third may be sufficient for a diagnosis of severe dysplasia, depending on individual features present, particularly bulbous rete processes, budding and disorganization of basal cells, and marked pleomorphism.

It has long been recognized that many cases of OED have a lichenoid immune response composed of a lymphohistiocytic infiltrate with T cell–mediated epithelial cell destruction {2397, 3110,4427}. This histopathological finding can be confused with oral lichen planus, in which the presence of dysplasia is an exclusion criterion {809,3109,4847}. More difficult to assess is dysplasia grading when primarily architectural features of OED are present in the absence of or with minimal cytological atypia. This combination is commonly found in papillary and verrucous lesions {3109,4427}. Carcinoma in situ in the oral cavity is considered synonymous with severe dysplasia, but the term is not recommended.

Although OED is considered to be an indicator of malignant transformation, there are important caveats to its clinical use. It has variable observer reproducibility (intraobserver and interobserver) {4181,3651}. Consensus grading after review by more than one pathologist may enhance diagnostic reliability {1409, 4181,4183}. To improve reproducibility, some authors advocate a binary system (low grade and high grade) for dysplasia grading {4735,3157}, but this still requires additional validation against malignant transformation.

Cytology
Not clinically relevant

Diagnostic molecular pathology
Not clinically relevant

Essential and desirable diagnostic criteria
Essential: cytological and/or architectural atypia; nuclear hyperchromasia; high N:C ratios.

Staging
Not relevant

Prognosis and prediction
Not all cases of OED progress to malignancy (3–50%) {92,2920, 4182,766}, and the results of studies on the prognostic value of

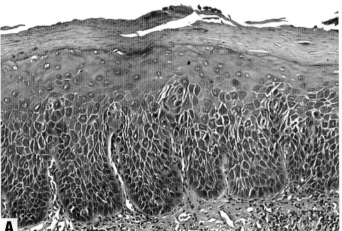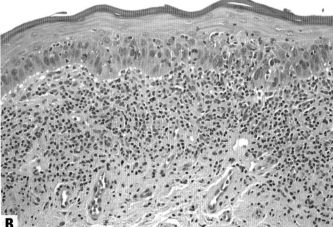

Fig. 5.19 Oral epithelial dysplasia, moderate. **A** Drop-shaped rete processes with increased mitotic figures, reduced keratinocyte cohesion, and abnormal variation in nuclear size, extending to the spinous layer. **B** Band-like inflammatory infiltrate at the epithelial–stromal interface imparts a lichenoid appearance, but loss of basal cell polarization, nuclear hyperchromasia, and mitoses extending to the mid-third of the atrophic epithelium excludes oral lichen planus.

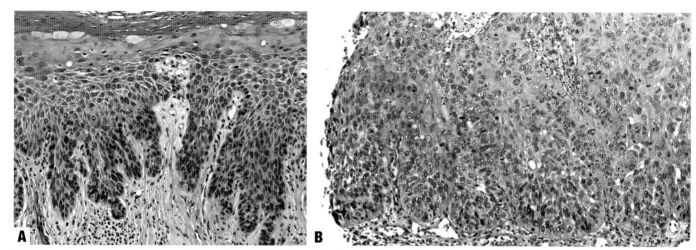

Fig. 5.20 Oral epithelial dysplasia, severe. **A** Increased keratinization, loss of cohesion in the prickle cell layer, and increased numbers of basaloid cells with mild hyperchromatism and anisonucleosis with budding and downward growth. **B** Loss of basal cell polarity, epithelial differentiation, increased mitotic figures, and abnormal variation in nuclear and cellular features extending throughout the full epithelial thickness.

dysplasia grade are ambivalent {2754,1393,4183}. OPMDs without evidence of OED can progress to squamous cell carcinoma. The predictive value of OED grading plays a significant role in stratifying malignant transformation risk. Although the absence of OED does not preclude malignant transformation {766}, a higher grade of OED is significantly associated with both earlier and higher risk of malignant transformation {2920,4182,2023,4907}. A recent population-based cohort study that included > 1800 patients showed that the overall hazard ratios for malignant transformation increased significantly with the grade of dysplasia, the overall hazard ratios being 4.9 and 15.8 for mild dysplasia and severe dysplasia, respectively {766}. This and other data {3265} support a three-grade system to both distinguish lesions with different risks of transformation and estimate time to transformation. The presence of low grades of OPMD carries a very long term risk of malignant transformation, extending for ≥ 18 years {766,3265} and apparently not reducing with time {1308}. There are no established biomarkers to aid dysplasia grading or malignant transformation prediction, although DNA ploidy and loss-of-heterozygosity assays have shown promising results {3266}.

HPV-associated oral epithelial dysplasia

Woo SB
Robinson M
Thavaraj S

Definition

HPV-associated oral epithelial dysplasia (HPVOED) is characterized by distinctive viral cytopathic changes caused by transcriptionally active high-risk HPV, with a risk of progression to squamous cell carcinoma.

ICD-O coding

8085/0 HPV-associated oral epithelial dysplasia, low grade
8085/2 HPV-associated oral epithelial dysplasia, high grade

ICD-11 coding

None

Related terminology

Not recommended: HPV-associated squamous intraepithelial neoplasia; koilocytic dysplasia; oral Bowen disease; oral bowenoid papulosis.

Subtype(s)

None

Localization

The ventral/lateral tongue and the floor of the mouth are the commonest sites, followed by the buccal mucosa. The palatal mucosa, gingiva, and labial mucosa are less commonly affected {2568,1837,236}.

Clinical features

Patients with HPVOED generally present with a white, red/white, or red patch, which is usually flat and demarcated but sometimes slightly raised or nodular {2568,1837}.

Epidemiology

There is a male predilection (M:F ratio: 6:1) and a wide age range, with a peak incidence in the sixth decade of life {2898, 2568,1837,142,236}.

Etiology

HPVOED is caused by epithelial infection by high-risk HPV subtypes, usually type 16, although other types may be detected {2568,2273,1051}. In limited series, most patients are tobacco smokers {2568} and some are immunosuppressed.

Pathogenesis

The pathogenesis is unclear in this context but is assumed to follow pathways causing uterine cervical dysplasia through E6/E7 transcription, p53 degradation, and p16 overexpression {627}. Lesions vary; some show viral integration through the downregulation of the HPV E2 protein {2272}, and others express the HPV proteins E4 and L1, indicating possible productive infection {1837}. *APOBEC3B*-associated mutagenesis has also been implicated in the pathogenesis of HPVOED {236}.

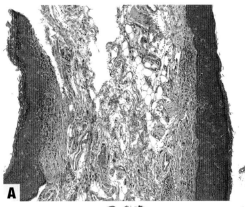

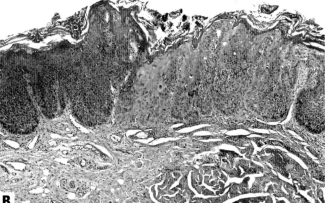

Fig. 5.21 HPV-associated oral epithelial dysplasia. **A** Marked architectural and cytological changes of dysplasia, with karyorrhectic and apoptotic cells. **B** Dysplastic epithelium with a brightly eosinophilic keratin surface and basaloid morphology.

Macroscopic appearance

None

Histopathology

The epithelial surface is covered by a brightly eosinophilic layer of parakeratin in most cases, although orthokeratosis may be seen. There are marked architectural and cytological changes of dysplasia, characterized by a monotonous population of keratinocytes exhibiting basaloid morphology and a high N:C ratio. Some cases show pleomorphic cells, and koilocytes may be present superficially {2568,142,2273,1837}. Two types of cells are characteristic of the cytopathic effect of HPV: karyorrhectic cells with condensed coarse chromatin resembling cells in mitosis, with a pericellular halo resulting from a loss of attachment to adjacent cells; and apoptotic cells with dense eosinophilic cytoplasm that in the initial stages contains residual chromatin {2568,142}. There is a continuum between these two cell types. The specificity of karyorrhectic and apoptotic keratinocytes as a surrogate for HPVOED increases as the number of such cells increases {2273,2272}.

Chapter 5

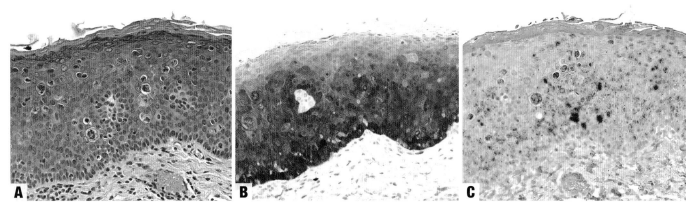

Fig. 5.22 HPV-associated dysplasia. **A** Marked architectural and cytological changes of dysplasia with karyorrhectic and apoptotic cells. **B** The epithelium shows full-thickness intense cytoplasmic and nuclear immunoreactivity for p16. **C** RNA in situ hybridization for high-risk HPV shows punctate, dot-like nuclear staining.

Immunohistochemistry

Although there is strong and diffuse nuclear and cytoplasmic positivity for p16 by immunohistochemistry, in a continuous band (block positivity) that is often sharply demarcated from the adjacent non-dysplastic epithelium, this feature is not yet validated for diagnosis in this setting {1837}. Most studies indicate that positivity in > 50% of the epithelial thickness, excluding the keratin layer, suggests HPV-associated dysplasia; however, studies have not defined a threshold for p16 interpretation {1837}.

Differential diagnosis

The combination of dysplasia, viral cytopathic changes, and the presence of high-risk HPV distinguishes HPVOED from conventional oral epithelial dysplasia, flat warts, and multifocal epithelial hyperplasia {4848,4237}.

Cytology

Not clinically relevant

Diagnostic molecular pathology

Strong and diffuse nuclear and cytoplasmic p16 immunohistochemical expression in the presence of oral epithelial dysplasia with viral cytopathic changes should be supported by testing for high-risk HPV by DNA or RNA in situ hybridization, or PCR {2273,2568,2272,142}. Standard consensus PCR alone, without a strong p16 reaction and supportive histopathological criteria, is insufficient for the diagnosis of HPVOED {1051}.

Essential and desirable diagnostic criteria

Essential: epithelial dysplasia with prominent karyorrhectic/apoptotic cells; presence of high-risk HPV.

Desirable: strong p16 immunohistochemical expression exceeding half of the epithelial thickness, excluding keratin.

Staging

None

Prognosis and prediction

According to limited data, the development of invasive squamous cell carcinoma occurs in 5– 15% of cases {2568,2273}. To date, there are no validated grading criteria to predict transformation. In the interim, it is recommended that HPVOED should be graded and managed similarly to conventional oral epithelial dysplasia, pending further evidence. In general, such HPVOEDs are amenable to surgical excision. The role of prophylactic vaccination in the management of HPVOED is unknown.

Oral squamous cell carcinoma

Lingen MW
Cheong SC
Fujii S
Gupta PC

Hille J
Hunter KD
Salo TA

Definition
Oral squamous cell carcinoma (OSCC) is a malignant epithelial neoplasm with squamous differentiation arising from the mucosal epithelium of the oral cavity.

ICD-O coding
8070/3 Squamous cell carcinoma
8074/3 Spindle cell squamous cell carcinoma
8083/3 Basaloid squamous cell carcinoma
8075/3 Acantholytic squamous cell carcinoma
8560/3 Adenosquamous carcinoma
8052/3 Papillary squamous cell carcinoma
8082/3 Lymphoepithelial carcinoma

ICD-11 coding
2B6E.0 Squamous cell carcinoma of other or ill-defined sites in the lip, oral cavity, or pharynx

Related terminology
None

Subtype(s)
Spindle cell squamous cell carcinoma; basaloid squamous cell carcinoma; acantholytic squamous cell carcinoma; adenosquamous carcinoma; papillary squamous cell carcinoma; lymphoepithelial carcinoma

Localization
OSCC can arise from any oral mucosal site. In European populations, the most commonly affected sites are the lateral/ventral tongue, floor of the mouth, posterior buccal mucosa, and gingiva / alveolar mucosa {2475,4498}. In southern and southeastern Asia, OSCC most commonly affects the buccal mucosa because of the prevalence of areca nut / betel quid chewing {4294}.

Clinical features
Patients with OSCC may be completely asymptomatic, particularly in the early stage of the disease, whereas advanced tumours are associated with pain, alteration in sensation, and restriction of tongue movement or swallowing {309}. OSCCs may appear as white, red, or mixed red and white, flat/nodular/mass lesions of varying size. When present, advanced ulcers

Chapter 5

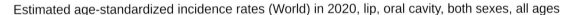

Estimated age-standardized incidence rates (World) in 2020, lip, oral cavity, both sexes, all ages

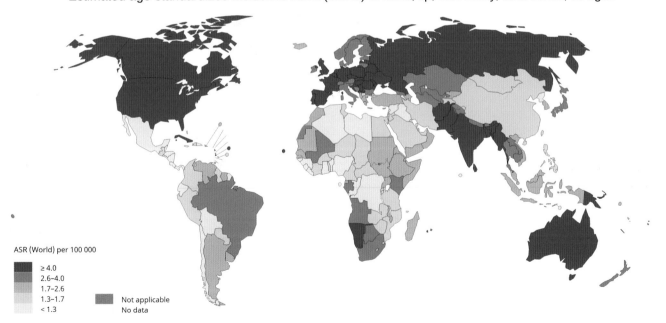

ASR (World) per 100 000

- ≥ 4.0
- 2.6–4.0
- 1.7–2.6
- 1.3–1.7
- < 1.3

Not applicable
No data

Data source: GLOBOCAN 2020
Graph production: IARC
(http://gco.iarc.fr/today)
World Health Organization

World Health Organization

© International Agency for Research on Cancer 2021

Fig. 5.23 Oral squamous cell carcinoma. Estimated age-standardized incidence rates (ASRs, World Standard Population), per 100 000 person-years, of lip and oral cavity cancer in 2020 among both sexes (all ages).

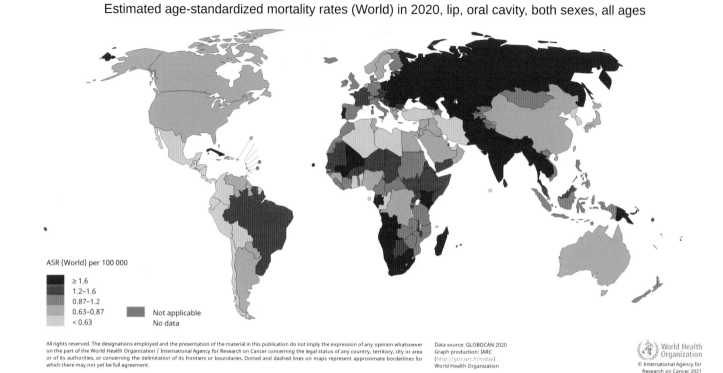

Estimated age-standardized mortality rates (World) in 2020, lip, oral cavity, both sexes, all ages

ASR (World) per 100 000

- ≥ 1.6
- 1.2–1.6
- 0.87–1.2
- 0.63–0.87
- < 0.63

Not applicable
No data

Data source: GLOBOCAN 2020
Graph production: IARC
(http://gco.iarc.fr/today)
World Health Organization

World Health Organization
© International Agency for Research on Cancer 2021

Fig. 5.24 Oral squamous cell carcinoma. Estimated age-standardized mortality rates (ASRs, World Standard Population), per 100 000 person-years, of lip and oral cavity cancer in 2020 among both sexes (all ages).

often have a raised and rolled margin; however, early OSCC can manifest as deceptively bland-appearing lesions. Other clinical findings may include tissue fixation and induration, mobility of teeth, trismus, bone destruction, and pathological fracture, depending on the localization of the neoplasm {309}. An unknown proportion (probably the majority) of OSCCs arise in oral potentially malignant disorders, although OSCC may arise in clinically normal mucosa {4733}. A thorough visual and tactile oral cavity examination remains the most effective method of screening. Several adjuncts to aid clinical inspection have been developed, but all have less than ideal sensitivity and specificity for routine clinical application {2758,1596,2668,2667}.

Epidemiology

Worldwide, oral cancer (including of the mucosal lips) is the 16th most common cancer, accounting for > 377 000 cases per annum; 70% of patients are male {4295}. However, these overall figures obscure a marked variation in incidence and mortality worldwide {2424}. The highest estimated age-standardized incidence rates have been reported in Melanesia (males: 22.2 cases per 100 000 person-years; females: 14.6 cases per 100 000) and southern/central Asia (males: 13.3 cases per 100 000; females: 4.6 cases per 100 000). In India and Thailand, the sex ratio is reversed, with M:F ratios of 1:2 and 1:1.5, respectively {2387}. The estimated age-standardized incidence rates in western Africa are much lower (in both sexes: ≤ 2.0 cases per 100 000 person-years). Trends in incidence are variable, with a marked reduction in lip cancers in the past decade, and although male oral cavity cancer rates are reducing overall, this is not the case in all populations, including India and

the UK. Furthermore, modest increases in incidence rates in females have been reported in many populations {2387}. Age-standardized rates of mortality have remained constant over many decades {3685}. The highest cumulative risk of mortality has been reported in Melanesia and in southern/central Asian populations {4295}. A worldwide increase in the incidence of oral tongue cancer, particularly in individuals aged < 45 years, has been reported {3196}.

Etiology

Globally, tobacco (smoked or smokeless) {266} is the main etiological factor, accounting (with alcohol) for > 70% of attributable risk in a European population {177}. The consumption of alcohol in combination with the use of tobacco (smoked or smokeless) results in a synergistic increase in odds ratio for the occurrence of OSCC {2933}. In some geographical regions, areca nut (the seed of the *Areca catechu* palm) is the primary carcinogen and is an independent risk factor {1716}. This is consumed in various forms and may be mixed with tobacco, various formulations of lime, *Piper betle* inflorescence, and spices, and wrapped in betel leaf {2633}. In practice, this may be combined with tobacco smoking, further increasing the risk of OSCC. Ultraviolet (UV) light is the principal etiological factor in actinic cheilitis and squamous cell carcinoma (SCC) of the cutaneous lip {1019}. Poor general oral health and diets lacking in fruits and vegetables may act as contributory factors to OSCC incidence and poor clinical outcomes {1340,3728}. Although it is important for oropharyngeal SCC, HPV has not been shown to be a significant etiological factor in OSCC {2669,4978,3168}. OSCC may arise in patients without known risk factors. The pattern

Table 5.03 Subtypes of squamous cell carcinoma (SCC) of the oral cavity and mobile tongue

OSCC subtype	Features	References
Acantholytic SCC	Squamous carcinoma with acantholysis in epithelial islands creating a gland or duct-like appearance Rare in the oral cavity, may occur on the lip, has a poor prognosis	{1175,1537,5051,2829}
Adenosquamous carcinoma	Carcinoma with both squamous and adenocarcinoma components Aggressive and infiltrative behaviour, frequent metastases, associated with a worse prognosis than conventional OSCC	{2205,2867,3944,3889}
Basaloid SCC	Carcinoma with islands composed of basaloid cells, often with comedonecrosis and a high mitotic rate High-grade carcinoma, which often metastasizes, with overall survival similar to conventional OSCC	{1480,4879,3931}
Carcinoma cuniculatum	Very well differentiated, lacking cytological malignancy, burrowing invasion pattern, keratin-containing crypts, abundant intraepithelial and stromal neutrophils Destructive bone invasion but no metastases	{4290,1335,3358}
Lymphoepithelial carcinoma	Carcinoma with minimal differentiation and numerous interspersed non-neoplastic lymphocytes 70% are associated with regional lymph node metastases, most are EBV-positive	{3792,4439,4802}
Papillary SCC	Exophytic carcinoma with multiple thin, filiform, finger-like papillary projections; keratinizing and non-keratinizing types; cytological atypia Better prognosis than conventional OSCC of a similar clinical stage, worse prognosis than verrucous carcinoma	{1136,2922}
Spindle cell SCC (sarcomatoid carcinoma)	Carcinoma without epithelial tissue architecture and composed of spindle cells; may develop by transformation from conventional OSCC, often after radiotherapy Aggressive, recurs and metastasizes easily; oral cavity lesions have a worse outcome than do conventional OSCCs	{3592,1571,4641}
Verrucous SCC	Low-grade, surface carcinoma with verrucous architecture that lacks atypia and shows pushing cohesive invasion Good prognosis; an indolent, mostly laterally spreading carcinoma that carries a long-term risk of development of OSCC	{2807,3261,1927}

OSCC, oral squamous cell carcinoma.

of incidence and clinical outcomes may be different in such patients {394,301}.

The evidence of an inherited genetic predisposition to OSCC is limited. A genome-wide association study reported the association of OSCC with 2p23.3 (rs6547741, *GPN1*), 9q34.12 (rs928674, *LAMC3*), 9p21.3 (rs8181047, *CDKN2B-AS1*), and 5p15.33 (rs10462706, *CLPTM1L*) {2572}. However, the strongest link to susceptibility is in individuals with inherited syndromes including Li–Fraumeni syndrome {3594}, Fanconi anaemia {507, 2434}, dyskeratosis congenita {147}, Bloom syndrome, Lynch syndrome, and Xeroderma pigmentosum {3876}.

Pathogenesis
The majority of OSCCs arise in areas of pre-existing epithelial dysplasia or are preceded by oral potentially malignant

disorders {1050,4847}. Most OSCCs are genetically unstable and characterized by significant chromosomal alterations and a high somatic mutation burden. Chromosomal losses at 3p, 8p, 9p, and 17p, with gains at 3q, 5p, 8q, and 11q, are reproducibly observed {653,778}. Several large-scale sequencing studies have defined the mutation landscape for OSCC with somatic mutations being observed in a number of genes, including *TP53*, *CDKN2A*, *FAT1*, *NOTCH1*, *KMT2D*, *CASP8*, *AJUBA*, *NSD1*, *HLA-A*, *TGFBR2*, *USP9X*, *KMT2D* (*MLL4*), *HRAS*, *UNC13C*, *ARID2*, and *TRPM3* {67,4244,653,2014, 3534,4262}.

Macroscopic appearance
OSCCs are exophytic and/or endophytic, often ulcerated, firm, indurated tumours, with a tan or white cut surface.

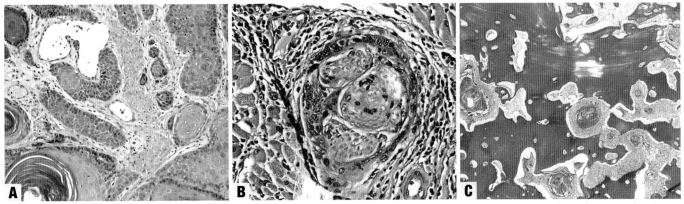

Fig. 5.25 Squamous cell carcinoma. **A** Well-differentiated, keratinizing conventional type. **B** Oral cavity squamous cell carcinoma demonstrating perineural invasion. **C** Mandibular medullary bone invasion by squamous cell carcinoma.

Table 5.04 Histological prognostic factors in oral cavity and tongue cancer – an overview of data derived from meta-analyses, depicted as hazard ratio (HR) or odds ratio (OR) for overall survival or for disease-specific survival (DSS)

Risk factor	HR or OR (95% CI)	Remarks	Reference
DOI	OR: 0.49 (0.10–2.34)	DOI > 5 mm compared with DOI < 5 mm	{645}
Tumour budding	HR: 1.88 (1.25–2.82)	Compared with no budding	{127}
Perineural invasion	HR: 2.01 (1.10–3.7)	Compared with no invasion	{767}
Lymphovascular invasion	HR: 1.55 (1.43–1.69)	Compared with no invasion	{1948}
Worst pattern of invasion 5	HR: 2.77 (1.66–4.64)	Compared with worst pattern of invasion 1–4	{4888}
Tumour-to-stroma ratio	DSS HR: 2.10 (1.56–2.84)	> 50% stroma in deeply invasive tumour	{126}
Bone invasion	HR: 2.14 (1.46–5.61)	Mandibular medullary invasion compared with no invasion	{2606}
	HR: 1.52 (1.02–2.25)	Any bone invasion compared with no invasion	
LNR	HR: 2.76 (1.90–3.99)	High LNR compared with low LNR	{1951}

DOI, depth of invasion; LNR, lymph node ratio (the ratio of the number of positive lymph nodes to the total number of lymph nodes removed).

Histopathology

Most cancers in the oral cavity and mobile tongue are conventional keratinizing SCC. However, other subtypes can rarely occur (see Table 5.03, p. 279). Well-differentiated neoplasms contain large nests, cords, and islands of cells with pink cytoplasm; prominent intercellular bridging; and round, often hyperchromatic nuclei. Squamous pearls and dyskeratotic cells are also prominent. Higher-grade neoplasms may demonstrate marked nuclear and cellular pleomorphism, nuclear hyperchromasia, and mitotic figures (including atypical forms), and small islands or individuals cells can be observed at the invasive front. A desmoplastic stroma with various degrees of inflammation can be found around invading tumour cell nests and islands. Perineural and lymphovascular invasion may occur, generally in poorly differentiated high-grade tumours. Adjacent mucosal epithelium may show various grades of dysplasia. Grading alone does not

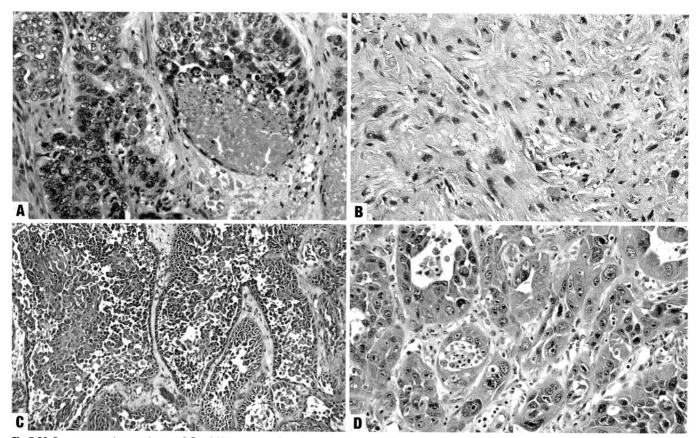

Fig. 5.26 Squamous carcinoma subtypes. **A** Basaloid squamous cell carcinoma. Well-rounded nests of basaloid cells with peripheral palisading, frequent mitoses, and comedonecrosis. **B** Spindle cell squamous cell carcinoma. A haphazard collection of atypical spindled and pleomorphic cells with hyperchromatic nuclei, lacking obvious epithelial differentiation. **C** Acantholytic squamous cell carcinoma. Pseudoglandular structures with dyskeratotic cells and prominent acantholysis that results from a loss of epithelial cohesion. **D** Adenosquamous carcinoma. A blending of epithelial and glandular components with necrosis, mitoses, and marked cellular and nuclear pleomorphism.

correlate well with prognosis. However, a number of specific features may have important biological relevance (see Table 5.04).

Immunohistochemistry
In less differentiated OSCC, immunohistochemical confirmation of epithelial differentiation (using keratins such as AE1/AE3) or squamous differentiation (using CK5/6, p63, and p40) may be needed {476}.

Cytology
Although confirmatory evaluation by histology of incisional or excisional biopsies of intraoral carcinomas remains the gold standard, brush cytology may be helpful for screening and for the diagnosis of early OSCC {1654,1104}. FNAB is useful for evaluating lymph node metastases.

Diagnostic molecular pathology
Not clinically relevant

Essential and desirable diagnostic criteria
Essential: infiltrating malignant epithelial cells with squamous differentiation.

Staging
Staging follows the eighth edition of the Union for International Cancer Control (UICC) / American Joint Committee on Cancer (AJCC) TNM staging system.

Prognosis and prediction
Conventional OSCC is aggressive, with a propensity for local invasion and early lymph node metastasis. The most significant prognostic factors are tumour size, depth of invasion, nodal status, and distant metastases. Stage at diagnosis and oral cancer mortality vary by site of cancer, with low stage at diagnosis in lip cancers and highest mortality in tongue cancers {4265}. Conventional histological grading corresponds poorly with clinical outcomes {564}. Histological factors associated with a worse prognosis include a non-cohesive pattern of invasion, tumour budding, perineural and lymphovascular invasion, and bone invasion (see Table 5.04). In addition, anatomical invasive depth (invasion into intrinsic muscles) is an independent predictive factor for delayed cervical lymph node metastasis after partial glossectomy for patients with clinically node-negative tongue

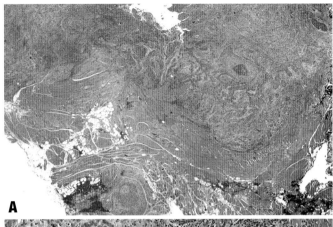

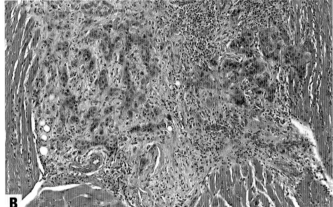

Fig. 5.27 Squamous cell carcinoma. **A** Although the tumour appears to have a cohesive invading front, a detached tumour satellite > 1 mm from the main tumour is a worst pattern of invasion 5 and an adverse prognostic factor (see Table 5.04). **B** Worst pattern of invasion 3, composed of small groups of > 15 tumour cells and single infiltrating tumour cells associated with a desmoplastic stroma (see Table 5.04).

SCC {3027}. Narrow tumour bed margins (≤ 4 mm) {107,3575A} and high-grade dysplasia at the mucosal margins have been reported to correlate with local recurrence {4755}. Surgical clearance taken from margins of the main resection specimen predicts local control better than sampling from the tumour bed {2889,4194,624}. Positive lymph nodes, particularly extranodal extension into the adjacent tissue {6} and involvement of levels IV and V, correlate with adverse outcome.

Verrucous carcinoma of the oral cavity and mobile tongue

Zidar N
Bishop JA
Vigneswaran N
Woo SB
Zain RB

Definition

Verrucous carcinoma (VC) is a well-differentiated non-metastasizing squamous cell carcinoma (SCC) that has a warty keratinized surface and specific architecture, lacks substantial cytological features of malignancy, and is characterized by slow lateral spread and pushing invasion below the level of the adjacent epithelium.

ICD-O coding

8051/3 Verrucous carcinoma, NOS

ICD-11 coding

2B66.0 & XH5PM0 Squamous cell carcinoma of other or unspecified parts of mouth & Verrucous carcinoma, NOS

Related terminology

Not recommended: Ackerman tumour; verrucous hyperplasia.

Subtype(s)

None

Localization

The oral mucosa is the most common site for VC, accounting for 50–75% of all VC cases in the head and neck {2348}. In the oral cavity, the buccal mucosa, gingiva, and tongue are most frequently involved {132}.

Clinical features

VC presents as a slowly growing and slightly exophytic white tumour. VC may erode bones and can cause extensive destruction if left untreated.

Epidemiology

VC is rare, accounting for 2–16% of oral carcinomas {3680}. It occurs predominantly in older people, usually in the sixth decade of life or later, with a strong male predilection.

Etiology

VC has been etiologically related to the use of chewing tobacco or snuff. The habitual use of areca nut / betel quid chew has been implicated in the high incidence of oral VC in India {1416}. VC is not associated with HPV infection {1079,3414,3262}.

Pathogenesis

Little is known about the pathogenesis of VC, but its molecular signature appears distinct from that of other oral SCCs {3843}. Gene expression {3260,3261,1095,4725} and differentiation markers {3263} differ from those of SCCs of the same head and neck sites.

Macroscopic appearance

VC presents as a broad-based exophytic tumour with a warty, white or red surface, depending on the amount of keratinization. On cut surface it is firm, tan to white, and may show keratin-filled clefts and a flat, well-defined pushing interface with underlying tissue.

Histopathology

VC consists of a broad-based, well-differentiated exophytic and endophytic squamous epithelial proliferation with marked surface keratinization and keratin plugging. VC invades the stroma evenly with well-defined pushing borders, extending below the level of adjacent epithelium that may be difficult to visualize on small biopsies. Bulbous rete processes often coalesce. A

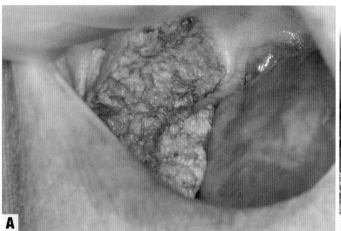 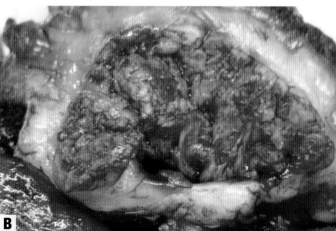

Fig. 5.28 Verrucous carcinoma. **A** A large exophytic tumour with verrucous architecture blanketing the edentulous mandibular alveolar ridge and extending to the involve the vestibule and buccal mucosa. **B** Verrucous carcinoma with minimal invasive carcinoma. Examination of the whole specimen showed verrucous carcinoma with a focus of conventional squamous cell carcinoma.

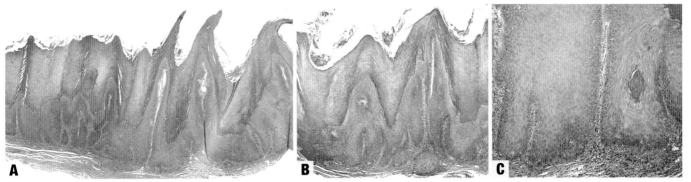

Fig. 5.29 Verrucous carcinoma. **A** A broad-based, well-differentiated epithelial proliferation with marked papillary parakeratosis and keratin plugging. Verrucous carcinoma invades the stroma evenly with well-defined pushing borders, extending below the level of the adjacent epithelium. **B** A bulbous, coalescing rete and an expanded spinous layer are present. A lichenoid immune response is often seen. **C** A lack of cytological atypia with normal maturation is usually seen in verrucous carcinoma. Rarely, mitoses may be present in the basal/parabasal layer, but without atypical mitotic forms.

sharply defined stromal–epithelial interface is generally seen, often associated with a lymphoplasmacytic inflammatory response {1036}. VC lacks substantial cytological features of malignancy, and it should have no more than mild/low-grade nuclear pleomorphism. Surface ulceration is uncommon and raises the concern for conventional SCC {3414}. Tumours with severe/high-grade dysplasia and limited carcinoma within VC should be termed "hybrid VC" or "invasive well-differentiated SCC with verrucous features".

Differential diagnosis
This includes conventional and papillary SCCs and condyloma acuminatum. Epithelial down-growth extending deeper than the adjacent normal epithelium distinguishes VC from dysplastic lesions with a verrucous morphology, but there are intermediate lesions that are difficult to classify {2151}. The term "verrucous hyperplasia" has been used for some of these lesions, but such lesions lack clear diagnostic criteria {2151}, appear dysplastic rather than hyperplastic, harbour copy-number variation, and carry a risk of malignant transformation {4870}, suggesting they are part of the wider spectrum of dysplastic verrucous lesions {4427}. A lack of substantial atypia distinguishes VC from conventional and papillary SCCs. VC is characterized by a high frequency of initial misdiagnosis {3326,670}. A full-thickness biopsy with adjacent normal epithelium (with sufficient stroma to evaluate for pattern of invasion) and thorough sampling of the specimen is needed to make the diagnosis of VC and to rule out coexisting SCC {2151,1626,1625,4981}.

Cytology
Not clinically relevant

Diagnostic molecular pathology
Not clinically relevant

Essential and desirable diagnostic criteria
Essential: a broad-based, well-differentiated epithelial proliferation with marked papillary parakeratosis, acanthosis, and keratin plugging, extending below the level of adjacent normal epithelium; mitoses limited to basal/parabasal layers; full-thickness biopsy to assess invasion; no or minimal cytological atypia; a pushing, even border without deep invasive growth.
Desirable: examination of the whole tumour to exclude SCC; dense lymphoplasmacytic submucosal chronic inflammation.

Staging
Staging follows the eighth edition of the Union for International Cancer Control (UICC) / American Joint Committee on Cancer (AJCC) TNM staging system.

Prognosis and prediction
VC has an excellent prognosis; the overall 5-year survival rate is 77–86% {132,2348,4682}. Surgery is the treatment of choice; irradiation is less effective but is accepted as an appropriate treatment for some VCs {4400,2134,2348,2363}. VC may be a precursor to SCC, and 20% of oral cavity VCs contain concomitant SCC {2914}. Carcinomas with both patterns behave as SCC. VCs with focal dysplasia and/or minimal invasive SCC (≤ 2 mm in depth) do not adversely affect outcomes and should be treated as VC {3413}.

Carcinoma cuniculatum

Thavaraj S
Bishop JA
Kaplan I
Morgan PR

Definition
Carcinoma cuniculatum (CC) is a rare, well-differentiated, locally destructive, non-metastasizing squamous cell carcinoma type, characterized by a burrowing invasive pattern, keratin-containing crypts, and minimal cytological atypia.

ICD-O coding
8051/3 Carcinoma cuniculatum

ICD-11 coding
2B6E.0 Squamous cell carcinoma of other or ill-defined sites in the lip, oral cavity, or pharynx

Related terminology
Not recommended: epithelioma cuniculatum.

Subtype(s)
None

Localization
The gingivo-alveolar complex of the mandible is the commonest site, followed by that of the maxilla. The tongue, buccal mucosa, and lower lip are rarely affected {1335}.

Clinical features
Pain, swelling, mucosal ulceration, tooth mobility, and induration are common {1335}. The presence of sequestra or yellow keratinaceous discharge from oral or cutaneous fistulae may lead to misdiagnosis as osteomyelitis or abscess {4301, 1431,3358}. Longstanding symptoms in some individuals may reflect diagnostic delay and/or the slow-growing nature of this tumour.

Imaging
On mucoperiosteal sites, CC presents radiologically as an osteolytic lesion with a poorly defined moth-eaten outline {1335}. Sequestration may be evident {4301}.

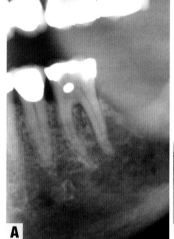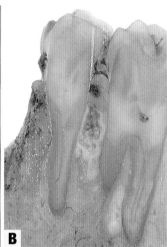

Fig.5.30 Carcinoma cuniculatum. **A** Panoramic radiograph showing a carcinoma cuniculatum in the posterior body of the mandible, producing a moth-eaten partial radiolucency with cortical preservation. The appearance can resemble osteomyelitis, particularly when sequestra are detected radiographically. **B** Macroscopic view of carcinoma cuniculatum infiltrating bone between tooth roots. The white tumour encloses necrotic bone. The apparently separate islands were contiguous in a different plane.

Epidemiology
CC presents most commonly in the seventh and eight decades of life. There is no sex predilection.

Etiology
None

Pathogenesis
The pathogenetic mechanisms are unknown, and there is no association with HPV {123,2396,4401}.

Macroscopic appearance
CC is predominantly endophytic with a white to yellow-white appearance. Infiltrative keratin-filled crypts may be seen.

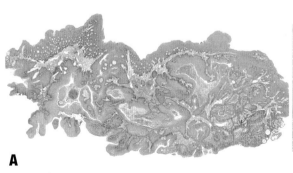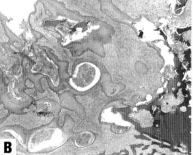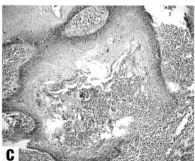

Fig.5.31 Carcinoma cuniculatum. **A** A characteristic infiltrative labyrinthine network of keratin-filled crypts. **B** Bone invasion with microsequestra. **C** No more than mild cytological atypia and keratin microabscess formation.

Histopathology

CC is characterized by a primarily endophytic growth pattern of a burrowing labyrinthine network of well-differentiated squamous epithelium forming interconnecting keratin-filled crypts communicating with the surface. A minor exophytic component may be present. There is no more than mild nuclear atypia. Intraepithelial and stromal neutrophils are abundant, often with keratin microabscesses. Microsequestra are frequently associated with bone invasion.

Differential diagnosis

Non-representative sampling may lead to misdiagnosis as cystic well-differentiated squamous cell carcinoma, verrucous carcinoma, osteomyelitis, odontogenic keratocyst, orthokeratinized odontogenic cyst, or abscess {1335}.

Cytology

Not clinically relevant

Diagnostic molecular pathology

None

Essential and desirable diagnostic criteria

Essential: correlation with imaging; well-differentiated, heavily keratinizing squamous epithelium; mild atypia; a labyrinthine, burrowing, cohesive invasive pattern.

Desirable: keratin microabscesses; stromal neutrophils; microsequestra; bone invasion at mucoperiosteal sites.

Staging

Staging follows the eighth edition of the Union for International Cancer Control (UICC) / American Joint Committee on Cancer (AJCC) TNM staging system.

Prognosis and prediction

The prognosis is excellent after complete excision. Local recurrence is uncommon after correct preoperative diagnosis, and no metastases develop despite multiple interventions {1335}. There are no known predictive factors.

Congenital granular cell epulis

Allon I
Fuller MY
McNamara K

Definition
Congenital granular cell epulis (CGCE) is a rare congenital benign tumour, occurring on the alveolar ridge of the newborn, composed of sheets of cells with abundant granular cytoplasm.

ICD-O coding
None

ICD-11 coding
KC23 Neonatal disorders of the oral mucosa

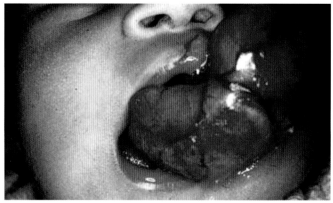

Fig. 5.32 Congenital granular cell epulis. A newborn girl with a sessile lobulated pink mass of the maxillary alveolar process measuring several centimetres in diameter. The mass interferes with feeding.

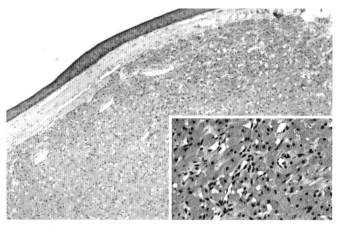

Fig. 5.33 Congenital granular cell epulis. A well-circumscribed lesion beneath an attenuated epithelium that lacks rete ridges. An uninvolved zone of lamina propria separates the lesion from the epithelium. The lesion is composed of tightly packed polygonal cells with abundant granular cytoplasm. Nuclei are eccentric and dark-staining, with inconspicuous nucleoli and no evidence of mitotic activity. Thin-walled vessels are distributed throughout the lesion (**inset**).

Related terminology
Acceptable: congenital epulis; congenital epulis of the newborn; congenital gingival granular cell tumour; Neumann tumour.
Not recommended: congenital granular cell myoblastoma.

Subtype(s)
None

Localization
Most lesions arise on the maxillary anterior alveolar process, with a maxillary-to-mandibular ratio of 2–3:1. As many as 20% are multifocal, and rare extra-alveolar involvement has been reported {3975,4910,4161,5060}.

Clinical features
Patients present with a pedunculated soft tissue mass. Masses range in size from several millimetres to several centimetres. Larger lesions may interfere with feeding and, to a lesser extent, respiration. The mass may sometimes be detected on ultrasonography from gestational week 26 {4975}.

Epidemiology
Newborns are affected with an estimated incidence of 0.0006% {535} and an M:F ratio of 1:7.7 {4161}.

Etiology
The etiology is unknown. CGCE develops primarily during the third trimester of pregnancy, with no relation to any risk factors such as premature delivery, maternal age, or pregnancy status {4161}.

Pathogenesis
The pathogenesis of CGCE is unknown, but it is thought to result from a degenerative metabolic process affecting mesenchymal stem cells {2447,3975,4625}.

Macroscopic appearance
CGCE is a firm soft tissue mass with a pedunculated base. The cut surface is typically tan-yellow, homogeneous, and smooth {2307,831}.

Histopathology
CGCE is a well-circumscribed lesion composed of sheets and nests of tightly packed polygonal cells with abundant granular cytoplasm and well-delineated cell membranes. Nuclei are eccentric and dark, with inconspicuous nucleoli without mitosis. Thin-walled vessels are distributed throughout the lesion. The overlying epithelium is atrophic without rete ridges. In addition, inflammation, odontogenic epithelial rests, fibrosis, and spindle cells may present.

Immunohistochemistry

The granular cells are positive for vimentin, NSE, and laminin; PAS-positive, diastase-resistant; and negative for muscle markers, SOX10, and S100. Histiocytic markers are variably positive {3722}.

Differential diagnosis

The entities include granular cell tumour, which shows S100 and SOX10 positivity and most frequently occurs on the dorsal tongue {5060,840}.

Cytology

Not clinically relevant

Diagnostic molecular pathology

None

Essential and desirable diagnostic criteria

Essential: a soft lump on the maxillary or mandibular alveolar ridge; neonatal presentation; sheets and nests of polygonal cells with eosinophilic, granular cytoplasm.

Desirable: attenuated to atrophic stratified squamous epithelium of uniform thickness; negative reaction for S100.

Staging

Not applicable

Prognosis and prediction

If progressive enlargement is not observed after birth, spontaneous regression may occur, and such lesions should be followed up without excision. Conservative excision is indicated if the tumour interferes with feeding or respiration. Recurrence has not been reported, even with incomplete excision {5060, 4625,98}. Malignant transformation has not been reported.

Granular cell tumour

Allon I
McNamara K

Definition
Granular cell tumour is a neuroectodermal tumour composed of large, round to oval cells with abundant and distinctly eosinophilic granular cytoplasm.

ICD-O coding
9580/0 Granular cell tumour, NOS
9580/3 Granular cell tumour, malignant

ICD-11 coding
2E89.1 & XH09A9 Benign tumours of uncertain differentiation, soft tissue & Granular cell tumour, NOS
2B5F.2 & XH90D3 Sarcoma, not elsewhere classified of other specified sites & Granular cell tumour, malignant

Related terminology
Not recommended: Abrikossoff tumour; granular cell myoblastoma; granular cell schwannoma.

Subtype(s)
None

Localization
Granular cell tumour occurs in any subcutaneous or submucosal site, but of the oral cases about 85% arise in the tongue {4464,2452}.

Clinical features
Patients with granular cell tumour present with a non-tender, slowly enlarging, sessile mucosal to yellowish-coloured submucosal mass, usually < 10 mm in diameter (but they can be as large as 20 mm). Multifocal tumours occur infrequently {3092, 3037,2827}.

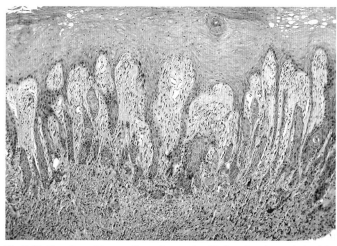

Fig. 5.34 Granular cell tumour. Dramatic pseudoepitheliomatous hyperplasia of the overlying mucosa should not be erroneously interpreted as squamous cell carcinoma, and the unencapsulated mass of granular cells immediately beneath the epithelium should not be overlooked.

Epidemiology
Granular cell tumours can present at any age, but most occur in the fourth to sixth decades of life, with an M:F ratio of 1:3 {2452, 343}.

Etiology
Unknown

Pathogenesis
Sporadic oral granular cell tumours do not contain the *PTPN11* and *PTEN* mutations {1450} associated with granular cell tumours in LEOPARD syndrome (multiple lentigines, electrocardiographic conduction abnormalities, ocular hypertelorism, pulmonic stenosis, abnormal genitalia, retardation of growth, and

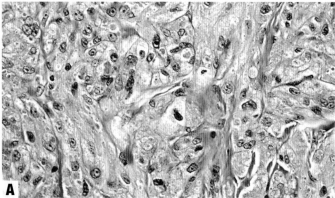
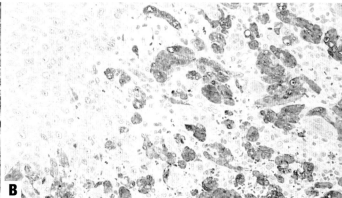

Fig. 5.35 Granular cell tumour. **A** Sheets of large polygonal cells intermingled with skeletal muscle fibres. The cells demonstrate abundant granular cytoplasm and small round nuclei either eccentrically or centrally located. **B** The granular cells are immunoreactive for S100.

sensorineural deafness), Noonan syndrome {3929,3640,327}, and *PTEN* hamartoma tumour syndrome {2825}. Whole-exome sequencing has revealed either mutations in the genes *ATP6AP1*, *ATP6AP2*, and *ATP6V1A* (components of the V-ATPase complex) {3397,1451} or mutations in genes for endosomal/lysosomal/autophagosomal networks {1451}. Overexpression of TFE3 is observed in skin lesions, but not in oral tumours {2686}.

Macroscopic appearance
Granular cell tumour is a pale-tan to yellowish-white homogeneous submucosal nodule on cut surface {2760,343}.

Histopathology
Granular cell tumour is an unencapsulated tumour composed of large polygonal cells with abundant eosinophilic granular cytoplasm and small round nuclei in the subepithelial tissue. Granular cell tumours can grow in a syncytial pattern or be arranged in sheets surrounding and replacing muscle fascicles or nerves. Occasionally, granular cell tumours may be granular cell–poor with extensive fibrosis. Pseudoepitheliomatous hyperplasia of the overlying mucosa is observed in 25–50% of cases {4624,3175}, raising a risk of erroneous diagnosis of squamous cell carcinoma in superficial biopsies. Criteria for malignancy in granular cell tumour include at least three of the following: nuclear pleomorphism, cell spindling, mitotic activity (> 2 mitoses/2 mm^2), prominent nucleoli, a high N:C ratio, and necrosis. Cases meeting one or two of the criteria are classified as atypical {1331A}.

Immunohistochemistry
The tumour cells are immunoreactive for S100, CD57, SOX10, inhibin, and calretinin. CD68 highlights the cytoplasmic granules composed of lysosomes {1760,2760,3120}. A rare non-neural granular cell tumour subtype is S100-negative and shows cell spindling, mitotic activity, rich vascularity, and an absence of pseudoepitheliomatous hyperplasia. Both subtypes are positive for NKI/C3 {3663}.

Differential diagnosis
Granular cell tumour is relatively characteristic, but the differential diagnosis of other granular cell lesions is aided by immunohistochemistry {2760,3037}.

Cytology
Smears are usually cellular, with sheets of large cells with usually central, round to mildly pleomorphic nuclei and abundant granular cytoplasm, as well as a small number of single cells often resembling histiocytes, in a granular background {1401A}.

Diagnostic molecular pathology
None

Essential and desirable diagnostic criteria
Essential: neoplastic sheets and nests of granular cells.
Desirable: pseudoepitheliomatous hyperplasia; S100 positivity.

Staging
Not relevant

Prognosis and prediction
Recurrence is rare after excision, even when the tumour is incompletely excised {2452,4624,3175,3092}. Malignant granular cell tumour is associated with metastases and poor survival {2388}.

Ectomesenchymal chondromyxoid tumour

Dickson BC
Koutlas IG

Definition

Ectomesenchymal chondromyxoid tumour (EMCMT) is a mesenchymal neoplasm characterized by spindle to polygonal cells within a myxoid to collagenous stroma and usually harbouring a *RREB1::MRTFB* fusion.

ICD-O coding

8982/0 Ectomesenchymal chondromyxoid tumour

ICD-11 coding

None

Related terminology

Not recommended: reticulated myxoid tumour.

Subtype(s)

None

Localization

EMCMT occurs in the tongue, particularly in the anterior dorsal aspect {4143,96,234,1128}. Less common locations include the palate {1666,4501} and mandible {610}.

Clinical features

Patients with EMCMT have a slow-growing, painless mass, with a duration ranging from months to years {4143}.

Epidemiology

There are < 100 reported cases in the English literature. EMCMTs occur over a broad age range, but most commonly in young adults. There is no sex predilection {4143,96,234,1128}.

Etiology

Unknown

Pathogenesis

Approximately 90% of tumours are defined by the fusion of *RREB1* to *MRTFB* (*MKL2*). This fusion product has molecular pleiotropy and is not disease-specific; it has been reported in other tumours, including biphenotypic sinonasal sarcoma {2913}, mediastinal mesenchymal neoplasms {2803}, and oropharyngeal sarcoma {4060}. A minority of cases may have alternate molecular drivers, including *EWSR1* {234,1128}.

Macroscopic appearance

Tumours are generally circumscribed, lobulated, and range from 5 to 30 mm in diameter {4143,1128}. On cut section they may be grey, tan, and/or yellow {4143}.

Histopathology

EMCMTs have a broad morphological spectrum. They are frequently multilobulated and comprise cells arranged in sheets, fascicles, and/or reticular patterns. Less commonly they may be microcytic to cystic, or papillary {4143,1128}. The margins are well demarcated but usually unencapsulated, with incorporation of surrounding muscle fibres at the periphery {4143,96,1128}. The cells range from spindle to stellate to polygonal, with variable eosinophilic cytoplasm and round to ovoid, monomorphic nuclei. Occasional atypia, binucleation, and pseudonuclear inclusions may be identified. Mitotic activity is usually inconspicuous. The intervening stroma may be myxoid to collagenous, and focally hyaline {4143,96,1128}.

Immunohistochemistry

Immunohistochemistry reveals polyphenotypic differentiation. Most tumours have diffuse expression of GFAP. Other stains, such as S100, desmin, SMA, myogenin, CD56, CD57, keratin, and EMA, are typically patchy and weak {4143,1128}.

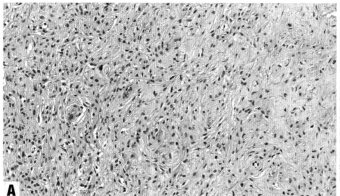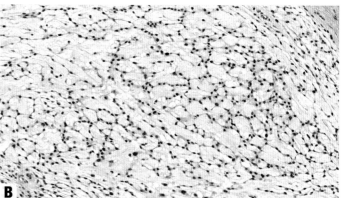

Fig. 5.36 Ectomesenchymal chondromyxoid tumour. **A** Spindle cells arranged in loose fascicles and whorls, with myxohyaline stroma. **B** Stellate cells with a reticular pattern and abundant myxoid stroma.

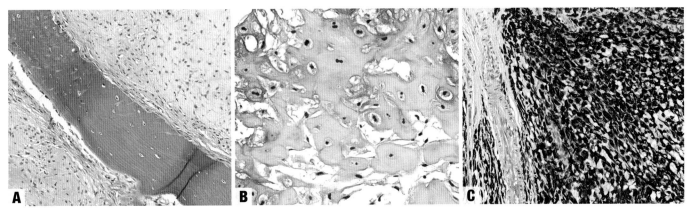

Fig. 5.37 Ectomesenchymal chondromyxoid tumour. **A** Locally aggressive features, such as bone involvement, are uncommon. **B** Hyaline cartilage matrix is paradoxically rare and, when present, is typically only focal. **C** Most tumours express GFAP.

Cytology
Not clinically relevant

Diagnostic molecular pathology
The presence of a *RREB1::MRTFB* gene fusion, in the appropriate context, may be diagnostically helpful.

Essential and desirable diagnostic criteria
Essential: sheets, cords, and/or a reticular arrangement of spindle to stellate to polygonal cells; variable stroma that may be myxoid, hyaline, or collagenous.
Desirable: consistent immunohistochemistry.

Staging
Not clinically relevant

Prognosis and prediction
Most tumours have an indolent clinical course, with occasional local recurrence {4143,3573}. Rarely, tumours may be locally aggressive {610}.

Melanotic neuroectodermal tumour of infancy

Prasad ML
Alaggio R
Sloan P
Thompson LDR

Definition
Melanotic neuroectodermal tumour of infancy (MNTI) is a biphasic tumour of small neuroblast-like cells and larger melanin-producing epithelial cells.

ICD-O coding
9363/1 Melanotic neuroectodermal tumour, NOS
9363/3 Melanotic neuroectodermal tumour, malignant

ICD-11 coding
2D42 & XH6C72 Malignant neoplasms of ill-defined sites & Melanotic neuroectodermal tumour

Related terminology
Not recommended: melanotic progonoma; retinal anlage tumour.

Subtype(s)
None

Localization
More than 90% of MNTIs occur in the craniofacial bones, most commonly affecting the maxilla (> 60%), followed by the skull (~15%) and mandible (~8%) {1511,3627,3065,3682}. Rarely, tumours develop in the genital tract, trunk, and extremities {128, 3627,1315}.

Clinical features
Typically, patients present with a sessile, painless, rapidly enlarging mass in the upper alveolus, causing facial deformity and feeding disruption. The mass is usually bluish-black owing to its melanin content. Some tumours produce circulating vanillylmandelic acid (VMA; 34%) and AFP {3627,3065,882}.

Imaging
Imaging shows destruction of cortical bone with entrapment of developing tooth buds and extension into the sinus, nasal cavity, or orbit {3172}.

Epidemiology
This rare tumour usually affects infants aged 3–6 months, although it has been diagnosed in utero, at birth, in older children, and in adults. There is a slight male predilection {1511, 3627,3065,882,3682}.

Etiology
Unknown

Pathogenesis
MNTI is thought to be of neural crest cell origin, and the pathogenesis is unknown {882}. MNTI shows morphological similarity to melanotic medulloblastoma, and more recently it has been shown to share a DNA methylation profile with high-grade medulloblastoma (MB G3) despite its low-grade behaviour {1209,2714}. Germline mutations in CDKN2A and somatic BRAF p.V600E pathogenic sequence variants are also reported {1640,344}.

Macroscopic appearance
Tumours are pigmented and firm, unencapsulated, and lobulated, without necrosis or ulceration. The mean size is 30 mm, but they may be as large as 200 mm, with larger tumours in the skull {3627,3213,882,3682}.

Histopathology
Tumour cells are arranged in alveolar nests, cords, and trabeculae, infiltrating into dense vascularized, fibrocollagenous stroma. Melanotic epithelial cells typically surround small neuroblast-like cells and may form tubuloglandular structures {1511}. The small cells may rarely produce a neurofibrillary matrix

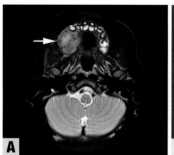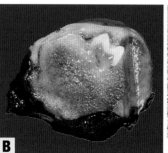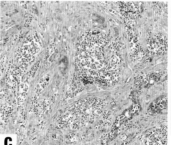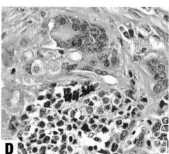

Fig. 5.38 Melanotic neuroectodermal tumour of infancy. **A** This CT image shows a large jaw mass expanding into the soft tissues (arrow). **B** A tooth is incorporated into the tumour mass. Note the blue-black pigmentation. **C** Aggregates of tumour cells separated by fibrous stroma. There are small blue cells, with larger epithelial cells at the periphery, some of which contain melanin pigment. **D** High-power view of the small neuroblast-like cells with hyperchromatic nuclei and scant cytoplasm associated with larger epithelial cells with vesicular nuclei and cytoplasmic pigment.

{3065}. The tumour frequently destructively infiltrates bone and contains entrapped odontogenic tissue. Mitoses and necrosis are generally absent.

Immunohistochemistry

Immunohistochemistry is seldom necessary for diagnosis. Both small and large tumour cells express vimentin and synaptophysin but are typically negative for chromogranin, neurofilaments, S100, and desmin. The large cells coexpress pancytokeratin, HMB45, and melan-A, confirming dual epithelial and melanocytic features, but are negative for other melanoma markers. Rarely, membranous expression of CD99, as well as focal rhabdomyoblastic and glial differentiation, may be seen {1511,1243, 3517,3065}.

Differential diagnosis

This includes other malignant small blue round cell tumours, usually with worse prognoses, such as Ewing sarcoma, rhabdomyosarcoma, and lymphoma. However, these alternatives lack the characteristic biphasic melanin-producing, keratin-positive epithelial cells and the synaptophysin-positive neuroblast-like cells.

Cytology

Smears are cellular with discrete, biphasic populations of tumour cells comprising monomorphic small cells with scant cytoplasm and round nuclei with fine chromatin, and large epithelioid cells with vesicular nuclei and intracytoplasmic melanin pigment {128,1621,2217}.

Diagnostic molecular pathology

Not clinically relevant

Essential and desirable diagnostic criteria

Essential: biphasic appearance with small neuroblast-like cells and large melanotic epithelial cells arranged in lobules separated by a fibrocollagenous stroma.
Desirable: patient aged < 1 year; jaw location; bone destruction; epithelial cells positive for keratin and HMB45.

Staging

Not clinically relevant

Prognosis and prediction

MNTI is a rapidly growing, locally destructive, paradoxically low-grade tumour of uncertain malignant potential. Approximately 20–30% of tumours recur, usually within 6 months {1511, 3065,882,3570,3697}, especially in patients aged < 5 months at diagnosis {3627,882}. Approximately 2% of MNTIs behave in a malignant fashion, with metastases of the neuroblast-like cells, and result in death {882}. Predictive factors are not well defined {3065}, but larger tumours, which usually affect the skull, have a worse prognosis {3213,3682}.

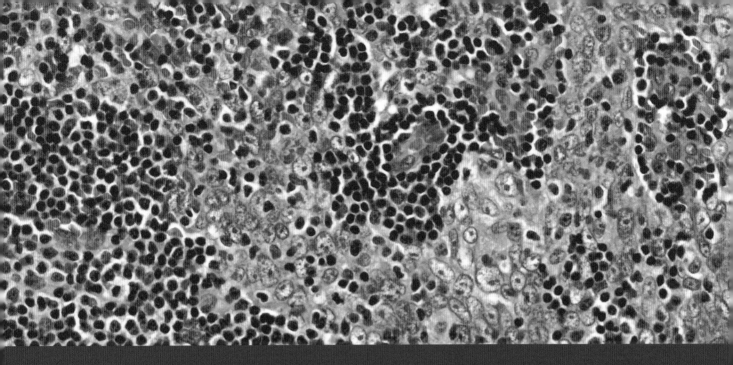

6

Oropharyngeal tumours

Edited by: Lewis JS Jr, Thompson LDR

Oropharyngeal tumours: Introduction

Lewis JS Jr
Bishop JA

The oropharynx comprises the palatine tonsils, soft palate, base of tongue (posterior to the circumvallate papillae), and lateral and posterior pharyngeal walls. It is an anatomical site rich in lymphoid tissue and harbouring the anatomically unique reticulated tonsillar crypt epithelium, is one of the major head and neck sites of virus-related carcinogenesis. The vast majority of oropharyngeal malignancies are squamous cell carcinoma (SCC), and almost all SCC subtypes occur here {1649}. It is now well established that a high fraction of all SCC cases, particularly those in the USA, Canada, and parts of northern Europe (but also to a lesser extent in most of the rest of the world) are driven by transcriptionally active high-risk HPV {700}. There is uniform agreement on the prognostic benefit of positive HPV status in these patients, and entirely specific staging systems from the International Collaboration on Cancer Reporting (ICCR), Union for International Cancer Control (UICC), and American Joint Committee on Cancer (AJCC) have been developed for them {2743}. These distinctions render the pathologist and p16/HPV testing critical in routine practice. To acknowledge this unique and extremely important tumour type, while drawing a clear distinction from SCC of the oral cavity, larynx, nasopharynx, and sinonasal tract, the fourth edition of the WHO classification of head and neck tumours created a separate chapter for the oropharynx, which has been retained in the current edition (topographically including the tonsils, base of the tongue, soft palate, uvula, and posterior wall).

Several topics are not duplicated in this chapter, even though the entities develop in the oropharynx with some regularity. Squamous papilloma is discussed in the chapters on laryngeal tumours (see *Squamous papilloma and papillomatosis*, p. 129) and oral cavity tumours (see *Squamous papilloma*, p. 261), pleomorphic adenoma and other salivary gland tumours are discussed in the chapter on salivary gland tumours (see *Pleomorphic adenoma*, p. 167), and extranodal lymphomas and haematopoietic tumours that develop in the Waldeyer ring are discussed in Chapter 10: *Haematolymphoid proliferations and neoplasia*. Neuroendocrine neoplasms (NENs; especially carcinomas), many HPV-associated, are discussed in the respective NEN sections (see Chapter 15: *Neuroendocrine neoplasms and paraganglioma*). Finally, a new section is included on hamartomatous polyps, a rare type of tonsillar tumour (*Hamartomatous polyps*, p. 297).

Hamartomatous polyps

Nelson BL
Altemani AM
Mehrad M

Definition

Hamartomatous polyps are lesions associated with the palatine tonsils composed of a haphazard proliferation of elements that are normally found in the oropharynx.

ICD-O coding

None

ICD-11 coding

DB35.3 Hamartomatous polyp

Related terminology

Acceptable: lymphangiectatic fibrous polyp; fibrovascular polyp; polypoid lymphangioma; papillary lymphoid polyp; benign hamartomatous polyp; lymphangiectatic fibrolipomatous polyp.

Not recommended: tonsillar lipoma.

Subtype(s)

None

Localization

Palatine tonsil

Clinical features

Patients with hamartomatous polyp may have dysphagia, sore throat, globus, or obstructive symptoms. Lesions may be present for weeks to years. The entity appears as a unilateral polypoid mass and may be clinically worrisome for a neoplasm {2189,1113,3014}.

Epidemiology

Hamartomas are rare, accounting ≤ 2% of all tonsillar tumours. Lymphangiectatic fibrous polyps account for the overwhelming majority of hamartomas. Even lesions with a predominance of lymphoid tissue (lymphoid polyp) and those with prominent adipose tissue (fibrolipomatous polyp) are thought to potentially belong to the overall spectrum of lymphangiectatic fibrous polyps. The age range of patients affected is broad (3–63 years, median: 25.5 years), and there is no sex predilection {2189,265, 355}.

Etiology

Unknown

Pathogenesis

Unknown

Macroscopic appearance

Hamartomatous polyp is a polypoid, often pedunculated, mucosal surface mass. The size is variable, ranging from very small to as large as 80 mm {2189,355}.

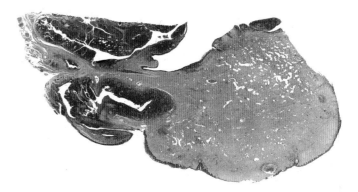

Fig. 6.01 Lymphangiectatic fibrous polyp. Low-power image shows the lymphoid and fibrous component.

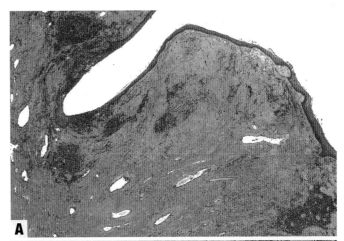

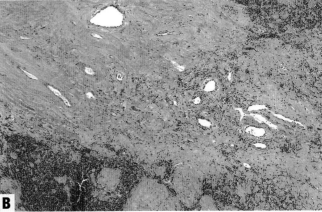

Fig. 6.02 Lymphangiectatic fibrous polyp – hamartoma. **A,B** Polypoid tumour from the palatine tonsil, with fibrous stroma and dilated vasculature intermixed with normal lymphoid stroma.

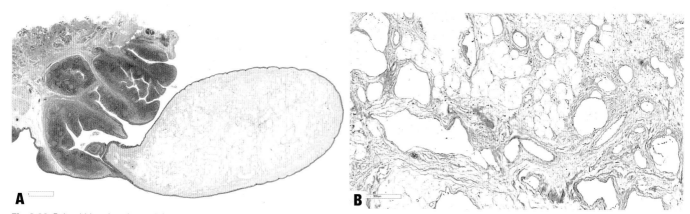

Fig. 6.03 Polypoid lymphangioma. **A** Low-power image shows the lymphoid and dilated vascular channels. **B** High-power image shows numerous small to medium-sized dilated vascular channels.

Histopathology

The lymphangiectatic fibrous polyp has numerous small to medium-sized dilated vascular channels containing proteinaceous fluid with lymphocytes. The overlying mucosa is generally intact, displaying respiratory or squamous epithelium without dysplasia. Small collections of intraepithelial lymphocytes can be seen. The stroma is variable and may consist of fibrous and lymphoid tissue. Adipose tissue and muscle may also be seen, in lesions termed "fibrolipomatous polyp" {2189}.

Cytology

Not applicable

Diagnostic molecular pathology

Not applicable

Essential and desirable diagnostic criteria

Essential: a polypoid tumour of the palatine tonsils; a submucosal proliferation of lymphovascular channels containing proteinaceous fluid with lymphocytes, in a background of lymphoid or connective tissue.

Staging

Not applicable

Prognosis and prediction

Recurrence is rare after surgical treatment. However, without treatment, the airway may become critically obstructed {2189}.

Squamous cell carcinoma, HPV-associated

Westra W
Badoual C
Bishop JA
Chernock RD
Faquin WC

Fujii S
Robinson M
Rooper LM
Yamamoto H

Definition

HPV-associated oropharyngeal squamous cell carcinoma (OPSCC) is a malignant epithelial tumour with squamous differentiation, caused by transcriptionally active high-risk HPV and usually arising from the tonsillar crypts.

ICD-O coding

8085/3 Squamous cell carcinoma, HPV-associated

8085/3 Non-keratinizing squamous cell carcinoma, HPV-associated

8085/3 Keratinizing squamous cell carcinoma, HPV-associated

8085/3 Papillary squamous cell carcinoma, HPV-associated

8085/3 Adenosquamous carcinoma, HPV-associated

8085/3 Ciliated adenosquamous carcinoma, HPV-associated

8085/3 Lymphoepithelial carcinoma, HPV-associated

8085/3 Spindle cell / sarcomatoid squamous cell carcinoma, HPV-associated

8085/3 Basaloid squamous cell carcinoma, HPV-associated

ICD-11 coding

2B6A.0 & XH0EJ7 Squamous cell carcinoma of oropharynx & Squamous cell carcinoma, HPV-positive

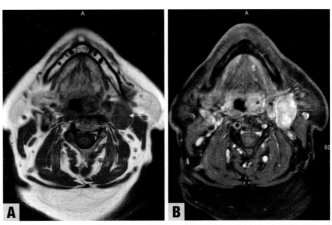

Fig. 6.04 Squamous cell carcinoma, HPV-associated. T1-weighted axial MRI (**A**) and T1-weighted, postcontrast, fat-suppressed/saturated axial MRI (**B**) showing a well-defined exophytic and enhancing soft tissue lesion of the left palatine tonsil (red arrows) with a metastatic, partially necrotic, level II lymph node (yellow arrows).

Related terminology

Acceptable: HPV-positive squamous cell carcinoma; HPV-related squamous cell carcinoma; p16-positive squamous cell carcinoma.

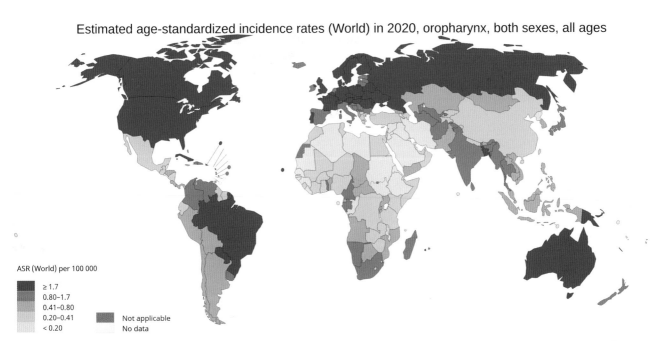

Estimated age-standardized incidence rates (World) in 2020, oropharynx, both sexes, all ages

ASR (World) per 100 000

- ≥ 1.7
- 0.80–1.7
- 0.41–0.80
- 0.20–0.41
- < 0.20
- Not applicable
- No data

Data source: GLOBOCAN 2020
Graph production: IARC
(http://gco.iarc.fr/today)
World Health Organization

World Health Organization

© International Agency for Research on Cancer 2021

Fig. 6.05 Squamous cell carcinoma, HPV-associated. Estimated age-standardized incidence rates (ASRs, World Standard Population), per 100 000 person-years, of oropharyngeal squamous cell carcinoma in 2020 among both sexes (all ages).

Chapter 6

Table 6.01 Comparison of HPV-associated and HPV-independent oropharyngeal squamous cell carcinoma (SCC)

Characteristics	HPV-associated	HPV-independent
Incidence trend	Increasing	Decreasing
Age	Younger (~3–4 years)	Older
Risk factors	Number of oral sex partners +/– smoking	Smoking +/– alcohol
Stage	Small primary, large nodal metastases	Variable
Site of origin	Crypt epithelium of palatine and lingual tonsils	Surface epithelium
Precancerous lesion	Not recognized	Squamous dysplasia
Predominant morphology	Non-keratinizing SCC	Keratinizing (conventional) SCC
Grading	Not applicable	Applicable
p16 immunostaining	Almost always positive	Typically negative
Survival	Better overall and progression-free survival	Worse overall and progression-free survival

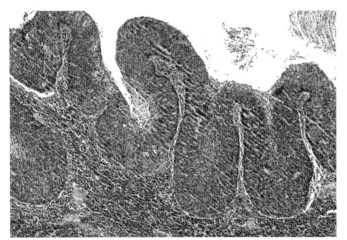

Fig. 6.06 Squamous cell carcinoma, HPV-associated. Oropharyngeal. Extensive surface growth mimicking an in situ process.

Subtype(s)

Non-keratinizing squamous cell carcinoma, HPV-associated; keratinizing squamous cell carcinoma, HPV-associated; papillary squamous cell carcinoma, HPV-associated; adenosquamous carcinoma, HPV-associated; ciliated adenosquamous carcinoma, HPV-associated; lymphoepithelial carcinoma, HPV-associated; spindle cell / sarcomatoid squamous cell carcinoma, HPV-associated; basaloid squamous cell carcinoma, HPV-associated

Localization

HPV-associated OPSCC arises from the tonsillar-bearing regions of the oropharynx (i.e. the lingual and palatine tonsils), where it takes origin from the specialized squamous epithelium lining the tonsillar crypts {1561}.

Clinical features

Patients may present with clinical signs related to local tumour effects, but most present with small primary tumours that have metastasized to the upper and mid jugular chain lymph nodes (levels II and III). Painless cervical lymphadenopathy is the most common presentation {2906}. HPV-associated OPSCC imaging differs from HPV-independent OPSCC imaging in that primary tumours are more commonly enhancing and exophytic, with well-defined margins. Patients also more commonly present with multiple positive nodes, and the metastases are more commonly cystic (see Table 6.01) {1631,657}.

Epidemiology

The incidence of HPV-associated OPSCC has risen over the past four decades globally, and particularly in North America and northern Europe. Patients with HPV-associated OPSCC are typically male (M:F ratio: 4:1), White, and of higher socioeconomic

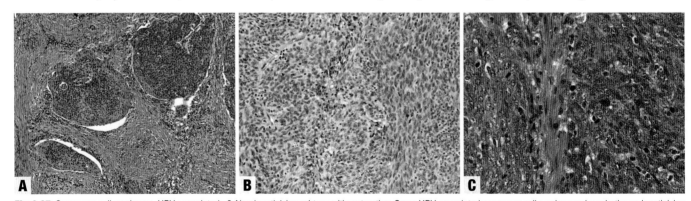

Fig. 6.07 Squamous cell carcinoma, HPV-associated. **A** Non-keratinizing subtype with maturation. Some HPV-associated squamous cell carcinomas have both non-keratinizing and keratinizing areas, which frequently show an unusual pattern of reverse maturation, where the keratinizing areas are peripheral with artefactual clefting. **B** Non-keratinizing subtype. This non-keratinizing HPV-associated squamous cell carcinoma has large nests with smooth edges in a lymphoid stroma and with tumour cells with high N:C ratios and round to oval nuclei. **C** Non-keratinizing subtype. Nests of cells with round to spindled, hyperchromatic nuclei, with abundant mitosis and apoptosis.

status. Over time, the prevalence of HPV in OPSCC has been increasing among older adults, causing an upward shift in the median patient age to 55–58 years and closing the age gap with HPV-independent OPSCC {3688,4832}.

Etiology

HPV-associated OPSCC is caused by high-risk HPV, with type 16 responsible for approximately 90% of all cases {2868}. Sexual behaviour is an established risk factor, with the lifetime number of oral sex partners as the most strongly associated factor {1181,1812,1591}. Individuals with HPV-associated OPSCC are less likely than patients with HPV-independent OPSCC to be smokers (see Table 6.01). However, a history of tobacco smoking is present in 60–75% of patients, and about 25% of patients are active smokers at presentation. Tobacco smoking is associated with a significantly higher risk of oral HPV infection and therefore may play a role in the progression from oral HPV infection to OPSCC {1320}.

Pathogenesis

HPV oncoproteins E6 and E7 inactivate p53 and RB1 by targeting them for protein degradation. The role of other viral oncoproteins, such as E5, is less clear, but they may play a role in escaping immunosurveillance {357}.

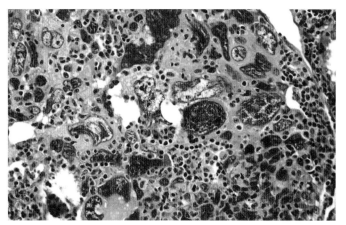

Fig. 6.08 Squamous cell carcinoma, HPV-associated. Example with nuclear anaplasia. Some HPV-associated squamous cell carcinomas show areas of tumour cell multinucleation and extreme nuclear pleomorphism, although this is not of clear prognostic significance.

Macroscopic appearance

The appearance of primary tumours is highly variable, ranging from small and imperceptible to occasionally large and bulky. Lymph node metastases are often large and cystic.

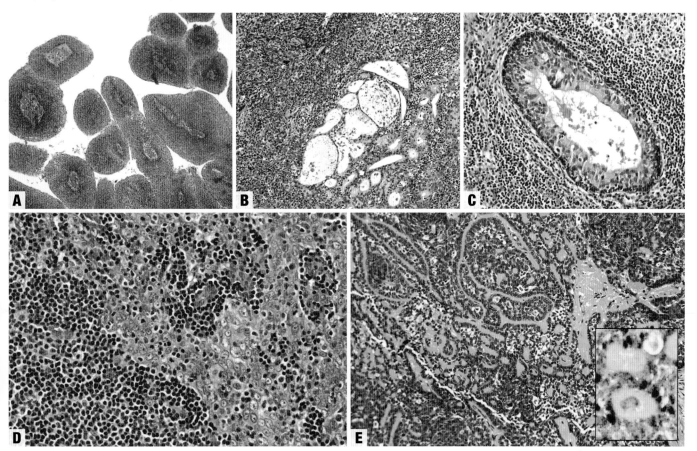

Fig. 6.09 Squamous cell carcinoma, HPV-associated. **A** Papillary subtype. This tumour shows prominent papillary surface growth, with papillae lined by non-keratinizing epithelium. **B** Oropharyngeal carcinoma, HPV-associated. Adenosquamous subtype. HPV-associated oropharyngeal carcinoma exhibiting a non-keratinizing squamous cell component and a glandular component. **C** Ciliated adenosquamous subtype. Rare HPV-associated carcinomas can have glands with cilia, seen here with rounded, smooth lumina and cells with terminal bar formation and prominent cilia. **D** Lymphoepithelial subtype. The tumour shows lymphoepithelial features including syncytial cytoplasm, vesicular nuclei with prominent central nucleoli, and an associated lymphoplasmacytic infiltrate. **E** Basaloid subtype. HPV detection (**inset:** DNA in situ hybridization) is needed to distinguish these tumours from the more aggressive basaloid variant of HPV-independent squamous cell carcinoma.

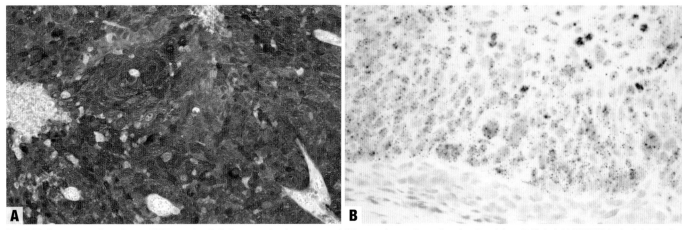

Fig. 6.10 Squamous cell carcinoma, HPV-associated. **A** A tumour showing strong and diffuse nuclear and cytoplasmic p16 staining. **B** High-risk HPV RNA in situ hybridization is positive in this HPV-associated carcinoma showing punctate, granular nuclear and cytoplasmic staining.

Histopathology

The histological progression through the sequential stages of surface dysplasia culminating in carcinoma in situ and invasive growth that characterizes HPV-independent squamous cell carcinoma (SCC) is not evident for HPV-associated OPSCC. Instead, tumours originate from the tonsillar crypts and infiltrate beneath the surface epithelium, growing as nests and lobules, often with central necrosis. Invasive growth may not elicit a desmoplastic stromal reaction, and because the reticulated tonsillar crypt epithelium is a poor barrier to spread, SCC adjacent to organized lymphoid tissue can metastasize, despite appearing histologically only in situ. The tumour nests tend to be surrounded by a lymphoid stroma that may permeate the tumour lobules. In the typical tumour, the tumour cells display high N:C ratios, oval to spindled nuclei, and syncytial cytoplasm (indistinct cell borders) without intercellular bridges, and they usually lack significant cytoplasmic keratinization. These cellular features are termed "non-keratinizing SCC". Histological grading has been shown to lack prognostic utility and is not advocated. Some tumours may show nuclear anaplasia or multinucleation {2598,3047}.

The morphological spectrum of HPV-associated OPSCC also includes subtypes with papillary {2922}, adenosquamous {2867}, ciliated adenosquamous {485}, lymphoepithelial (undifferentiated) {4089}, sarcomatoid / spindle cell {476}, and basaloid features {396}. The clinical behaviour of these subtypes mirrors that of HPV-associated OPSCC with typical morphology. HPV-associated neuroendocrine carcinomas (NECs) (i.e. small cell and large cell NECs) can arise in the oropharynx, sometimes in association with an HPV-associated OPSCC {4407,4798,527}. Despite the presence of HPV, NECs have aggressive clinical behaviour necessitating distinction from HPV-associated OPSCC (see the sections on neuroendocrine carcinomas). Recognition of a high-grade neuroendocrine component is facilitated by immunohistochemistry showing absent or diminished expression of the squamous markers p63 and p40 and positive expression of neuroendocrine markers (synaptophysin, chromogranin, INSM1).

Cytology

FNABs of metastatic lesions show cohesive and more loosely arranged tissue fragments of cells with scant cytoplasm and hyperchromatic nuclei without prominent nucleoli. A cystic component of inflammatory cells and keratinized debris is common. Because of cystic degeneration and possibly fixation effects in cytology preparations, p16 immunostaining of cell blocks is not always reliable for determining HPV status of the tumour {332,1254}.

Diagnostic molecular pathology

Diffuse (nuclear and cytoplasmic) immunohistochemical staining for p16 that is of moderate to strong intensity is a highly reliable surrogate marker for high-risk HPV and is widely advocated as a standalone test for determining HPV status of primary and metastatic SCCs of oropharyngeal origin {2591}. In some scenarios, direct HPV detection assays (e.g. RNA/DNA in situ hybridization and/or PCR) may be appropriate, such as when required by clinical trials, in geographical regions with a low overall HPV-attributable fraction, when p16 immunostaining is equivocal, or when there is a discrepancy between p16 staining and morphology (e.g. p16-positive keratinizing SCC) {1253}.

Essential and desirable diagnostic criteria

Essential: SCC (usually non-keratinizing); positivity for high-risk HPV as determined by surrogate marker p16 immunohistochemistry alone (70% nuclear and cytoplasmic cut-off point) or by p16 immunohistochemistry plus HPV-specific testing.

Desirable: p40/p63 (positive) and neuroendocrine marker (negative) immunohistochemistry (in selected cases).

Staging

Staging follows the eighth edition of the Union for International Cancer Control (UICC) / American Joint Committee on Cancer (AJCC) TNM staging system. OPSCC staging is predicated upon p16/HPV status.

Prognosis and prediction

Patients with HPV-associated OPSCC have significantly better survival outcomes than those with HPV-independent OPSCC (see Table 6.01, p. 300). Approximately 20% of patients experience disease recurrence after treatment, with 3- and 5-year overall survival rates of 86% and 80%, respectively {3334}. The favourable prognosis may be tempered by the adverse effects of active cigarette smoking {1322,200}.

Squamous cell carcinoma, HPV-independent

Chernock RD
Badoual C
Kiss K
Thavaraj S
Westra W
Yamamoto H

Definition

HPV-independent oropharyngeal squamous cell carcinoma (OPSCC) is a malignant epithelial tumour with squamous differentiation that lacks transcriptionally active HPV.

ICD-O coding

8086/3 Squamous cell carcinoma, HPV-independent
8086/3 Keratinizing squamous cell carcinoma, HPV-independent
8086/3 Verrucous carcinoma, HPV-independent
8086/3 Basaloid squamous cell carcinoma, HPV-independent
8086/3 Papillary squamous cell carcinoma, HPV-independent
8086/3 Spindle cell / sarcomatoid squamous cell carcinoma, HPV-independent
8086/3 Adenosquamous carcinoma, HPV-independent
8086/3 Lymphoepithelial carcinoma, HPV-independent

ICD-11 coding

2B6A.0 & XH4CR9 Squamous cell carcinoma of oropharynx & Squamous cell carcinoma, keratinizing, NOS

Related terminology

Acceptable: HPV-negative or p16-negative squamous cell carcinoma.

Subtype(s)

Keratinizing squamous cell carcinoma, HPV-independent; verrucous carcinoma, HPV-independent; basaloid squamous cell carcinoma, HPV-independent; papillary squamous cell carcinoma, HPV-independent; spindle cell / sarcomatoid squamous cell carcinoma, HPV-independent; adenosquamous carcinoma, HPV-independent; lymphoepithelial carcinoma, HPV-independent

Localization

HPV-independent OPSCC is more common in tonsillar sites than in non-tonsillar sites, but it represents a much greater fraction of non-tonsillar OPSCCs, because HPV-associated tumours predominate in tonsillar tissue {2840,1561,686}. Most non-tonsillar tumours are located in the soft palate.

Clinical features

Patients typically present with pain / sore throat, dysphagia, and/or a neck mass {4220,686}.

Epidemiology

Patients are slightly older and less likely to be male and White than patients with HPV-positive OPSCC {4220}. Recent data indicate that the age differences between HPV-independent and HPV-associated OPSCC may be decreasing {4832,4486}.

Etiology

HPV-independent OPSCC is caused by tobacco use and alcohol use, which have a synergistic effect. See also the discussion of squamous cell carcinomas in Chapter 3: *Hypopharyngeal, laryngeal, tracheal, and parapharyngeal tumours* and Chapter 5: *Oral cavity and mobile tongue tumours*.

Pathogenesis

HPV-independent OPSCC is caused by the accumulation of DNA damage in surface mucosa from exposure to carcinogens, mainly from tobacco and alcohol use. *TP53* is commonly mutated (see Chapter 3: *Hypopharyngeal, laryngeal, tracheal, and parapharyngeal tumours* and Chapter 5: *Oral cavity and mobile tongue tumours*). Hypoxia signatures may be increased compared with HPV-independent squamous cell carcinoma at other head and neck sites {2288}.

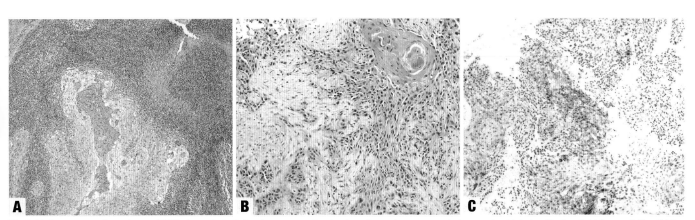

Fig. 6.11 Squamous cell carcinoma, HPV-independent. **A** Carcinomas usually arise from the surface mucosa but may extend into tonsillar lymphoid tissue. **B** Keratinizing subtype. The tumour shows irregular, angulated nests of cells with dense, eosinophilic cytoplasm with rare keratin pearls and associated desmoplastic stromal reaction. **C** Keratinizing subtype, p16-negative. Immunohistochemistry for p16 shows that the tumour cells have only patchy, moderate-intensity reactivity in much less than 70% of tumour cells, a negative result (as a surrogate of high-risk HPV).

Macroscopic appearance

Primary tumours are larger (higher T stage) and nodal disease burden is lower than in HPV-associated OPSCC {4220}.

Histopathology

Most tumours exhibit a keratinizing morphology {1248,813}. Therefore, tumour nests are infiltrative and angulated, and often surrounded by prominent stromal desmoplasia. The cells are polygonal with distinct cell borders. Squamous maturation, including keratinization and intercellular bridges, is usually present. Other squamous cell carcinoma subtypes are rare (for descriptions, see Chapter 3: *Hypopharyngeal, laryngeal, tracheal, and parapharyngeal tumours).* Tumours are traditionally graded as well, moderately, or poorly differentiated, on the basis of their resemblance to normal squamous epithelium. Well-differentiated OPSCC may be difficult to distinguish from benign mucosa, whereas poorly differentiated OPSCC may require immunohistochemistry (p40/p63 and CK5/6) to confirm a squamous epithelial origin {476}. Surface squamous dysplasia is often present in the background, similar to in other head and neck sites (see *Laryngeal and hypopharyngeal epithelial dysplasia*, p. 132, and *Oral epithelial dysplasia*, p. 272).

Cytology

Smears of neck metastases show keratinizing squamous cell carcinoma with polygonal to spindle to tadpole cells showing dense sky-blue (Giemsa stain) to dark-green to orangeophilic (Pap) cytoplasm. Considerable keratinized debris and necrosis is usually present, with a granulomatous inflammatory reaction in some cases. Occasional cases have features that overlap with non-keratinizing squamous cell carcinoma.

Diagnostic molecular pathology

Transcriptionally active HPV is absent. p16 is typically not over-expressed but can be positive in a small subset {3169,2096, 4043}.

Essential and desirable diagnostic criteria

Essential: squamous cell carcinoma (usually keratinizing); negative HPV status (p16 negativity, using a nuclear and cytoplasmic cut-off point of 70% as an acceptable surrogate).

Staging

Staging follows the eighth edition of the Union for International Cancer Control (UICC) / American Joint Committee on Cancer (AJCC) TNM staging system.

Prognosis and prediction

The 3-year overall and progression-free survival rates are 55–60% and 40–45%, respectively {200}. The number of positive lymph nodes and presence of extranodal extension may be prognostic {3539,1886}.

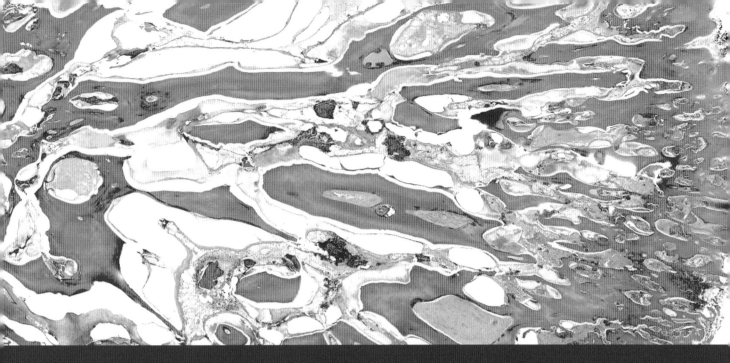

7

Odontogenic and maxillofacial bone tumours

Edited by: Muller S, Odell EW, Tilakaratne WM

Odontogenic and maxillofacial bone tumours: Introduction

Odell EW
Muller S

The principles of the classification of individual odontogenic cysts, odontogenic tumours, and tumours of the jaws are unchanged from previous editions of the WHO classification of head and neck tumours, but there has been a major reorganization. The classification now follows the new WHO classification structure, in which more aggressive lesions appear at the end of each chapter. New definitions of what should constitute an entity and subtype have required several changes, and the bone-related lesions have been more logically divided into fibro-osseous tumours and dysplasias, benign neoplasms, and malignant neoplasms.

The relatively short time since the last edition has resulted in only one completely novel entity being included. However, several other conditions that have been established in the literature for long periods are new to the WHO classification. The rationale for adding these conditions varies. Some, such as the cysts, are included for completeness of classification. Others are included to prevent misdiagnosis as conditions with different treatment or clinical implications. For some, the intention has been to propose consensus definitions and clear diagnostic criteria because the descriptions in the literature are heterogeneous. Although a consensus has been achieved on these diagnostic criteria, they must be regarded as proposals to be tested, and they may need to be adapted in future editions. Differentiating these poorly defined lesions will be critical in selecting them for molecular analysis and interpreting the data.

Since the last edition, there has been a marked increase in the availability of molecular data. Although these data have clarified the relationships between different lesions, they are not yet detailed enough to dictate changes to the WHO classification. Only one lesion in this chapter is defined by its molecular change: rhabdomyosarcoma with *TFCP2* rearrangement {1034}. Characteristic molecular changes are present in several bone and odontogenic tumours but are not defining criteria.

The common hotspot mutations found in other human neoplasms do not seem to be present in the odontogenic cysts and tumours, reflecting the fact that many are hamartomas, benign, or low-grade malignant neoplasms. However, some common themes are emerging {1137,1187}. Dysregulated MAPK signalling caused by *BRAF* p.V600E mutations is a likely driver for ameloblastoma and is found in conventional, unicystic, and peripheral subtypes, as well as in many ameloblastic carcinomas. *BRAF* pathogenic variants seem common to other epithelial and mixed odontogenic tumours that have ameloblastic differentiation. They can be found in both the epithelial and mesenchymal components of ameloblastic fibroma and lesions previously classified as ameloblastic fibrodentinoma and fibro-odontoma, and in the mesenchymal component of some odontogenic sarcomas. PTCH1 and sonic hedgehog pathway alterations are associated with odontogenic keratocyst and ameloblastoma. WNT pathway signalling is implicated in odontoma formation, and mutations in *CTNNB1* (encoding β-catenin) are associated with ghost cell differentiation in cysts and benign and malignant neoplasms. *FOS* rearrangement and FOS overexpression in cementoblastoma confirm its relationship with osteoblastoma. MAPK/ERK pathway activation may drive odontogenic myxoma. However, the pathogenetic role of each of these changes remains to be elucidated. Although such changes are often associated with neoplasia or malignancy in other tissues, most of these pathways are key to odontogenesis {4404,321} and may act in a context-specific manner.

Oncogene and tumour suppressor gene alterations continue to raise the possibility that some odontogenic cysts and hamartomas might be neoplasms. In the absence of a molecular definition of neoplasia and in recognition of this situation in other benign conditions {2212}, the classification has been maintained on the basis of progressive growth pattern and metastasis. As an example, the status of odontogenic keratocyst remains contentious, but it is molecularly similar to other conditions with alterations in oncogenes or tumour suppressor genes that promote growth but fail to cause a neoplastic phenotype, such as fibrous dysplasia caused by *GNAS* (*GNAS1*) mutation, simple bone cyst with *NFATC2* fusion, and adenomatoid odontogenic tumour with *KRAS* mutation.

Odontogenic tumours

It has not proved possible to clarify the complex overlap between lesions variously termed "amyloid-rich subtype of odontogenic fibroma" and "non-calcifying subtype of calcifying epithelial odontogenic tumour", and their Langerhans cell–rich subtypes. Although some features favour classification as odontogenic fibroma, both potential parent entities lack defined molecular markers to allow a definitive classification to be made.

The new classification principles have required the addition of the descriptor "conventional" to ameloblastoma, because this is not a grouping of subtypes and must be distinguished from other ameloblastoma entities. The term "solid/multicystic" previously performed this function but was removed in the 2017 WHO classification and is now replaced by "conventional", to follow WHO practice in other fifth-edition volumes.

Adenoid ameloblastoma {2725} has been accepted as an entity in the category of benign odontogenic tumours. It has been recognized for several decades and has a distinctive appearance, but there is variation in the diagnostic criteria in the literature and a lack of clarity about its behaviour. This lesion may lack the *BRAF* mutations found in other ameloblastomas, although data are limited and preliminary, and the nuclear β-catenin immunostaining is consistent with this lesion's ghost cell differentiation and may suggest a relationship with the ghost cell tumour group. A small number of cases with a high proliferative fraction and aggressive behaviour are difficult to distinguish from ghost cell odontogenic carcinoma and ameloblastic carcinoma with ghost cells. Further reporting and molecular analysis of this and similar entities is encouraged, to clarify their relationships and classification.

The reclassification of ameloblastic fibro-odontoma as a developing odontoma was a contentious change in the previous edition. Sufficient molecular data have not yet been accrued to clarify the situation, and so the classification has remained unchanged, pending further evidence. The change in 2017 was made because the literature suggested that many developing odontomas were misdiagnosed as ameloblastic fibro-odontoma, risking patient harm through overtreatment. Although the existence of a neoplastic ameloblastic fibro-odontoma was not disputed, it was thought to be very rare and it was felt that the great majority of lesions with the histological appearance of ameloblastic fibro-odontoma were destined to mature into odontomas. Molecular analysis suggests these intermediate lesions are mixed, with some lesions previously diagnosed as ameloblastic fibrodentinoma or ameloblastic fibro-odontoma bearing *BRAF* p.V600E mutations. However, any histological differences between mutation-positive and -negative lesions has not been defined, and it remains difficult or impossible to differentiate these possible entities from the much more common developing odontomas on histological grounds alone. A review of the literature for the WHO classification suggested that a significant number of lesions published as ameloblastic fibroma are also developing odontomas, and it seems likely that reclassification including some ameloblastic fibromas may be required in the future. In the meantime, the requirement is that, without evidence to change it, the classification must remain unchanged.

No changes have been made to the classification of the malignant odontogenic tumours, retaining the simplified structure from the previous edition. Odontogenic carcinoma with dentinoid {3085} has not been included, because of a possible overlap with other carcinomas and the aggressive end of the behaviour spectrum of adenoid ameloblastoma. The possibility of clear cell carcinoma with dentinoid has been removed because of a lack of evidence of a relationship to clear cell odontogenic carcinoma. Odontogenic carcinosarcoma remains contentious and extremely rare. Confusion over its status as an entity has centred on whether a specific line of sarcoma differentiation must be present. Because none is present in odontogenic sarcomas, this condition cannot apply and the entity has been retained, accepting its extreme rarity.

Giant cell lesions and bone cysts

Since the last edition of the WHO classification of head and neck tumours it has been found that the central giant cell granuloma is driven by MAPK pathway activation caused by mutation in one of several genes {1639}. Somewhat surprisingly, peripheral giant cell granuloma harbours the same changes despite its limited growth potential and occasional spontaneous involution. Both are retained as separate entities in view of their differing presentations, growth patterns, and treatment. In line with the classification of bone and soft tissue tumours, the concept of secondary aneurysmal bone cyst has now been replaced by one of cystic haemorrhagic degeneration, because the cystic changes frequently found associated with fibro-osseous lesions of the jaw lack the *USP6* rearrangement and are unrelated to the aneurysmal bone cyst.

Fibro-osseous tumours and dysplasias

The fibro-osseous lesions have long been an area of diagnostic difficulty, caused primarily by the fact that it has been considered impossible to differentiate them on histological grounds alone. The current classification attempts to differentiate these lesions more clearly, but it must be appreciated that the clinical presentation, radiographic appearance, and growth pattern are essential factors in diagnosis.

Molecular analysis of fibro-osseous lesions is in its early stages and does not yet define any entity. This edition of the classification introduces the subtype of familial florid cemento-osseous dysplasia on the basis of its earlier age of onset and frequency of marked expansion {3178}. Very early data have identified *ANO5* (*GDD1*) mutation in one family, distinct from the mutation found in gnathodiaphysial dysplasia and its associated cemento-ossifying fibromas, but suggesting a related pathogenesis. One further reason for defining the familial type as a separate subtype is to better define familial gigantiform cementoma. This controversial and extremely rare disorder has been retained in the WHO classification, separate from florid cemento-osseous dysplasia and syndromes with multiple cemento-ossifying fibromas, pending molecular characterization.

Segmental odontomaxillary dysplasia {4804} is a relatively well-defined condition that may be underdiagnosed and is prone to misdiagnosis as fibrous dysplasia. For this reason, it is included in the WHO classification for the first time.

Benign maxillofacial bone and cartilage tumours

In the previous edition, cemento-ossifying fibroma was grouped with juvenile trabecular ossifying fibroma and juvenile psammomatoid ossifying fibroma as three subtypes of the entity ossifying fibroma. An additional paragraph noted its odontogenic nature in the benign mesenchymal odontogenic tumours. In the current edition, changes to the definition of entity and subtype have abolished the category of ossifying fibroma, making it necessary for cemento-ossifying fibroma to take its place in the sections on benign mesenchymal odontogenic tumours.

Early molecular evidence suggests that cemento-ossifying fibromas are heterogeneous {378,2750}, meaning that reclassification may be required in future. Lesions resembling cemento-ossifying fibroma can arise from a variety of causes including *CDC73* (*HRPT2*) {3545} or *ANO5* (*GDD1*) mutation or deregulation of the WNT pathway {3468}. The number of entities, clinical features, localization, and classification of this group may have to be reconsidered in the light of molecular evidence, which is not yet sufficiently well defined to justify changes. Both psammomatoid ossifying fibroma and juvenile trabecular ossifying fibroma appear to have a distinct molecular pathogenesis, although this is based on limited data.

The term "juvenile" has been removed from psammomatoid ossifying fibroma because the age range is broad, with a peak incidence in the second to fourth decades of life. Juvenile trabecular ossifying fibroma retains its "juvenile" descriptor. Although the literature includes many cases in older patients, stricter diagnostic criteria suggest that this remains a lesion that arises primarily in children.

Malignant maxillofacial bone and cartilage tumours

The only completely novel entity in the WHO classification is rhabdomyosarcoma defined by *TFCP2* rearrangement {1034}. This rhabdomyosarcoma has a predilection for craniofacial bones. Its variable morphology includes epithelioid and spindle cells with a confusing immunoprofile of a positive reaction for cytokeratins; sometimes positivity for p63 and ALK together with desmin, myogenin, and MYOD1; and occasionally positivity for S100. Although the appearances are suggestive in routine stains, it is recommended that the diagnosis is confirmed by molecular methods, because this entity may be easily confused with completely unrelated malignant neoplasms.

Radicular cyst

Speight P
Soluk Tekkeşin M

Definition
Radicular cyst (RC) is an inflammatory odontogenic cyst associated with the root of a non-vital tooth.

ICD-O coding
None

ICD-11 coding
DA09.8 Radicular cyst

Related terminology
Acceptable: periapical cyst; apical cyst.
Not recommended: (apical) periodontal cyst; inflammatory dental cyst; dental cyst.

Subtype(s)
Residual cyst (residual radicular cyst)

Localization
RCs are located at the apex of a tooth root, or on the lateral aspect of the root associated with a lateral root canal. The most common site is the anterior maxilla, where 40–50% arise, followed by the lower molar area {2121,4385}.

Clinical features
RCs are always associated with a non-vital tooth. Patients may report swelling, but RCs are often symptomless and found incidentally on radiological investigation. There may be a history of dental pain or abscess.

Imaging
RCs form a round or oval, well-demarcated, corticated radiolucency, usually 10–20 mm in diameter but occasionally larger. Residual cysts are found at a site of previous tooth extraction.

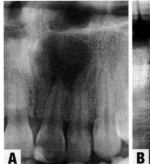 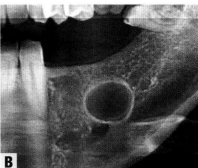

Fig. 7.01 Radicular cyst. **A** Periapical radiograph showing a well-demarcated, corticated radiolucency at the apex of an upper incisor tooth. **B** Panoramic radiograph showing a residual radicular cyst at a site of a previous tooth extraction. It appears as a corticated radiolucency.

Epidemiology
RC is the most common jaw cyst, accounting for about 60% of all odontogenic cysts. There is a peak incidence in the fourth and fifth decades of life and a slight male predilection {2121, 4385}.

Etiology
RC is caused by chronic inflammation at the apex of a non-vital tooth, after pulp necrosis, usually due to dental caries.

Pathogenesis
Inflammation stimulates cell rests of Malassez to proliferate and form a cystic cavity that enlarges as a result of osmotic pressure, causing peripheral bone resorption.

Macroscopic appearance
RC is usually a sac-like cystic mass.

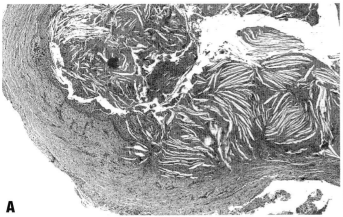 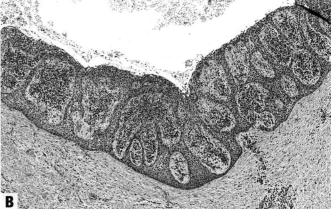

Fig. 7.02 Radicular cyst. **A** Cholesterol clefts disrupt the epithelial lining and protrude into the cyst lumen. **B** The cyst is lined by hyperplastic epithelium showing a characteristic arcading pattern.

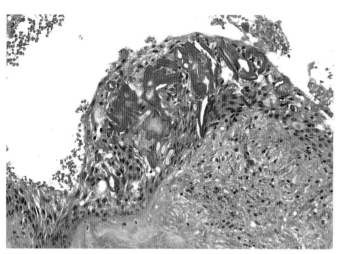

Fig. 7.03 Radicular cyst. A cluster of hyaline (Rushton) bodies forms a small nodule in the epithelial lining, indicating an odontogenic cyst.

Histopathology

RC is lined by non-keratinized stratified squamous epithelium that is proliferative with a characteristic arcading pattern. Hyaline (Rushton) bodies, mucous (goblet) cells, or small areas of keratinization are not uncommon {4510,298}. The wall is composed of inflamed fibrous tissue, often with foamy histiocytes. Deposits of cholesterol crystals (clefts) with foreign body giant cells are often seen and may form luminal nodules. Residual and longstanding cysts are less inflamed and have a more regular thin epithelium. Residual cyst (residual radicular cyst) is a radicular cyst that is retained in the jaw after removal of the causative tooth.

Cytology

Smears of aspirated cysts may show squamous cells but more commonly show degenerative cyst fluid with cholesterol crystals and debris.

Diagnostic molecular pathology

Not clinically relevant

Essential and desirable diagnostic criteria

Essential: non-vital tooth; cyst lined by non-keratinizing epithelium.

Staging

Not relevant

Prognosis and prediction

Extraction of the causative tooth or root canal treatment remove the cause, and enucleation of the cyst is rarely followed by recurrence {3203}. Residual cyst may follow extraction alone.

Inflammatory collateral cysts

Speight P
Soluk Tekkeşin M

Definition
Inflammatory collateral cysts (ICCs) are inflammatory cysts on the buccal or distobuccal aspect of the roots of partially or recently erupted teeth.

ICD-O coding
None

ICD-11 coding
DA05.Y Other specified cysts of oral or facial-neck region

Related terminology
Acceptable: mandibular infected buccal cyst; inflammatory paradental cyst.

Subtype(s)
Paradental cyst (PC); mandibular buccal bifurcation cyst (MBBC)

Localization
PCs account for 60% of all ICCs and are found on the distobuccal aspect of mandibular third molars. MBBCs (35%) are found on the buccal aspect of mandibular first or second molars and are often bilateral (in as many as 25% of cases). Rare cases of ICC (4%) arise at other sites {3524,4613}.

Clinical features
PCs are associated with chronic pericoronitis but are often symptomless at presentation. MBBCs may be infected with pain, tenderness, and suppuration. The tooth is vital and often tilted buccally with deep periodontal pockets.

Imaging
ICCs appear as corticated radiolucencies overlying the buccal or distobuccal aspect of the tooth. The lamina dura is intact, and the follicular space surrounding a partially erupted tooth is normal {927}.

MBBCs may extend to the lower border of the mandible {3524}, and they often show a periosteal reaction, with laminated new bone formation.

Epidemiology
ICCs account for 5% of odontogenic cysts and have a male predilection (70%). The average age is 30 years for PC and 9 years (first molar) or 17 years (second molar) for MBBC {966, 3524}.

Etiology
ICCs are caused by inflammation in the pericoronal tissues. Cyst formation may be exacerbated by food impaction or by an enamel projection on the buccal aspect of the tooth {966, 927}.

Pathogenesis
ICCs are pocket cysts caused by dilation of the pericoronal tissues and lined by sulcular or junctional epithelium derived from the reduced enamel epithelium {966,2865}.

Macroscopic appearance
If removed intact, the cyst appears as a sac-like mass attached to the buccal or distobuccal aspect of the coronal third of the tooth root.

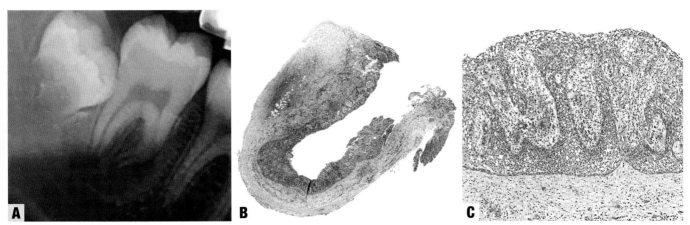

Fig. 7.04 Inflammatory collateral cyst. **A** A mandibular buccal bifurcation cyst overlies the buccal aspect of a mandibular second molar tooth. It appears as a well-demarcated, corticated radiolucency. Note that the periodontal space and lamina dura are intact and normal. **B** This paradental cyst is composed of an inflamed fibrous wall lined by hyperplastic epithelium. The cyst appears as an open pocket. **C** The epithelial lining is squamous and non-keratinized and shows secondary inflammatory changes with arcading rete hyperplasia and has no specific features.

Histopathology

ICC is indistinguishable from radicular cyst. It has an inflamed wall lined by hyperplastic non-keratinized epithelium. Cholesterol deposition and foamy histiocytes are common. The cyst may be open and continuous with the pericoronal or gingival tissues.

Cytology

Not relevant

Diagnostic molecular pathology

Not relevant

Essential and desirable diagnostic criteria

Essential: associated with partially or recently erupted vital tooth; radiolucency distinct from dental follicle; intact lamina dura; non-keratinized epithelium.

Staging

Not relevant

Prognosis and prediction

Cysts are enucleated. Third molars associated with PC are removed. Molars associated with MBBC can be conserved and usually erupt normally.

Surgical ciliated cyst

Nelson BL
Speight P

Definition
Surgical ciliated cyst is a benign cyst caused by the traumatic implantation, usually surgical, of respiratory epithelium in the gnathic bones.

ICD-O coding
None

ICD-11 coding
DA05.Y Other specified cysts of oral or facial-neck region

Related terminology
Acceptable: surgical ciliated cyst of the maxilla; postoperative maxillary cyst (if maxillary location); (respiratory) implantation cyst.

Subtype(s)
None

Localization
Surgical ciliated cysts arise in the gnathic bones, most commonly in the posterior maxilla {2162,168}. They are very rare in the mandible.

Clinical features
Surgical ciliated cysts may be asymptomatic or present with swelling, pain, or tenderness {365,3216}.

Imaging
Radiographs show a well-demarcated unilocular radiolucency of the jaws. Approximately 60% of cases are at least partially surrounded by a corticated margin. Occasional large lesions in the maxilla may fill the sinus or be multilocular {4902,2162}.

Epidemiology
Surgical ciliated cysts are rare {3216,1628}. There is no sex predilection, and the most common age range is the fifth to sixth decades of life.

Etiology
Cysts develop from entrapped sinus or nasal mucosa in the jawbones after trauma or surgery. These inciting factors include, but are not limited to, Caldwell–Luc and Le Fort 1 procedures, sinus surgery, maxillary fracture, midface osteotomy, or traumatic tooth extraction {2378,545,2608}. Mandibular cases are generally caused by implantation of sinus epithelium by contaminated instruments, or transfer of epithelium with autologous nasal osteocartilaginous grafts for chin augmentation {2378,545,2608,4403}. The cyst usually develops after a long latent period, the reported delay being as long as 20 years after the causative surgery {3216}.

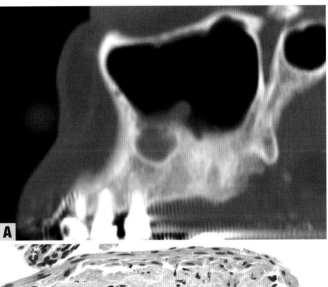

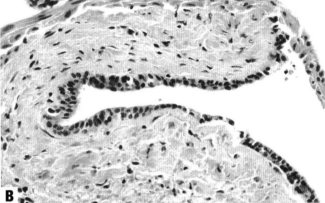

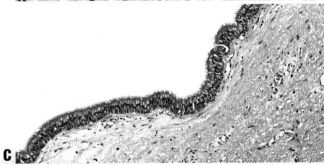

Fig. 7.05 Surgical ciliated cyst. **A** Sagittal CT of a surgical ciliated cyst of the maxilla, from a patient with a history of traumatic tooth extraction. **B** Cyst lined by bilaminar cuboidal epithelium with focal cilia. **C** Cyst lined by fully differentiated respiratory epithelium.

Pathogenesis
It is thought that the implanted epithelium forms a cyst cavity due to persistent mucous secretion. In this respect, some regard the lesion as a type of mucous retention cyst {4902}.

Chapter 7

Macroscopic appearance

Lesions are often fragmented but show a cyst wall of variable thickness. The lumen may contain mucinous material.

Histopathology

The cyst is lined by pseudostratified ciliated columnar (respiratory-type) epithelium. Areas of squamous metaplasia or simple cuboidal cells may be seen {2770}. Mucous (goblet) cells are common. The cyst wall is composed of loose fibrous connective tissue, which may be inflamed. Areas of subepithelial fibrosis or hyalinization are frequent {365,4902}.

Cytology

Not relevant

Diagnostic molecular pathology

Not relevant

Essential and desirable diagnostic criteria

Essential: a history of previous surgery; a radiolucent, well-demarcated cyst; respiratory epithelial lining.

Staging

Not relevant

Prognosis and prediction

Treatment is simple enucleation and recurrences are rare.

Nasopalatine duct cyst

Rich AM
Neville BW

Definition
Nasopalatine duct cyst (NDC) is a developmental non-odontogenic cyst arising in the incisive canal.

ICD-O coding
None

ICD-11 coding
DA05.1 Developmental non-odontogenic cysts of oral region

Related terminology
Acceptable: incisive canal cyst.

Subtype(s)
None

Localization
NDCs present in the midline of the anterior hard palate.

Clinical features
Most NDCs present as sessile swellings posterior to the maxillary incisors, or they may be entirely asymptomatic. More deeply sited cysts present as a swelling on the labial alveolus or bulging into the nasal floor {722,356}. Rarely, an NDC will develop within the soft tissue of the incisive papilla. The typical diameter is 10–20 mm, but they may reach several centimetres {4305,1278,4300}.

Imaging
Radiology shows a corticated, symmetrical radiolucency in the anterior hard palate between the roots of the incisors, which may be displaced. Unless there are other reasons for loss of vitality, adjacent teeth are vital with intact lamina dura. Radiographic superimposition of the anterior nasal spine often produces a characteristic heart- or pear-shaped radiolucency in occlusal view. Diagnosis requires a size of > 6 mm (the diameter of the normal incisive canal {4305}), slightly more in older patients {4529}.

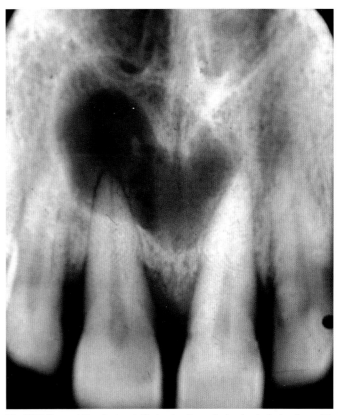

Fig. 7.06 Nasopalatine duct cyst. Occlusal radiograph showing typical radiographic appearances of a corticated radiolucency just behind and around the apices of the upper central incisors.

Epidemiology
Fewer than 5% of all cysts of the jaws are NDCs, but they account for as many as 80% of all non-odontogenic cysts {1009,2123}. NDC occurs most frequently in patients aged 30–60 years, with an M:F ratio of about 3:1 {356}.

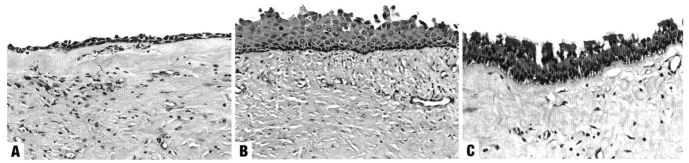

Fig. 7.07 Nasopalatine duct cyst. **A–C** Three areas of the wall from the same cyst showing a range of lining epithelium, from bilaminar cuboidal to low squamous and respiratory. Intermediate appearances are often seen.

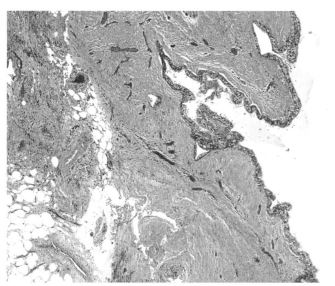

Fig. 7.08 Nasopalatine duct cyst. The cyst wall is lined by respiratory-type epithelium with thick-walled vessels, fat, and nerves.

Etiology

NDC is categorized as a developmental cyst and arises from respiratory and squamous epithelial vestigial remnants of an embryonic nasopalatine duct present in some individuals {2294}.

Pathogenesis

In one third of cases, inflammation from non-vital teeth or periodontal ligament may be a factor, by stimulating the epithelial remnants to proliferate {1278,4300}.

Macroscopic appearance

Fibrous curettings and cyst lining

Histopathology

About 90% of NDCs are lined by non-keratinized stratified squamous epithelium, with focal cuboidal, columnar, or ciliated areas. About half contain respiratory epithelium, but < 10% are lined entirely by it {4305,356}. Cysts with respiratory-type epithelium tend to be more superiorly placed in the incisive canal {1278}. The cyst wall contains prominent neurovascular bundles and occasionally mucous glands or cartilage.

Cytology

Smears of aspirated cysts show degenerative cyst fluid with debris and macrophages, some of which contain haemosiderin. Epithelium is absent or scant. However, these findings are nonspecific.

Diagnostic molecular pathology

Not relevant

Essential and desirable diagnostic criteria

Essential: epicentre in the incisive canal; lining of non-keratinized squamous or respiratory epithelium.
Desirable: a neurovascular bundle in the cyst wall.

Staging

Not relevant

Prognosis and prediction

NDCs do not normally recur after enucleation.

Gingival cysts

Vargas PA
Gomez RS

Definition
Gingival cysts are developmental odontogenic cysts arising in the attached gingiva or alveolar ridge mucoperiosteum.

ICD-O coding
None

ICD-11 coding
DA05.0 Developmental odontogenic cysts

Related terminology
Acceptable: in infants: gingival cyst of the newborn, Bohn nodules; in adults: gingival cyst of adult.
Not recommended: Bohn nodules (in adults); alveolar cysts.

Subtype(s)
None

Localization
In adults, most cysts arise in the gingiva of the mandibular premolar/canine region {4667,878} or (less frequently) in the anterior maxillary gingiva, almost always on the buccal aspect of the alveolus. In infants, the cysts occur anywhere on the edentulous alveolar ridge of the mandible or maxilla {3066,3891}.

Clinical features
Gingival cyst of the adult (GCA) usually forms a single painless, well-circumscribed nodule of the attached gingivae, sometimes with a bluish-grey translucent appearance. Radiographs are not helpful in detecting GCA, despite occasional superficial erosion of the underlying alveolar bone. Gingival cyst of the infant

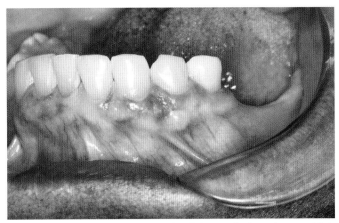

Fig. 7.09 Gingival cyst of the adult. A small, well-circumscribed, translucent nodule in the left lower attached gingiva, buccal to the first premolar.

(GCI) presents as small (< 2 mm) white nodules on the alveolar mucosa, which are often multiple {3054}.

Epidemiology
GCA accounts for < 0.5% of odontogenic cysts {4353}. The majority of patients are in their fifth or sixth decade of life {1599, 878,4353}. GCI is found in as many as 90% of neonates but is rare after the age of 3 months {2010}.

Etiology
Unknown

Pathogenesis
Unknown

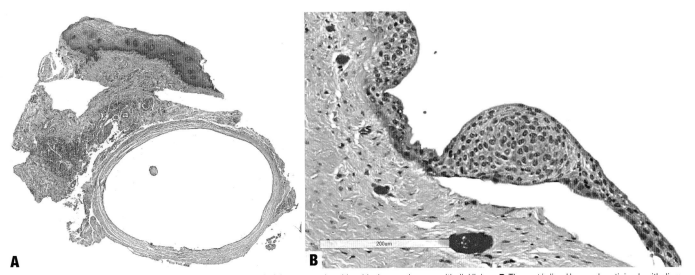

Fig. 7.10 Gingival cyst of the adult. **A** Gingival mucosa with an underlying cyst cavity with a thin, inconspicuous epithelial lining. **B** The cyst is lined by non-keratinized epithelium with two plaque-like thickenings that protrude into the lumen.

Chapter 7

Macroscopic appearance

Nodular mucosa with a smooth surface; whitish or translucent

Histopathology

GCA is lined by a thin, flat or cuboidal squamous epithelium, 1–3 cells thick, without rete ridges. Plaque-like thickenings that protrude into the lumen or the connective tissue wall and clear cells are usually present. The connective tissue wall may contain islands of epithelium resembling the epithelial plaques. GCIs are rarely biopsied, but they are lined by thin keratinized epithelium that may have a connection to the surface epithelium.

Cytology

Not relevant

Diagnostic molecular pathology

Not relevant

Essential and desirable diagnostic criteria

Essential: for GCA: site in attached gingiva; thin epithelial lining; for GCI: site in alveolar ridge; patient aged < 3 months.

Staging

None

Prognosis and prediction

GCAs do not recur after conservative excision {878}. GCIs rupture or involute and resolve spontaneously.

Dentigerous cyst

Nelson BL
White SJ

Definition
Dentigerous cyst is a developmental odontogenic cyst of the jaws surrounding the crown of an unerupted tooth, with the lining attached to the cementoenamel junction.

ICD-O coding
None

ICD-11 coding
DA05.0 Developmental odontogenic cysts

Related terminology
Acceptable: follicular cyst.

Subtype(s)
Eruption cyst; inflammatory follicular cyst

Localization
Dentigerous cysts develop most frequently on third molars and maxillary canines, but any unerupted tooth or odontoma may be affected {2653,453,1941,2156}. An eruption cyst is a superficial dentigerous cyst over an erupting tooth, usually a deciduous first molar, in a child {3978}.

Clinical features
Most dentigerous cysts are small and asymptomatic and are discovered on routine dental radiographs or when investigating the failure of a tooth to erupt. Larger cysts cause expansion of the jaw and may reach several centimetres in diameter. Infection, generally associated with oral communication, may result in symptoms of pain and swelling.

Imaging
Radiographically, the cyst forms a well-defined, unilocular radiolucency with a corticated border. Large cysts may appear pseudoloculated, expand the jaw, or displace or resorb adjacent teeth. The cyst is closely associated with the crown of an unerupted tooth and appears to originate from its cementoenamel junction, although the cyst may surround the tooth crown, lie lateral to it, or surround parts of the root in addition, depending on the direction of enlargement {2653,453,1941,2156,287}.

Epidemiology
Dentigerous cysts are the most common developmental cysts of the jaws, representing about 25% of all jaw cysts. The age range is broad (5–83 years), with a peak incidence in the second and third decades of life. There is a male sex predilection (M:F ratio: 1.7:1) {2653,453,1941,2156}.

Etiology
Dentigerous cysts develop by the accumulation of fluid between reduced enamel epithelium and the crown of a tooth {3714,453, 1941}. The great majority are considered developmental, but some are induced by adjacent inflammation in pericoronitis or at the apices of deciduous teeth {2848}.

Pathogenesis
The pathogenesis is unknown. Dentigerous cysts do not harbour the *BRAF* p.V600E mutations found in ameloblastomas {3467,990}.

Macroscopic appearance
The macroscopic appearance is that of a fibrous, tan, friable cyst wall and an extracted tooth. Although the relationship to tooth is usually lost with the extraction of the associated tooth, adherent tags of cyst lining often remain at the cementoenamel junction.

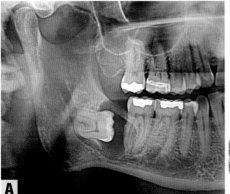
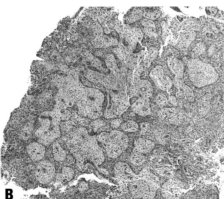
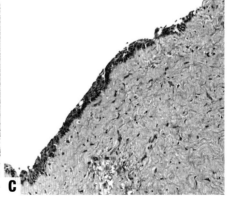

Fig. 7.11 Dentigerous cyst. **A** Typical pericoronal radiolucency around the lower third molar, with attachment of the cyst lining at the cementoenamel junction. The associated tooth is displaced posteriorly. **B** The thick and hyperplastic epithelial lining of an inflamed dentigerous cyst in relationship to the dense acute and chronic inflammation. **C** Thin, regular squamous epithelial lining.

Histopathology

The dentigerous cyst has a thin, non-keratinized stratified squamous epithelial lining, which is often bilaminar in areas. Cuboidal, columnar, and ciliated cells may be present, as can mucous or sebaceous metaplasia {4345,2653,3714}. Hyaline (Rushton) bodies and focal keratinization may also occur {2785, 298}. When not inflamed, the cyst wall is composed of loose, often myxoid, fibrous connective tissue and may contain occasional odontogenic epithelial rests {2653}.

Differential diagnosis

Inflamed dentigerous cysts show hyperplasia and thickening of the lining epithelium and often foamy macrophages and cholesterol clefts associated with foreign body giant cells {2653,1941}, and they come to resemble radicular cysts histopathologically.

Cytology

Not clinically relevant

Diagnostic molecular pathology

None

Essential and desirable diagnostic criteria

Essential: a well-defined radiolucency associated with the crown of an unerupted tooth; epithelium and cyst wall attached to the cementoenamel junction of the unerupted tooth.

Staging

None

Prognosis and prediction

Dentigerous cyst does not recur after enucleation and removal of the associated unerupted tooth. Decompression before enucleation may be indicated for large lesions {2690}. Some may be treated conservatively, preserving the associated tooth, by marsupialization or extraction of associated non-vital deciduous teeth, depending on the location {2848}.

Orthokeratinized odontogenic cyst

Speight P
Neville BW

Definition
Orthokeratinized odontogenic cyst (OOC) is a developmental cyst lined by orthokeratinized stratified squamous epithelium.

ICD-O coding
None

ICD-11 coding
DA05.0 Developmental odontogenic cysts

Related terminology
Not recommended: orthokeratinized variant of odontogenic keratocyst.

Subtype(s)
None

Localization
Most OOCs (80%) are found in the mandible and 65% are found in the posterior body and ramus region {4861,1159,2757}.

Clinical features
OOC usually presents as a painless swelling {1159,2757}, but many are incidental findings during radiographic examination. Rare cases of multiple or bilateral OOC have been reported, but there is no evidence of any association with naevoid basal cell carcinoma syndrome (Gorlin syndrome) {810,968}.

Imaging
OOCs are well-demarcated spherical, unilocular, radiolucent lesions, often with a corticated margin. Occasional cases (< 10%) are multilocular {2757}. As many as 70% of all lesions are associated with an impacted tooth, with a radiological similarity to dentigerous cyst {1159}.

Epidemiology
OOC is rare and accounts for ≤ 1% of odontogenic cysts {227, 4353}. It arises over a wide age range, with an average of about 35 years and a peak in the third and fourth decades of life. About 65% of patients are male {4861,1159,2757}.

Etiology
Unknown

Pathogenesis
OOC is a developmental cyst that most likely arises from remnants of dental lamina {2625}.

Macroscopic appearance
Multiple fragments of cyst wall. The contents are cream or yellow in colour, with a cheesy or buttery texture.

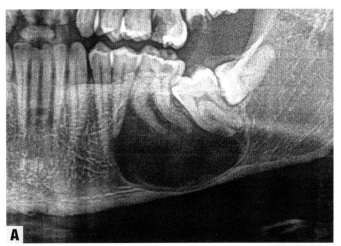
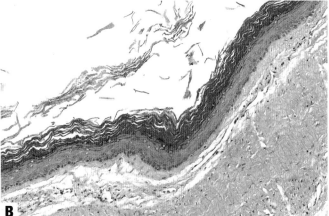

Fig. 7.12 Orthokeratinized odontogenic cyst. **A** Radiology shows a well-demarcated and corticated unilocular radiolucency. **B** A thin, regular lining of orthokeratinized stratified squamous epithelium. The keratin is lamellated and extends into the lumen.

Histopathology
OOC is lined by thin regular orthokeratinized stratified squamous epithelium with a prominent granular cell layer and inconspicuous or low cuboidal basal cells. It is heavily keratinized, often with lamellae of keratin filling the lumen. The wall is fibrous and may show areas of inflammation. There may be parakeratinized or non-keratinized areas, but these form a small part of the lining and are often associated with inflammation {4861}. Rare examples include sebaceous glands in the lining {836}. Microcysts may be seen in the wall in 5% of cases {4861,2625}.

Cytology
Examination of an aspirate may show lamellae and fragments of orthokeratin.

Diagnostic molecular pathology
Not relevant

Essential and desirable diagnostic criteria
Essential: site in a tooth-bearing area of the jaw; thin, regular epithelial lining with orthokeratinization.
Desirable: prominent granular cell layer; flat basal cells.

Staging
Not relevant

Prognosis and prediction
Recurrence is rare (< 5%) after enucleation {2757}.

Lateral periodontal cyst and botryoid odontogenic cyst

Vargas PA
White SJ

Definition
Lateral periodontal cyst (LPC) is a developmental odontogenic cyst lined by non-keratinized epithelium with characteristic thickenings.

Botryoid odontogenic cyst (BOC) is a less common multilocular subtype of LPC.

ICD-O coding
None

ICD-11 coding
DA05.0 Developmental odontogenic cysts

Related terminology
None

Subtype(s)
Botryoid odontogenic cyst (BOC)

Localization
The cysts are mainly localized in the mandibular canine / premolar alveolar bone, with 70% of LPCs and 85% of BOCs arising here; the remaining cases usually arise in the maxilla {4667, 878}. Multifocal occurrence has been reported.

Clinical features
LPC and BOC are asymptomatic in almost 90% of cases and usually identified incidentally on radiographs. They cause buccal alveolar bone expansion in 50% of cases {878}.

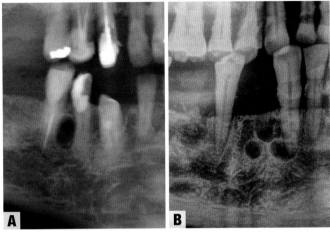

Fig. 7.13 Lateral periodontal and botryoid odontogenic cysts. **A** A typical lateral periodontal cyst producing a unilocular radiolucency between the right lower premolar roots. **B** A typical botryoid odontogenic cyst showing a similar but multilocular cyst in the right mandibular canine/premolar region.

Imaging
LPC is a well-demarcated, often corticated unilocular radiolucency, closely related to the lateral surface of the root of an erupted tooth {4875}. Cortical bone expansion and perforation may be evident on cone-beam imaging in half of all cases. Tooth roots are almost never resorbed. Most lesions are < 10 mm in size. BOC has a multilocular appearance.

Epidemiology
LPCs and BOCs are rare, accounting for < 1% of odontogenic cysts {151,4353}. The majority present in the fifth to seventh decades of life {878} with a male preponderance {878}.

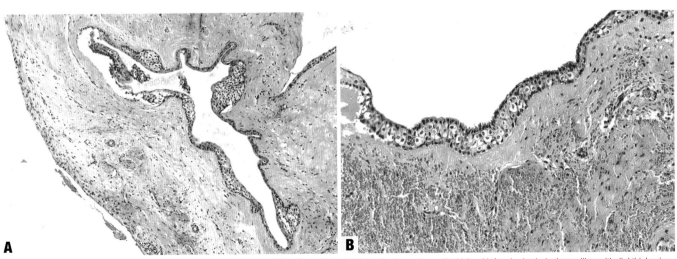

Fig. 7.14 Lateral periodontal cyst. **A** A cyst with uninflamed fibrous wall lined by a thin cuboidal epithelium a few cells thick, with focal, whorled, plaque-like epithelial thickenings containing clear cells. **B** High-power view showing clear cells in the epithelium.

Chapter 7

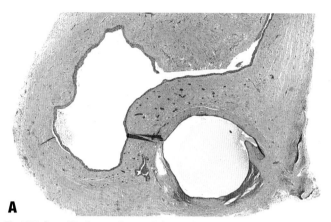 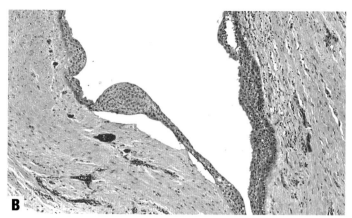

Fig. 7.15 Botryoid odontogenic cyst. **A** A cyst showing multiple cystic spaces, with the same histology as lateral periodontal cyst. **B** Uninflamed fibrous wall lined by a thin, non-keratinized squamous epithelium, and focal plaque-like epithelial thickening.

Etiology
Unknown

Pathogenesis
LPC and BOC are developmental and thought to arise from odontogenic epithelial rests of dental lamina, reduced enamel epithelium, or rests of Malassez.

Macroscopic appearance
Intact LPC presents as a small, tan, soft tissue cystic sac containing clear fluid. BOC is multilocular. The luminal surface of both may show focal thickenings {453}.

Histopathology
LPC has an uninflamed fibrous wall lined by a thin, non-keratinized squamous or cuboidal epithelium 1–3 cells thick. Focal, whorled, plaque-like epithelial thickenings are present, identical to those found less frequently in gingival cyst of the adult. Clear cells are often found in the thickenings {453}. BOC is multilocular with otherwise the same appearance {3866}.

Cytology
Not relevant

Diagnostic molecular pathology
Not relevant

Essential and desirable diagnostic criteria
Essential: site on the lateral aspect or between the roots of vital erupted teeth; characteristic whorled epithelial plaques; multilocular (BOC only).

Staging
None

Prognosis and prediction
Recurrence of LPC is exceedingly rare after enucleation. BOC recurs after enucleation in about 22% of cases and additional treatment may be indicated for recurrent BOC {878}.

Calcifying odontogenic cyst

Wright JM
Soluk Tekkeşin M

Definition
Calcifying odontogenic cyst (COC) is a developmental odontogenic cyst characterized histologically by ghost cells, which often calcify.

ICD-O coding
None

ICD-11 coding
DA05.0 & XH3R33 Developmental odontogenic cysts & Calcifying odontogenic cyst

Related terminology
Acceptable: calcifying cystic odontogenic tumour; Gorlin cyst.

Subtype(s)
None

Localization
COC usually arises in the tooth-bearing segments of the jaws, almost equally in the maxilla and mandible. In the maxilla there is a strong predilection for the anterior segments, whereas mandibular lesions are more evenly distributed {612,2503,1043}. Approximately 10% of cases are extraosseous with a predilection for the anterior mandibular gingiva {884}.

Clinical features
Most patients are asymptomatic, although intrabony lesions typically cause cortical expansion. Extraosseous lesions present as submucosal swellings {1043,3176}.

Imaging
COCs generally form well-defined unilocular lesions; about one third are uniformly radiolucent, and the remainder are of mixed radiolucency. Cortical expansion is common {1043,3176}.

Epidemiology
COC shows a worldwide distribution {1043} but is rare, accounting for < 1% of odontogenic cysts {2121}. There is no sex predilection, and the peak incidence is in the second and third decades of life.

Etiology
Unknown

Pathogenesis
COC has mutations in *CTNNB1* (which encodes β-catenin), a feature shared with adamantinomatous craniopharyngioma and pilomatrixoma {738,1060,1637} and implicating the WNT pathway {3969,4973}. No other pathogenic variants in oncogenes or tumour suppressor genes were detected in a 50-gene panel {1060}. WNT is also involved in odontomas, with which COC

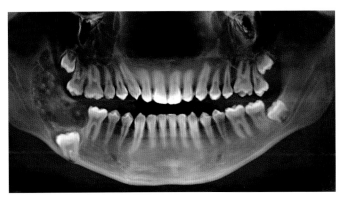

Fig. 7.16 Calcifying odontogenic cyst. Typical radiographic presentation as a pericoronal mixed radiolucent/radiopaque lesion of the right posterior mandible and ramus.

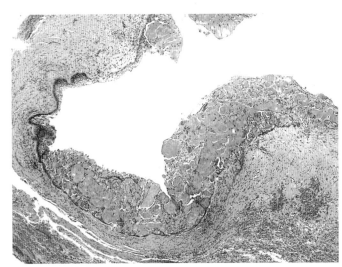

Fig. 7.17 Calcifying odontogenic cyst. Cystic architecture with prominent basal cells and numerous homogeneous eosinophilic ghost cells.

is often associated. It is not yet known whether the mutations cause a replication error phenotype.

Macroscopic appearance
There is a cystic cavity architecturally, unless the cyst is curetted.

Histopathology
COC is a unilocular cyst with a stratified epithelial lining of varying thickness, often loose, resembling stellate reticulum, and with palisaded and hyperchromatic columnar ameloblast-like basal cells. Cysts may show intraluminal and/or mural epithelial proliferation producing ameloblastoma-like areas. Ghost cells are characteristic rounded or stacked flattened pale eosinophilic cells within the epithelium, with distinct outlines and karyolysis resulting in a ghost-like appearance. These are variable in morphology

Chapter 7

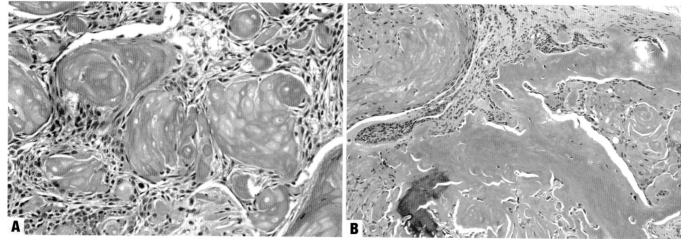

Fig. 7.18 Calcifying odontogenic cyst. **A** Cytological detail of ghost cells devoid of nuclei but with maintenance of cell outlines. **B** Areas of the cyst wall containing ghost cells and a homogeneous eosinophilic dentinoid product with cell inclusions.

and number, and they often calcify. Masses of ghost cells often pass into the connective tissue of the cyst wall, eliciting a foreign body reaction and inducing dentinoid (dentine-like matrix or mineralized tissue without a tubular structure) {612,2503}. Although characteristic, ghost cells form in other odontogenic tumours and do not alone justify a diagnosis of COC. COCs can occur with odontomas or other mixed odontogenic tumours {2650}.

Differential diagnosis
The differential diagnosis includes dentinogenic ghost cell tumour {884} and ghost cell odontogenic carcinoma.

Cytology
Not clinically relevant

Diagnostic molecular pathology
Not clinically relevant

Essential and desirable diagnostic criteria
Essential: cystic architecture; numerous ghost cells.
Desirable: palisaded hyperchromatic basal cells; dentinoid.

Staging
None

Prognosis and prediction
COCs are treated by conservative surgical removal, enucleation, and/or curettage. A systematic review reported an 8% recurrence rate {1043}.

Glandular odontogenic cyst

Speight P
Rautava J

Definition
Glandular odontogenic cyst (GOC) is a developmental cyst in which the epithelial lining resembles glandular tissue.

ICD-O coding
None

ICD-11 coding
DA05.0 Developmental odontogenic cysts

Related terminology
Not recommended: sialo-odontogenic cyst; mucoepidermoid odontogenic cyst.

Subtype(s)
None

Localization
GOC arises in tooth-bearing areas of the jaws. About 75% of cases are in the mandible. Mandibular and maxillary lesions have a propensity for the anterior regions.

Clinical features
GOC usually presents as a slowly expanding, painless swelling.

Imaging
GOCs are well-defined, corticated, unilocular or multilocular radiolucencies. Tooth displacement or root resorption is seen in as many as 25% of cases. Lesions may reach a large size and cross the midline in the mandible {2819,879}.

Epidemiology
GOCs account for < 0.5% of odontogenic cysts {2121}. There is no sex predilection. The average age at presentation is about 50 years, with a peak in the fifth to seventh decades of life {879}.

Etiology
Unknown

Pathogenesis
GOC is a developmental cyst thought to arise from cell rests of the dental lamina. No pathogenic variants were detected in a

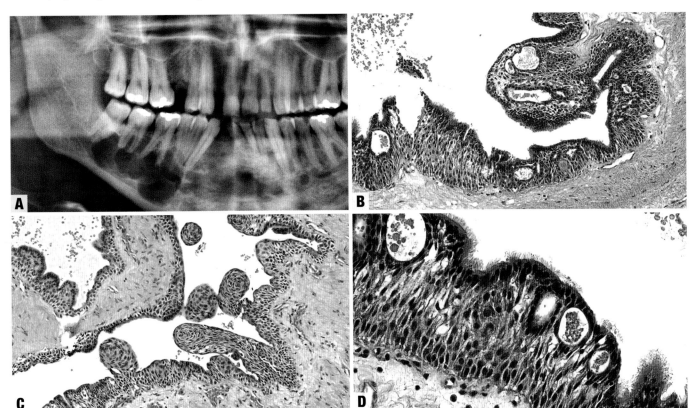

Fig. 7.19 Glandular odontogenic cyst. **A** An extensive multilocular lesion filling the entire body of the mandible and crossing the midline. **B** The epithelial lining shows microcysts and duct-like structures. There is a superficial layer of columnar cells, with cilia in places. **C** The lining shows whorled epithelial thickenings and papillary projections. Superficial columnar cells can also be seen. **D** A thickening in the epithelium containing glands and with a ciliated surface.

Chapter 7

panel of 50 oncogenes and tumour suppressor genes screened by next-generation sequencing {4092}.

Macroscopic appearance

GOCs are often multicystic or lobular. The cyst wall may have thickenings or papillary projections.

Histopathology

GOCs are often multilocular cysts and are lined by epithelium of variable thickness, from a thin layer of flattened squamous or cuboidal cells to stratified squamous epithelium, often with whorled epithelial thickenings, or plaques similar to those in lateral periodontal cyst. Cuboidal or low columnar cells on the luminal surface (hobnail cells) are found in all cases. Other typical features include intraepithelial microcysts, apocrine metaplasia, clear cells, papillary projections (tufting), cilia, and mucous cells {2180,1445,879}. Not all features are present in every case, and a higher number of features allows more confident diagnosis {1445}.

Differential diagnosis

GOC may show similar features to central mucoepidermoid carcinoma and this must be considered in the differential diagnosis {1445,2179}.

Cytology

Not clinically relevant

Diagnostic molecular pathology

GOC is generally considered to be negative for *MAML2* gene rearrangements {491}. However, recent studies have shown rearrangements in lesions that meet the histological criteria for GOC. These lesions may have been central mucoepidermoid carcinoma at the outset, but it raises the possibility that some central mucoepidermoid carcinomas might develop from a pre-existing GOC, and *MAML2* rearrangement studies must be interpreted with caution {1687}.

Essential and desirable diagnostic criteria

Essential: a radiolucent cystic lesion in a tooth-bearing area of the jaw; often multilocular.

Desirable: a lining of variable thickness with epithelial thickenings, plaques, or papillary projections; luminal columnar or cuboidal (hobnail) cells; microcysts or duct-like structures; mucous or clear cells.

Staging

None

Prognosis and prediction

GOCs, especially large and multilocular lesions, recur after enucleation in about 22% of cases {2181,879}.

Odontogenic keratocyst

Wright JM
Li TJ

Definition

Odontogenic keratocyst (OKC) is a developmental odontogenic cyst that is characterized histologically by a thin, parakeratinized stratified squamous epithelial lining with palisaded and hyperchromatic basal cells.

ICD-O coding

None

ICD-11 coding

DA05.0 Developmental odontogenic cysts

Related terminology

Acceptable: keratocystic odontogenic tumour.

Subtype(s)

None

Localization

OKCs are unique to the jaws, with a mandible-to-maxilla incidence ratio of 4:1. There is a strong predilection for the posterior mandible and ramus {565,2121,2756}.

Clinical features

Most patients are asymptomatic, and just under half have detectable swelling. The insidious growth pattern of OKC produces large cysts at diagnosis with significant bony destruction but minimal bone expansion {565,2504,2121,2756,4385}. Pathological fracture is often a risk. OKCs are a component of naevoid basal cell carcinoma syndrome, which is autosomal dominant and most often results from mutation of *PTCH1*. Syndromic OKCs are typically multiple and occur in younger patients {4853}. Occasionally OKCs can arise extraosseously in the gingiva, where they can be distinguished from gingival cysts by their distinct histological features {1345}.

Imaging

OKCs form well-circumscribed radiolucencies, with just over half showing cortication in the border. Approximately three quarters are unilocular and one quarter are multilocular. Most show at least some cortical expansion radiographically but tend to grow anteriorly and posteriorly initially, producing only minor expansion for their total length. Root resorption is occasionally observed. Approximately 35% are associated with unerupted teeth {2756}.

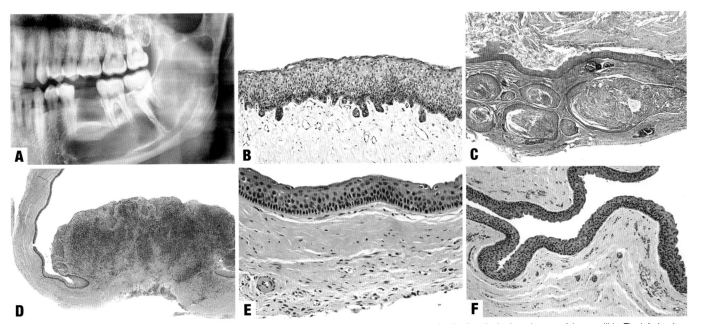

Fig. 7.20 Odontogenic keratocyst. **A** Panoramic radiograph of a large, multilocular odontogenic keratocyst enlarging into the body and ramus of the mandible. The inferior dental nerve canal is displaced inferiorly, but despite the longitudinal extent there is minimal expansion and displacement of teeth. **B** Some odontogenic keratocysts display basal budding. **C** Microcysts or satellite cysts in the wall. **D** In areas of inflammation, metaplastic change obscures the characteristic diagnostic features of odontogenic keratocyst epithelium, often preventing diagnosis in inflamed areas or small samples. **E** The epithelial cyst lining displays surface parakeratosis, cuboidal to columnar basal cells with hyperchromatic nuclei, and focal reverse nuclear polarity. **F** Cyst wall lined by uniform stratified squamous–type epithelium without rete ridges but with hyperchromatic palisaded basal cell nuclei and characteristic corrugated surface parakeratin.

Chapter 7

Epidemiology

OKCs are the third most commonly diagnosed odontogenic cyst and they have a worldwide distribution {2756}. They occur in all ages but show a dominant peak in the second or third decade of life and a second smaller peak in old age. There is a slight male predominance {565,2504,2121,2756,4385}.

Etiology

Unknown

Pathogenesis

OKCs arise from remnants of the dental lamina. The most notable molecular finding in OKCs is frequent mutations of the tumour suppressor gene *PTCH1* (9q22.3-q31) in syndromic OKCs and in as many as 80% of sporadic OKCs {2577,2623,3616}. A next-generation sequencing panel for the members of the sonic hedgehog pathway revealed an inactivating mutation rate of 93%, with biallelic inactivation in 80% {3615}. Other genetic alterations, including mutations in *PTCH2* and *SUFU*, as well as *BRAF* p.V600E, have also been reported, but at a much lower frequency and not always confirmed {3615,5019,1449}, and sequencing showed no pathogenic changes in commonly mutated oncogenes and tumour suppressor genes {1449}. These findings indicate that constitutive activation of sonic hedgehog signalling plays a major role in OKC pathogenesis, raising the possibility of treatment with small-molecule inhibitors of sonic hedgehog signalling {5002}. The possible role of fibroblasts in OKC fibrous capsules in promoting or regulating cyst growth via interaction with epithelial cells has also been reported {1913,4696}.

Macroscopic appearance

OKCs are architecturally cystic unless submitted as multiple smaller curetted fragments. The lumen may contain yellowish-white thick keratin.

Histopathology

The histological features of OKC are diagnostic, unlike the more common odontogenic cysts. The cyst is lined by a thin stratified squamous epithelium, approximately 4–8 cells thick, typically without rete ridges. The surface typically shows corrugation with parakeratin; a small proportion shows focal orthokeratosis. The characteristic basal cells are hyperchromatic, palisaded, and range from cuboidal to columnar, with some limited reverse nuclear polarity but rarely subnuclear vacuolization. Cysts are usually uninflamed, but when they are secondarily inflamed the inflammatory reaction induces metaplastic change in the epithelium and these characteristic features are lost. Nonspecific changes can be seen, including cholesterol deposition, Rushton bodies, mucous or sebaceous cells, and even cartilage in the wall of the cyst {566,1437}. Some OKCs display basal budding with small rounded rete ridges. Many also have remnants of dental lamina and microcysts in their walls, and this tends to be more prominent in syndromic OKCs {4852}. OKCs have an increased proliferative capacity, as evidenced by increased mitoses and other indexes of cell proliferation {1752}. A controversial solid subtype of OKC has been reported, but care must be taken to distinguish this from keratin-producing ameloblastoma and well-differentiated squamous cell carcinoma {4623}. Rarely, odontogenic carcinoma can arise from the epithelial lining of OKCs, and this should be considered if solid areas have developed. OKCs treated by decompression before enucleation develop metaplastic changes and lose their unique diagnostic features {284}.

Cytology

Smears show polygonal, anucleate squamous cells with well-defined cytoplasmic margins; squamous cells with pyknotic nuclei; and fragments of keratinous debris that may appear lamellar {3541,3369,2149}.

Diagnostic molecular pathology

Molecular analysis is not normally required, but finding *PTCH1* mutations may help in differentiating ambiguous cystic lesions or possible malignant neoplasms that may mimic OKCs.

Essential and desirable diagnostic criteria

Essential: site in the jaws; stratified squamous epithelial lining with surface parakeratin; palisaded hyperchromatic basal cells.

Staging

None

Prognosis and prediction

OKCs have a risk of recurrence (20–30%, although a wide range is reported) after traditional enucleation {497,1049,2316}. This risk can be greatly reduced by more aggressive or adjunctive treatment, including curettage, resection, peripheral ostectomy, cryotherapy, or chemical cautery of the cavity, as well as excision of the overlying mucosa. Before definitive cystectomy, many cysts are decompressed/marsupialized. This has led to a significantly diminished recurrence rate {1049,3565}. Recurrence rates are comparable for syndromic and non-syndromic OKCs {1390}.

Adenomatoid odontogenic tumour

Vargas PA
Gomes CC
Upadhyaya J
van Heerden WFP

Definition
Adenomatoid odontogenic tumour (AOT) is a benign encapsulated epithelial odontogenic tumour that contains rosette- or duct-like structures.

ICD-O coding
9300/0 Adenomatoid odontogenic tumour

ICD-11 coding
2E83.0 & XH2SD0 Benign osteogenic tumours of bone or articular cartilage of skull or face & Adenomatoid odontogenic tumour

2E83.1 & XH2SD0 Benign osteogenic tumours of bone or articular cartilage of lower jaw & Adenomatoid odontogenic tumour

Related terminology
None

Subtype(s)
None

Localization
AOT appears almost exclusively within the jawbones, with two thirds of cases in the maxilla, most commonly in the anterior regions. Three quarters of cases are associated with an unerupted permanent tooth, usually the maxillary canine, and expand the follicle. The rarer extraosseous lesion occurs mainly in the anterior maxillary gingiva {875}.

Clinical features
Most cases are asymptomatic and all have limited growth potential. Large AOTs present as bone-hard swellings with cortical expansion but not perforation. Peripheral/extraosseous AOTs appear as small gingival nodules {3696}.

Imaging
AOTs arising in a tooth follicle form well-defined, unilocular radiolucencies around or alongside the crown of an unerupted tooth, often extending apically past the cementoenamel junction. Extrafollicular AOT appears as a unilocular radiolucency located between, above, or superimposed upon the roots of erupted teeth {1667}. Tooth displacement and root resorption have been reported, and two thirds of cases exhibit discrete radiopaque foci {3526,3696,875,3778}. Extraosseous lesions may cause superficial erosion of the underlying alveolar bone.

Epidemiology
AOT accounts for < 10% of odontogenic tumours. Two thirds of cases are in female patients. Although AOTs have been reported over a wide age range, > 80% are diagnosed in the second and third decades of life {3526,3696,875}.

Etiology
The etiology is unknown. Multiple AOTs can occur in patients with Schimmelpenning syndrome (MIM number: 163200) {1275, 772}, caused by postzygotic RAS mutations {1691}.

Pathogenesis
KRAS p.G12V and p.G12R mutations are detected in approximately 70% of sporadic AOTs and are independent of the clinicopathological features {1636,956}. MAPK pathway activation occurs in AOT irrespective of *KRAS* mutations {514, 956}. Additionally, copy-number loss at 6p15 and 7p15.3 has been detected in 1 case of AOT {1636}. No other pathogenic variants in oncogenes or tumour suppressor genes have been detected in AOTs {1636}.

Macroscopic appearance
Most AOTs are smooth, rounded, symmetrical masses with a firm consistency {1667}. On cut surface, the lesions are brownish or yellowish, and the growth patterns range from solid to cystic. Follicular AOTs may be removed with the affected tooth.

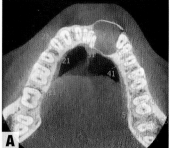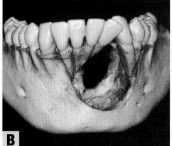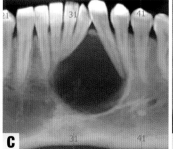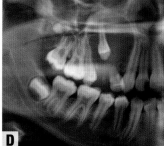

Fig. 7.21 Adenomatoid odontogenic tumour. **A–C** Cone-beam imaging of an adenomatoid odontogenic tumour showing a relatively well-defined radiolucency containing small speckles of mineralization: axial (**A**), 3D reconstruction (**B**), and panoramic reconstruction (**C**). **D** Cropped panoramic radiograph showing an adenomatoid odontogenic tumour with cyst formation on the upper first premolar. The corticated radiolucency is associated with tooth root displacement. There is no visible internal mineralization.

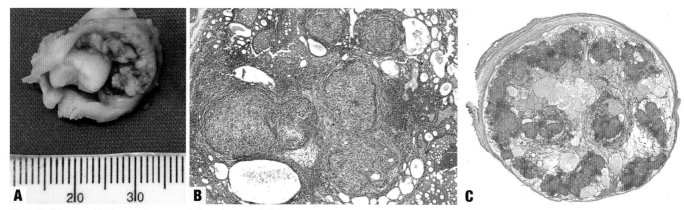

Fig. 7.22 Adenomatoid odontogenic tumour. **A** Gross features of a follicular adenomatoid odontogenic tumour showing a thick fibrous capsule around the crown of a permanent premolar, with intraluminal proliferation. **B** Tumour showing prominent epithelial proliferation organized in solid nodules and strands formed by cuboidal odontogenic epithelial cells, with round arrays of back-to-back columnar cells. **C** Extrafollicular example. A fibrous capsule encloses odontogenic epithelium organized in solid nodules and strands of varying size containing duct-like structures and focal calcification in a haemorrhagic stroma.

Histopathology

AOTs are encapsulated and contain variably sized nodules of spindle, cuboidal, and columnar epithelial odontogenic cells, with minimal stroma {1667}. Within the nodules are rosette- or duct-like structures, which when frequent produce the adenomatoid or gland-like appearance. In some tumours, the duct-like spaces can be inconspicuous. Between the epithelial cells and in the centre of the rosette-like structures, eosinophilic amorphous secretory material similar to enamel matrix is present {3696}. Anastomosing strands of epithelial cells in a plexiform pattern are often present and are more prominent at the periphery. Small foci of calcification, dentinoid matrix, and haemorrhage are variably seen {3696,3778}. AOTs may contain cysts lined by non-keratinizing stratified epithelium, resembling a dentigerous cyst when AOT develops in a dental follicle {3778}.

Differential diagnosis

AOT-like areas have been recognized within other odontogenic tumours, including odontomas, adenomatoid odontogenic hamartoma, adenomatoid dentinoma, and adenoid ameloblastoma {117,4601,2725}, and AOT may contain areas resembling calcifying epithelial odontogenic tumour with clear cells {3083}. These histological overlaps make radiological and clinical correlation essential for definitive diagnosis.

Cytology

Not relevant

Diagnostic molecular pathology

Not relevant

Essential and desirable diagnostic criteria

Essential: site in alveolar processes of jaws; epithelial nodular structure; rosettes of spindled to columnar epithelial cells; duct-like structures; minimal stroma.

Desirable: encapsulation; young patient; association with tooth follicle.

Staging

None

Prognosis and prediction

AOT has almost no risk of recurrence after conservative enucleation.

Squamous odontogenic tumour

Gomez RS
Hunter KD
Upadhyaya J

Definition
Squamous odontogenic tumour (SOT) is a benign epithelial odontogenic tumour with squamous differentiation.

ICD-O coding
9312/0 Squamous odontogenic tumour

ICD-11 coding
2E83.0 & XH4PV9 Benign osteogenic tumours of bone or articular cartilage of skull or face & Squamous odontogenic tumour
2E83.1 & XH4PV9 Benign osteogenic tumours of bone or articular cartilage of lower jaw & Squamous odontogenic tumour

Related terminology
None

Subtype(s)
None

Localization
SOT affects the tooth-bearing parts of the jaws. Most are solitary lesions with a predilection for the anterior maxilla and posterior mandible. Multifocal and peripheral SOTs have been reported {2554,303,1249}.

Clinical features
SOT usually present as an asymptomatic swelling. A minority are associated with pain, tenderness, mobility of teeth, or bone expansion.

Imaging
SOT typically presents as a triangular or semicircular unilocular radiolucency with well-defined borders along one or more tooth roots. Cortication of margins is variable. Root displacement is common, but root resorption is rare. Cortical bone perforation is seen in less common multilocular and aggressive lesions.

Epidemiology
The mean age at diagnosis is 34.8 years, with an almost equal prevalence in men and women {885,4541}. Multifocal SOTs tend to present in a younger age group and show a marked predilection for African Americans {1249}.

Etiology
The etiology is unknown, but a familial incidence has been reported {2554,976}.

Pathogenesis
A role for NOTCH receptors and their ligands in the cytodifferentiation of SOT has been proposed {4056}, and mutations in *AMBN* have been found {3463}.

Macroscopic appearance
Most SOTs are submitted as tan-grey or brown curettings of soft tissue.

Histopathology
SOT comprises variably sized and shaped islands of cytologically bland well-differentiated squamous epithelium in a fibrous or myxoid stroma. The peripheral cells of the islands are flat to cuboidal, with very infrequent mitoses. The central cells have a tendency for cystic degeneration, individual cell keratinization, and calcification. Mucous metaplasia, sebaceous differentiation, and ghost cell–like areas may be present as minor changes {1249,4541}. SOT does not exhibit peripheral palisading, reverse nuclear polarity, cellular atypia, or pleomorphism.

Differential diagnosis
The entities should include acanthomatous ameloblastoma, desmoplastic ameloblastoma, and well-differentiated squamous cell carcinoma. SOT-like proliferation of epithelium may develop in the lining of odontogenic cysts and is a close histological mimic of SOT {4860}.

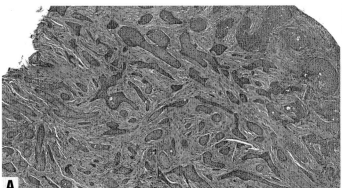
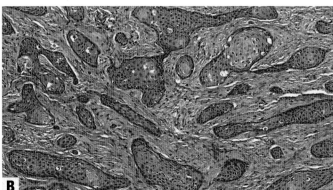

Fig. 7.23 Squamous odontogenic tumour. **A** Islands of benign squamous epithelium in a mature fibrous stroma. **B** The peripheral cells are flattened, and central cells show areas of microcystic degeneration and individual cell keratinization.

Chapter 7

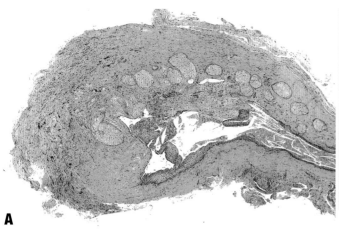

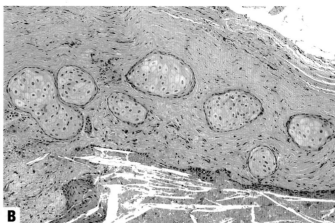

Fig. 7.24 Squamous odontogenic tumour-like proliferation in the wall of an odontogenic cyst. **A,B** Proliferation of epithelium in the wall of an odontogenic cyst can be a close mimic for squamous odontogenic tumour, but the context is not compatible with that diagnosis.

Cytology
Not clinically relevant

Diagnostic molecular pathology
Not relevant

Essential and desirable diagnostic criteria
Essential: location in tooth-bearing areas of jaw; closely packed islands of cytologically bland epithelium; uniform squamous differentiation without significant keratinization; no peripheral palisading or stellate reticulum.

Staging
None

Prognosis and prediction
Unifocal SOT rarely recurs after conservative surgery. Multifocal or recurring SOT, especially of the maxilla, may require a more radical approach.

Calcifying epithelial odontogenic tumour

Hunter KD
Gomez RS
Siriwardena BSMS

Definition
Calcifying epithelial odontogenic tumour (CEOT) is a benign epithelial odontogenic tumour characterized by amyloid, which may calcify.

ICD-O coding
9340/0 Calcifying epithelial odontogenic tumour
9340/0 Clear cell calcifying epithelial odontogenic tumour
9340/0 Cystic/microcystic calcifying epithelial odontogenic tumour
9340/0 Non-calcifying / Langerhans cell–rich calcifying epithelial odontogenic tumour

ICD-11 coding
2E83.0 & XH4PT4 Benign osteogenic tumours of bone or articular cartilage of skull or face & Calcifying epithelial odontogenic tumour
2E83.1 & XH4PT4 Benign osteogenic tumours of bone or articular cartilage of lower jaw & Calcifying epithelial odontogenic tumour

Related terminology
Acceptable: Pindborg tumour.

Subtype(s)
Clear cell CEOT; macrocystic/microcystic CEOT; non-calcifying / Langerhans cell–rich CEOT

Localization
CEOTs arise in tooth-bearing areas of the jaws. Approximately 60% occur in the mandible, with a predilection for the body. Over 85% of CEOTs arise centrally, the remainder occurring at adjacent extraosseous sites {876}.

Clinical features
Many CEOTs are asymptomatic. Larger examples cause slow-growing localized expansion of the jaw and tooth mobility.

Imaging
Radiographically, 75% of CEOTs have mixed radiodensity, but the extent of calcification increases with age. About 30% of CEOTs appear multilocular, and about half have cortical

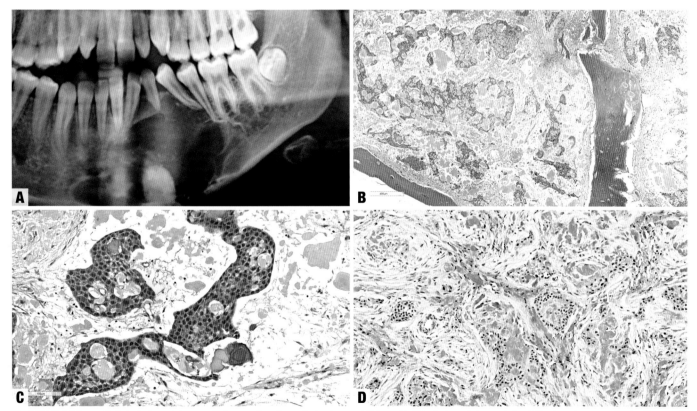

Fig. 7.25 Calcifying epithelial odontogenic tumour. **A** Panoramic radiograph showing a calcifying epithelial odontogenic tumour in the left body and parasymphysis of the mandible, generally a well-defined radiolucency with some small internal mineralizations. **B** Islands of odontogenic epithelium, with amyloid and focal calcification. **C** High-power view of the epithelial islands, including the polygonal cells, intercellular prickles, and mild nuclear pleomorphism. **D** Congo red stain demonstrating the amyloid material.

perforation. Cortication is variable. About half of all cases are associated with an unerupted tooth. On CT, the lesion has diffuse high attenuation. On MRI, the lesion is hypointense on T1-weighted images and hyperintense on T2-weighted images {977}.

Epidemiology
Central lesions occur across a wide age range (8–83 years), with a maximum incidence in the fourth decade of life and with an equal sex distribution {876}.

The clear cell subtype arises in a slightly older patient population, with a female predominance.

Etiology
Unknown

Pathogenesis
The pathogenesis is unknown. Mutations in the tumour suppressor genes *PTEN* and *CDKN2A*, in the oncogenes *JAK3* and *MET* {1059}, and in *AMBN* {3462,172} and *PTCH1* {3445} have been reported in CEOT.

Macroscopic appearance
Lesions are solid with variable calcification and, rarely, cystic spaces.

Histopathology
The histological features are variable. There are clear cell, macrocystic/microcystic, and non-calcifying / Langerhans cell–rich histological subtypes. Lesions with mixed CEOT and adenomatoid odontogenic tumour features should be classified as adenomatoid odontogenic tumour subtypes.

Most CEOTs comprise sheets, cords, or nests of polyhedral epithelial cells with distinct cell borders and prominent intercellular bridges. Nuclear pleomorphism may be present, and sometimes extreme, but mitoses are very rare. Classic CEOTs contain deposits of amorphous, lightly eosinophilic amyloid composed of ameloblast-associated proteins including odontogenic ameloblast-associated protein (ODAM). This stains with Congo red and is birefringent on polarization. The amyloid may calcify, forming large masses or small, round, concentric, densely basophilic calcifications with Liesegang rings. CEOT may extend into adjacent medullary spaces in an infiltrative pattern, which is worrisome for malignancy. Foci resembling CEOT may be found in odontomas and the follicles of unerupted teeth.

Subtypes
The clear cell subtype contains a variable proportion of cells with PAS-positive, diastase-labile glycogen accumulation. Stains for mucins are negative. Most also contain areas of more

conventional CEOT {876,4096}. Macrocystic and microcystic subtypes have been reported, some with areas of focal pseudoglandular change in an otherwise conventional CEOT {3851}. The natural history of these subtypes is not known.

The non-calcifying / Langerhans cell–rich subtype is an area of diagnostic uncertainty, with morphological and molecular features suggesting it is a subtype of odontogenic fibroma rather than CEOT {5031}. Although the lack of calcification could reflect relative immaturity of the lesions, this subtype appears to be distinct, because such tumours often contain significant numbers of Langerhans cells. Some cases have other features of CEOT focally, but the majority consist of small, scattered islands of epithelium in a collagenous and amyloid-rich background, resembling the amyloid-rich subtype of odontogenic fibroma {5031,3781}.

Cytology
Smears are paucicellular, with scattered tissue fragments of mildly pleomorphic squamous cells with abundant eosinophilic (Pap) amorphous material and often plentiful concentric calcifications in a cystic or bloody background {4016,1720}. Nuclear pleomorphism may result in a misleading suggestion of a malignant neoplasm. The role of FNAB cytopathology is contentious, with some arguing it assists in distinguishing benign from malignant lesions and often specific diagnoses in the jaw when used in concert with clinical/site and radiological findings {3541}.

Diagnostic molecular pathology
EWSR1 gene rearrangement may aid in the differentiation of the clear cell subtype of CEOT from clear cell odontogenic carcinoma {456}.

Essential and desirable diagnostic criteria
Essential: radiology: a unilocular or (less commonly) multilocular lesion, which may be radiolucent or of mixed radiodensity; histology: sheets, islands, and cords of polyhedral cells with distinct cell borders and very few or no mitoses; presence of amyloid.
Desirable: prominent intercellular bridges; pleomorphism.

Staging
None

Prognosis and prediction
The recurrence rate is about 13% and varies with treatment modality, being much higher in those treated by curettage {876}. No histological parameters predict recurrence. Malignant transformation develops rarely {4324}. The non-calcifying / Langerhans cell–rich subtype behaves like odontogenic fibroma, with minimal or no risk of recurrence {5031}.

Ameloblastoma, unicystic

Vered M
Heikinheimo K
Nagatsuka H
Siriwardena BSMS

Definition
Unicystic ameloblastoma (UAM) is an intraosseous ameloblastoma with a single cyst cavity.

ICD-O coding
9310/0 Ameloblastoma, unicystic
9310/0 Luminal ameloblastoma, unicystic
9310/0 Intraluminal ameloblastoma, unicystic
9310/0 Mural ameloblastoma, unicystic

ICD-11 coding
2E83.0 & XH1SV4 Benign osteogenic tumours of bone or articular cartilage of skull or face & Ameloblastoma, NOS
2E83.1 & XH1SV4 Benign osteogenic tumours of bone or articular cartilage of lower jaw & Ameloblastoma, NOS

Related terminology
None

Subtype(s)
Luminal UAM; intraluminal UAM; mural UAM

Localization
Most UAMs develop in the posterior body and the ramus of the mandible {24,3522,4097}.

Clinical features
UAM is usually an asymptomatic jaw swelling.

Imaging
Most UAMs are unilocular, well-demarcated radiolucencies, often accompanied by unerupted teeth (frequently mandibular third molars) {1304,3522}. Root resorption and cortical bone perforation are often present {3760}.

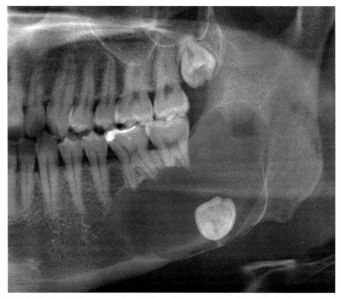

Fig. 7.26 Ameloblastoma, unicystic. Part of a panoramic radiograph showing a typical corticated unilocular radiolucency with resorption of roots of the adjacent molar teeth.

Epidemiology
UAM accounts for 5–22% of all ameloblastomas {3522}. For UAM associated with impacted teeth, the mean patient age is 16 years, versus 35 years for UAM in the absence of tooth impaction {3522}. Approximately 50% of cases are diagnosed in the second decade of life {24,4097}, and there is a slight male predominance.

Etiology
Unknown

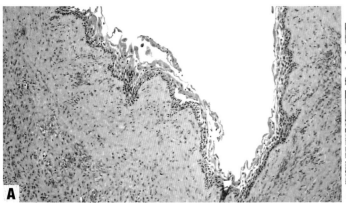
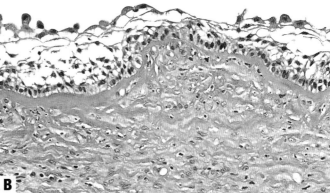

Fig. 7.27 Ameloblastoma, unicystic. **A** Low-power view of the cyst wall, showing regular epithelium that appears to be dyscohesive and no islands in the wall. There is a prominent hyperchromatic basal cell layer, palisaded focally. **B** High-power view showing the lining epithelium in one of the zones with elongate or palisaded basal cells, reverse polarity, and cytoplasmic vacuolation. The surface cells, sometimes called "parachute cells" because of their shape, are distinctive. Subepithelial hyalinization in a narrow band is a common finding.

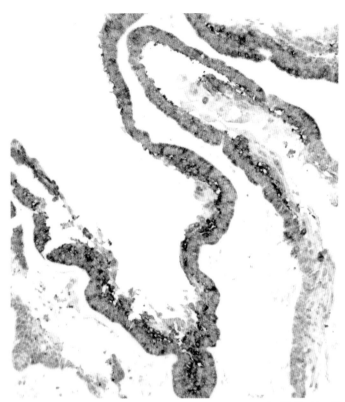

Fig. 7.28 Ameloblastoma, unicystic. Positive cytoplasmic staining for BRAF p.V600E by immunohistochemistry.

Pathogenesis
UAM is probably caused by dysregulated MAPK signalling pathways, with *BRAF* p.V600E being the most common activating mutation in all subtypes {3467,1821}. *SMO* mutation activating the hedgehog pathway also occurs {1821}.

Macroscopic appearance
UAM is a single cyst. Substantial extensions of the lining epithelium may fill the lumen.

Histopathology
A single cyst lined by epithelium, with a palisaded columnar basal layer with reverse polarity and stellate reticulum–like upper layers in most of the lining, constitutes the luminal subtype. Additional plexiform epithelial masses may extend into the lumen only, constituting the intraluminal type. Additional islands of epithelium extending into the wall constitute the mural subtype {3522}. Extensive sampling is required for accurate definition of subtype. Similar but focal changes may be seen in dentigerous and radicular cysts, especially in areas of inflammation.

Cytology
Not clinically relevant

Diagnostic molecular pathology
BRAF p.V600E immunohistochemistry and genetic testing have potential but are not yet validated for diagnosis {1821,3862}.

Essential and desirable diagnostic criteria
Essential: a single cyst; an ameloblastic epithelial lining.
Desirable: detection of luminal and mural extension for subtype diagnosis.

Staging
None

Prognosis and prediction
As many as 30% of UAMs may recur after enucleation {2483}, because a definitive diagnosis before initial treatment is not possible. Conservative marsupialization followed by enucleation is proposed for luminal and intraluminal UAM but carries a risk of recurrence, demanding long-term follow-up {3315,3072}.

Mural UAM appears to be intermediate between UAM and conventional ameloblastoma. A diagnosis of mural UAM might require consideration of more extensive surgery (like for conventional ameloblastoma), depending on size, extent of intramural proliferation, and radiological findings {3315,5055}. However, an accurate diagnosis often only follows definitive removal, allowing a period of follow-up to confirm recurrence before more aggressive treatment. *BRAF* p.V600E mutations confer a lower risk of recurrence than other MAPK pathway–related mutations {600,1710,1821} and may be a better predictor than division into unicystic and conventional types {5055}. The mutation status of all UAM subtypes is similar. Early data suggest BRAF-targeted therapy is effective in mutation-positive UAM {1877} and conventional ameloblastoma {4359}.

Ameloblastoma, extraosseous/peripheral

Chi A
Vered M

Definition
Extraosseous ameloblastoma (EA) is the soft tissue counterpart of intraosseous ameloblastoma.

ICD-O coding
9310/0 Ameloblastoma, extraosseous/peripheral

ICD-11 coding
2E83.0 & XH1SV4 Benign osteogenic tumours of bone or articular cartilage of skull or face & Ameloblastoma, NOS
2E83.1 & XH1SV4 Benign osteogenic tumours of bone or articular cartilage of lower jaw & Ameloblastoma, NOS

Related terminology
Not recommended: soft tissue ameloblastoma; ameloblastoma of mucosal origin; ameloblastoma of the gingiva.

Subtype(s)
None

Localization
EA occurs only in soft tissues overlying tooth-bearing areas or edentulous ridges of the jaws, with a mandible-to-maxilla ratio of 1.6:1 to 3.3:1 {3523,1725,617,616}. The most frequent subsites are the mandibular premolar and maxillary molar regions {617, 1725,3523,616,5023}; the lingual aspect of the alveolar ridge is often involved.

Clinical features
EA is an asymptomatic, slow-growing, firm epulis with a mean diameter of < 20 mm {3523,5023}.

Imaging
On imaging, superficial erosion of the underlying bone may be seen, but a central component precludes a diagnosis of EA.

Epidemiology
EA accounts for as many as 10% of all ameloblastomas {3523}. The mean patient age is 52 years (range: 9–92 years), with 64% of cases occurring during the fifth to seventh decades of life {3523}. The M:F ratio is 1.4:1 {3523}; however, a greater male predilection has been reported in some Asian series {3523, 5023}.

Etiology
Like other ameloblastomas, EA is probably caused by dysregulated MAPK signalling pathways.

Pathogenesis
BRAF p.V600E mutations have been reported in 10 of 16 peripheral ameloblastoma cases {4973,1710,2245,3346,517}, with *NRAS* p.Q61R occurring in 1 of 3 cases {4973}.

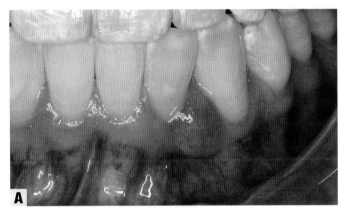

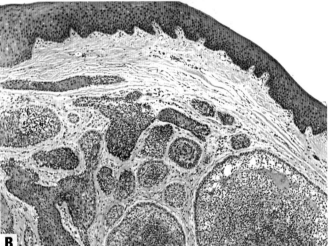

Fig. 7.29 Ameloblastoma, extraosseous. **A** A nodule on the gingiva, without radiographic evidence of underlying bone involvement. **B** Mucosa with ameloblastic tumour islands within the lamina propria, characterized by hyperchromatic peripheral basal cells and looser epithelium centrally.

Macroscopic appearance
EA is a firm to somewhat spongy mucosal mass, solid or with tiny cystic spaces {3523,5023}.

Histopathology
The histopathological features and growth patterns are the same as in conventional ameloblastoma {3523}.

Immunohistochemistry
BerEP4 expression on immunohistochemistry may aid in distinguishing intraoral basal cell carcinoma from EA {4542}.

Differential diagnosis
The differential diagnosis includes peripheral odontogenic fibroma, peripheral squamous odontogenic tumour, odontogenic gingival epithelial hamartoma, and intraoral basal cell carcinoma {3523}.

Cytology
Not clinically relevant

Diagnostic molecular pathology
Not relevant

Essential and desirable diagnostic criteria
Essential: site in the gingiva or edentulous alveolar mucosa; no intraosseous component; histopathological features of conventional ameloblastoma.

Staging
Not applicable

Prognosis and prediction
EA has a more indolent behaviour than conventional ameloblastoma {3523}. Recurrence rates after conservative supraperiosteal excision range from 9% to 20%, although some recurrences may result from incomplete removal {204} and long-term follow-up is recommended. Malignant transformation is exceedingly rare {304}.

Ameloblastoma, conventional

Vered M
Adebiyi KE
Heikinheimo K

Definition
Ameloblastoma (AM) is a benign but locally infiltrative epithelial odontogenic neoplasm of the jawbones characterized by ameloblast-like cells and stellate reticulum.

ICD-O coding
9310/0 Ameloblastoma, NOS
9310/0 Follicular ameloblastoma
9310/0 Plexiform ameloblastoma
9310/0 Acanthomatous ameloblastoma
9310/0 Granular cell ameloblastoma
9310/0 Basal cell ameloblastoma
9310/0 Desmoplastic ameloblastoma

ICD-11 coding
2E83.0 & XH1SV4 Benign osteogenic tumours of bone or articular cartilage of skull or face & Ameloblastoma, NOS
2E83.1 & XH1SV4 Benign osteogenic tumours of bone or articular cartilage of lower jaw & Ameloblastoma, NOS

Related terminology
Acceptable: solid/multicystic ameloblastoma.
Not recommended: classic intraosseous ameloblastoma.

Subtype(s)
Follicular AM; plexiform AM; acanthomatous AM; granular cell AM; basal cell AM; desmoplastic AM

Localization
As many as 87% of AMs arise in the mandible, predominantly in the posterior molar area {1838,5055}. Maxillary AMs are usually posteriorly sited. The exception is the desmoplastic subtype, which has an almost equal jaw distribution and a preponderance for the anterior regions {873}. Extremely rarely, AMs are also found in the sinonasal region {354,3907}.

Clinical features
AM presents as a painless, slow-growing mass that, if untreated, reaches a large size, displaces and loosens teeth, expands and perforates the cortices, may cause paraesthesia, and ultimately causes disfigurement and risks adjacent vital structures {1218, 3011}.

Imaging
On 2D radiographs, AM usually presents as a multilocular radiolucency showing a soap-bubble or honeycomb pattern (72%) and well-defined corticated margins (54%) {5055}; 3D imaging (preferably contrast-enhanced CT) reveals the internal bony architecture, content, size, expansion, and cortical perforation more accurately {222,152}. Impacted teeth are associated with 18% of AMs {5055}.

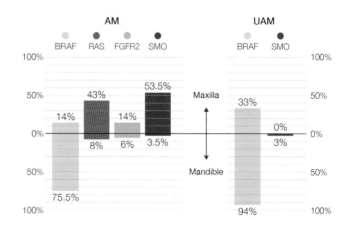

Fig. 7.30 Ameloblastoma, conventional. The most commonly identified oncogenic mutations and their relative frequencies in ameloblastoma (AM) and unicystic ameloblastoma (UAM) located in the mandible or maxilla {2422,600,4307,1821}.

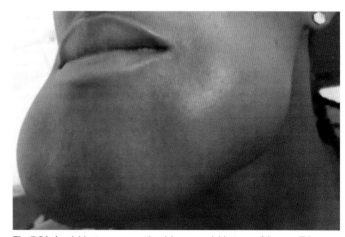

Fig. 7.31 Ameloblastoma, conventional. Large ameloblastoma of the mandible, causing facial deformity.

Bone formation in desmoplastic AMs may produce a fine honeycomb, mixed radiolucent appearance resembling a fibro-osseous lesion {873}.

Epidemiology
AM is the most common odontogenic neoplasm in all ethnic groups, representing approximately 1% of all head and neck neoplasms in Europe and the USA, probably with the highest incidence in African and Afro-Caribbean populations {3070}. The incidence of AM is approximately 0.052–0.092 new cases per 100 000 person-years worldwide, and there is no sex predilection. The peak incidence of diagnosis is in the fourth and

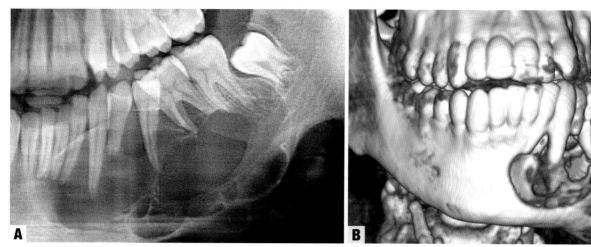

Fig. 7.32 Ameloblastoma, conventional. **A** Panoramic radiograph of an ameloblastoma forming a typical radiolucent, multilocular, soap bubble–pattern lesion with cortical expansion, tooth displacement, and root resorption. **B** 3D CT reconstruction highlights expansion and the multilocularity of the tumour.

fifth decades of life, with a patient age range of 8–92 years {615, 1504,1854}. The diagnosis is generally made at a somewhat lower age in women, especially in populations of African heritage {3313}. For *BRAF* p.V600E–mutant cases, the reported mean patient age at diagnosis is about 34 years, compared with about 54 years for *BRAF* wildtype cases {600}.

Etiology
Unknown

Pathogenesis
AM is caused by dysregulated MAPK and hedgehog signalling pathways, probably in SOX2-positive dental epithelial stem cells / ameloblast progenitor cells {3405,3963,1655,2133,1823}. *BRAF* p.V600E mutations are the most common activating mutations in the MAPK pathway, followed by mutually exclusive mutations in RAS genes (*KRAS*, *NRAS*, *HRAS*) and *FGFR2* {2422,4307, 600,1821}. Dysregulation of the hedgehog signalling pathway may participate, especially in maxillary AMs, where mutation of

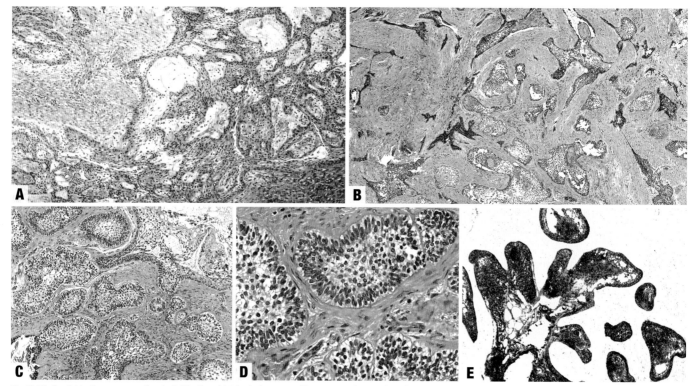

Fig. 7.33 Ameloblastoma, conventional. **A** Plexiform histological pattern with anastomosing cords and strands of tumour. **B** Mixed pattern, with larger, rounded, pale-staining areas characteristic of the follicular histological pattern and focally acanthomatous, spiky, darker-staining islands with more cellular central areas, characteristic of the desmoplastic pattern. **C** Follicular pattern, with acanthomatous change in the large cyst. Peripheral epithelial cells in the islands have hyperchromatic nuclei in a palisading pattern, reverse polarity, and often cytoplasmic vacuolation. **D** High-power view of the follicular pattern showing peripheral ameloblast-like cells with palisaded nuclei, reverse polarity, and cytoplasmic vacuolation; and looser, stellate reticulum–like cells in the centre of the follicles. **E** Positive immunohistochemical staining for p.V600E-mutant BRAF in ameloblastoma epithelium. The staining is cytoplasmic.

SMO is the most frequent mutation to co-occur with the MAPK pathway mutation {4307,600}. Epigenetic factors are largely unknown, but mutation signatures in mandibular AM appear to correlate with smoking {1699}.

Macroscopic appearance
AMs range from solid and yellowish-white tumours to multicystic tumours with little intervening solid tissue {3962}. AM may extend into adjacent cancellous bone.

Histopathology
In the commonest histological subtype, the follicular subtype, there are islands of epithelium resembling the epithelial component of the enamel organ in a fibrous stroma. Peripheral cells are columnar to cuboidal (ameloblast-like), with hyperchromatic nuclei arranged in a palisading pattern with reverse polarity, and often subnuclear vacuolation {4630,3515}. The central epithelium is reminiscent of stellate reticulum, with loosely arranged angular cells, and often undergoes cystic change. The second commonest subtype is the plexiform subtype, composed of anastomosing strands of ameloblastomatous epithelium with an inconspicuous stellate reticulum, less prominent ameloblast-like cells, and cyst-like degeneration in the stroma rather than the epithelium. Mitoses are usually scattered but posterior maxillary AM may have high cellularity and frequent mitoses.

Several other subtypes are recognized {1854}. The acanthomatous subtype has squamous differentiation centrally in islands but maintains the reverse polarization of the nuclei in peripheral columnar cells. In the granular cell subtype the central epithelium develops abundant eosinophilic granular cytoplasm. The basal cell subtype comprises islands and strands of basaloid cells with scant cytoplasm and peripheral palisading, reminiscent of basal cell carcinoma {3012}. The desmoplastic subtype has more widely dispersed islands with spiky outlines, cuboidal to flat peripheral cells, and central spindle-shaped cells in a densely collagenous stroma, sometimes with osteoplasia. Many AMs contain more than one histological subtype {3084}.

Cytology
Not clinically relevant

Diagnostic molecular pathology
BRAF p.V600E immunohistochemistry and genetic testing have potential but are not yet validated for diagnosis {600,1821}.

Essential and desirable diagnostic criteria
Essential: location in jaws; islands/strands of odontogenic epithelium bounded by cuboidal/columnar cells with palisaded, hyperchromatic nuclei; reverse polarity (less marked in the plexiform pattern); loose central epithelium resembling stellate reticulum; no cytological atypia.

Staging
None

Prognosis and prediction
AM recurs if inadequately removed. The standard of care is complete excision with negative margins {3515}, irrespective of the histopathological subtype {3566}. This requires removal of a bone margin of ≥ 10 mm beyond the radiographic margin to ensure removal of AM permeating medullary bone, usually by a segmental resection, mandibulectomy, or maxillectomy, depending on size {3012}. More conservative surgery has a high recurrence rate (60–80%), and long follow-up (1–2 decades) is mandatory {3675}. Mandibular tumours are more likely to harbour *BRAF* p.V600E mutations, and AM with these mutations is associated with a later recurrence than wildtype AM {2422, 4307,600,1821}. Furthermore, single versus multiple mutations and geographical regions also seem to stratify patients for recurrence risk {1710}.

BRAF inhibitor treatment has been proposed, alone or in combination with MEK inhibitors, which also inhibit the MAPK/ERK pathway {1642,1822,3346,1487}. Early data show effectiveness in selected cases {1877} and in disseminated AM {2233}.

Chapter 7

Adenoid ameloblastoma

Thavaraj S
Bilodeau EA

Definition
Adenoid ameloblastoma (AA) is an epithelial odontogenic neoplasm characterized by a cribriform architecture and duct-like structures, often with dentinoid.

ICD-O coding
9310/0 Adenoid ameloblastoma

ICD-11 coding
2E83.0 & XH1SV4 Benign osteogenic tumours of bone or articular cartilage of skull or face & Ameloblastoma, NOS
2E83.1 & XH1SV4 Benign osteogenic tumours of bone or articular cartilage of lower jaw & Ameloblastoma, NOS

Related terminology
Acceptable: adenoid ameloblastoma with dentinoid.

Subtype(s)
None

Localization
No site predilection defined

Clinical features
There is usually a painless swelling, with a mean diameter of 40 mm {2725}. Sometimes there is pain and paraesthesia {1044}.

Imaging
Most AAs are radiolucent and unilocular with well-defined boundaries, but multilocularity, internal mineralization, cortical perforation, root resorption, and paranasal sinus involvement may occur {31,4171}.

Epidemiology
Incidence peaks in the fourth decade of life, with a slight male predilection (M:F ratio: 1.3:1), but there is a wide age range (15–82 years) {2066}. Most AAs have occurred in South America and Asia {2725,3274A,2265A,4893A,4009A}.

Etiology
Unknown

Pathogenesis
AAs harbour *CTNNB1* mutations {364A}, whereas *BRAF* p.V600E mutations, typical of other ameloblastomas, appear to be absent {958}. The *KRAS* p.G12V and p.G12R mutations typical of adenomatoid odontogenic tumour also appear to be absent {958}.

Macroscopic appearance
AA is predominantly multicystic, with solid zones and variable hard tissue.

Histopathology
AA is characterized by a partly cribriform arrangement of basal ameloblast-like cells demonstrating reversed nuclear polarity and a minor component of suprabasal stellate reticulum–like epithelium. Basal cells may be multilayered, with a transition to a round or ovoid morphology. Distinctive features are duct-like structures formed by cuboidal to columnar cells, some of which contain mucin, and focal whorled cellular condensations reminiscent of morules. Two thirds of cases contain varying amounts of dentinoid. Clear cells are often closely associated with dentinoid, and ghost cell keratinization may be a minor feature {2066}.

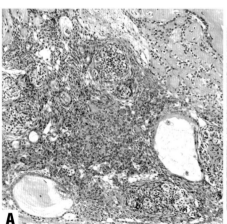 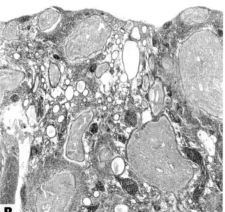 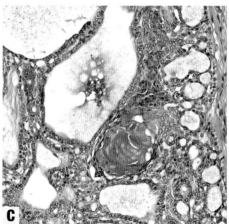

Fig. 7.34 Adenoid ameloblastoma. **A** Duct-like structures, epithelial whorls, and clear cells in close approximation to dentinoid. **B** Characteristic cribriform architecture with pseudocysts, duct-like structures, and whorls or morules. **C** Focal ghost cell keratinization.

Immunohistochemistry
There is variable staining for CK14, CK19, p40, p16, and p53. CK7 is weak to negative {31}. Nuclear β-catenin positivity colocalizes with morules, and Ki-67 indexes are usually high {2725,2266,455}.

Differential diagnosis
There are overlapping histomorphological features with adenomatoid odontogenic tumour and dentinogenic ghost cell tumour, but AA is distinguished by the combination of cribriform pattern, duct-like structures, whorls/morules, and dentinoid. A lack of *EWSR1* rearrangement aids the exclusion of clear cell odontogenic carcinoma when clear cells are prominent. Criteria to distinguish aggressive AA from odontogenic carcinoma with dentinoid are not yet defined {2725}.

Cytology
Not clinically relevant

Diagnostic molecular pathology
Not clinically relevant

Essential and desirable diagnostic criteria
Essential: an ameloblastoma-like component; duct-like structures; whorls/morules; cribriform architecture.
Desirable: dentinoid; clear cells; focal ghost cell keratinization.

Staging
None

Prognosis and prediction
AA is locally infiltrative, with a recurrence rate as high as 70% {1290,1999,3899,2725,2066}. Cytological atypia, hypercellularity, p53 positivity, and high Ki-67 proliferation index are associated with recurrence, but the border line with ameloblastic carcinoma {3085} is not yet defined.

Metastasizing ameloblastoma

Chi A
Franchi A
Sarode SC

Definition

Metastasizing ameloblastoma (MA) is an ameloblastoma that has metastasized despite a benign histopathological appearance in the primary and metastatic foci.

ICD-O coding

9310/3 Ameloblastoma, metastasizing

ICD-11 coding

2E83.0 & XH96J9 Benign osteogenic tumours of bone or articular cartilage of skull or face & Ameloblastoma, metastasizing
2E83.1 & XH96J9 Benign osteogenic tumours of bone or articular cartilage of lower jaw & Ameloblastoma, metastasizing

Related terminology

Acceptable: benign metastasizing ameloblastoma.
Not recommended: malignant ameloblastoma; malignant adamantinoma; metastatic ameloblastoma; atypical ameloblastoma.

Subtype(s)

None

Localization

The primary tumour develops more frequently in the mandible than in the maxilla {1921,3380}. The most common sites of metastasis are the lungs, followed by the cervical lymph nodes {3380}, with distant metastasis in approximately 68% of MAs {1921}. Infrequently reported metastatic sites include bone, brain, liver, and pericardium {3204,3225,436,3823,3380}.

Clinical features

Symptoms vary by site; some patients are asymptomatic. Pulmonary metastases may cause dry cough, haemoptysis, and dyspnoea {4563,3820}. Metastasis may be diagnosed concurrently with the primary tumour or after a variable, often long, latent period (range: 0–45 years; mean: 11 years) {4586, 3380}. Metastases retain the benign ameloblastoma growth pattern.

Epidemiology

Incidence data are only available combined with ameloblastic carcinoma, which is more common; the combined annual cumulative incidence is 1.79 cases per 10 million person-years {3708}. MA has a mean age at diagnosis of 45 years and a slight male predominance {1921,3380}.

Etiology

MA harbours *BRAF* p.V600E mutations {2233}. Risk factors for metastasis include large size, rapid enlargement, protracted clinical course, inadequate removal, and multiple recurrences at the primary site {1921}.

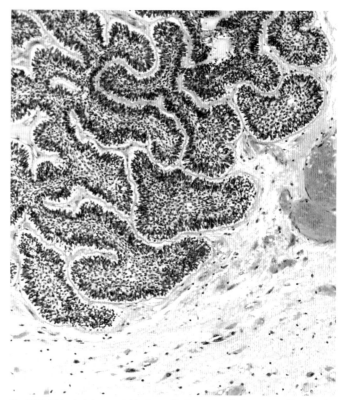

Fig. 7.35 Metastasizing ameloblastoma. Brain metastasis from a maxillary ameloblastoma.

Pathogenesis

Metastasis may result from haematogenous spread during surgical treatment of the primary {1921}. Alternatively, metastasis could be driven by additional genetic alterations without histopathological changes {1921}, but no putative molecular markers of metastatic behaviour have been identified {1530}.

Macroscopic appearance

Features are identical to those of conventional ameloblastoma.

Histopathology

MA exhibits identical histopathological features to conventional ameloblastoma, with no specific features predicting metastasis. Among reported MA cases, the plexiform histological pattern is most common {4586,3380}.

Cytology

FNAC has been employed in some cases for evaluating metastatic deposits, although cytological features alone are not sufficient for conclusive diagnosis {651A,670A}.

Diagnostic molecular pathology

Not relevant

Essential and desirable diagnostic criteria

Essential: benign conventional ameloblastoma in the primary tumour and metastasis; no cytological atypia or features of malignancy in the primary tumour or metastasis.

Staging

None

Prognosis and prediction

MA has an overall mean survival time of 5 years on systematic review {3380}. Surgery is the mainstay of treatment; radiotherapy and chemotherapy have no proven benefit {1140,1921}. BRAF-targeted therapy has been reported in limited cases {2233,597}. Recurrence occurs in about one quarter of cases and is associated with increased mortality {1921}.

Odontoma

Vered M
Gomes CC
Soluk Tekkeşin M

Definition
Odontomas are mixed odontogenic hamartomas that mature from soft tissue to predominantly dental hard tissues with a small amount of residual odontogenic epithelium and ectomesenchyme.

ICD-O coding
9280/0 Odontoma, NOS
9280/0 Complex odontoma
9280/0 Compound odontoma

ICD-11 coding
2E83.0 & XH4QJ8 Benign osteogenic tumours of bone or articular cartilage of skull or face & Odontoma, NOS
2E83.1 & XH4QJ8 Benign osteogenic tumours of bone or articular cartilage of lower jaw & Odontoma, NOS

Related terminology
None

Subtype(s)
Complex odontoma (CxO); compound odontoma (CdO)

Localization
CxOs develop mainly in the posterior body of the mandible, CdOs in the anterior maxilla {4163,3882}.

Clinical features
Odontomas are asymptomatic, slow-growing lesions, often associated with unerupted teeth. The diameter is typically 10–30 mm; larger lesions expand the jaws, displace and resorb teeth, and prevent tooth eruption. Odontomas as large as 80 mm in diameter can be encountered {4473,2549}. Odontomas occasionally erupt or sustain trauma and may become infected. Odontomas may be multiple.

Imaging
Radiographically, developing odontomas are predominantly radiolucent with a corticated periphery, sometimes with small radiopacities. Small lesions resemble a developing tooth crypt. With maturation, CxO slowly develops irregular disorganized masses of calcified material of enamel and dentine radiodensity. CdO develops into tooth-like structures of varying size and shape. Mixed patterns may occur. Both types retain a narrow peripheral radiolucent zone with a smooth or lobular outline.

Epidemiology
Among referral series of odontogenic tumours, odontoma is the second most common lesion, frequently occurring in the second and third decades of life, without a distinct sex predilection {4163,4094,4095,4164}, but many small odontomas are treated outside hospital or left untreated.

Etiology
Unknown

Genetic factors
Multiple odontomas arise in odontoma-dysphagia syndrome (MIM number: 164330), Schimmelpenning–Feuerstein–Mims syndrome (MIM number: 163200), familial

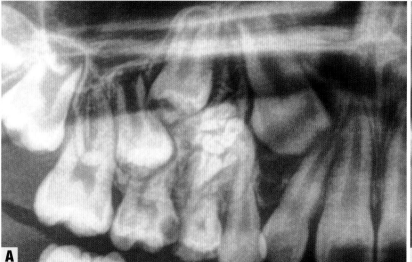
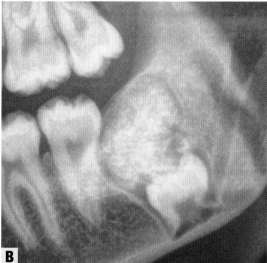

Fig. 7.36 Odontoma. **A** Compound subtype. Cropped panoramic radiograph showing a mass composed of several small, radiopaque tooth-like structures, displacing the first maxillary premolar upwards. **B** Complex subtype. Cropped panoramic radiograph showing a well-defined radiopaque mass associated with the mandibular third molar, which was displaced downwards to the lower border of the mandible with the inferior alveolar nerve canal.

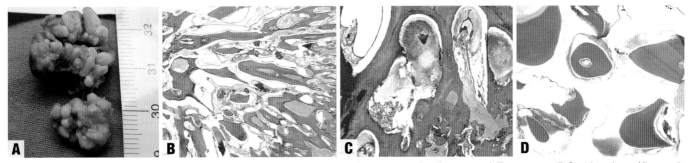

Fig. 7.37 Odontoma. **A** Compound subtype. Macroscopic view showing a conglomerate of numerous small, rudimentary tooth-like structures. **B** Complex subtype. Microscopic section showing radiating sheets of dentine enclosing spaces containing enamel matrix where mature enamel has been removed by decalcification. **C** Complex odontoma at high magnification, highlighting the keyhole spaces containing basophilic enamel matrix, which has a prismatic structure. Residual odontogenic epithelium is also present around matrix. **D** Compound subtype. Microscopic view of multiple small, tooth-like structures.

adenomatous polyposis (MIM number: 175100), and encephalocraniocutaneous lipomatosis (MIM number: 613001).

Pathogenesis

WNT/β-catenin pathway activation in embryonic SOX2-positive dental stem cells can drive odontoma formation {4876,1494}.

Odontoma does not harbour *BRAF* p.V600E mutations {957, 3273}, unlike ameloblastic fibroma {600,607,3273,957} and histopathologically similar lesions, previously classified as ameloblastic fibro-odontoma (AFO) {607,3273,957} and ameloblastic fibrodentinoma (AFD) {600,957}.

Macroscopic appearance

CxO comprises amorphous masses of dentine and enamel; CdO comprises multiple tooth-like structures of varying size. Both may be surrounded by capsule-like soft tissue with a smooth surface.

Histopathology

CxO consists of a disorganized mass of mature tubular dentine intermixed with rounded zones of enamel matrix where enamel has been lost on decalcification, with areas of dental pulp and cementum. CdO contains multiple rudimentary teeth exhibiting dentine and enamel matrix. Dentine in odontomas usually shows some irregularity of tubule structure. A variable amount of loose connective tissue and capsule may be present, resembling dental papilla or follicle. These may contain varying amounts of immature odontogenic epithelium in islands and strands {4163, 3882}. These epithelial residues may be prominent and may contain ghost cells, granular cells, and other features resembling other odontogenic tumours, but these are hamartomatous and of no significance.

Developing odontomas are initially soft tissue, mostly dental papilla–like with prominent epithelial strands, and there may be limited or no evidence of dental hard tissue induction. They resemble ameloblastic fibroma closely and may be difficult to differentiate histologically. Lesions previously diagnosed as AFD and AFO also resemble ameloblastic fibroma, with less prominent and less well organized induction of dental hard tissue matrix or hard tissue than in odontomas. Radiographic appearance, patient age, and lesion size may help distinguish these lesions {4166}.

AFD and AFO were previously classified as developing odontomas. However, a proportion of AFDs {600,957} and fewer AFOs {607,3273,957} harbour *BRAF* p.V600E mutations, suggesting a relationship with ameloblastic fibroma, rather than with odontomas, which lack this mutation. Histological and molecular overlap makes it unclear whether AFD and AFO are separate entities, intermediate lesions with a spectrum of behaviour that ultimately result in the formation of odontoma, or a mixture of developing odontomas and ameloblastic fibromas.

Odontomas are occasionally the origin of cysts of the dentigerous type.

Cytology

Not clinically relevant

Diagnostic molecular pathology

None

Essential and desirable diagnostic criteria

Complex odontoma
Essential: consistent radiographic features; a conglomerate mass of enamel and dentine.
Desirable: dental pulp; cementum.

Compound odontoma
Essential: consistent radiographic features; multiple small, tooth-like structures.

Staging

None

Prognosis and prediction

Odontomas do not recur after enucleation, although recurrence may follow incomplete removal of growing lesions {4473}.

Primordial odontogenic tumour

Mosqueda-Taylor AA
Bilodeau EA

Definition
Primordial odontogenic tumour (POT) is composed of variably cellular fibrous tissue with areas similar to dental papilla, surrounded by epithelium resembling the internal epithelium of the enamel organ.

ICD-O coding
None

ICD-11 coding
2E83.1 & XH43L1 Benign osteogenic tumours of bone or articular cartilage of lower jaw & Odontogenic tumour, benign

Related terminology
None

Subtype(s)
None

Localization
POT arises in the tooth-bearing segments of the jaw and occurs 2–3 times as frequently in the mandible as in the maxilla.

Clinical features
Most cases are asymptomatic. Some POTs produce marked cortical expansion.

Imaging
POT appears as a well-defined radiolucency associated with unerupted teeth, most commonly the mandibular third molar, producing an apparent pericoronal radiolucency. POT may displace and resorb roots of adjacent teeth {515}.

Epidemiology
The age range is 2–19 years (mean: 11.4 years) and there is a slight male predilection {515,4997,1085,2232,3140}.

Etiology
The etiology is unknown. No mutations were identified in 151 cancer-associated genes and 42 odontogenesis-associated genes in 3 POTs studied with next-generation sequencing {2999}.

Pathogenesis
The expression profile of dentinogenesis-associated genes suggests an inhibition of dentine formation. No BRAF p.V600E mutations were found {2999}.

Macroscopic appearance
POT is a solid, well-circumscribed, sometimes multilobulated, whitish mass. The crown of a tooth may be embedded but is easily detached {3086}.

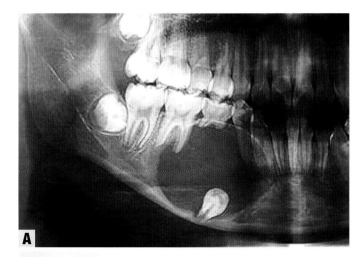

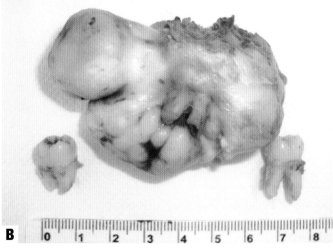

Fig. 7.38 Primordial odontogenic tumour. **A** A well-defined unilocular radiolucency surrounding and displacing the second premolar and producing slight root resorption of the first permanent molar. **B** Macroscopic appearance. A solid, white mass displacing the enclosed molar towards the periphery, visible just below the surface centrally, and closely associated with two further teeth.

Histopathology
POT comprises loose or myxoid fibrous tissue containing variable numbers of fusiform and stellate fibroblasts and areas with the appearance of cellular odontogenic mesenchyme. The periphery is covered by a single layer of columnar or cuboidal epithelium, with scant superficial layers of stellate reticulum–like cells partially enclosed by a thin fibrous capsule. Epithelial cords may appear to be within the lesion as a result of lobular infolding. Extracellular concentric mineralized structures within the epithelium have been reported, but there is no evidence of odontoblastic differentiation or mature dentine.

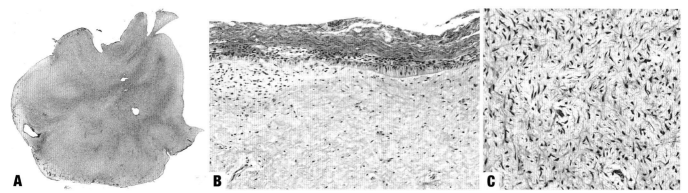

Fig. 7.39 Primordial odontogenic tumour. **A** Macroscopic appearance, with a lobular outline and thin odontogenic epithelial covering. **B** The outer layer, with epithelial cells and palisaded cells and a thin fibrous outer capsule. **C** Cellular loose mesenchyme.

Immunohistochemistry

Mesenchymal cells are positive for vimentin, and subepithelial expression of CD34 and CD138 have been demonstrated in several cases. The Ki-67 index is low (< 5%). The epithelial component is positive for pancytokeratins (AE1/AE3), CK5, and CK14, whereas CK19 is usually expressed by the columnar cells. Amelogenin, ameloblastin, and DSPP have also been detected. Other markers are variably expressed {3086,513,185, 3000,2999}.

Differential diagnosis

POT resembles a mesenchymal proliferation very similar to the dental papilla of a developing tooth.

Cytology

Not clinically relevant

Diagnostic molecular pathology

Not relevant

Essential and desirable diagnostic criteria

Essential: a mass of myxoid dental papilla–like tissue; entire periphery covered by columnar or cuboidal enamel epithelium.

Desirable: focal stellate reticulum–like cells externally; lobular clefted surface.

Staging

None

Prognosis and prediction

POT does not recur after conservative excision {515,4997,1085, 2232,3140}.

Ameloblastic fibroma

Vered M
Gomes CC
Gomez RS

Definition

Ameloblastic fibroma (AF) is a rare, benign, mixed odontogenic tumour comprising cellular mesenchymal tissue resembling dental papilla and an epithelial component resembling early developing enamel organ, without dental hard tissue or matrix.

ICD-O coding

9330/0 Ameloblastic fibroma

ICD-11 coding

2E83.0 & XH06Y3 Benign osteogenic tumours of bone or articular cartilage of skull or face & Ameloblastic fibroma

2E83.1 & XH06Y3 Benign osteogenic tumours of bone or articular cartilage of lower jaw & Ameloblastic fibroma

Related terminology

None

Subtype(s)

None

Localization

AFs are 3 times as frequent in the mandible as in the maxilla {618,870}. The posterior mandible is the most common location, with lesions in the incisor–canine region being infrequent in both jaws, although large lesions (~10%) can occupy as much as a jawbone quadrant.

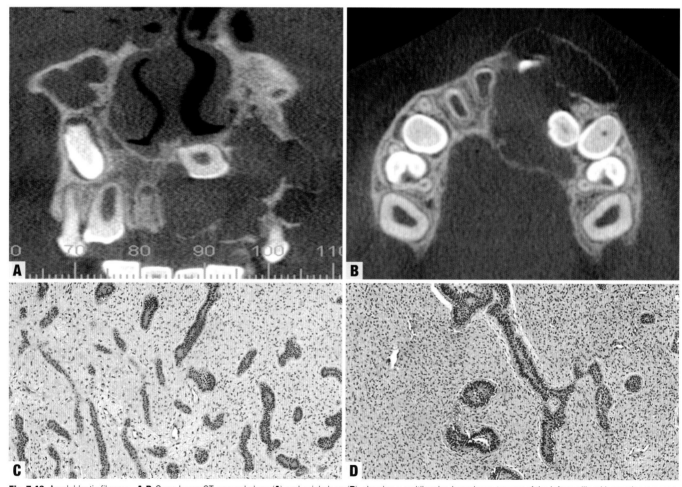

Fig. 7.40 Ameloblastic fibroma. **A,B** Cone-beam CT, coronal plane (**A**) and axial plane (**B**), showing a multilocular, hypodense tumour of the left maxilla with prominent expansion, cortical thinning, and tooth root displacement. **C** Ameloblast-like epithelial cells with tall, hyperchromatic, palisading nuclei with reverse polarity arranged in bilayered, parallel strands in a hypercellular stroma that resembles dental papilla. **D** Some of the epithelial strands widen into rounded expansions, the larger of which may contain a small amount of loose, stellate reticulum–like epithelium. Occasionally, if these enlargements are wide enough, they resemble an early enamel organ.

Clinical features

Most AFs (78%) are slow-growing and eventually cause asymptomatic jawbone expansion. Rare cases range from an incidental radiological finding to large enough to cause facial deformity {618,870}.

Imaging

Radiographically, AFs are well-defined and corticated, with a mean diameter of 50 mm. About 60% are unilocular; larger lesions are multilocular. AFs are usually associated with unerupted and displaced teeth (80%), most frequently the first or second permanent molars. Cortical perforation and tooth root resorption occur in a minority (22%) {870}.

Epidemiology

AF accounts for up to 2% of all odontogenic tumours {1527, 2115}. The mean patient age is 15 years (range: 7 weeks to 61 years) {618,870}, with 80% of cases occurring in patients aged < 22 years {618}. The M:F ratio is 1.4:1.

Etiology

Unknown

Pathogenesis

AF has been considered a neoplasm of both epithelial and mesenchymal components. AF harbours *BRAF* p.V600E mutations in 46% of cases {600,607,3273,957}, which are usually limited to the mesenchymal component and only occasionally identified in both components {957}.

These mutations are also detected in cases previously classified as ameloblastic fibro-odontoma (AFO) (34%) {607,3273, 957} and ameloblastic fibrodentinoma (AFD) (60%) {600,957}, suggesting that at least some cases may be related to AF or other *BRAF*-mutated odontogenic tumours. Although mutations at other oncogenes and tumour suppressor genes have not been detected {957}, AF shows allelic loss at 17p13 {1527}.

Macroscopic appearance

AF is a solid, well-circumscribed, slightly myxoid mass with a smooth outer surface.

Histopathology

The mesenchymal component is myxoid and evenly hypercellular and resembles the dental papilla of the tooth bud. The epithelial component forms long, narrow cords and strands of bilaminar cuboidal to columnar palisaded cells with occasional thickenings. These may contain a minor component of stellate reticulum–like tissue, resembling the follicular stage of the enamel organ. A collagenous capsule may be present. No dental hard tissue is normally present but extensive sampling may reveal small foci.

From histopathological features alone, it may not be possible to distinguish between the neoplastic AF and early-stage hamartomatous odontomas before they differentiate and mature {618,614}. In general, AF lacks architectural organization and is more evenly and densely hypercellular.

Lesions previously diagnosed as AFD and AFO are histologically intermediate between AF and odontomas and have previously been classified as developing stages of odontoma. The status of these tumours has been debated for decades, and the current classification as odontoma is not consistent with the *BRAF* p.V600E mutations, occasional cases with locally aggressive biological behaviour, large size, and recurrence, which appear neoplastic {2318}. AFD and AFO resemble AF but with the additional induction of dental hard tissue matrix (AFD) or dentine and enamel (AFO). It is unclear whether these intermediate lesions are a mixture of odontomas and AFs with hard tissue induction or if they form a spectrum of behaviour, and currently this cannot be resolved histopathologically.

Cytology

Not clinically relevant

Diagnostic molecular pathology

The diagnostic relevance of *BRAF* mutation is not yet defined, but it appears useful for excluding developing odontoma in selected cases.

Essential and desirable diagnostic criteria

Essential: consistent radiographic features; bland, hypercellular, dental papilla–like mesenchyme; dispersed bilaminar strands of cuboidal or columnar odontogenic epithelium.

Staging

None

Prognosis and prediction

AF does not recur after meticulous enucleation, applied to small, asymptomatic tumours in young patients {3525,618}. Recurrence occurs in 19% of cases with more conservative removal {870}. Extensive, destructive, and recurrent tumours should be treated radically. BRAF-targeted inhibitors for selected cases have not yet been assessed. Long-term follow-up is required.

Sarcomatous transformation is rare, but 24% of ameloblastic fibrosarcomas arise in benign AF or recurrent AF {870}. Carcinosarcoma develops even more rarely {1080}.

Dentinogenic ghost cell tumour

Carlos R
Vered M

Definition

Dentinogenic ghost cell tumour (DGCT) is a benign but locally infiltrative odontogenic tumour characterized by ameloblastoma-like sheets and islands of epithelium with prominent ghost cell keratinization and varying amounts of dentinoid in the stroma. Both the ghost cells and dentinoid may mineralize.

ICD-O coding

9302/0 Dentinogenic ghost cell tumour

ICD-11 coding

2E83.0 & XH12N4 Benign osteogenic tumours of bone or articular cartilage of skull or face & Dentinogenic ghost cell tumour
2E83.1 & XH12N4 Benign osteogenic tumours of bone or articular cartilage of lower jaw & Dentinogenic ghost cell tumour

Related terminology

Not recommended: calcifying ghost cell odontogenic tumour; (epithelial) odontogenic ghost cell tumour; dentinoameloblastoma; solid/neoplastic variant of calcifying odontogenic cyst.

Subtype(s)

None

Localization

DGCT arises with almost equal incidence in the mandible and maxilla, with a predilection for the posterior region in both jaws {613,1043}. As many as 25% of all DGCTs are peripheral, located in the gingiva or alveolar ridge mucosa {2503,884,1043}.

Clinical features

DGCT presents as a slow-growing tumour with cortical expansion and occasional cortical perforation {613,1043}. The mean diameter at presentation is 40 mm, but occasional DGCTs reach 100 mm and cause gross facial deformity {4156}. Mild pain can be present. Peripheral DGCT presents as a gingival nodule.

Imaging

Radiographically, the majority of DGCTs are unilocular, well-defined, mixed radiolucent tumours; about a quarter appear multilocular, and about one third have focally irregular or poorly

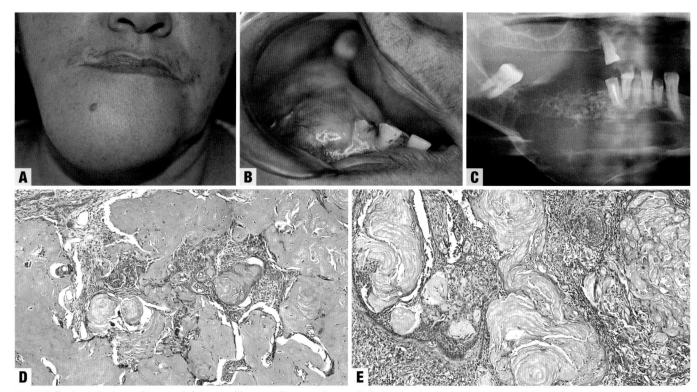

Fig. 7.41 Dentinogenic ghost cell tumour. **A** A 59-year-old woman with an anterior mandibular tumour, showing facial asymmetry. **B** Intraoral view of the same patient shows the tumour with gross cortical bone expansion. **C** Panoramic radiograph from the same patient, showing a markedly expansile multilocular lesion with cortical thinning, partial cortication, and multiple internal radiopacities in the body and anterior mandible. **D** An ameloblastoma-like epithelial proliferation with ghost cells entrapped within masses of dentinoid. Aggregates of ghost cells devoid of epithelium are being integrated within the dentinoid. **E** Large aggregates of flattened, pale eosinophilic ghost cells surrounded by a thin hyperchromatic epithelium resembling ameloblastoma.

defined borders {613,1043}. Tooth displacement and root resorption are frequent in larger tumours. A few cases have been reported in association with odontoma {2503,613}.

Epidemiology

DGCT is rare, and the second most common of the ghost cell–rich odontogenic tumours, all of which have a predilection for Asian men {2503,1043}. In Asia, DGCT accounts for 0.3–0.5% of all odontogenic tumours {2093,4094}. There are almost twice as many male patients as female patients {613,1043}. The mean age at presentation is between 40 and 47 years (range: 1–84 years) and most cases are diagnosed between the third and fifth decades of life {613,1043}.

Etiology

Unknown

Pathogenesis

BRAF p.V600E mutations, found in other ameloblastoma-like odontogenic tumours, are absent from DGCT {5019}. Mutation in *CTNNB1* (encoding β-catenin) has been associated with calcifying odontogenic cysts and ghost cell keratinization, but the *CTNNB1* mutation status of DGCT is unclear {2299,3275}.

Macroscopic appearance

DGCTs are solid and friable, with variable amounts of mineralization, focal areas of haemorrhage, and occasional small cysts. Cortical plates may be perforated.

Histopathology

DGCTs are composed of nests, islands, and sheets of odontogenic epithelium resembling conventional ameloblastoma, with cuboidal to columnar hyperchromatic basal cells that have reverse nuclear polarity at least focally {613}. Tissue resembling stellate reticulum usually lies centrally in islands and may undergo cystic degeneration. Frequently, nests or eddies of basaloid cells are observed within the cellular areas, and occasional aggregates of clear cells may be present. DGCT is characterized by epithelial cells with aberrant ghost cell keratinization, forming large rounded or stacked flattened cells with homogeneous pale eosinophilic cytoplasm with a pale or clear central hole where the nucleus is missing. The number of ghost cells is variable, ranging from scattered individual cells to small clusters and to large masses, but they are a prominent feature and ghost cells can replace the epithelial islands entirely. Ghost cells often undergo mineralization. Clusters of ghost cells frequently pass into the fibrous connective tissue, where they may induce a foreign body giant cell reaction. Dentinoid material is frequent and characteristic, especially in close association with the epithelial component {3754}. The dentinoid forms irregular eosinophilic masses that often entrap individual or groups of epithelial cells and ghost cells. Mineralization of dentinoid is frequent and may be followed by remodelling to produce a mixed dentinoid and bone-like appearance. Mineralization of dentinoid, and to a lesser degree that of the ghost cells, defines the radiological features of the tumour. The relative amounts of ameloblastomatous epithelium, ghost cells, and dentinoid material vary from tumour to tumour. In general, mitotic figures are scarce, but cellular pleomorphism can be present; however, it should not be interpreted as evidence of malignant transformation. The proliferation fraction on Ki-67 immunohistochemistry ranges from 2% to 29%.

Immunohistochemistry

Immunohistochemical stains for CK14 and CK19 highlight the epithelial component {3754}.

Differential diagnosis

This includes calcifying odontogenic cyst, adenoid ameloblastoma, ghost cell carcinoma, and the poorly defined odontogenic carcinoma with dentinoid {3085}.

Cytology

Not clinically relevant

Diagnostic molecular pathology

Not clinically relevant

Essential and desirable diagnostic criteria

Essential: a solid tumour; conventional ameloblastoma-like epithelium; ghost cells; dentinoid.
Desirable: scarce mitotic figures; mild cellular pleomorphism in a minority.

Staging

None

Prognosis and prediction

DGCT has a recurrence rate as high as 73% after conservative surgery (enucleation or curettage) and 33% after radical surgery (marginal or segmental resection), occurring from 1 to 20 years after treatment. Long-term follow-up is recommended. It is unclear whether multiple recurrences might be associated with malignant transformation in view of other histologically similar entities in the differential diagnosis.

Peripheral DGCTs have a much more indolent behaviour and rarely recur after conservative excision {2503,655}.

Odontogenic fibroma

van Heerden WFP
Hunter KD
Li TJ
Vargas PA

Definition

Odontogenic fibroma (OdF) is a neoplasm of mature fibrous or fibromyxoid connective tissue with variable amounts of inactive-appearing odontogenic epithelium, with or without associated mineralization.

ICD-O coding

9321/0 Odontogenic fibroma, NOS
9321/0 Odontogenic fibroma, amyloid subtype
9321/0 Odontogenic fibroma, granular cell subtype
9321/0 Hybrid odontogenic fibroma with central giant cell granuloma

ICD-11 coding

2E83.0 & XH1MT3 Benign osteogenic tumours of bone or articular cartilage of skull and upper face & Odontogenic fibroma, NOS

2E83.1 & XH1MT3 Benign osteogenic tumours of bone or articular cartilage of lower jaw & Odontogenic fibroma, NOS

Related terminology

Acceptable: central odontogenic fibroma.
Not recommended: central odontogenic fibroma WHO/non-WHO types.

Subtype(s)

Odontogenic fibroma, amyloid subtype; odontogenic fibroma, granular cell subtype; hybrid odontogenic fibroma with central giant cell granuloma

Localization

Although conflicting results have been reported, the maxilla appears slightly more frequently affected {3779}. Most maxillary central OdFs occur anterior to the first molar, whereas slightly

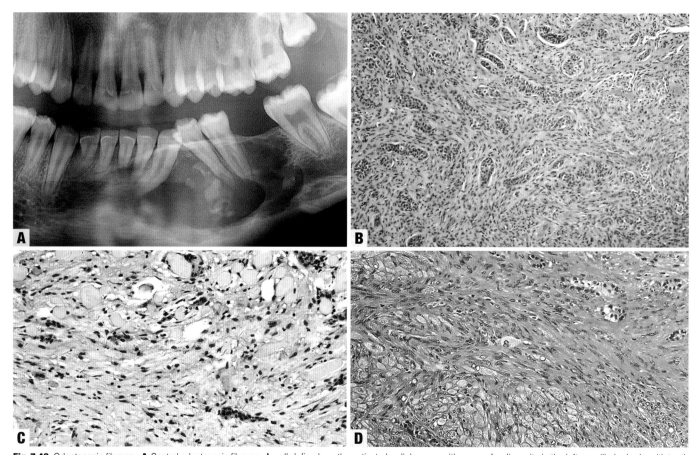

Fig. 7.42 Odontogenic fibroma. **A** Central odontogenic fibroma. A well-defined, partly corticated radiolucency with areas of radiopacity in the left mandibular body, with tooth displacement. **B** Central odontogenic fibroma. Appearance of the conventional pattern, cellular connective tissue associated with strands of odontogenic epithelium. **C** Central odontogenic fibroma, amyloid subtype. Fibrous tissue with scattered odontogenic epithelial islands associated with amyloid deposits presenting as homogeneous eosinophilic ovoid masses. **D** Odontogenic fibroma, granular cell pattern. Granular stromal cells associated with odontogenic epithelial islands.

more than half of all mandibular tumours are found posterior to the first molar {3779}.

Clinical features
Small OdFs are usually asymptomatic, whereas larger tumours present with localized swelling, loosening of teeth, and associated pain. OdFs on the anterior maxillary alveolus often have a characteristic depression rather than expansion.

Imaging
Small OdFs typically present as well-defined corticated radiolucencies closely associated with roots of erupted teeth. Larger tumours may have a multilocular appearance and produce divergence or resorption of associated tooth roots. About 10% of tumours have a mixed radiolucent/radiopaque appearance {3779}.

Epidemiology
Central OdFs have a female predilection (M:F ratio: 1:2.2) and develop over a wide age range, with a mean age at presentation of 34 years {3779}.

Etiology
Unknown

Pathogenesis
Unknown

Macroscopic appearance
Consistency varies from soft to firm depending on the collagen content. Internal mineralizations may produce a gritty consistency on section.

Histopathology
OdFs are composed of moderately cellular, bland fibrous tissue with moderate to dense collagen content, accompanied by varying amounts of dispersed, inactive-appearing odontogenic epithelial nests and cords, which are sometimes completely absent. There may be minor hard tissue formation in the form of mineralized dentinoid, or round, dense, basophilic, cementum-like mineralizations, both associated with the odontogenic epithelium.

Several rare subtypes of central OdF have been described.

The amyloid subtype is characterized by amyloid deposits, with Langerhans cells often present in the epithelial elements {5031}. This subtype accounts for approximately 16% of all cases {3779}. These non-calcifying Langerhans cell–rich lesions have also been considered to be part of the spectrum of calcifying epithelial odontogenic tumour, and their correct classification remains unclear. The site, sex predilection, and

biological behaviour of this subtype more closely resemble those of OdF {5031,3781}.

The granular cell subtype is composed of granular cells with variable amounts of odontogenic epithelium and accounts for about 5% of lesions. Completely granular central OdFs are sometimes referred to as granular cell odontogenic tumours but are best regarded as a subtype of OdF {3779}.

An ossifying subtype, demonstrating OdF components intermingled with ossifying fibroma–like tissue, has also been reported {1300,3779}.

OdFs with hybrid features of central giant cell granuloma and OdF {3267,1300,3779} have been described.

Differential diagnosis
The differential diagnosis should include sclerosing odontogenic carcinoma. This shows infiltration, but diagnosis can be challenging because of epithelial neurotropism of benign odontogenic epithelium in OdF {1998}. Small radiolucent lesions surrounding the crowns of impacted teeth and showing histological features of OdF should be diagnosed as hyperplastic dental follicles and are not neoplasms. Peripheral OdF arises extraosseously on the gingiva, usually anteriorly, and shares some histological features and its name with OdF {3706}, but there is little evidence that peripheral OdFs are neoplastic {203}, and they appear to be unrelated to intraosseous OdF. Peripheral OdFs are much more common than OdF, with a similar female predominance and a peak incidence in the second to fourth decades of life {1300}. Peripheral OdFs are treated by surgical excision. A recurrence rate as high as 50% has been reported {3706}, but this is almost abolished if excision extends to the periodontal ligament.

Cytology
Not clinically relevant

Diagnostic molecular pathology
Not clinically relevant

Essential and desirable diagnostic criteria
Essential: site in a tooth-bearing segment of the jaws; a well-defined lesion radiologically; bland fibrous connective tissue of varying cellularity.
Desirable: odontogenic epithelial nests or cords.

Staging
None

Prognosis and prediction
OdFs almost never recur after enucleation and curettage.

Cementoblastoma

Rich AM
Collins LHC

Definition
Cementoblastoma (CB) is a benign odontogenic neoplasm that forms a rounded mass of cementum on the root of a tooth.

ICD-O coding
9273/0 Cementoblastoma

ICD-11 coding
2E83.0 & XH4VL1 Benign osteogenic tumours of bone or articular cartilage of skull or face & Cementoblastoma, benign
2E83.1 & XH4VL1 Benign osteogenic tumours of bone or articular cartilage of lower jaw & Cementoblastoma, benign

Related terminology
Acceptable: benign cementoblastoma.
Not recommended: true cementoma; cementoma.

Subtype(s)
None

Localization
CB develops on the apical third of a tooth root, most frequently in the posterior mandible, usually on the permanent first molar. Teeth in the mandibular premolar and maxillary molar regions are the second most frequently affected. Involvement of deciduous teeth is rare.

Clinical features
CB causes a slow-growing, characteristically painful expansion of the jaw. The associated tooth is vital in about 80% of cases. Root resorption occurs in about two thirds of cases. Cortical bone perforation and tooth displacement are rare {567,877}.

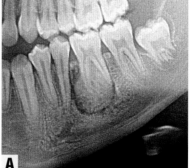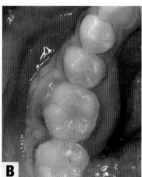

Fig. 7.43 Cementoblastoma. **A** Panoramic radiograph showing a cementoblastoma attached to the root of the first permanent molar, a typical radiopaque lesion with a radiolucent rim in continuity with the periodontal ligament. **B** Buccal and lingual expansion in a patient with a cementoblastoma affecting the mandibular fist molar tooth.

Imaging
Radiographically, there is a well-defined, circumscribed, radiopaque or mixed-density mass expanding from the root of the associated tooth. A characteristic radiolucent rim continuous with the periodontal ligament is usually present {567}.

Epidemiology
CB is a relatively rare tumour, accounting for about 3% of all odontogenic tumours. There is a wide age range, with the highest incidence in the second and third decades of life. There is no sex predilection {567,877,4164}.

Etiology
Unknown

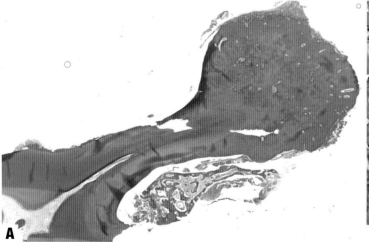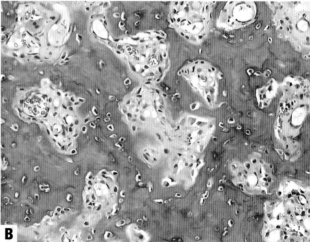

Fig. 7.44 Cementoblastoma. **A** A low-power photomicrograph showing a cementoblastoma arising from and fused to a resorbed tooth root. **B** Dense bone showing prominent resting and reversal lines with small medullary spaces partly or completely filled by multilayered eosinophilic and slightly enlarged osteoblasts.

Pathogenesis

CB harbours *FOS* rearrangement and shows FOS overexpression {2458}, features it has in common with osteoid osteoma and osteoblastoma {155}, with which it also shares histological similarity. FOS would be expected to affect the maturation and proliferation of cementoblasts in the same way as it does osteoblasts, but CB appears to have a more indolent growth pattern than osteoblastoma.

Macroscopic appearance

CB is a calcified mass, usually 20–30 mm in diameter, adherent to and fused with a tooth root.

Histopathology

CB resembles osteoblastoma histologically. The bulk of the lesion is composed of a mass of dense cellular cementum resembling bone, often with prominent reversal lines, fused with the resorbed surface of the tooth root. At the periphery there are radiating finger-like trabeculae of newly formed matrix, often associated with plump cementoblasts and cementoclasts and vascular immature fibrous tissue.

Differential diagnosis

This should include cemento-osseous dysplasia.

Cytology

Not clinically relevant

Diagnostic molecular pathology

Not clinically relevant

Essential and desirable diagnostic criteria

Essential: a mass fused to a tooth root; dense mineralization; radiating peripheral matrix; plump cementoblasts; no fibro-osseous component.

Staging

None

Prognosis and prediction

CB does not usually recur after extraction of the associated tooth and curettage. Recurrence follows incomplete removal or attempted conservation of the tooth {567}.

Cemento-ossifying fibroma

Chi A
Collins LHC

Definition
Cemento-ossifying fibroma (COF) is a benign odontogenic fibro-osseous neoplasm arising in the jaws and characterized by the production of bone and cementum-like calcifications in a fibrous stroma.

ICD-O coding
9274/0 Cemento-ossifying fibroma

ICD-11 coding
2E83.0 & XH52T0 Benign osteogenic tumours of bone or articular cartilage of skull or face & Cemento-ossifying fibroma

2E83.1 & XH52T0 Benign osteogenic tumours of bone or articular cartilage of lower jaw & Cemento-ossifying fibroma

Related terminology
Not recommended: cementifying fibroma; ossifying fibroma; ossifying-odontogenic fibroma; periodontoma.

Subtype(s)
None

Localization
The mandible is involved much more frequently than the maxilla, with a predilection for the mandibular premolar and molar region {4493,1747,1303}. Whether non-odontogenic lesions with similar histology that arise in craniofacial bones outside the jaws are related is unclear {378}.

Clinical features
COF typically causes painless jaw expansion. Growth is slow, but COF can reach a considerable size if left untreated {4493, 17,1747}. Most patients have a solitary lesion, but rare cases of multiple lesions can arise sporadically or as a component of hyperparathyroidism–jaw tumour syndrome, a rare autosomal dominant disorder characterized by COF, parathyroid adenoma,

or carcinoma. COFs present in up to 20% of patients with this syndrome {1996,4718}.

Imaging
Radiographs show a well-defined corticated radiolucency in the early stages. Variable degrees of central opacification develop with time; some COFs become densely sclerotic, but all retain an unmineralized periphery {4493,1303}. Mandibular lesions may cause characteristic downward bowing of the inferior border. Maxillary lesions may displace the sinus floor {2791}. Other findings include cortical thinning, tooth displacement, and root resorption {4493,72}.

Epidemiology
COF occurs over a broad age range, with a peak in the third to fourth decades of life, and has a female predilection (M:F ratio: as low as 1:5) {1246,2791,1747,4165}. The tumour arises in White patients primarily, followed by patients of African descent {2791}.

Etiology
COF is presumed to be odontogenic in origin, on the basis of its almost exclusive location in tooth-bearing areas of the jaws {3135} and its variable production of dense cementum-like bone, although the latter is not specific to COF or other types of ossifying fibromas {1755}.

Genetic factors
COFs, often multiple and in young patients, are a feature of hyperparathyroidism–jaw tumour syndrome (MIM number: 145001) {687,1053} and gnathodiaphysial dysplasia (MIM number: 166260) {2579,3699,1246}.

Pathogenesis
Inactivating mutations in the tumour suppressor gene *CDC73* (*HRPT2*) have been identified in a few sporadic cases of COF {3545}, and mutations in this gene are the underlying cause

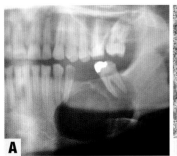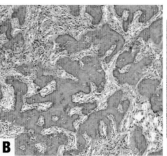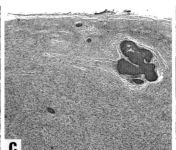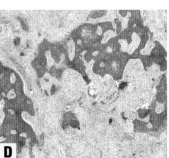

Fig. 7.45 Cemento-ossifying fibroma. **A** Panoramic radiograph showing a well-defined, expansile radiolucency in the posterior mandible with associated cortical thinning and tooth root displacement. **B** Trabeculae of heavily mineralized but sparsely cellular woven bone in a fibrous stroma. **C** Well-defined tumour mass with cellular fibrous stroma and focal cementum-like dense bone calcifications. This particular example shows abundant stroma and only a focal mineralized component. **D** A lesion in mid-phase maturation, with less-cellular fibrous stroma and dense lamellar bone mineralization.

of hyperparathyroidism–jaw tumour syndrome (MIM number: 145001) {687,1053}. *CDC73* encodes parafibromin, which exerts antiproliferative activity via interaction with cyclin D1 {1053}. Because *CDC73* mutations occur in only some COFs, they may play a role in tumour progression rather than in initiation {1053}. Assessment of hotspot mutations in 50 oncogenes and tumour suppressor genes by next-generation sequencing did not reveal any pathogenic variants in the COFs evaluated {3468}. COFs show copy-number variation, mostly on chromosomes 7 and 12, but with considerable heterogeneity {2750}.

COF in gnathodiaphysial dysplasia (MIM number: 166260) accompanies long bone fragility and cortical thickening of tubular bones {3699} caused by *ANO5* (*GDD1, TMEM16E*) mutations. These mutations are different from those in familial florid cemento-osseous dysplasia {2090,2826,197}.

In addition, gene transcription studies have implicated deregulation of the WNT/β-catenin pathway in the molecular pathogenesis of COF {3468}, and a number of other probably non-pathogenic genetic changes have been detected {1219,3468}.

Macroscopic appearance
COF is a single rounded mass or multiple large pieces of bony tissue, with some smooth surfaces {4165}.

Histopathology
COF consists of variable proportions of fibrous and mineralized tissue, more heavily mineralized centrally, and with a thin fibrous capsule or well-demarcated margin from the surrounding normal bone. The fibroblastic stroma may have areas of hypercellularity and show nuclear hyperchromasia but no pleomorphism, and mitoses are infrequent {1747}. Stromal vascularity is generally low.

A fibro-osseous appearance of condensation of woven bone from stroma must be present at least focally. COF exhibits considerable variation in the amount and type of mineralization, even within a single lesion. Woven to lamellar bone and osteoid may be present, as well as dense, acellular or paucicellular, basophilic, rounded, cementum-like calcifications {1246} that form round droplets, irregular bulbous forms, and fine brush-stroke forms {1747}. The bony trabeculae may form thick anastomosing strands or fuse into large sheets centrally. Osteoblastic rimming is frequent and there is bone remodelling in the lesion, with infrequent osteoclasts {4165}. Haemorrhagic cystic degeneration resembling aneurysmal bone cyst formation occurs rarely {4165, 3135}. Histological features alone are not diagnostic and areas resembling COF may be seen in psammomatoid and (less frequently) in trabecular ossifying fibroma, and COF may contain ossicles like psammomatoid ossifying fibroma as a minor feature.

COFs in syndromes have the same features as non-syndromic COFs. COFs in gnathodiaphysial dysplasia are at the more fibrous end of the spectrum, with predominantly basophilic rounded islands and droplets of acellular bone {2579,3699, 1246}.

Differential diagnosis
The differential diagnosis includes fibrous dysplasia, which has a more uniform woven or lamellar architecture but may contain islands of basophilic bone and, in the jaws, shows osteoblast rimming. However, the sharp demarcation of COF and the cortical expansion rather than replacement distinguish it from fibrous dysplasia. Histologically COF also resembles focal cemento-osseous dysplasia, and COF-like expansion may occur in florid cemento-osseous dysplasia, particularly its familial form.

It should be noted that the so-called peripheral ossifying fibroma is not regarded as an extraosseous ossifying fibroma but an unrelated reactive gingival hyperplasia with mineralization that shows only some histological similarity to neoplastic COFs {2251,588}.

Cytology
Not clinically relevant

Diagnostic molecular pathology
There is no diagnostic molecular pathology for sporadic COF. Syndromic forms can be identified clinically or by *CDC73* (*HRPT2*) mutations in COF or other tissues {687,3545,799, 1996}. COF does not exhibit the *GNAS* mutations seen in fibrous dysplasia.

Essential and desirable diagnostic criteria
Essential: location in a tooth-bearing region of the jaws; benign fibro-osseous histology; well demarcated.
Desirable: slow, continuous growth; cementum-like calcifications.

Staging
None

Prognosis and prediction
COF is usually treated by enucleation and curettage because it shells out readily and recurs rarely {4461}. There is a single reported case of possible malignant transformation {2543,4666}.

Odontogenic myxoma

Fitzpatrick SG
Adebiyi KE

Definition

Odontogenic myxoma (OM) is a benign neoplasm histologically resembling odontogenic ectomesenchyme and characterized by sparse spindle or stellate cells in a myxoid stroma.

ICD-O coding

9320/0 Odontogenic myxoma

ICD-11 coding

2E83.0 & XH48L4 Benign osteogenic tumours of bone or articular cartilage of skull or face & Odontogenic myxoma

2E83.1 & XH48L4 Benign osteogenic tumours of bone or articular cartilage of lower jaw & Odontogenic myxoma

Related terminology

Acceptable: odontogenic fibromyxoma.

Subtype(s)

None

Localization

OM arises in the jaws {871,3796}. Two thirds of OMs are located in the mandible and one third in the maxilla {2857}, usually in relation to a tooth, typically a premolar or molar {2626}. Maxillary lesions tend to obliterate the maxillary sinuses as an early feature, and expansion is an early and consistent feature. Rare cases have been reported to occur extraosseously in the gingiva {3023}.

Clinical features

OM is characterized by insidious and oligosymptomatic, slow, permeative growth, causing bone destruction, expansion {2626,2556}, mobility or absence of tooth, and eventual cortical perforation and soft tissue infiltration {4082,2168}. On palpation, OM is firm in consistency and not tender {4729}.

Imaging

Radiographically OMs are unilocular or multilocular radiolucencies with defined or diffuse borders, better defined by CT or MRI {2278}. Unilocular OMs are more frequent in children and in the anterior region of the jaw {3878,3668}. Fine straight internal trabeculation is characteristic {3232}. OM of the maxilla is less frequent and has a tendency to spread to the maxillary sinus {883}. Root displacement and resorption may occur, but as late features.

Epidemiology

OM accounts for < 10% of all odontogenic tumours and is the third most frequent after odontoma and ameloblastoma {615, 2857,4328,3270}. OM affects mostly young adults between the second and third decades of life, but with a wide age range {1460}. In many studies, OM is as much as twice as common in females as males, but not in all populations {3232,2857,1168}.

Etiology

Unknown

Pathogenesis

The pathogenesis is unknown. No pathogenic mutations were found in 50 oncogenes and tumour suppressor genes commonly mutated in human cancers {3865}. OMs show MAPK/ERK pathway activation, and its inhibition may reduce tumour growth {3466}. OM is not associated with Carney syndrome {1641} but has been reported occasionally with familial adenomatous polyposis, naevoid basal cell carcinoma syndrome, and tuberous sclerosis {4006,442,3834}.

Macroscopic appearance

OM appears as unencapsulated, gelatinous, white-grey loose tissue {328}.

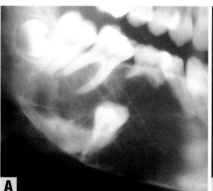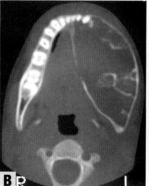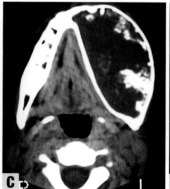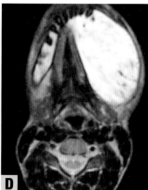

Fig. 7.46 Odontogenic myxoma. **A** This deliberately slightly underexposed panoramic radiograph shows the characteristic straight criss-crossing internal bony septa found in some lesions. **B–D** This example in the body of the mandible shows thin, expanded cortex and bony septa in the CT bone window (**B**) and low soft tissue density (**C**). The high proton density resulting from the high water content in the myxoid tissue gives a hyperintense signal on T2-weighted MRI (**D**).

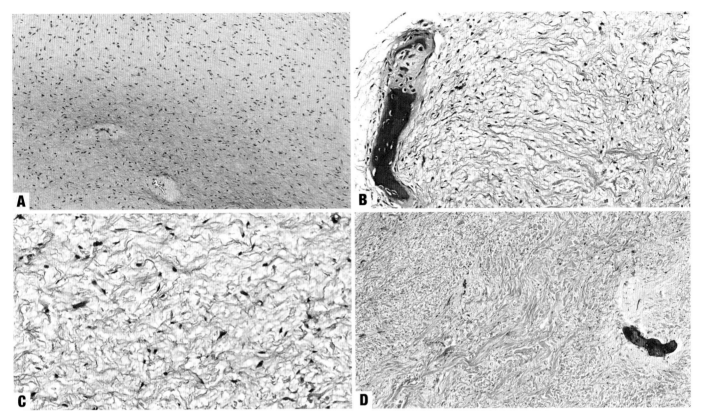

Fig. 7.47 A Normal dental follicle resembling odontogenic myxoma. Histologically, dental follicle and papilla are almost identical to odontogenic myxoma, but a clue may be given by the size, shape, and presence of epithelial remnants running along some surfaces. **B-D** Odontogenic myxoma. **B** An odontogenic myxoma from the mandible, comprising loose myxoid tissue with a sparse cell population. **C** High-magnification view of an odontogenic myxoma from the mandible, showing loose myxoid tissue stroma with scattered spindle and stellate cells without atypia and forming minimal or no collagen. **D** This myxoma has prominent collagen formation, but excess basophilic ground substance remains between the fibres. Such lesions are sometimes termed "fibromyxoma".

Histopathology

OM is composed of predominantly loose myxoid stroma with a sparse population of stellate to spindle cells. Small inactive rests of odontogenic epithelium are present in a small minority of OMs and are few in number {883}. The tumour is generally unencapsulated with permeative spread in medullary bone {1168}. Lesions with more collagenous stroma are often referred to as odontogenic fibromyxomas. Immunohistochemistry does not aid diagnosis.

Differential diagnosis

The most significant differential diagnosis for OM is dental follicle or developing dental papilla, which are histologically identical but clinically and radiographically distinct {104}. Myxoid neurofibroma may have overlapping histology but will generally show positive immunohistochemical staining for S100 {104}. Other differential diagnoses include chondromyxoid fibroma, odontogenic fibroma, and low-grade myxofibrosarcoma, particularly in OM with a more collagenized stroma {104}.

Cytology

Not clinically relevant

Diagnostic molecular pathology

Not relevant

Essential and desirable diagnostic criteria

Essential: arising in tooth-bearing segments of jaws; myxoid stroma with variable collagenization; sparse stellate or spindle-shaped cells.

Desirable: scattered inactive odontogenic rests.

Staging

None

Prognosis and prediction

The lack of capsule and the permeative spread produce uncertainty over extent, and account for recurrence rates for OM ranging from 10% to 43% {3796}. It is unclear whether recurrence increases with more conservative treatment methods {3796,1168}. OMs in the maxilla appear to be more likely to recur than mandibular lesions {3796}. MAPK/ERK pathway inhibition may have the potential to reduce tumour growth {3466}. If malignant transformation is possible in OM, it is exceedingly rare and may represent misdiagnosis of low-grade myxoid malignancies {3362}.

Sclerosing odontogenic carcinoma

Koutlas IG

Definition
Sclerosing odontogenic carcinoma (SOC) is a primary intra-osseous carcinoma of the jaws with bland cytology, markedly sclerotic stroma, and local aggressive infiltration, but no metastatic potential.

ICD-O coding
9270/3 Sclerosing odontogenic carcinoma

ICD-11 coding
2B5J & XH4M89 Malignant miscellaneous tumours of bone or articular cartilage of other or unspecified sites & Odontogenic tumour, malignant

Related terminology
None

Subtype(s)
None

Localization
Most cases affect the posterior mandible. Maxillary SOCs tend to lie anteriorly.

Clinical features
SOC presents as swelling that occasionally grows rapidly. Most cases are asymptomatic, with only a few mandibular examples characterized by paraesthesia.

Imaging
Radiographically, SOC is a poorly defined radiolucency with cortical bone destruction and occasional tooth mobility. Tumour extension beyond radiographic margins has been reported in many cases.

Epidemiology
There is a very slight female predilection. The age at diagnosis ranges from 31 to 73 years, with the majority of cases arising in the fifth to seventh decades of life {2646}. SOC may be underrecognized or may have been described under another name {1997}.

Etiology
Unknown

Pathogenesis
Unknown

Macroscopic appearance
Dense fibrous tissue fragments

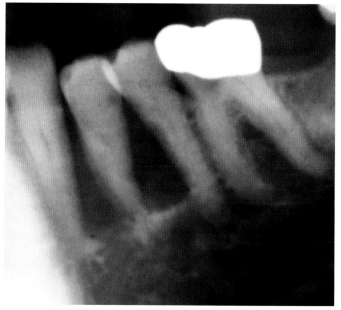

Fig. 7.48 Sclerosing odontogenic carcinoma. Radiographic image showing a relatively low-grade tumour appearance, with a well-defined and partly corticated outline.

Histopathology
A dense, fibrocollagenous sclerotic stroma is the hallmark of SOC, containing malignant epithelial cells forming single-file thin cords, strands, small nests, and infrequent islands of more epidermoid cells {2377}. Only mild cellular atypia has been observed in most cases. SOCs are infiltrative and lack encapsulation. Perineural or intraneural invasion is frequently seen, but lymphovascular invasion is rare. Mitotic activity is inconspicuous and necrosis is rare. Mucus-negative clear cells may be present, but glandular differentiation has also been reported {2646}. Calcifications including cementum-like bone, bone, or dentinoid have been observed in half of the cases.

Immunohistochemistry
There is no specific immunohistochemical marker for SOC. The epithelial component is highlighted by CK5/6, CK14, CK19, and p63.

Cytology
Not clinically relevant

Diagnostic molecular pathology
All cases studied have been negative for *EWSR1* rearrangement.

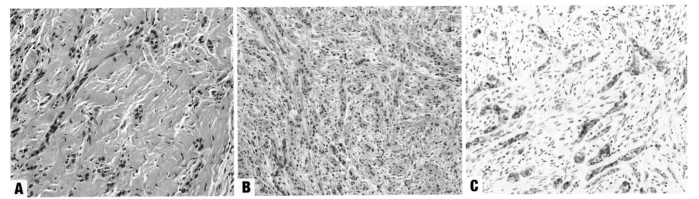

Fig. 7.49 Sclerosing odontogenic carcinoma. **A** Typical appearance, with extensive sclerosis of the stroma and dispersed, sometimes inconspicuous, epithelial islands and strands. **B** A cellular example with less sclerotic stroma showing haphazardly arranged thin cords, strands, and small nests of epithelium blending with loose and dense collagenous stroma. Mild inflammation is present in the background, which can cause some difficulty in distinguishing the epithelial component. **C** CK19 immunostain highlights the epithelial component.

Essential and desirable diagnostic criteria

Essential: malignant odontogenic carcinoma with infiltrating thin cords and nests of epithelium; sclerotic stroma.

Desirable: mild atypia; perineural/intraneural infiltration (often prominent).

Staging

There is no defined eighth-edition Union for International Cancer Control (UICC) / American Joint Committee on Cancer (AJCC) TNM staging system staging guidance, but the use of International Collaboration on Cancer Reporting (ICCR) minimum data set reporting is encouraged {4138}.

Prognosis and prediction

To date, the prognosis has been excellent, with only local recurrence in a few cases despite perineural invasion. Exceedingly rare recurrence and metastasis have been reported {1500A}.

Ameloblastic carcinoma

Magliocca K
Yoon HJ

Definition
Ameloblastic carcinoma (AC) is a primary odontogenic carcinoma histologically resembling ameloblastoma.

ICD-O coding
9270/3 Ameloblastic carcinoma

ICD-11 coding
2B5J & XH4M89 Malignant miscellaneous tumours of bone or articular cartilage of other or unspecified sites & Odontogenic tumour, malignant

Related terminology
Not recommended: malignant ameloblastoma; dedifferentiated ameloblastoma.

Subtype(s)
None

Localization
AC is an intraosseous jaw carcinoma with a mandibular predilection, usually arising posteriorly {1597,1429,1094}. Most ACs arise de novo, but there may be pre-existing ameloblastoma {4137,81,4553}. Extraosseous AC is extremely rare {3523}.

Clinical features
Patients present with jaw or orofacial swelling, sometimes with pain and paraesthesia {1597,1094}, and later with tooth mobility and extension into the oral mucosa and trismus {4943, 1429,1094}. Rarely, AC is associated with hypercalcaemia of malignancy {961}.

Imaging
Contrast-enhanced CT shows a poorly defined expanding lesion with medullary and cortical bone destruction {4943}. MRI delineates soft tissue or marrow extension. Moderate FDG uptake on PET-CT helps detect metastasis {1109,4553}.

Epidemiology
AC accounts for ≤ 2% of all odontogenic tumours {2451,2093, 4095} and 30% of malignant odontogenic tumours {731}. A wide age range is affected, with a median age of 49 years {1597}, and there is a male predilection {1738,2613,1597}.

Etiology
The etiology is unknown. Some ACs develop in longstanding untreated ameloblastoma {1429} or in locally recurrent ameloblastoma after surgery and/or irradiation {4137,3228,961}.

Pathogenesis
BRAF p.V600E mutations have been reported in up to 40% of ACs {1138,607,3274,3226}.

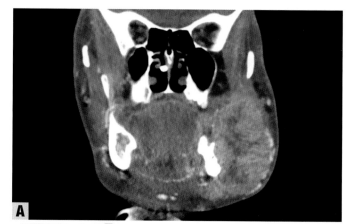

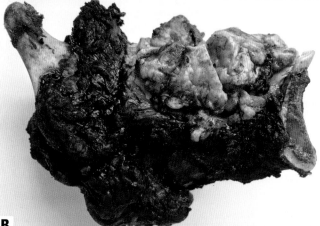

Fig. 7.50 Ameloblastic carcinoma. **A** CT showing a solid mass with heterogeneous enhancement related to tumour necrosis in the left mandible, with marked expansion, cortical destruction, and soft tissue extension. **B** Composite mandibular segmental resection with temporomandibular joint disarticulation. The mass expands beyond cortical bone, with a large exophytic component.

Macroscopic appearance
AC is a solid mass with irregular borders and limited cystic change {1109,2880}.

Histopathology
AC resembles ameloblastoma and has variable features of malignancy. The architecture ranges from ameloblastoma-like follicular or plexiform patterns to solid, compact sheets of basaloid epithelium or anastomosing strands with a loss of stellate reticulum. Peripheral palisading, nuclear reverse polarity, and stellate reticulum must be evident, at least focally. The threshold for diagnosis of malignancy is poorly defined, but ACs usually show some of the following: at least moderate cellular or nuclear atypia, increased mitotic activity, increased N:C ratio, hyperchromatic vesicular nuclei, crowding of basal cells and expansion of the basal cell compartment with

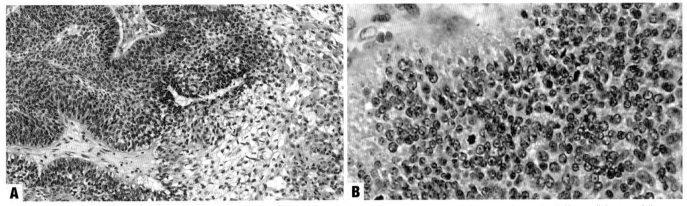

Fig. 7.51 Ameloblastic carcinoma. **A** Hypercellular peripheral epithelial compartment with overlapping cells, clear cell change, and necrosis. **B** Hypercellular area of disorganized and overlapping epithelial cells, exhibiting a high mitotic rate at the periphery of follicles and sheets.

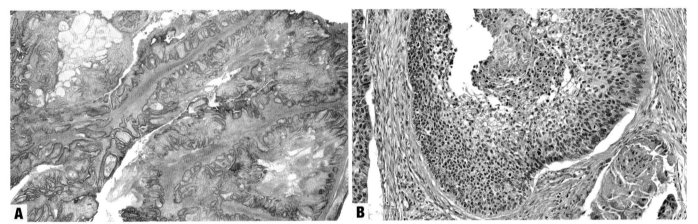

Fig. 7.52 Ameloblastic carcinoma. **A** A low-power image demonstrating thick, multilobulated ribbons of tumour in dense fibrous tissue. Extensive necrosis is present in the upper-left corner, with comedonecrosis in the lower-right corner. **B** Cellular atypia and apoptotic necrosis in the centre of the follicle.

disordered polarity, and expansion of atypical cells into stellate reticulum. Central necrosis in islands is a helpful finding, but it may be subtle with apoptosis. Extension into the mucosa and infiltration into the medullary space do not distinguish benign ameloblastoma from AC. Increased mitotic activity or Ki-67 proliferative fraction cannot define AC, and emphasis is placed on identifying a combination of architectural and cytomorphological abnormalities.

Minor differentiation patterns include squamous, clear cell, spindle cell, and pseudosarcomatous morphology. Combinations are possible, and these features vary in extent {1738,4943, 3228,2726,2909}. Dispersed invasion and perineural infiltration are uncommon in AC {2726,4138,3226}, in contrast to other odontogenic malignant neoplasms {2377,456}.

Benign ameloblastoma may be present as a precursor lesion {4950,3228}.

Immunohistochemistry
Unlike ameloblastoma, AC shows expression of p53 {2726}, SMA, and SOX2 {415,2551}, but these are not validated as arbiters of malignancy.

Differential diagnosis
This includes benign ameloblastoma, especially maxillary examples that can show high cellularity. Basaloid AC must be separated from basal cell ameloblastoma, basaloid squamous

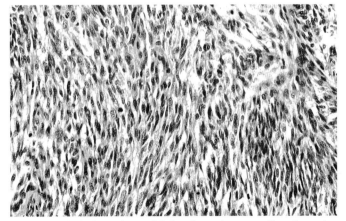

Fig. 7.53 Ameloblastic carcinoma. Spindle cell growth pattern, with stellate reticulum–like cells and less evident peripheral palisading.

cell carcinoma, and adamantinoma-like Ewing tumour {466, 2344}. AC with spindle cell changes warrants the exclusion of spindle cell / sarcomatoid squamous cell carcinoma, carcinosarcoma, and other spindle cell malignancies {2880,2909}. AC with clear cell features must be separated from clear cell odontogenic carcinoma {456}. A primary intraosseous carcinoma lacking ameloblastoma features is better categorized as primary intraosseous carcinoma.

Chapter 7

Cytology

FNAB may detect possible metastasis in known cases {1109}.

Diagnostic molecular pathology

BRAF p.V600E mutations {1138,3226} and *TP53* mutation {3228} are of undefined diagnostic value. *EWSR1* translocation indicates clear cell odontogenic carcinoma rather than AC with clear cell phenotype {456}.

Essential and desirable diagnostic criteria

Essential: a histological resemblance to ameloblastoma; cytological atypia.

Desirable: an intraosseous jaw tumour; tumour necrosis; *BRAF* mutations (in a subset); an associated ameloblastoma precursor.

Staging

Although there is no defined eighth-edition Union for International Cancer Control (UICC) / American Joint Committee on Cancer (AJCC) TNM staging system staging guidance, the use of International Collaboration on Cancer Reporting (ICCR) minimum data set reporting is encouraged {4138}.

Prognosis and prediction

Radical surgical resection is the treatment of choice, with radiotherapy for non-surgical candidates, recurrent/metastatic disease, and/or inadequate surgical margins {221, 2250}. AC recurs locally in up to 40% of cases {4943,4553}, and metastases to cervical nodes occur in up to 13% of patients {1597,2786,3226}. Distant metastasis develops in one third of cases, most commonly in the lung, followed by the brain, liver, and bone {423,1597}, worsening the prognosis {4943,1094}. The 5-year overall survival rate is 70%, better after complete surgical resection {1597}. Origin in a benign precursor {4137,81,4553} and histopathological patterns do not affect the clinical course {3835}. Novel treatment considerations include proton beam therapy {4899} and BRAF-targeting agents {2250}.

Clear cell odontogenic carcinoma

Bilodeau EA
Maiorano E
Neville BW

Definition
Clear cell odontogenic carcinoma (CCOdC) is an odontogenic carcinoma characterized by sheets, nests, or cords of clear cells in a fibrocellular or hyalinized stroma.

ICD-O coding
9341/3 Clear cell odontogenic carcinoma

ICD-11 coding
2B5J & XH5DZ4 Malignant miscellaneous tumours of bone or articular cartilage of other or unspecified sites & Clear cell odontogenic carcinoma

Related terminology
Not recommended: clear cell odontogenic tumour; clear cell ameloblastoma.

Subtype(s)
None

Localization
All CCOdCs develop in the jaws. Three quarters of cases arise in the mandible, most frequently in the posterior body and lower ramus {2681}.

Clinical features
The clinical manifestations are nonspecific, with destructive jaw swelling with or without pain, paraesthesia, and tooth mobility, and later with ulceration to the mucosa. Less commonly, patients develop lymphadenopathy (19%) or distant metastases (11%).

Imaging
Radiographically, CCOdCs are expansile, poorly defined radiolucencies often exhibiting tooth root resorption {2681}.

Epidemiology
More than 100 cases of CCOdC have been reported in the literature, with a mean age at presentation of 53 years, and with 63% of cases in female patients {1700}.

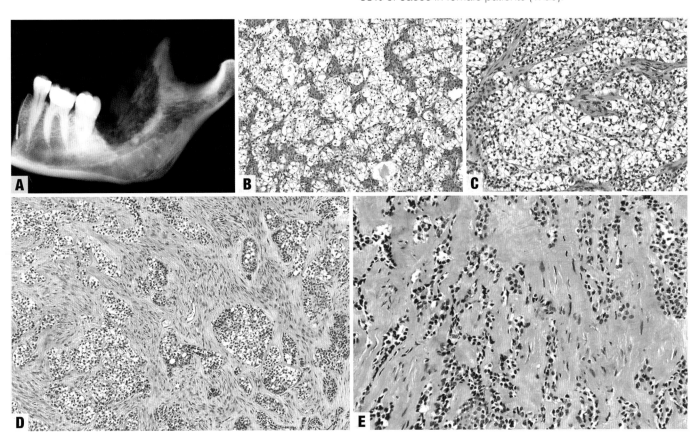

Fig. 7.54 Clear cell odontogenic carcinoma. **A** Resection specimen showing a poorly defined, destructive radiolucency in the posterior body and ramus of the mandible. **B** The tumour shows a solid biphasic pattern. **C** The tumour is composed predominantly of optically clear cells. **D** Clear cell tumour nests in a prominent fibrocellular stroma. **E** The tumour demonstrates cords of cells with clear to faintly eosinophilic cytoplasm in a hyalinized stroma.

Chapter 7

Etiology

Unknown

Pathogenesis

EWSR1 rearrangements have been reported in > 80% of cases {456}. ATF1 is the most common fusion partner, and CREB1 and CREM are less frequent {456,4646,581}. CCOdCs are morphologically and immunohistochemically similar to salivary gland hyalinizing clear cell carcinomas, which share the EWSR1 translocation, suggesting a common pathogenesis {213}.

Macroscopic appearance

CCOdC is an intraosseous tumour with a homogeneous, tan-white cut surface; indistinct borders; and sometimes soft tissue extension.

Histopathology

CCOdCs are composed of lobular sheets, nests, or trabeculae of monomorphic, polygonal cells with clear to slightly eosinophilic cytoplasm and eccentric nuclei embedded in a hyalinized or fibrocellular stroma {1764}. Peripheral palisading may or may not be present, and the tumour may have a heterogeneous appearance, with areas of more basaloid epithelium without cytoplasmic clearing. The clear cells are negative for mucin, but they are PAS-positive and diastase-sensitive, indicating glycogen. The mitotic index is low, and some CCOdCs are bland and relatively indolent. Necrosis and angiolymphatic invasion are uncommon, but perineural invasion is reported in one third of tumours {454}.

Immunohistochemistry

CCOdCs are positive for cytokeratins (AE1/AE3, CK5/6, CK19), p63, and EMA, but they are negative for myoepithelial markers (SMA, calponin, and S100 {454,2681}).

Differential diagnosis

The differential diagnosis includes other clear cell–rich gnathic neoplasms, including other odontogenic tumours (clear cell calcifying epithelial odontogenic tumour, amyloid subtype of odontogenic fibroma), salivary tumours, both metastatic and intraosseous primary neoplasms (mucoepidermoid carcinoma, epithelial-myoepithelial carcinoma), and metastatic neoplasms (renal cell carcinoma, melanoma) {4096}. Odontogenic carcinoma with dentinoid has overlapping morphological features, with some cases having a clear cell phenotype, but these form dentinoid and appear to be a distinct entity {3085}.

Cytology

Not clinically relevant

Diagnostic molecular pathology

EWSR1 rearrangement facilitates diagnosis but is technically challenging due to specimen decalcification.

Essential and desirable diagnostic criteria

Essential: location in jaws; prominent clear cell phenotype; infiltrative margin; hyalinized or fibrocellular stroma.
Desirable: EWSR1 translocation.

Staging

Although there is no defined eighth-edition Union for International Cancer Control (UICC) / American Joint Committee on Cancer (AJCC) TNM staging system staging guidance, the use of International Collaboration on Cancer Reporting (ICCR) minimum data set reporting is encouraged {4138}.

Prognosis and prediction

Primary management is complete surgical resection. The role of adjuvant therapy is not clearly defined. The prognosis is variable, with a local recurrence rate of nearly 40% {2681}. Metastases have been reported to cervical lymph nodes, and (uncommonly) to the lungs and bone, and may occur after many years. Approximately 11% of patients succumb to the disease {1700}.

Ghost cell odontogenic carcinoma

van Heerden WFP
Gomes CC

Definition

Ghost cell odontogenic carcinoma (GCOC) is an odontogenic carcinoma with ghost cells and sometimes with dentinoid deposition.

ICD-O coding

9302/3 Ghost cell odontogenic carcinoma

ICD-11 coding

2B5J & XH2BX2 Malignant miscellaneous tumours of bone or articular cartilage of other or unspecified sites & Ghost cell odontogenic carcinoma

Related terminology

Not recommended: dentinogenic ghost cell carcinoma; malignant calcifying ghost cell odontogenic tumour; malignant calcifying odontogenic cyst; calcifying ghost cell odontogenic carcinoma.

Subtype(s)

None

Localization

GCOC arises within the jaws and is almost twice as common in the maxilla as in the mandible. The ramus and molar areas are the most affected regions in the mandible {1043,2082}.

Clinical features

GCOC may present with nonspecific signs and symptoms suggestive of malignancy, including pain, swelling, ulceration,

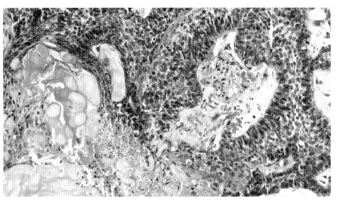

Fig. 7.55 Ghost cell odontogenic carcinoma. Malignant odontogenic epithelium with some peripheral palisading associated with ghost cells and apoptotic necrosis.

tooth mobility, and paraesthesia. Soft tissue infiltration may be present {2082}.

Imaging

GCOC typically presents as a poorly demarcated radiolucency, and half of all cases are associated with internal mineralization. Root resorption and displacement are common.

Epidemiology

GCOC is a rare tumour, with < 50 cases reported, of which about half occurred in people of Asian descent {2082}. GCOC is more common in men than women (M:F ratio: 3.2:1). It can arise at any age (range: 10–89 years), with a peak incidence in patients aged 30–60 years {2082}.

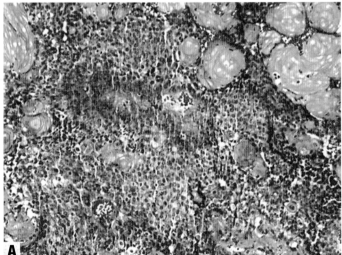
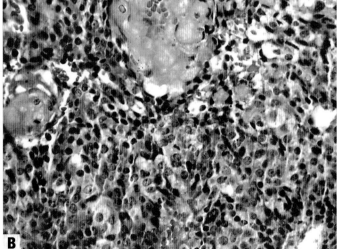

Fig. 7.56 Ghost cell odontogenic carcinoma. **A,B** A solid carcinoma, comprising sheets of malignant hyperchromatic epithelium with scattered clusters of ghost cells. There is no epithelial architecture, peripheral palisading, or evidence of ameloblastic differentiation.

Etiology
Unknown

Pathogenesis
GCOC may arise de novo or in a calcifying odontogenic cyst (COC) or a dentinogenic ghost cell tumour (DGCT) benign precursor {2503,3177}.

Mutation of *CTNNB1* (β-catenin) has been reported in GCOC {3655}, similar to that found in other tumours with ghost cells and/or dentinoid material and clear cells, including odontogenic carcinoma with dentinoid {1647}, DGCT {2299}, and calcifying cystic odontogenic tumours {3969,1060}. Notably, mutations in *APC* (also part of the WNT/β-catenin pathway) have also been reported in 1 case of GCOC {537}, in similarity with odontogenic carcinoma with dentinoid {1647}. Additional mutations in genes in the sonic hedgehog and ATM pathways, as well as losses of the *RB1*, *FHIT*, *PTEN*, *ATM*, and *CHEK2* gene regions, are reported, among other changes {537}.

Macroscopic appearance
Appearances of GCOC vary from solid to multicystic, often with a gritty consistency on section.

Histopathology
The histological features are those of DGCT and COC with cytological evidence of malignancy. The main component is odontogenic epithelial sheets, islands, and strands, resembling an ameloblastoma with palisaded columnar hyperchromatic basal cells with reverse polarity, at least focally, and additional aberrant keratinization as ghost cells. Ghost cells may mineralize. The ghost cells may be dispersed, isolated, or present in clusters {2503,2082}. In higher-grade lesions, the malignant epithelial cells are basaloid or nondescript, and ameloblastoma-like features may be absent. Dentinoid may be present adjacent to the epithelial cells. The amount of dentinoid and ghost cells are variable. Evidence of malignancy includes mitotic activity, pleomorphism, hyperchromatism, necrosis, and an infiltrative growth pattern. Benign precursor COC or DGCT may be present.

Differential diagnosis
Differential diagnosis
GCOC should be differentiated from similar but benign odontogenic tumours, including DGCT and COC, and other odontogenic tumours that may contain ghost cells as a minor component, such as ameloblastoma and adenoid ameloblastoma. The diagnosis of GCOC requires cytological evidence of malignancy, which is not present in these other tumours. There is histological overlap with adenoid ameloblastoma and odontogenic carcinoma with dentinoid {3085}. It is possible these entities are related, and the differentiating criteria are not well defined.

Cytology
Not clinically relevant

Diagnostic molecular pathology
Not clinically relevant

Essential and desirable diagnostic criteria
Essential: a poorly demarcated lesion radiologically; ameloblastoma-like epithelium; prominent ghost cells; cytological evidence of malignancy.

Desirable: mixed radiolucency; root resorption; dentinoid formation.

Staging
Although there is no defined eighth-edition Union for International Cancer Control (UICC) / American Joint Committee on Cancer (AJCC) TNM staging system staging guidance, the use of International Collaboration on Cancer Reporting (ICCR) minimum data set reporting is encouraged {4138}.

Prognosis and prediction
Complete surgical excision is the treatment of choice. The aggressive nature of GCOC is reflected by a high recurrence rate of about 63%, reported in 44 patients. Distant metastases developed in 3 patients, and 9 patients died {1043}. Long-term follow-up is required.

Primary intraosseous carcinoma NOS

Koutlas IG
Sloan P

Definition
Primary intraosseous carcinoma NOS (PIOC) is a central jaw carcinoma that cannot be categorized as any other type of carcinoma and derives from odontogenic cysts, rests of odontogenic epithelium, the reduced enamel epithelium surrounding impacted teeth, or other benign precursors.

ICD-O coding
9270/3 Primary intraosseous carcinoma, NOS

ICD-11 coding
2B5J & XH4M89 Malignant miscellaneous tumours of bone or articular cartilage of other or unspecified sites & Odontogenic tumour, malignant

Related terminology
Not recommended: primary intraosseous squamous cell carcinoma, cystogenic type; primary intraosseous squamous cell carcinoma, solid type; primary intra-alveolar epidermoid carcinoma; primary odontogenic carcinoma.

Subtype(s)
None

Localization
PIOC is more frequent in the posterior body and ramus of the mandible and less frequent in the anterior maxilla. Cases arising in cysts are more frequent in the mandible. An intraosseous origin must be established for the diagnosis, excluding extension of gingival or alveolar squamous cell carcinoma or antral carcinoma into the jaws {4855}. Metastases must be

excluded. In the mandible these usually localize below the inferior alveolar nerve, in contrast to PIOC, which develops above it {4854}.

Clinical features
PIOC may be asymptomatic, discovered incidentally on radiographs, with or without tooth root resorption and cortical erosion. More advanced lesions are characterized by painful cortical expansion, loosening of teeth, non-healing extraction sites, labial or facial paraesthesia, and pathological fractures. Approximately 40% of patients have metastasis at the time of presentation {5063}.

Imaging
Poorly defined osteolytic area with or without tooth root resorption and cortical erosion. There may be radiological evidence of a benign precursor, and PIOC arising in cysts may produce a multilocular or scalloped radiolucency.

Epidemiology
PIOC is rare, and data are mostly in case reports. A systemic review identified 257 reported cases in 2020, the majority apparently arising from odontogenic cysts, more frequently residual and radicular cysts and less often dentigerous and odontogenic keratocysts {1054}. There is a male predilection (M:F ratio: 2:1), and the mean age at diagnosis is 55–60 years, although a wide age range is described, with occasional cases in young patients.

Etiology
Unknown

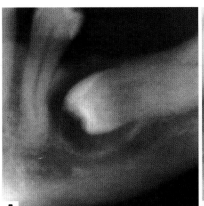
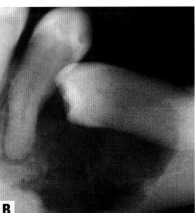
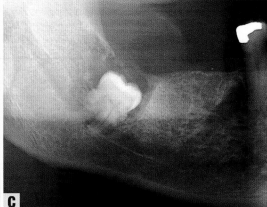

Fig. 7.57 Primary intraosseous carcinoma NOS. **A** Subtle early signs of intraosseous carcinoma in the dental follicle of an unerupted lower premolar, with slight expansion and loss of cortication. **B** Two years later, there is extensive poorly localized destruction and pathological fracture. **C** This radiolucency associated with the lower third molar presented in an 82-year-old man and had increased in size when compared with a panoramic radiograph taken 7 years earlier, and it had developed a poorly defined periphery. There was complete bony destruction of buccal cortex, root resorption, and paraesthesia along the distribution of the right inferior alveolar nerve.

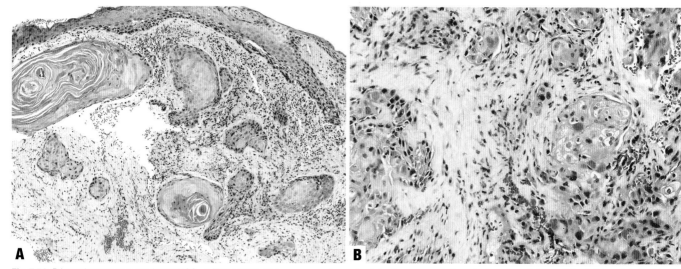

Fig. 7.58 Primary intraosseous carcinoma NOS. **A** This primary intraosseous carcinoma is arising from a pre-existing odontogenic cyst. A search for definite cytological atypia, mitotic activity, and invasion may be required, because hyperplastic islands of epithelium often develop in the walls of odontogenic cysts, and those primary intraosseous carcinomas that arise in cysts are often well differentiated. **B** Typical squamous carcinoma that arose in an odontogenic cyst.

Pathogenesis

Those that arise in odontogenic cysts may be preceded by dysplasia.

Macroscopic appearance

The macroscopic appearance is nonspecific unless a cyst or other precursor is present.

Histopathology

PIOCs are squamous carcinomas, comprising islands and small nests of atypical squamous epithelium with prickle cells and minimal keratinization. Cytological atypia ranges from quite bland to severe. Most PIOCs are moderately differentiated, and necrosis is rare.

Immunohistochemistry

CK19 positivity on immunohistochemistry supports an odontogenic epithelial origin but has low specificity.

Differential diagnosis

Peripheral palisading or plexiform patterns may occur, but if prominent they suggest ameloblastic carcinoma. Imaging, histopathology, and clinical information are essential to exclude metastasis (which is considerably more common), other malignant odontogenic tumours, mucosal and sinonasal primary carcinomas invading bone, and intraosseous salivary gland cancers.

Cytology

Not clinically relevant

Diagnostic molecular pathology

None

Essential and desirable diagnostic criteria

Essential: epicentre in jaws; destructive central jaw lesion; absence of a communication with the surface mucosa or antrum; exclusion of other primaries and metastatic disease by staging and immunohistochemistry.

Desirable: CK19 positivity on immunohistochemistry; historic radiological evidence of an odontogenic precursor.

Staging

Although there is no defined eighth-edition Union for International Cancer Control (UICC) / American Joint Committee on Cancer (AJCC) TNM staging system staging guidance, the use of International Collaboration on Cancer Reporting (ICCR) minimum data set reporting is encouraged {4138}.

Prognosis and prediction

Prognosis is generally poor. Outcomes are similar to stage IV oral squamous cell carcinoma, with an overall 5-year survival rate of about 45%. Radical resection with neck dissection is the most frequent treatment, with adjunctive radiotherapy providing a benefit. Recurrence is frequent (occurring in as many as 60% of cases) and is associated with a poor outcome. Distant metastasis is rare but is typically to the lung. Cases arising in cysts have a more prolonged clinical course, but the 5-year survival rate is about 40%. If dysplasia is found incidentally in a cyst after enucleation, close follow-up is appropriate.

Odontogenic carcinosarcoma

Wright JM

Definition
Odontogenic carcinosarcoma is a malignant mixed odontogenic tumour in which the epithelial component and the ectomesenchymal component show features of malignancy.

ICD-O coding
9342/3 Odontogenic carcinosarcoma

ICD-11 coding
2B5J & XH4LP1 Malignant miscellaneous tumours of bone or articular cartilage of other or unspecified sites & Odontogenic carcinosarcoma

Related terminology
Not recommended: malignant odontogenic mixed tumour; ameloblastic carcinosarcoma.

Subtype(s)
None

Localization
All cases have involved the posterior mandible, with 1 equivocal case in the maxilla {4361,1166}.

Clinical features
Most patients present with pain and swelling. The mean tumour diameter at diagnosis is approximately 60 mm. Paraesthesia or anaesthesia has been reported.

Imaging
Radiographically, most patients present with highly destructive, poorly margined radiolucencies. Cortical perforation is common, followed by soft tissue extension {2293}.

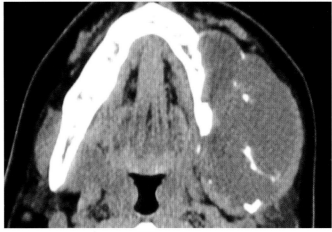

Fig. 7.59 Odontogenic carcinosarcoma. Axial CT shows a large, expansile, radiolucent lesion of the left mandible, with cortical destruction.

Epidemiology
Cases have been reported from Japan, Saudi Arabia, the Bolivarian Republic of Venezuela, the Republic of Korea, France, Germany, Brazil, and the USA. Age incidence has not been defined, although the mean age of female patients is significantly lower than that of male patients. There are twice as many male patients as female patients {3930}.

Etiology
Unknown

Pathogenesis
Most cases have been associated with a previously existing odontogenic neoplasm, often ameloblastic fibroma or ameloblastic fibrosarcoma {1080,3930}.

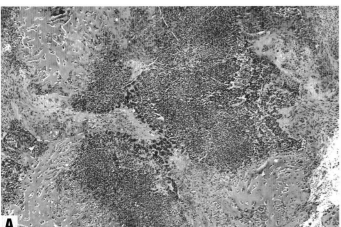 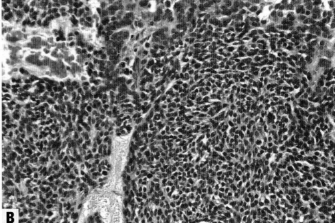

Fig. 7.60 Odontogenic carcinosarcoma. **A** Islands of highly cellular and poorly differentiated epithelium lying in a stromal component producing abundant dentinoid. **B** The epithelial component shows high cellularity, some pleomorphism and hyperchromatism, and frequent mitoses.

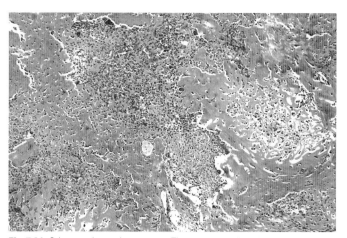

Fig. 7.61 Odontogenic carcinosarcoma. The ectomesenchymal component shows hypercellularity, some pleomorphism, hyperchromatism, increased mitoses, and extensive dentinoid.

Macroscopic appearance
The neoplasm is often tan, lobulated, and fleshy {1080,839}.

Histopathology
Histopathological features are based on few cases, but they resemble those of ameloblastic fibroma or fibrosarcoma. Both the epithelial and ectomesenchymal components must show convincing cytological features of malignancy. The epithelial component ranges from fine strands to larger islands, often with peripheral palisading. The ectomesenchymal component is hypercellular with cytological atypia. Mesenchymal hard tissues such as dentinoid, bone, and cartilage may be produced, but the histological appearances do not mimic osteosarcoma or other defined sarcomas. Both components show a high mitotic count and Ki-67 proliferative index {1080,1166}.

Immunohistochemistry
The epithelial component is reactive for a variety of cytokeratins, particularly CK19. The ectomesenchymal component is invariably positive for vimentin but may also show reactivity for desmin and MSA {1166}.

Differential diagnosis
This must exclude a malignant epithelial odontogenic tumour with a spindle cell component of epithelial origin, such as ameloblastic carcinoma, a significant diagnostic pitfall {2909}. The formation of matrix or hard tissue in an odontogenic carcinoma does not necessarily indicate sarcoma {239, 3085}. A spindle cell squamous carcinoma usually demonstrates epithelial differentiation histologically and/or immunohistochemically.

Cytology
Not clinically relevant

Diagnostic molecular pathology
Not relevant

Essential and desirable diagnostic criteria
Essential: origin in a tooth-bearing segment of the jaws; carcinoma and sarcoma components; significant cytological atypia in both components; exclusion of spindle cell squamous carcinoma.
Desirable: evidence of a pre-existing odontogenic tumour.

Staging
Although there is no defined eighth-edition Union for International Cancer Control (UICC) / American Joint Committee on Cancer (AJCC) TNM staging system staging guidance, the use of International Collaboration on Cancer Reporting (ICCR) minimum data set reporting is encouraged {4138}.

Prognosis and prediction
The treatment of choice is wide surgical excision. Almost two thirds of patients experience recurrence and just over 40% have metastasis, most often to lung. Disease-associated mortality is about 50% {3930}.

Odontogenic sarcomas

Wright JM
Chi A

Definition
The odontogenic sarcomas (OSs) are a group of malignant mixed odontogenic neoplasms in which only the ectomesenchymal component shows microscopic features of malignancy.

ICD-O coding
9330/3 Odontogenic sarcomas
9330/3 Ameloblastic fibrosarcoma
9330/3 Ameloblastic fibrodentinosarcoma
9330/3 Ameloblastic fibro-odontosarcoma

ICD-11 coding
2B5J & XH0XD5 Malignant miscellaneous tumours of bone or articular cartilage of other or unspecified sites & Ameloblastic fibrosarcoma

Related terminology
None

Subtype(s)
Ameloblastic fibrosarcoma; ameloblastic fibrodentinosarcoma; ameloblastic fibro-odontosarcoma

Localization
Approximately 75–80% arise in the mandible with a predilection for the posterior region {3983,3639}.

Clinical features
Patients present with locally aggressive expansile lesions, with or without pain. Many OSs arise from malignant transformation of a benign precursor.

Imaging
Early lesions may appear benign radiographically, features reflecting a benign precursor. However, with time, the lesions typically develop poorly defined margins with cortical destruction. Most lesions are unilocular or multilocular radiolucencies, but are occasionally mixed radiolucent/radiopaque {2789,870}. Tooth displacement, impaction, and root resorption are also possible {870}.

Epidemiology
Only about 100 cases have been reported {870,3639}. The M:F ratio is about 1.5:1. The average age at diagnosis is in the third decade of life {84,870}.

Etiology
The etiology is unknown; however, more than half of all OSs arise from malignant transformation of a pre-existing benign neoplasm, such as ameloblastic fibroma.

Pathogenesis
OSs have *BRAF* p.V600E activating mutations {54} in the mesenchymal component {957}. Single cases have shown *NRAS* p.Q61K mutation (mutually exclusive with *BRAF* p.V600E mutation), *EGFR* exon 20 insertions, *MDM2* amplification, or aneuploidy {3113,54,4393}.

Macroscopic appearance
Not reported

Histopathology
OSs contain an epithelial component and an ectomesenchymal component. The epithelial component is cytologically bland and benign. It varies considerably in quantity and morphology, ranging from thin dental lamina–like strands to larger islands of odontogenic epithelium, with peripheral cells showing nuclear palisading and reverse polarity but not stellate reticulum. The malignant ectomesenchymal component is characterized by hypercellularity, varying degrees of cytological atypia, and

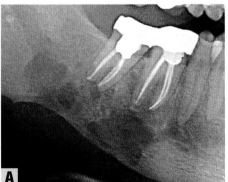 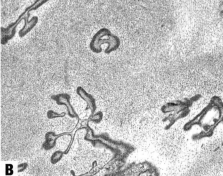 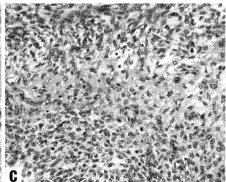

Fig. 7.62 A Odontogenic sarcoma. Radiographic image showing a poorly marginated osteolytic radiolucency of the right posterior mandible. **B** Ameloblastic fibrosarcoma. Mixed odontogenic tumour in which the epithelial component is cytologically bland but the ectomesenchymal component displays hypercellularity. **C** Odontogenic sarcoma. At high magnification, the ectomesenchymal component is hypercellular, with cytological atypia and a high mitotic index.

Chapter 7

increased mitotic activity {3571,3983}. In approximately 10% of cases, dysplastic dentine with or without enamel matrix is produced (amcloblastic fibrodentinosarcoma or ameloblastic fibro-odontosarcoma).

Cytology
Not clinically relevant

Diagnostic molecular pathology
The mutations identified (see *Pathogenesis*, above) are not yet clinically relevant.

Essential and desirable diagnostic criteria
Essential: origin in a tooth-bearing segment of the jaws; a mixed odontogenic neoplasm; a cytologically bland epithelial component; a cytologically malignant ectomesenchymal component.
Desirable: evidence of a benign precursor.

Staging
Although there is no defined eighth-edition Union for International Cancer Control (UICC) / American Joint Committee on Cancer (AJCC) TNM staging system staging guidance, the use of International Collaboration on Cancer Reporting (ICCR) minimum data set reporting is encouraged {4138}.

Prognosis and prediction
Most cases are treated by surgical resection, with an overall recurrence rate of 35% and a disease-related mortality rate of 21% {870}. Metastases are usually distant but affect < 5% of cases {3639}.

Central giant cell granuloma

Jordan RC
Gomes CC
Gomez RS

Definition
Central giant cell granuloma (CGCG) is a localized, benign but sometimes aggressive osteolytic jaw lesion consisting of a proliferation of osteoclasts in a mononuclear and fibrous vascular stroma.

ICD-O coding
None

ICD-11 coding
DA01.20 Giant cell granuloma, central

Related terminology
Not recommended: central giant cell lesion; reparative giant cell granuloma.

Subtype(s)
None

Localization
CGCG develops almost exclusively in the jaws and is more frequent in the anterior mandible.

Clinical features
CGCGs generally present as well-defined, asymptomatic, slow-growing, expansile radiolucencies. A minority of lesions are aggressive and may exhibit rapid growth, root resorption, tooth displacement, cortical perforation, and recurrence after curettage {894,2136}.

Imaging
CGCG appears as a corticated unilocular or multilocular radiolucency, sometimes with fine honeycomb or wispy trabecular opacity. Cortical expansion is often prominent, with

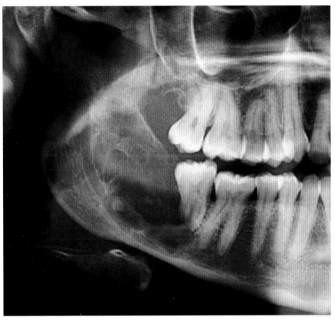

Fig. 7.63 Central giant cell granuloma. A typical giant cell granuloma in the posterior body and ramus of the mandible, showing a well-delineated but variably corticated, apparently multilocular radiolucency. Faint internal septa of osteoid and thin bone are present posteriorly, producing a honeycomb appearance.

perforation. Tooth root resorption is infrequent. MRI is helpful in delineating soft tissue involvement, and multicentricity can be verified with fusion PET-CT.

Epidemiology
The incidence of CGCG is 1.1 cases per 1 million person-years in Europe {1081}. Most patients are female, and most cases occur in patients aged < 30 years {872}.

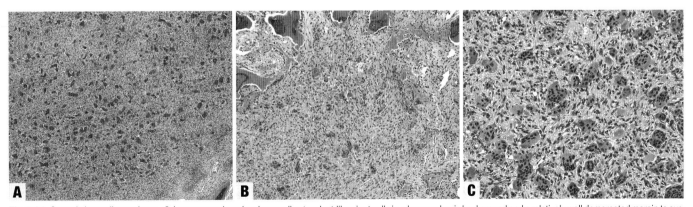

Fig. 7.64 Central giant cell granuloma. **A** Low-power view showing small osteoclast-like giant cells in a haemorrhagic background and a relatively well demarcated margin to surrounding bone. **B** Osteoclast-like giant cells and mononuclear cells in a vascular stroma that also contains trabecular bone and osteoid. **C** High-power image showing relatively small multinucleated osteoclast-type giant cells intermixed with mononuclear cells.

Chapter 7

Etiology
Unknown

Genetic factors
Multiple giant cell granulomas occur in syndromes including neurofibromatosis type 1, osteoglophonic dysplasia, Noonan syndrome, cardiofaciocutaneous syndrome, oculoectodermal syndrome, LEOPARD syndrome, Schimmelpenning–Feuerstein–Mims syndrome, and Jaffe–Campanacci syndrome, most of which are caused by MAPK pathway gene mutations {1639}.

Pathogenesis
CGCGs arise from osteoclast precursors in the mononuclear stroma, induced by RANKL, VEGF, and bFGF; the last of these amplifies the resorptive action of PTH.

Sporadic CGCG have a low tumour mutation burden, lack fusions {1643}, and are driven by mutually exclusive somatic mutations in *KRAS* (more often affecting codon 12), *FGFR1* (either p.C381R or p.N330I), and *TRPV4* (p.M713V/I) that occur in 70% of cases, leading to MAPK pathway activation {1643}. *TRPV4* codes a polymodal Ca^{2+}-permeable channel and is mutated in hereditary channelopathies characterized by peripheral nervous system and skeletal changes. Recently, CGCGs have been described as one feature of a polysystemic syndrome due to germline *TRPV4* mutation, expanding the spectrum of *TRPV4* channelopathies {3631}. Unlike in conventional giant cell tumours of long bones, *H3-3A* (*H3F3A*) mutations are not present {1638,1643}.

Macroscopic appearance
CGCGs have a fleshy, reddish-brown, haemorrhagic appearance.

Histopathology
CGCG is an unencapsulated proliferation of mononuclear spindle-shaped and polygonal cells intermingled with osteoclast multinucleated giant cells in a vascular background, with haemorrhage and haemosiderin pigment. The lesion may have a lobular architecture, lobules separated by fibrous septa that may contain thin osteoid and woven bone. The giant cells in CGCGs show reactivity for osteoclast and macrophage markers {4622,4478,1403}. The mononuclear stromal cells are the proliferating component, and mitoses may be readily found.

Differential diagnosis
The differential diagnosis includes cherubism in young patients and cystic haemorrhagic degeneration producing an aneurysmal bone cyst–like appearance in fibro-osseous lesions. Brown tumour of hyperparathyroidism is a close histological mimic and is only definitively excluded by serology.

Cytology
Mononuclear and osteoclast-type multinucleated giant cells; haemosiderin pigment

Diagnostic molecular pathology
None

Essential and desirable diagnostic criteria
Essential: location in the jaws; clustered osteoclast giant cells; haemorrhage; spindle cell stroma.
Desirable: a lobular structure.

Staging
None

Prognosis and prediction
Most CGCGs do not recur after thorough curettage. A more radical surgical approach may be necessary for aggressive or recurrent lesions. To limit the extent of resection of large lesions, intralesional or systemic pharmacological agents such as corticosteroids, calcitonin, interferon, or denosumab may be considered, but the effects are inconsistent {872}.

Peripheral giant cell granuloma

Jordan RC
Gomes CC
Gomez RS

Definition
Peripheral giant cell granuloma (PGCG) is a reactive localized proliferation of mononuclear cells and osteoclasts in a vascular stroma located in the soft tissues of the gingiva or alveolar ridge mucosa.

ICD-O coding
None

ICD-11 coding
DA0D.Y Other specified disorders of gingival or edentulous alveolar ridge

Related terminology
Acceptable: giant cell epulis.
Not recommended: peripheral reparative giant cell granuloma.

Subtype(s)
None

Localization
PGCG arises in the gingiva or alveolar ridge, more commonly in the mandible than the maxilla {874,2573,3091}.

Clinical features
A sessile or pedunculated lump with a smooth, ulcerated, or nodular surface and often a characteristic red, maroon, or purple colour. PGCG may reach several centimetres in diameter, and

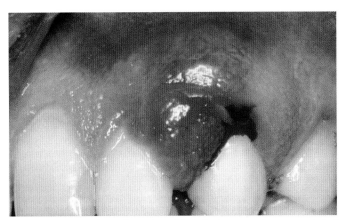

Fig. 7.65 Peripheral giant cell granuloma. The lesion forms a red or maroon gingival enlargement in the left maxilla between two teeth.

erosion of the underlying bone is found in almost one third of all cases {3091,2573}.

Imaging
Radiographic assessment should exclude a central giant cell granuloma.

Epidemiology
The epidemiology is unknown. PGCG is the commonest oral giant cell lesion. It is slightly more prevalent in women than in men (M:F ratio: 1:1.2) and arises over a wide age distribution.

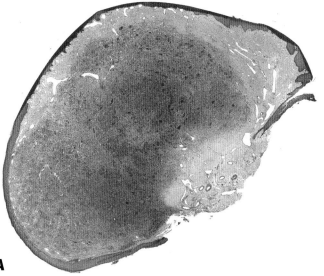

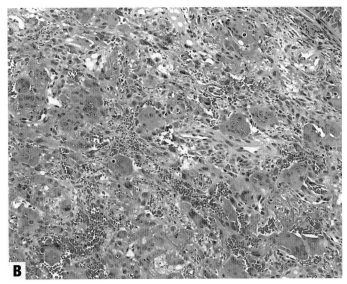

Fig. 7.66 Peripheral giant cell granuloma. **A** A complete lesion. A pedunculated polyp containing a cellular lobular mass of giant cells with haemorrhage. **B** Mononuclear and osteoclast-type multinucleated giant cells in a vascular stroma containing some haemosiderin, all covered by oral epithelium. The lesion is microscopically identical to a central giant cell granuloma.

Chapter 7

Etiology

PGCG is caused by local irritation of the mucoperiosteum or the coronal part of the periodontal ligament by dental calculus, plaque deposits, retained tooth roots, or other chronic irritation.

Pathogenesis

Similarly to central giant cell granulomas, about 70% of PGCGs harbour *KRAS* mutations, mainly in codons 146 and 12, and 10% have *FGFR1* p.C381R or *FGFR1* p.N330I mutations {1643}. Notably, when associated with dental implants, PGCG also harbours *KRAS* mutations {2861}. MAPK pathway activation is observed in PGCG irrespective of the presence of mutations {1643}.

Macroscopic appearance

PGCG appears as fleshy red-brown tissue due to vascularity and haemorrhage. When formalin-fixed, it has a solid consistency with a dark-brown coloration.

Histopathology

PGCG resembles central giant cell granuloma, with an unencapsulated proliferation of mononuclear spindle-shaped and polygonal cells with osteoclast multinucleated cells in a vascular loose fibrous tissue. Foci of haemorrhage, haemosiderin pigment, and scattered deposits of immature bone are frequent. An inflammatory component of fibrous or pyogenic granuloma–like hyperplasia may be present, reflecting local irritant causes.

Cytology

Not clinically relevant

Diagnostic molecular pathology

None

Essential and desirable diagnostic criteria

Essential: location on the gingiva or alveolar ridge; cellular mononuclear stroma; clustered osteoclasts; haemorrhage; no origin from underlying intraosseous giant cell granuloma.

Desirable: exclusion of hyperparathyroidism (very rarely associated with localized lesions).

Staging

None

Prognosis and prediction

The rate of recurrence after conservative surgical removal may be 16%. Curettage to periodontal ligament or peripheral osteotomy reduce recurrence, especially when the underlying bone is eroded {874}. Any source of irritation should be removed.

Cherubism

Gomez RS
Flanagan AM

Definition
Cherubism is a rare autosomal dominant–inherited bone disorder characterized by symmetrical expansion of the mandible, maxilla, or both, by an osteoclast-like giant cell–rich lesion.

ICD-O coding
None

ICD-11 coding
LD24.22 Cherubism

Related terminology
Not recommended: familial fibrous dysplasia; juvenile fibrous dysplasia.

Subtype(s)
None

Localization
Both jaws are affected bilaterally, with the mandible more commonly affected than the maxilla {3586}.

Clinical features
Slow, symmetrical expansion of the jaws develops in early childhood, usually before 6 years of age. Maxillary expansion in severe cases may cause orbital displacement with scleral exposure, producing the characteristic facial appearance similar to that of putti or cherubs in Renaissance paintings. Female patients are usually more severely affected. Tooth displacement and impaction, root resorption, and agenesis are typical. Partial or complete regression occurs by adulthood {1403}.

An association with odontogenic tumours is reported {235}.

Imaging
Radiologically, affected bones show a symmetrical, well-defined, radiolucent/hypodense, multilocular, soap bubble–like

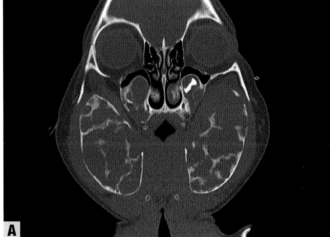
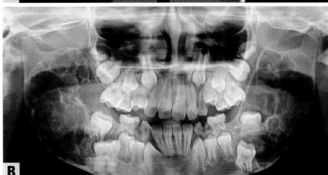

Fig. 7.67 Cherubism. **A** CT coronal reformat showing massive bilateral enlargement of both mandibular rami, with cortical thinning and perforation and an internal honeycomb structure of osteoid or woven bone trabeculae. **B** Panoramic radiograph showing bilateral multilocular radiolucencies in the posterior mandible.

appearance, with thinned cortex {886}. The fibrous tissue is progressively replaced by new bone, leading to sclerosis.

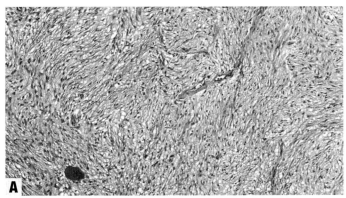
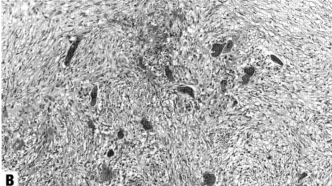

Fig. 7.68 Cherubism. **A** Much of the lesion is oedematous fibrous tissue with sparse giant cells and sometimes prominent vessels. **B** Vascular fibrous tissue with scattered multinucleated osteoclast-like giant cells, haemorrhage, and haemosiderin deposits.

Chapter 7

Epidemiology

The incidence is unknown. Two thirds of cases are familial, with complete penetrance in males and 60–70% penetrance in females, and with variable expressivity; the remaining cases arise as de novo germline alterations {886,2764}.

Etiology

Autosomal dominant *SH3BP2* mutations, located on chromosome 4p16.3 {2813,4462}, have been identified in about 90% of cases {886}. The majority of mutations occur in exon 9, within a proline-rich sequence six amino acids long {4531}.

Pathogenesis

The *SH3BP2* mutations result in the excessive generation of abnormally large osteoclasts with constitutive activity {2140}.

Macroscopic appearance

The macroscopic appearance is similar to that of other giant cell lesions, with red and haemorrhagic tissue and areas of cystic change.

Histopathology

The microscopic features are not specific and resemble those of other giant cell–rich lesions of the jaws, including giant cell granuloma, giant cell lesions in Noonan and Jaffe–Campanacci syndromes {1639}, and brown tumour of hyperparathyroidism. Typically, abnormally large multinucleated osteoclast-like giant cells lie in a monotonous loose or oedematous spindle cell stroma with eosinophilic cuff-like perivascular deposits {1403}.

Cytology

Not clinically relevant {1716A}

Diagnostic molecular pathology

Not relevant

Essential and desirable diagnostic criteria

Essential: only the posterior jaws affected; bilateral symmetrical lesions; giant cell lesion on histology.
Desirable: detection of *SH3BP2* germline mutation (in selected cases).

Staging

Not relevant

Prognosis and prediction

Most cases regress after puberty, but some show continued growth with little regression. Surgery should be performed only in severe cases, where it will provide a functional benefit {3586}.

Aneurysmal bone cyst

Jordan RC
Koutlas IG

Definition
Aneurysmal bone cyst (ABC) is a cystic or multicystic, expansile, osteolytic neoplasm composed of blood-filled sinusoidal spaces lined by fibrous septa that contain osteoclast-type giant cells.

ICD-O coding
9260/0 Aneurysmal bone cyst

ICD-11 coding
FB80.6 & XH23E0 Aneurysmal bone cyst & Aneurysmal bone cyst

Related terminology
Not recommended: primary aneurysmal bone cyst; secondary aneurysmal bone cyst.

Subtype(s)
None

Localization
More than 60% of jaw ABCs occur in the mandible, usually posteriorly. Maxillary lesions have a more uniform anatomical distribution. Other sites in the craniofacial complex can be affected {2525}.

Clinical features
ABC presents as an enlargement of the jaw that is frequently painful. Teeth remain vital; however, tooth mobility and displacement are common. ABCs can cause root resorption. Maxillary tumours can extend to the sinuses and nose, and orbital involvement can lead to exophthalmos.

Imaging
Radiographically, there is a well-delineated, unilocular or multilocular radiolucency, characteristically markedly expansile. CT may show bone septa compartmentalizing the lesion. CT and MRI studies may demonstrate characteristic fluid levels,

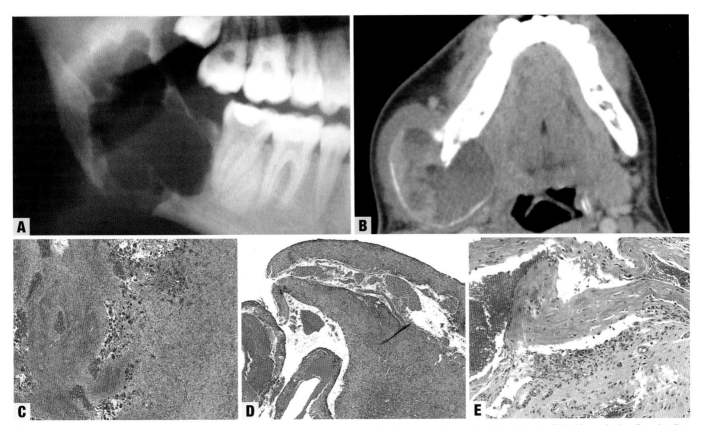

Fig. 7.69 Aneurysmal bone cyst. **A** Panoramic radiograph showing an aneurysmal bone cyst in the posterior body and ramus of the mandible with a typical scalloped outline, cortical erosion, and limited cortication. **B** Axial CT showing a circumscribed, partially fluid-filled mass with prominent expansion in the right posterior mandible. **C** Solid type, containing clusters of multinucleated giant cells set in a fibroblastic stroma. **D** Low-power image showing blood-filled sinusoidal spaces. **E** Higher-magnification view of a blood-filled sinusoidal space lined by multinucleated giant cells. The features are relatively nonspecific, but the diagnosis was supported by cytogenetic analysis showing rearrangement of *USP6*.

sometimes with perforation of the cortex and extension to adjacent soft tissue {2525}.

Epidemiology
ABC is rare, with an estimated incidence of approximately 0.15 cases per 1 million person-years {2557}, 1.5% of which arise in the jaws. All age groups are affected, but > 80% of cases occur in younger patients, usually during the first two decades of life. Both sexes are equally affected; however, a male predilection has been reported in jaw ABCs {3090}.

Etiology
Unknown

Pathogenesis
Fusion of *USP6* and *CDH11* is seen in 70% of cases {3289}, affecting the stromal fibroblast population only. Other fusion partners include *CNBP, COL1A1, CTNNB1, EIF1, FOSL2, OMD, PAFAH1B1, RUNX2, SEC31A, SPARC, STAT3, THRAP3,* and *USP9X* {376}. Fusion with any partner leads to upregulation of the *USP6* coding region that regulates several cellular processes such as intracellular trafficking, matrix degradation, and cell transformation {2525,3970}. *USP6* translocation is not present in jaw giant cell granuloma {58}.

Macroscopic appearance
ABC appears as haemorrhagic spongy tissue comprising multiple cysts separated by fibrous septa of various thickness. Solid areas may be present, and a rare completely solid form of ABC is recognized.

Histopathology
ABC is composed of blood-filled or empty sinusoidal spaces lined by macrophages and bland fibroblasts that are separated by fibrous septa containing scattered multinucleated osteoclastic giant cells. Woven bone in septa can appear prominently basophilic and has been referred to as blue bone, and if present this is characteristic, but not diagnostic. The solid pattern can feature cellular areas, which can be mitotically active, along with limited, inconspicuous cystic spaces.

Differential diagnosis
The entities include ABC-like cystic haemorrhagic degeneration in a range of other neoplasms including osteoblastoma, fibrous dysplasia, cemento-ossifying fibroma, other fibro-osseous lesions, and osteosarcoma.

Cytology
Not clinically relevant

Diagnostic molecular pathology
A translocation involving *USP6* and several 5' partners including *CDH11* is helpful in the diagnosis of the solid pattern (in selected cases).

Essential and desirable diagnostic criteria
Essential: compatible radiological features; multicystic; fibrous septa with haemorrhage and osteoclasts.
Desirable: woven bone in septa; *USP6* gene rearrangement (in selected cases).

Staging
None

Prognosis and prediction
There is a risk of recurrence after curettage, and en bloc resection may be necessary for large destructive tumours {2938}. The recurrence rate is approximately 10% with soft tissue extension.

Simple bone cyst

Gopalakrishnan R

Definition
Simple bone cyst (SBC) is an intraosseous cystic cavity lined by a fibrous membrane without epithelium, either empty or containing serosanguineous fluid.

ICD-O coding
None

ICD-11 coding
FB80.5 Solitary bone cyst

Related terminology
Acceptable: solitary bone cyst.
Not recommended: traumatic bone cyst; haemorrhagic bone cyst; unicameral bone cyst.

Subtype(s)
None

Localization
The mandible is most frequently affected, with a predilection for the body {880}. Bilateral or multiple SBCs are fairly frequent {880,943}.

Clinical features
The vast majority of cases are asymptomatic and discovered on routine examination. Expansion is unusual and limited.

Imaging
Radiographically, SBCs are well-delineated unilocular radiolucencies that scallop between the roots of associated vital teeth {943,3687}. A multilocular presentation is rare and typically only present in larger lesions. Cortical perforation, displacement of teeth, and root resorption are not observed, and expansion is rare.

Epidemiology
SBCs are found predominantly in patients in their second or third decade of life, with no sex differences {880}.

Etiology
Unknown

Pathogenesis
More than half of SBCs in the peripheral skeleton have been shown to harbour either *FUS::NFATC2* or *EWSR1::NFATC2* fusion {3557,1962}, one of the genetic changes seen in round cell sarcoma with *EWSR1*::non-ETS fusions {3310}. Jaw SBCs have not yet been analysed.

Macroscopic appearance
Sparse scrapings of fibrous tissue with bone fragments

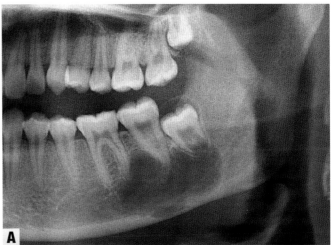

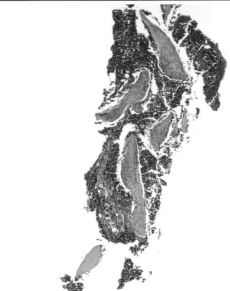

Fig. 7.70 Simple bone cyst. **A** Typical presentation of a simple bone cyst affecting the body of the mandible on the left. Note the lesion extending up in a rounded pattern between the roots of the associated teeth. **B** Scrapings from the wall of a simple bone cyst featuring bland fibrous tissue and bone fragments.

Histopathology
SBC has no epithelial lining, and samples contain nondescript thin strips of loosely collagenous or myxoid connective tissue with thin, lace-like fragments of immature bone at the periphery. Haemosiderin, cholesterol, and sparse osteoclasts may be present. Spiky, needle-like collagen fibres may lie peripherally and can become densely mineralized, a useful diagnostic feature when biopsy tissue is sparse {379}.

Cystic haemorrhagic degeneration in florid cemento-osseous dysplasia has been termed "SBC" and may account for as many as one third of apparent jaw SBCs {4273}, but the age

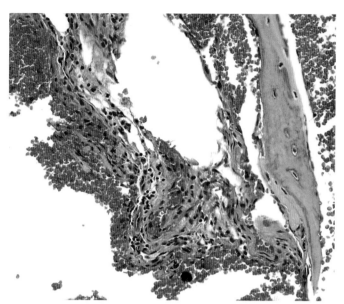

Fig. 7.71 Simple bone cyst. Scraping from the wall of a simple bone cyst featuring delicate connective tissue and irregular fragments of bone.

group is older and shows a female predilection {5053}, and these cysts are typically more expansile and may recur after treatment. Such cysts are probably not conventional SBC, but their mutation status is not defined.

Cytology
Not clinically relevant

Diagnostic molecular pathology
None

Essential and desirable diagnostic criteria
Essential: typical radiological features; empty cavity at operation.

Staging
None

Prognosis and prediction
Healing is induced by bleeding after surgical exploration and curettage {3687}. Occasional spontaneous healing is reported {3687,1017}. Occasional cases recur.

Cemento-osseous dysplasia

Boy S
Soluk Tekkeşin M

Definition
Cemento-osseous dysplasia (COD) is a non-neoplastic fibro-osseous lesion arising only in the tooth-bearing areas of the jaws.

ICD-O coding
None

ICD-11 coding
DA07.3 Disturbances in tooth formation & Florid cemento-osseous dysplasia

2E83.1 Benign osteogenic tumours of bone or articular cartilage of lower jaw & Periapical cemento-osseous dysplasia of lower jaw

Related terminology
Not recommended: osseous dysplasia; cemental dysplasia; cementoma.

Subtype(s)
Periapical cemento-osseous dysplasia (PCOD); focal cemento-osseous dysplasia (FocCOD); florid cemento-osseous dysplasia (FCOD); familial florid cemento-osseous dysplasia (FFCOD)

Localization
PCOD predominantly involves the periapical bone of the anterior mandibular teeth; FocCOD involves a single, usually posterior, mandibular tooth; and FCOD involves multiple tooth-bearing quadrants {3286,717}. FFCOD almost always has the same distribution as FCOD {3178}.

Clinical features
CODs are usually asymptomatic, non-expansile lesions associated with the roots of vital teeth. Some cases of FocCOD and as many as 25% of FCOD cases may expand the jaw, either directly or after cyst formation, sometimes markedly {3658}. Patients with FocCOD, FCOD, and FFCOD are prone to developing osteomyelitis in their late sclerotic stage, with pain and discharge {3658,3465}. COD may remain in edentulous jaw after tooth extraction. FFCOD has an earlier age of onset than FCOD, often affecting tooth eruption, and is prone to marked expansion, usually in the anterior mandible but sometimes multifocally {3178}, leading to confusion with familial gigantiform cementoma.

Imaging
Radiographic features are characteristic and often diagnostic. The early stage of all subtypes of COD produces well-defined periapical radiolucencies continuous with periodontal ligament, enlarging slowly before developing internal, usually central, radiopacities and patchy sclerosis beyond a well-defined radiolucent rim. Later, lesions become radiodense with lobulated dense mineralization {3286,717}. FocCOD is more variable {4260}.

Epidemiology
COD is the most common benign fibro-osseous lesion of the jaws, with a strong predilection for middle-aged women {1246, 4165}, most commonly African and African-American women, but with a significant incidence in Asian women {3520} and White women {3286}. FFCOD has a less marked racial and sex predilection {3178}.

Etiology
Unknown

Pathogenesis
The pathogenesis is unknown for PCOD, FocCOD, and FCOD. The members of one family with FFCOD have been shown to carry a mutation in *ANO5* that is proposed to destabilize this transmembrane ion channel {2742}. The mutated locus is

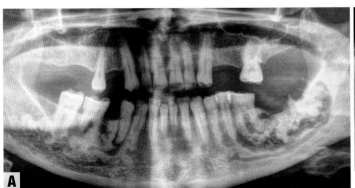
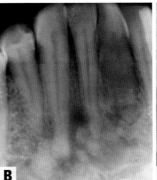
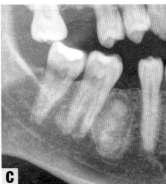

Fig. 7.72 Cemento-osseous dysplasia. **A** Florid subtype. A mixture of radiopaque and radiolucent lesions involving the anterior and posterior mandibular alveolar bone centred on tooth root apices. **B** Periapical form, with discrete mixed radiopaque and radiolucent lesions involving the anterior tooth root apices. **C** Focal subtype, similar to the periapical form, but solitary and surrounded by a well-defined osteolytic rim.

Chapter 7

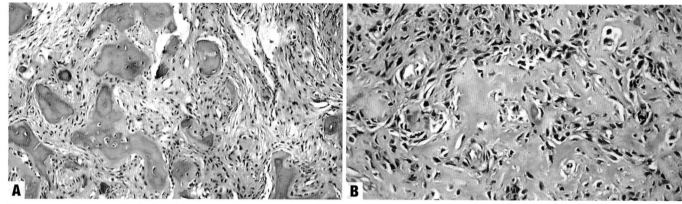

Fig. 7.73 Cemento-osseous dysplasia. **A** Irregular woven bone trabeculae and cementum-like particles in a cellular fibrovascular connective tissue background. **B** Woven bone and osteoid in a focally hypercellular stroma.

distinct from that in gnathodiaphysial dysplasia, in which there are multiple cemento-ossifying fibromas {1201}.

Macroscopic appearance
Multiple variably sized, gritty fragments of haemorrhagic bone and soft tissue

Histopathology
All COD subtypes exhibit identical microscopic features dependent on the degree of maturation. There are varying proportions of osteoid and woven bone; mature lamellar bone; and rounded, densely basophilic, cementum-like mineralizations; these appear in a cellular fibrous connective tissue stroma of loosely arranged collagen and prominently dilated, thin-walled vessels. Osteoblastic rimming is rare. There is often focal high cellularity. Maturing lesions show increasing calcification with often prominent reversal lines and reduced vascularity. Late-stage lesions are characterized by the coalescence of calcified tissue that forms hypocellular, sclerotic masses with limited stroma {4261,3183,3286,4165}.

Differential diagnosis
Approximately 10% of cases may develop expansile cystic degeneration resembling solitary bone cyst {145}, usually in the

mandible in late-stage disease. Expansile areas in FFCOD may be difficult to distinguish from cemento-ossifying fibroma {3178} if the background disease is not appreciated.

Cytology
Not clinically relevant

Diagnostic molecular pathology
Not relevant

Essential and desirable diagnostic criteria
Essential: radiological features are almost always diagnostic; benign fibro-osseous lesion histologically.

Staging
None

Prognosis and prediction
Radiological diagnosis is usual, with periodic follow-up for expansion, cyst formation, and osteomyelitis. Surgical intervention is indicated exclusively for symptomatic cases {3286,3465}, because osteomyelitis is a common complication of biopsy or tooth extraction. Cysts may recur after surgery.

Segmental odontomaxillary dysplasia

Koutlas IG
Lopes MA

Definition

Segmental odontomaxillary dysplasia (SOD) is a non-hereditary unilateral developmental disorder characterized by segmental maxillary and soft tissue enlargement with dento-osseous abnormalities and occasionally homolateral cutaneous manifestations.

ICD-O coding

None

ICD-11 coding

DA07.3 Disturbances in tooth formation

Related terminology

None

Subtype(s)

None

Localization

SOD is a unilateral maxillary enlargement, occurring almost equally on the right or left side, in the premolar/molar region of the maxilla.

Clinical features

Patients present with a painless maxillary buccal and palatal enlargement, usually in the first or second decade of life, with a failure of tooth eruption and with dental abnormalities clinically and radiographically. Enlargement appears stable and non-progressive, starting in childhood and continuing until puberty. Frequently there is associated fibrous gingival hyperplasia {1022}. The maxillary overgrowth extends to the sinus, reducing its volume radiographically {3601}.

Dental abnormalities include missing permanent teeth (usually premolars), retained primary molars beyond the normal time of exfoliation, enamel and dentine hypoplasia, and altered tooth shape and size. Facial manifestations, often subtle, include hypertrichosis, hyperpigmentation or hypopigmentation (including Becker naevus), an increased frequency of melanocytic naevi, erythema, and lip clefting {4147,698}.

There is a poorly defined overlap of features with some related presentations and syndromes including hemimaxillofacial dysplasia {3002} and HATS syndrome (hemimaxillofacial enlargement, asymmetry of the face, tooth abnormalities, and skin findings) {143}.

Imaging

Panoramic and periapical radiographs show a poorly defined area of abnormal bone, often with a characteristic vertical trabeculation, and coarse radiopacities.

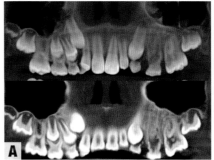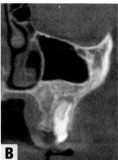

Fig. 7.74 Segmental odontomaxillary dysplasia. **A** Sequential tomograms reveal an absence of premolars, retained primary molars with root resorption of the second molar, and vertical trabeculation in the affected area of the maxilla. **B** Coarse radiopacities affecting the left side of the maxilla extending to the zygomatic bone and floor of the orbit.

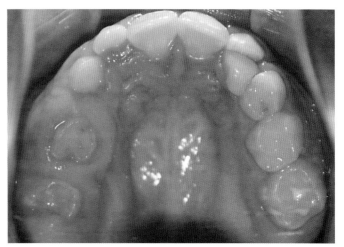

Fig. 7.75 Segmental odontomaxillary dysplasia. Fibrous and bony enlargement of the maxillary alveolar mucosa (left side of image). Retained primary molar on the same side.

Epidemiology

SOD is rare and has a slight male predilection.

Etiology

The etiology is unknown. Proposed causes include prenatal trauma, endocrine abnormalities, and bacterial or viral infection.

Pathogenesis

The possibility that somatic *PIK3CA* or *ACTB* mutations contribute to the overgrowth has been raised {1582}.

Macroscopic appearance

Bone trephine or sample with tooth fragments

Chapter 7

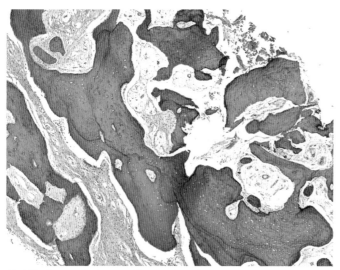

Fig. 7.76 Segmental odontomaxillary dysplasia. Abnormal woven and lamellar bone architecture with accentuated and multiple reversal and prominent resting lines associated with fibromyxoid tissue. Note the retraction artefact and lack of bone deposition.

Histopathology
Gingival biopsies may reveal fibrous hyperplasia with occasional dystrophic calcifications. Bone biopsies reveal irregular bone spicules with multiple accentuated reversal lines. The bone appears inert, without osteoblastic or osteoclastic activity, and histological features are probably the end stage of a much earlier developmental process. External root resorption of teeth, with dysplastic dentine and fibrosis of the pulp, has been described {4147}.

Cytology
Not relevant

Diagnostic molecular pathology
Not clinically relevant

Essential and desirable diagnostic criteria
Essential: localized swelling; abnormal soft tissues, bone, and teeth; characteristic radiographic features.
Desirable: inert bone histologically, with defects of tooth formation (only if fibrous dysplasia requires exclusion).

Staging
None

Prognosis and prediction
SOD shows slow or minimal enlargement until puberty. Surgery may be required for cosmetic and functional purposes.

Fibrous dysplasia

Nelson BL
Fitzpatrick SG
Flanagan AM

Definition
Fibrous dysplasia is a genetically based disorder of bone growth (usually involving *GNAS* mutation), in which bone is replaced by abnormal bone and fibrous tissue.

ICD-O coding
8818/0 Fibrous dysplasia
8818/0 Monostotic fibrous dysplasia
8818/0 Polyostotic fibrous dysplasia
8818/0 Craniofacial fibrous dysplasia

ICD-11 coding
FB80.0 Fibrous dysplasia of bone

Related terminology
Acceptable: craniofacial fibrous dysplasia (extending across more than one bone).

Subtype(s)
Monostotic fibrous dysplasia; polyostotic fibrous dysplasia; craniofacial fibrous dysplasia

Localization
Monostotic fibrous dysplasia affects a single bone (the term is not usually employed for the maxilla or facial bones), whereas polyostotic fibrous dysplasia affects multiple bones. The term "craniofacial fibrous dysplasia" applies when multiple adjacent bones in the craniofacial region are affected, extending across suture lines. The craniofacial bones are affected most commonly, typically involved in approximately 10% of patients with monostotic fibrous dysplasia and in as many as 100% of patients with polyostotic fibrous dysplasia. The maxilla and paranasal regions are more frequently affected than the mandible {1055}.

Clinical features
Patients generally present with painless swelling of bones, or the disease may be detected incidentally. Fibrous dysplasia of the jaws causes orofacial asymmetry. Tooth eruption is normal and teeth remain aligned but with arch distortion as the jaw expands. Tooth structure is normal. Maxillary fibrous dysplasia may cause nasal obstruction and chronic sinusitis. Skull base fibrous dysplasia may compress cranial nerves, resulting in visual impairment or hearing loss. The growth of fibrous dysplasia tends to slow or stop with skeletal maturation. Survey for extent and possible syndromic association may be necessary {2063}. In McCune–Albright syndrome, café-au-lait skin pigmentation and endocrine abnormalities are present {1199}.

Imaging
The radiological appearance varies with the stage of development and the age of the patient. Early lesions may appear radiolucent, gradually becoming more radiopaque over time, merging almost imperceptibly with unaffected bone at the periphery. Abnormal bone extends around tooth roots with minimal displacement. The lesions of fibrous dysplasia are characteristically described as having a ground-glass or, in the late stage, a fingerprint appearance {2755,3183,2063}.

Epidemiology
Fibrous dysplasia is an uncommon disease and is usually diagnosed in children and young adults. The monostotic form accounts for 80–85% of all cases and shows no sex predilection. Polyostotic fibrous dysplasia has a female predilection {2755}.

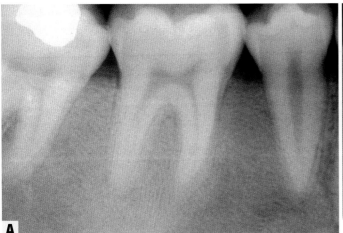
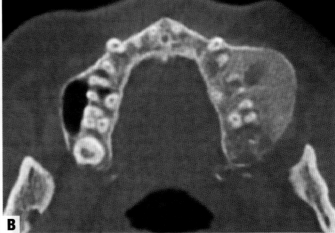

Fig. 7.77 Fibrous dysplasia. **A** Radiograph of an area affected by fibrous dysplasia. Note the ground-glass appearance, and the loss of lamina dura and cortex definition without tooth displacement. **B** CT, axial view, shows an even, mixed-radiolucency lesion of fibrous dysplasia, with marked expansion of the maxilla but no tooth displacement.

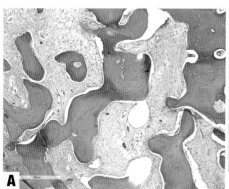 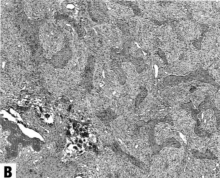 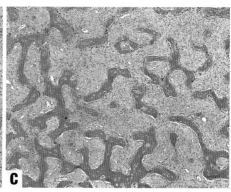

Fig. 7.78 Fibrous dysplasia. **A** Late-stage disease showing lamellar maturation but retaining irregularly shaped trabeculae and often lacking osteoblastic rimming. **B** Early-stage or active area of the disease with a hypercellular fibrous tissue and condensing woven bone trabeculae, with a focus of giant cells. **C** Maturing area of the lesion with a less cellular stroma and woven bone. Note the osteoblast rimming, which is common in maturing fibrous dysplasia of the jaws, unlike fibrous dysplasia of long bones.

Etiology

Genetic factors

Fibrous dysplasia occurs with endocrinopathies in McCune–Albright syndrome {4673,1055} and with myxomas in Mazabraud syndrome {1154}.

Pathogenesis

Fibrous dysplasia is caused by postzygotic activating missense mutations in *GNAS* (20q13.32), which encodes $G_s\alpha$ {2536}. The result is arrest of differentiation of proliferating cells of osteoblastic lineage to mature osteoblasts {5025}.

Macroscopic appearance

The sample type depends on the sampling method. Lesional bone resembles normal bone but may be compressible and is gritty on sectioning {3183}.

Histopathology

A lesion consists of bone with variable amounts of fibrous tissue. The fibrous component is composed of spindle cells without atypia; it can be quite cellular but becomes less so and more fibrous with age. Mitoses are uncommon, but small numbers may be observed in children. The bone is woven and forms irregular curvilinear trabeculae, commonly likened to Chinese characters or described as C-, S-, and Y-shaped trabeculae, which are not rimmed by osteoblasts. The immature bone merges almost imperceptibly with the surrounding lamellar bone, and it may be difficult to distinguish lesional from non-lesional bone. Jaw fibrous dysplasia develops osteoblast rimming and lamellar differentiation as it matures. Cartilage may form, but it is rare in the jaws {4136}. Subtypes are defined by number and location of affected bone(s).

Differential diagnosis

The histological appearances are characteristic but not completely specific, and the differential diagnosis includes other jaw fibro-osseous lesions including juvenile trabecular, psammomatoid, and cemento-ossifying fibromas; cemento-osseous dysplasias; and, in small specimens, aneurysmal bone cyst or giant cell lesions. Low-grade central osteosarcoma may resemble fibrous dysplasia closely but is rare in the jaws {1087}.

Cytology

Not clinically relevant

Diagnostic molecular pathology

Confirmation of fibrous dysplasia requires detection of somatic *GNAS* mutation by next-generation or Sanger sequencing {2063} or by mutation-specific restriction enzyme digestion PCR {2001}.

Essential and desirable diagnostic criteria

Essential: clinical, radiological, and histomorphological correlation; bone replaced by fibrous tissue and woven bone.
Desirable: GNAS mutation analysis (in selected cases).

Staging

Not relevant

Prognosis and prediction

Fibrous dysplasia follows a benign course, and growth reduces in adulthood. Treatment is focused on preventing loss of function from complications such as optic neuropathy or hearing loss, as well as on minimizing disfigurement, pathological fracture risk, and pain {628,2063}. Hypophosphataemia may be used to measure the activity and extent of skeletal lesions {2063}. Fibrous dysplasia carries a low risk of sarcomatous transformation, and the development of cystic haemorrhagic degeneration resembles aneurysmal bone cyst and giant cell lesions {4306}. Patients with fibrous dysplasia who take bisphosphonates have an elevated risk of medication-related osteonecrosis of the jaw {628,2063}.

Juvenile trabecular ossifying fibroma

Chi A
Collins LHC

Definition
Juvenile trabecular ossifying fibroma (JTOF) is a benign fibro-osseous neoplasm characterized by trabeculae of cellular osteoid and woven bone, rapid growth, and a predilection for the jaws of children and adolescents.

ICD-O coding
9262/0 Juvenile trabecular ossifying fibroma

ICD-11 coding
LD24.2Y & XH6M86 Other specified bone diseases with disorganized development of skeletal components & Ossifying fibroma

Related terminology
Acceptable: trabecular ossifying fibroma; trabecular juvenile ossifying fibroma.
Not recommended: juvenile (active or aggressive) ossifying fibroma.

Subtype(s)
None

Localization
JTOF predominantly affects the jaws, with almost equal distribution between the maxilla and mandible {1245,881}. There is variation in diagnosis, and it is not clear whether JTOF in extragnathic craniofacial bones {881} is the same entity.

Clinical features
Patients usually present with painless jaw expansion with rapid growth and tooth displacement {4135,881}. Maxillary lesions may cause nasal obstruction and epistaxis {1246}.

Imaging
Radiographic examination shows a well-defined radiolucency or mixed radiolucent/radiopaque lesion, often with focal cortication {881,4165}. The radiolucency is more often unilocular than multilocular {881}. Tooth displacement occurs in over half of all cases {881}. Less frequent findings include cortical perforation and tooth root resorption {881}.

Epidemiology
JTOF is rare {1747} and arises predominantly in children and adolescents (mean age: 11.3 years), with < 20% of cases affecting individuals aged > 15 years {881,1747}. However, variation in diagnosis may distort the age distribution, and most typical cases of JTOF probably arise before the age of 10 years. There is no sex predilection {881,1747}.

Etiology
Unknown

Pathogenesis
MDM2 and *RASAL1* amplification has been detected in 7 of 10 JTOFs {4325}.

Macroscopic appearance
JTOF appears as yellowish-white, gritty fragments of variable size or as an intact tumour mass; the cut surface may exhibit brown curvilinear strands {1246,4135}.

Histopathology
Histopathology shows an unencapsulated tumour with elongate strands (so-called "brush strokes"), trabeculae, and sheets of osteoid densely rimmed by osteoblasts and in a fibroblastic stroma {1246}. Newly formed osteoid blends imperceptibly with the surrounding stroma. Over time, the osteoid strands undergo

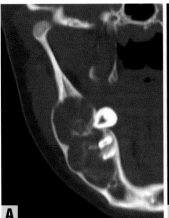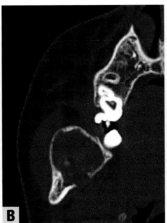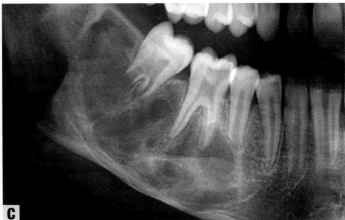

Fig. 7.79 A mandibular juvenile trabecular ossifying fibroma in a 12-year-old child. Coronal (**A**) and axial (**B**) reformatted CT images and panoramic radiograph (**C**), showing a well-defined scalloped margin, focally perforated cortex, and internal mineralization, with no root resorption but early root growth deflection of the second premolar.

Chapter 7

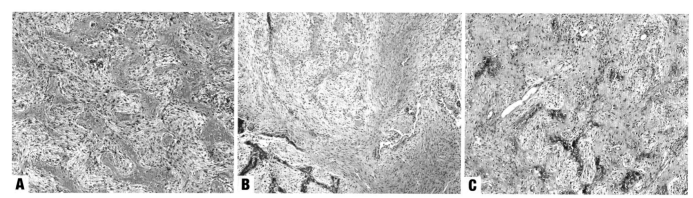

Fig. 7.80 Juvenile trabecular ossifying fibroma. **A** Anastomosing trabeculae of woven bone containing plump osteocytes and lying in a very cellular fibroblastic stroma. **B** A more fibrous area of cellular plump fibroblasts with thin trabeculae of woven bone. **C** In actively growing lesions, disorganized sheets of osteoid may raise concern for osteosarcoma.

central mineralization to form anastomosing trabeculae of woven bone. The stroma exhibits zones of variable cellularity, often hypercellular, and scattered aggregates of osteoclastic giant cells are usually evident.

Differential diagnosis

Appearance may be worrisome for osteosarcoma. Garland-like, curvilinear strands of oedema, haemorrhage, osteoclasts, and pseudocystic degeneration form the characteristic brown curvilinear strands seen macroscopically in JTOF; this feature has not been noted in cemento-ossifying or psammomatoid ossifying fibromas {4135}. Haemorrhagic cystic degeneration may resemble aneurysmal bone cyst {4066,4549,881}. A trabecular woven bone pattern may be seen in cemento-ossifying fibroma and other fibro-osseous lesions; this feature alone is insufficient for diagnosis.

Cytology

Not clinically relevant

Diagnostic molecular pathology

Not relevant

Essential and desirable diagnostic criteria

Essential: onset in childhood or adolescence; rapid expansion; well demarcated radiographically; a cellular benign fibro-osseous lesion with prominent osteoid.
Desirable: site in the jaws.

Staging

None

Prognosis and prediction

Approximately 21% of cases recur {881}, from 4% after resection to 53% after enucleation or curettage. Enucleation plus curettage or peripheral ostectomy may mitigate recurrence risk while avoiding surgical disfigurement {881}. JTOF may attain a large size {3135}, but malignant transformation has not been reported {1246,1756,4279}.

Psammomatoid ossifying fibroma

Chi A
Collins LHC

Definition
Psammomatoid ossifying fibroma (PsOF) is a benign fibro-osseous neoplasm of the craniofacial skeleton, characterized histologically by spherical ossicles set in a hypercellular bland stroma.

ICD-O coding
9262/0 Psammomatoid ossifying fibroma

ICD-11 coding
LD24.2Y & XH6M86 Other specified bone diseases with disorganized development of skeletal components & Ossifying fibroma

Related terminology
Acceptable: juvenile psammomatoid ossifying fibroma.
Not recommended: juvenile (active or aggressive) ossifying fibroma.

Subtype(s)
None

Localization
PsOF arises in the jaws and craniofacial bones, with 90% of cases occurring around the paranasal sinuses and orbit {4790, 2113,1245,881}.

Clinical features
PsOF is usually an asymptomatic, rapidly enlarging bony swelling, although pain is possible {881}. Additional findings may include nasal obstruction, epistaxis, proptosis, and visual disturbance, depending on site {1756,1747}.

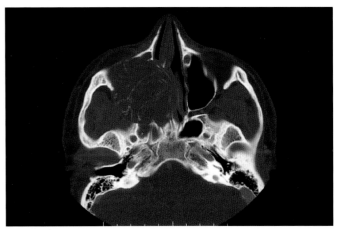

Fig. 7.81 Psammomatoid ossifying fibroma. Typical facial bone lesion showing early maturation with minimal internal mineralization, marked expansion, and cortical thinning.

Imaging
Radiographically, PsOF is a well-defined mass with variable opacification, with lesions being predominantly radiolucent in early-stage disease and later developing ground-glass opacification with central radiolucency, homogeneous ground-glass opacification, or discrete calcifications {3345,1756,1747}. The radiolucent component is more often unilocular than multilocular {881}. There may be tooth displacement, cortical thinning or perforation, and intracranial extension {2113,881}.

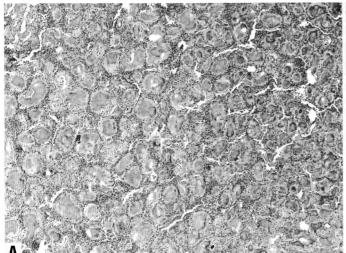

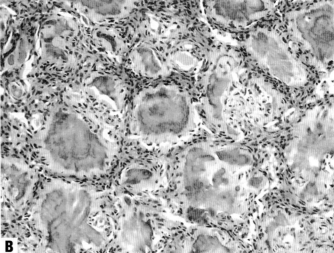

Fig. 7.82 Psammomatoid ossifying fibroma. **A** Numerous closely packed spherical ossicles or psammomatoid mineralizations in a cellular fibrous stroma. **B** Spherical ossicles with a wispy eosinophilic collagenous periphery.

Epidemiology

PsOF is rare {1747}. The peak incidence is in the second to fourth decades of life, with a broad age range {1245,1246,881} and an M:F ratio of approximately 1.4:1 {881}.

Etiology

Unknown

Pathogenesis

PsOFs carry *SATB2* gene rearrangements {907A}. Breakpoints at Xq26 and 2q33 with reciprocal translocation or insertion were reported in 3 apparent PsOFs (reported as "cemento-ossifying fibromas of the orbit") {3898}. *MDM2* and *RASAL1* amplification was present in 2 of 3 cases {4325}.

Macroscopic appearance

Large, intact bone pieces with a yellow, gritty cut surface {2113, 1246,4165}

Histopathology

PsOF is an unencapsulated lesion containing multiple spherical ossicles in a hypercellular stroma of bland ovoid and spindle cells. The spherules are usually small and relatively uniform, with osteoid rims and wispy eosinophilic collagen fibres at the periphery and no osteoblastic rimming {4165}. Ossicles fuse together in late disease, forming lumpy trabeculae. Although described as psammomatoid, the ossicles are much larger than psammoma bodies, not as sharply defined, and not lamellar. Mitotic figures may be seen occasionally, and multinucleated giant cells are an infrequent finding.

Differential diagnosis

The small, densely basophilic, cementum-like droplet calcifications in cemento-ossifying fibroma are more similar to psammoma bodies than the ossicles in PsOF {2113} and should not lead to the misdiagnosis of cemento-ossifying fibroma as PsOF. PsOF may contain minority areas of more typical fibro-osseous architecture with woven bone trabeculae and dense basophilic bone. Secondary changes include myxoid change and haemorrhagic cystic degeneration resembling aneurysmal bone cyst {1245,3877,881}.

Cytology

Cytology has not been shown to be specific.

Diagnostic molecular pathology

None

Essential and desirable diagnostic criteria

Essential: well demarcated radiographically; site in craniofacial bone or jaw; benign fibro-osseous lesion histologically; predominant ossicle pattern.
Desirable: onset in the second to fourth decades of life.

Staging

None

Prognosis and prediction

PsOF recurs in approximately 30% of cases after surgical excision {2113,881}, but no features predict recurrence. Malignant transformation has not been reported {1246,3626}.

Familial gigantiform cementoma

Chi A
Collins LHC

Definition
Familial gigantiform cementoma (FGC) is a rare benign fibro-osseous lesion of the jaws, characterized by an early onset and multifocal grossly expansile growth.

ICD-O coding
None

ICD-11 coding
2E83.0 & XH6W94 Benign osteogenic tumours of bone or articular cartilage of skull or face & Gigantiform cementoma
2E83.1 & XH6W94 Benign osteogenic tumours of bone or articular cartilage of lower jaw & Gigantiform cementoma

Related terminology
Acceptable: gigantiform cementoma.
Not recommended: florid osseous dysplasia, expansive osseous dysplasia.

Subtype(s)
None

Localization
The disease affects the jaws, with multifocal involvement in two to four quadrants {1246}.

Clinical features
There is rapidly progressive, painless expansion, resulting in significant deformity, orbital distortion, and possible airway compromise {1392,9,1246}. Many cases of florid cemento-osseous dysplasia have been diagnosed as FGC, particularly cases of the familial form {3178}, but the degree of expansion is usually less marked and patients are generally older {3658}. Presentations of gnathodiaphysial dysplasia and large cemento-ossifying fibromas are also often mistaken for FGC.

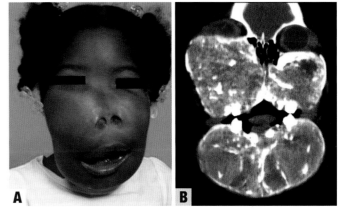

Fig. 7.83 Familial gigantiform cementoma. **A** A tumour in a 3-year-old girl. A massive expansion of the jaws, causing marked facial deformity. **B** CT showing markedly expansile masses with well-circumscribed borders and mixed density in the mandible and maxilla bilaterally.

Imaging
Radiographic examination shows well-defined, markedly expansile radiolucencies with associated calcifications; lesions often cross the midline {9,3997,1246}. Features of cemento-osseous dysplasia should be absent.

Epidemiology
FGC is extremely rare {2748}. Onset is in early childhood, with continuous growth into early adulthood {1246}. Cases have been described in various countries, with 55% from Asia.

Etiology
The etiology is unknown. Autosomal dominant inheritance with a high level of penetrance and variable expressivity {1246} has been proposed; other cases are sporadic {9,4699}.

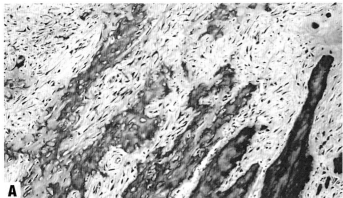
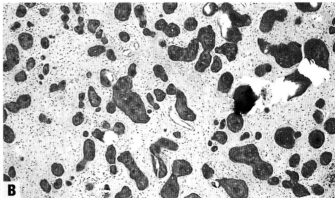

Fig. 7.84 Familial gigantiform cementoma. **A** Mineralized osteoid and immature bone within a background of cellular fibrous connective tissue. **B** Cementum-like calcifications appearing as spheroidal to curvilinear deposits of hypocellular, basophilic material.

Pathogenesis
Unknown

Macroscopic appearance
Lobular mineralized masses {3231}.

Histopathology
The histopathological features are similar to those of cemento-ossifying fibroma and other fibro-osseous lesions. Immature bony trabeculae and cementum-like calcifications are seen within a hypercellular fibroblastic stroma. The cementum-like calcifications appear as hypocellular, spheroidal to curvilinear structures, which may be surrounded by radiating Sharpey fibres as visualized under polarized light {1246}.

Cytology
Not clinically relevant

Diagnostic molecular pathology
None

Essential and desirable diagnostic criteria
Essential: onset in childhood or adolescence; multifocal/multiquadrant involvement; very marked expansion; benign fibro-osseous histology analogous to cemento-ossifying fibroma.

Desirable: rapid progression followed by slower growth later in life; family history.

Staging
None

Prognosis and prediction
Surgical management is complicated by extensive disease and rapid regrowth; complete resection is often not practical {2748}. Surgical recontouring or partial excision typically results in regrowth, which may occur at an accelerated rate. Although the condition is characterized by a rapidly progressive growth phase, spontaneous stabilization may occur later in life {4699}.

Osteoma

Toner ME
Gupta R

Definition
Osteoma is a benign bone-forming neoplasm consisting of mature bone, restricted almost exclusively to the jaws and craniofacial bones.

ICD-O coding
9180/0 Osteoma
9180/0 Surface (periosteal) osteoma
9180/0 Central (endosteal) osteoma

ICD-11 coding
2E83.Z & XH4818 Benign osteogenic tumours of unspecified site & Osteoma, NOS

Related terminology
Not recommended: exostosis.

Subtype(s)
Surface (periosteal) osteoma; central (endosteal) osteoma

Localization
In the jaws, the mandible is more often affected than the maxilla {2474}. Sinuses are a site of predilection, most commonly the frontal sinus followed by the other sinuses {509,2894,2474}.

Clinical features
Central osteomas are often asymptomatic, whereas surface osteomas may present with a slow-growing swelling, facial distortion, or altered dental occlusion. Osteomas in familial adenomatous polyposis often arise near the mandibular angle and may be multiple. Sinus/orbital tumours may present with headache or pain {509,1086}.

Imaging
Osteomas are dense radiopacities with well-defined margins.

Epidemiology
Osteomas occur over a wide age range but mostly in the third to fifth decades of life, with an equal sex distribution {2894,1086}.

Etiology
Unknown

Genetic factors
Osteomas may be a manifestation of familial adenomatous polyposis, an autosomal dominant disorder associated with a germline mutation in *APC* {1134,376A}, and they may be the first manifestation.

Pathogenesis
Osteomas predominantly affect bone formed by membranous ossification {2474}, and they have a simple karyotype {1452}.

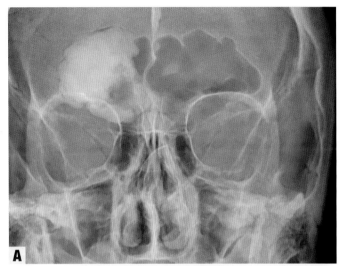

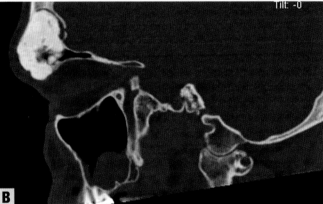

Fig. 7.85 Osteoma of the right frontal sinus. Frontal radiograph (**A**) and sagittal reformatted CT (**B**) demonstrating a heavily ossified mass in the sinus, arising from the bone surface.

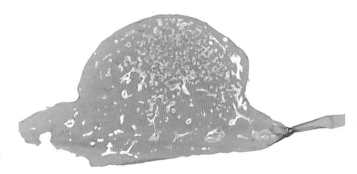

Fig. 7.86 Osteoma, surface type. Osteoma of the maxillary sinus, with a dense, smooth swelling of compact mature bone with focal more cellular osteoblast-like areas centrally.

Macroscopic appearance

Osteoma appears as a bony mass. Surface osteomas may be widely pedunculated to underlying bone. Central osteomas merge with surrounding intramedullary bone.

Histopathology

Osteomas are composed mostly of lamellar bone, compact or trabecular, in which osteoblasts and osteoclasts are usually inconspicuous. Some contain osteoblastoma-like areas that are thought to represent a reactive remodelling process and do not imply more aggressive behaviour {2905}. As many as 40% of sinus/orbital osteomas contain such areas {2894}. Fibro-osseous lesions, sclerosing osteomyelitis, and ossification in a fibrous epulis may mimic an osteoma {1086}.

Lesions of the central (endosteal) subtype of osteoma are also known as bone islands. Unlike surface osteomas, bone islands arise more frequently in long bones and are a mixture of hamartomas and true neoplasms. Rare extraosseous osteoma occurs in soft tissue {1086}.

Cytology

Not clinically relevant

Diagnostic molecular pathology

Not clinically relevant

Essential and desirable diagnostic criteria

Essential: compatible radiological features; surface origin (surface type); mature lamellar bone with solid cortical or medullary patterns.

Staging

None

Prognosis and prediction

Growth is slow. Resection is performed for symptomatic osteomas; recurrence is unusual {2474,509}.

Osteochondroma

Toner ME
Gupta R

Definition
Osteochondroma is a benign neoplasm forming a bony projection with a cartilaginous cap, with continuity between the marrow cavity of the tumour and underlying bone.

ICD-O coding
9210/0 Osteochondroma

ICD-11 coding
2E83.Y & XH5Y87 Benign osteogenic tumour of other specified site & Osteochondroma

Related terminology
Not recommended: osteochondromatous exostosis.

Subtype(s)
None

Localization
Osteochondromas are rare in the craniofacial bones, usually involving the mandibular condyle and coronoid process {2940}.

Clinical features
Craniofacial osteochondromas often cause swelling, asymmetry, trismus, and temporomandibular joint dysfunction {3777, 2940}, but they may be chance radiographic findings. Osteochondromas may be multiple, but multiple lesions usually affect long bones.

Imaging
Radiographic imaging shows an uneven enlargement or protrusion from the condyle {2940,2080}, unlike the diffuse condylar enlargement of condylar hyperplasia.

Epidemiology
Osteochondroma of the jaw manifests in the second to fourth decades of life, slightly later than at other sites, and unlike at other sites it often continues to grow slowly after puberty {4629}. A slight female predominance is seen {3777}.

Etiology
Trauma and (rarely) prior radiotherapy may be etiological factors {3777}.

Pathogenesis
Homozygous deletions of *EXT1* are associated with sporadic osteochondromas, suggesting a neoplastic rather than developmental condition {4392}. Heterozygous germline mutations of *EXT1* and *EXT2* are associated with hereditary multiple osteochondroma, but the facial bones are not usually affected {546, 4392}.

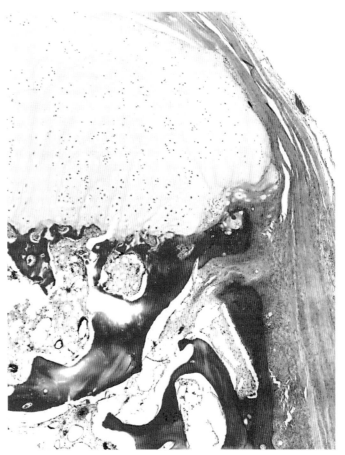

Fig. 7.87 Osteochondroma. Cartilaginous cap covered by periosteum at the surface, merging with underlying trabecular bone.

Macroscopic appearance
Osteochondroma is a bony mass, sessile or pedunculated, with a cartilage cap.

Histopathology
Osteochondroma is a cartilage-capped bony projection from the external bone surface, showing cortical and medullary continuity with the parent bone. There is a surface layer of fibrous tissue and a middle layer that mimics growth plate cartilage with endochondral ossification, merging with underlying mature trabecular bone {2080,4961}. Binucleated cells, nodularity, and cystic/mucoid changes may be present, but neither mitoses nor marked pleomorphism are seen {1041}.

Differential diagnosis
Although a cartilaginous cap > 20 mm in thickness in adults must raise the suspicion of secondary chondrosarcoma,

occurrence in the facial bones is very rare {4392}. Criteria for the histological distinction of osteochondroma from condylar hyperplasia are poorly defined {2080,4961}.

Cytology

Not clinically relevant

Diagnostic molecular pathology

Not clinically relevant

Essential and desirable diagnostic criteria

Essential: pedunculated or broad-based bony exostosis; a cartilaginous cap with a growth plate–like architecture; continuity with underlying bone cortex and marrow.

Staging

Not applicable

Prognosis and prediction

Recurrence after excision is rare, unless the lesion is incompletely removed {2940,4392}.

Osteoblastoma

Toner ME

Definition

Osteoblastoma is a benign but locally aggressive bone-forming tumour ≥ 20 mm in diameter, morphologically similar to osteoid osteoma, with sheets of large osteoblasts and woven bone with prominent osteoblastic rimming.

ICD-O coding

9200/1 Osteoblastoma, NOS

ICD-11 coding

2E83.Z & XH4316 Benign osteogenic tumour of unspecified site & Osteoblastoma, NOS

Related terminology

None

Subtype(s)

None

Localization

About 10% of osteoblastomas are found in the craniofacial bones, most often in the body of the mandible. They may be intraosseous or periosteal {3662}.

Clinical features

Osteoblastoma may be asymptomatic or present with localized swelling and pain {2118}.

Imaging

Radiographs show a circumscribed round to oval lesion ≥ 20 mm in diameter, varying from radiolucent to radiopaque, and usually without a sclerotic border or periosteal reaction {2118}. The clinical and radiological appearance is sometimes more aggressive and may mimic malignancy {1777}.

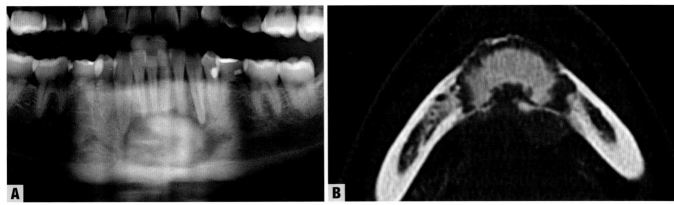

Fig. 7.88 Osteoblastoma. **A** Radiographic appearance of an osteoblastoma in a panoramic radiograph. **B** CT showing a well-defined but irregular outline and radiolucent rim with dense patchy mineralization centrally.

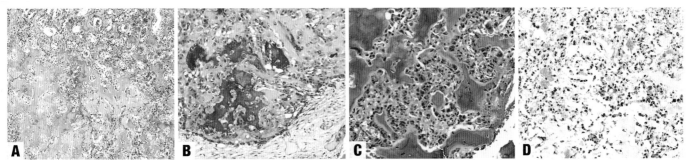

Fig. 7.89 Osteoblastoma. **A** Irregular interconnected trabeculae of osteoid, partially mineralized and with resting and reversal lines. There is a prominent, sometimes multilayered osteoblast rim with scattered osteoclasts. **B** Circumscribed edge and characteristic blue-bone appearance. The spaces in osteoid are filled by multilayered large eosinophilic osteoblasts. **C** Prominent osteoblastic rimming with a layer of large osteoblasts several cells thick on the bone surface. **D** Immunohistochemistry showing strong nuclear positivity for the transcription factor FOS.

Epidemiology

Osteoblastoma is a rare tumour that occurs mostly in the second to third decades of life, with a slight female predominance (unlike long bone lesions) {2118}.

Etiology

Unknown

Pathogenesis

Recurrent rearrangements of *FOS* or (less frequently) *FOSB* define osteoblastoma and osteoid osteoma {1400} and are also found in cementoblastoma, suggesting a pathogenetic relationship {2458}.

Macroscopic appearance

Curettings show red to tan tissue, reflecting vascularity. If resected, bone expansion with well-defined borders is typical {2733}.

Histopathology

Osteoblastoma is composed of anastomosing trabeculae of bone and osteoid, rimmed by plump osteoblasts, sometimes with densely mineralized foci, and set in a loose, richly vascular fibrous stroma. Mitoses are rare {3662}. A lack of nuclear atypia, permeative growth into surrounding bone, and atypical mitoses distinguish osteoblastoma from osteosarcoma {2733}. In some cases, the osteoblasts may appear larger and epithelioid, but this does not indicate a clinically aggressive course. A tumour size of > 40 mm and an anatomical site that makes removal difficult are better predictors of aggressive clinical behaviour {1777,4229}.

Differential diagnosis

The differential diagnosis includes osteoid osteoma for a lesion < 20 mm in diameter and cementoblastoma if on a tooth root.

Cytology

Not clinically relevant

Diagnostic molecular pathology

The translocations of *FOS* and *FOSB* identified in osteoblastoma are extremely rare in osteosarcoma, and FOS immunohistochemistry may be a helpful diagnostic tool in this setting, but only if there has been short decalcification {2459}.

Essential and desirable diagnostic criteria

Essential: a radiologically well-demarcated tumour; ≥ 20 mm diameter; bone tumour with trabeculae of woven bone; prominent plump osteoblasts; vascular stroma.

Staging

None

Prognosis and prediction

Recurrence may follow curettage or incomplete removal {4229}.

Chondroblastoma

van Heerden WFP
Baumhoer D

Definition
Chondroblastoma is a benign tumour of bone composed of chondroblasts forming sheets and islands of eosinophilic chondroid matrix.

ICD-O coding
9230/0 Chondroblastoma, NOS

ICD-11 coding
2E82.Z & XH4NK2 Benign osteogenic tumour of unspecified site & Chondroblastoma, NOS

Related terminology
None

Subtype(s)
None

Localization
Chondroblastomas predominantly involve the epiphysis of long bones. When occurring in the head and neck, chondroblastomas are located mainly around the temporomandibular joint and the squamous part of the temporal bone {446,1795}.

Clinical features
The most frequent clinical symptom is pain. Hearing loss, tinnitus, and vertigo may be present when tumours are located in the temporal bone, and trismus may be present if tumours are around the temporomandibular joint {446,2022}.

Imaging
Chondroblastomas of the temporal bone have a well-demarcated, lobulated, radiolucent appearance with foci of

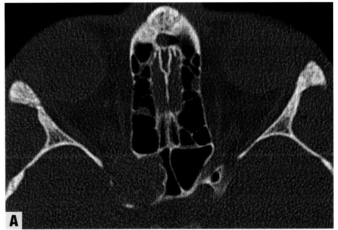
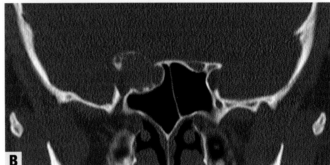

Fig. 7.90 Chondroblastoma. Expansile and well-delineated tumour in the wall of the right sphenoidal sinus. CT, axial (**A**) and lower coronal reconstruction (**B**).

calcifications {446}. Cystic haemorrhagic degeneration may produce aneurysmal bone cyst–like changes with fluid levels on MRI {3623,4742}.

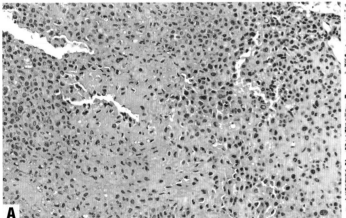
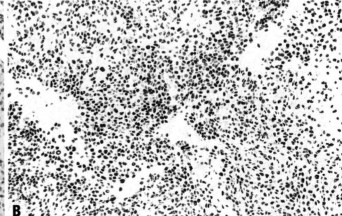

Fig. 7.91 Chondroblastoma. **A** Oval to polygonal chondroblasts associated with an eosinophilic cartilaginous matrix. **B** H3.3B diffuse nuclear expression in the chondroblastic cells (H3.3B immunostain).

Epidemiology

Chondroblastomas of the head and neck region are rare, with about 100 cases reported in the literature {3302}. Although most chondroblastomas occur in the second decade of life, patients with skull tumours are slightly older, presenting in their third or fourth decade of life {2022}. A slight male predominance (M:F ratio: 1.3:1) has been reported for temporal chondroblastomas {3302}.

Etiology

Unknown

Pathogenesis

H3-3A and *H3-3B* mutations drive chondroblastoma, with the *H3-3B*:c.110A>T p.K37M (K36M) mutation being most common {398,2728,2571}.

Macroscopic appearance

Chondroblastomas are well-defined lesions with a thin sclerotic rim and a soft to gritty consistency. Haemorrhagic areas may be present.

Histopathology

The tumour cells are uniform, eosinophilic, and polygonal, with well-defined borders and nuclear grooves. The cells are intermingled with an amorphous eosinophilic matrix with osteoclast-like giant cells and varying amounts of chicken-wire calcification {1004,4564}. Cystic haemorrhagic degeneration is frequent. Tumours harbouring mutations in *H3-3A* or *H3-3B* resulting in the expression of H3 p.K37M (K36M) mutant protein, show consistent nuclear immunoreactivity with a mutant-specific antibody K36M {158,2571}.

Differential diagnosis

The differential diagnosis includes aneurysmal bone cyst, clear cell chondrosarcoma, chondromyxoid fibroma, and Langerhans cell histiocytosis.

Cytology

Not clinically relevant

Diagnostic molecular pathology

Detection of the *H3-3B*:c.110A>T p.K37M (K36M) mutation is highly specific for chondroblastoma {906,2571} and may be useful in selected cases.

Essential and desirable diagnostic criteria

Essential: sheets of chondroblasts; scattered osteoclasts; eosinophilic chondroid matrix.

Desirable: a fine network of chicken-wire calcification; histone H3 mutation or H3 p.K37M (K36M) immunopositivity (in selected cases).

Staging

None

Prognosis and prediction

As many as 50% of cases recur. Metastasis has been reported only rarely (< 1% of cases) {434}.

Chondromyxoid fibroma

Purgina B
Baumhoer D

Definition
Chondromyxoid fibroma (CMF) is a benign lobulated cartilaginous neoplasm with a zonal architecture composed of chondroid, myxoid, and myofibroblastic areas.

ICD-O coding
9241/0 Chondromyxoid fibroma

ICD-11 coding
2E82.Z & XH89S0 Benign osteogenic tumour of unspecified site & Chondromyxoid fibroma

Related terminology
None

Subtype(s)
None

Localization
Most craniofacial CMFs occur in the jaw and sinonasal bones, but any craniofacial bone can be affected {1751,4864,2752,294, 1385,2897,4895,2949}.

Clinical features
Depending on the site, there may be tinnitus, visual disturbances, headaches, hearing loss, and sinonasal congestion {4864,4895,1230,1255}.

Imaging
Radiographically, craniofacial CMFs are similar in appearance to CMFs in other locations. They are primarily lytic, often with a sclerotic rim, and they frequently demonstrate cortical thinning or erosion {4864,2022}. Matrix mineralization occurs in approximately 10% of cases and is usually focal {4864}. A subset of craniofacial CMFs develop on the surface of bone {2949}.

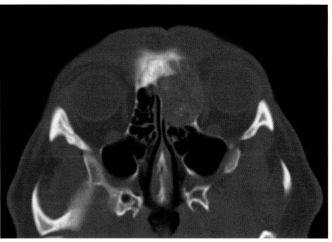

Fig. 7.92 Chondromyxoid fibroma. Head CT, axial view, showing an expansile, osteolytic tumour with matrix mineralization, a sclerotic margin, and cortical thinning, involving the ethmoid bone and left frontal sinus.

Epidemiology
CMF is rare, and 5% of all cases involve craniofacial bones {4864,2022}.

Etiology
Unknown

Pathogenesis
The majority of CMFs harbour a recombination of the glutamate receptor gene *GRM1* with one of several 5′ partner genes, which represent strong promoters, leading to high GRM1 expression. This is considered the driver event for approximately 90% of CMFs {3238}. GRM1 expression is absent or very low in other cartilaginous tumours {3238}.

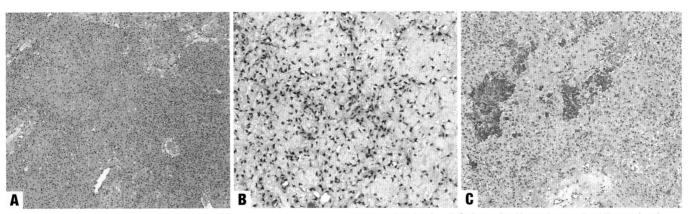

Fig. 7.93 Chondromyxoid fibroma. **A** Lobular tumour with cellular condensation at the periphery of the lobules. **B** Stellate cells with prominent eosinophilic cytoplasmic processes embedded in a myxoid matrix. **C** Foci of coarse calcification.

Chapter 7

Macroscopic appearance

CMF is a lobular, grey-white tumour with a smooth surface.

Histopathology

CMF consists of a lobular proliferation of spindled and stellate cells with abundant eosinophilic cytoplasm and a chondromyxoid background {4864}. The lobules show a hypocellular centre and a hypercellular periphery with intermingled osteoclast-like giant cells. In a third of cases there are scattered coarse calcifications, but hyaline cartilage is only occasionally seen {4864}. Cytological atypia may occur; however, mitoses are uncommon {4864}. In approximately 10% of cases, cystic haemorrhagic degeneration produces aneurysmal bone cyst–like changes {4864}.

Immunohistochemistry

Immunohistochemistry is typically not required. CMF shows variable staining for SMA, S100, EMA, and SOX9 and is negative for cytokeratins and GFAP {502,2369,2949}.

Cytology

Not clinically relevant

Diagnostic molecular pathology

Molecular pathology is not usually needed for diagnosis. If required, upregulation of GRM1 expression can help distinguish CMF from its mimics {3238}.

Essential and desirable diagnostic criteria

Essential: radiographic lytic lesion with sharp margins, a lobulated lesion; zonal distribution of spindled and stellate cells; chondromyxoid matrix; condensation of lesional cells at the periphery of lobules, admixed with multinucleated giant cells.

Staging

None

Prognosis and prediction

The prognosis is excellent, even for recurrent tumours. Recurrence is more common in craniofacial CMFs because it is challenging to obtain clear surgical margins {2022,439,4895,2949}.

Desmoplastic fibroma of bone

Hicks MJ
Baumhoer D
Günhan Ö

Definition
Desmoplastic fibroma of bone (DFB) is a locally aggressive fibroblastic/myofibroblastic tumour composed of benign spindle cells embedded in a collagenous background, mimicking desmoid-type fibromatosis.

ICD-O coding
8823/1 Desmoplastic fibroma

ICD-11 coding
2F7B & XH6YK5 Neoplasms of uncertain behaviour of bone and articular cartilage & Desmoplastic fibroma

Related terminology
Not recommended: desmoid tumour of bone; fibromatosis of jaw.

Subtype(s)
None

Localization
The jaws are a site of predilection. In the jaws, 82% of DFBs affect the mandible, 70% affecting the posterior body and angle {3809,4851,2277,2192,2142}. The remainder involve the maxilla, usually anteriorly.

Clinical features
Most individuals (66%) present with asymptomatic swelling or facial asymmetry. Other signs and symptoms include pain (15%), trismus with limited mouth opening (11%), mobile teeth (7%), infection (3%), and bleeding (3%) {3809,4851,2277,2192, 2142}.

Imaging
Radiography shows a well-defined radiolucency without mineralization, either unilocular or multilocular, with pushing borders, expansion, cortical erosion, tooth displacement, and root resorption, often with soft tissue extension {3809,4851,2277, 2192,2142}.

Epidemiology
DFB presents over a wide age range (0.5–70 years) {3809, 4851,2277,2192,2142}, with 35% occurring in the first decade of life and almost 70% occurring before the age of 30 years (mean age at diagnosis: 20 years). DFB in the jaws has a slight female predilection (M:F ratio: 1:1.3) and is more prevalent in non-Hispanic White people (51%) than in people of African (24%), Hispanic (16%), or Asian (9%) descent.

Etiology
Unknown

Genetic factors
DFB occurs in tuberous sclerosis, more commonly involving the maxilla (60%) {4603,1318}.

Pathogenesis
Unknown

Macroscopic appearance
DFB is a firm white tumour with a coarse, whorled architecture; focal myxoid areas; and no necrosis. Soft tissue extension may be present.

Chapter 7

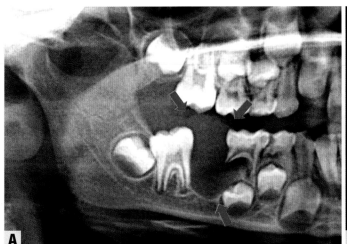 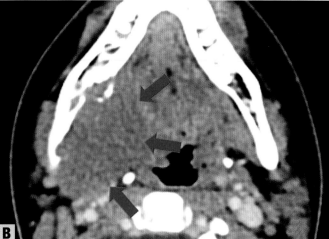

Fig. 7.94 Desmoplastic fibroma of bone. **A** Panoramic radiograph shows a desmoplastic fibroma of bone (arrows) with marked bone erosion, extension into the oral cavity, loss of the first permanent molar, resorption of the second primary molar root, and a pushing margin. **B** CT shows loss of the lingual cortical bone with soft tissue extension (arrows).

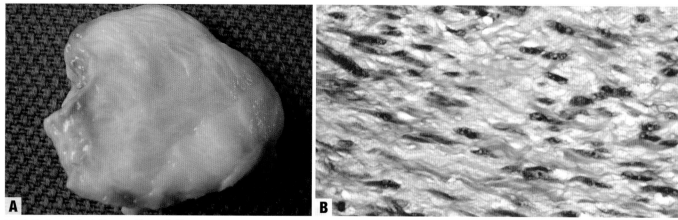

Fig. 7.95 Desmoplastic fibroma of bone. **A** Macroscopic appearance of the cut surface, showing the white, whorled banding. **B** Moderately cellular proliferation of bland spindle cells lacking atypia and pleomorphism, with interspersed collagen fibres.

Histopathology

DFB is composed of uniform benign spindle cells with slender, tapering nuclei, arranged in intertwining fascicles, without atypia or pleomorphism and with only rare mitoses. The cells often have indistinct cytoplasmic borders that blend with adjacent collagen, which can become keloid-like. Myxoid areas, cysts, and osteoclasts are present rarely. Thin-walled vessels interposed between spindle cell fascicles may be present. Because of the infiltrative margin, entrapped residual bone trabeculae may be present.

Immunohistochemistry

DFBs express vimentin (92%), SMA (80%), MSA (63%), and S100 (7%), and they have low Ki-67 expression {3809,4851,2277,2192, 2142}. Almost all DFBs lack nuclear β-catenin expression; only 2 cases with *CTNNB1* mutation have been reported.

Differential diagnosis

Differential diagnosis is by exclusion of desmoid fibromatosis (nuclear β-catenin; *CTNNB1* or *APC* mutation), fibrous dysplasia (*GNAS* mutation), low-grade central osteosarcoma (MDM2, CDK4), low-grade myofibroblastic sarcoma (SMA, desmin, nuclear β-catenin), synovial sarcoma (*SS18* rearrangement),

spindle cell rhabdomyosarcoma of the jaw (*TFCP2* rearrangement), and myoepithelial tumours (S100, CAM5.2; *EWSR1* rearrangement, SMARCB1 [INI1] loss).

Cytology

Not clinically relevant

Diagnostic molecular pathology

None

Essential and desirable diagnostic criteria

Essential: intraosseous site; benign spindle cell lesion; no cytological atypia or pleomorphism; dense collagenous background; exclusion of alternative fibrous tumours.

Staging

None

Prognosis and prediction

DFB frequently recurs after curettage (31%) or enucleation (25%) {3809,4851,2277,2192,2142}. The recurrence rate after resection is approximately 10%.

Osteosarcoma of the jaw

Lopes MA
Baumhoer D
Jay A

Definition

Osteosarcoma constitutes a group of malignant bone neoplasms in which the cells produce immature bone.

ICD-O coding

9180/3 Osteosarcoma, NOS
9186/3 Conventional osteosarcoma
9185/3 Small cell osteosarcoma
9183/3 Telangiectatic osteosarcoma
9187/3 Low-grade central osteosarcoma
9192/3 Parosteal osteosarcoma
9193/3 Periosteal osteosarcoma
9194/3 High-grade surface osteosarcoma
9184/3 Radiation-induced osteosarcoma

ICD-11 coding

2B51.0 Osteosarcoma of bone or articular cartilage of jaw

Related terminology

None

Subtype(s)

Conventional osteosarcoma; small cell osteosarcoma; telangiectatic osteosarcoma; low-grade central osteosarcoma; parosteal osteosarcoma; periosteal osteosarcoma; high-grade surface osteosarcoma; radiation-induced osteosarcoma

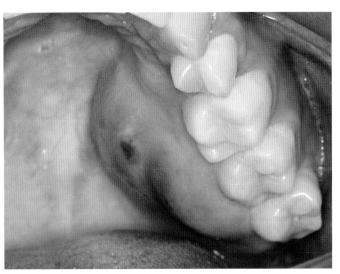

Fig. 7.96 Osteosarcoma. A painful swelling on the hard palate around the posterior teeth in a 33-year-old woman, a typical expansion without clinical features of malignancy.

Localization

Conventional osteosarcoma most commonly arises in the metaphysis of long bones, but the fourth most common site of origin is the jawbones (particularly the mandible), accounting for about 6% of cases. However, any craniofacial bone can be involved {4587,377}.

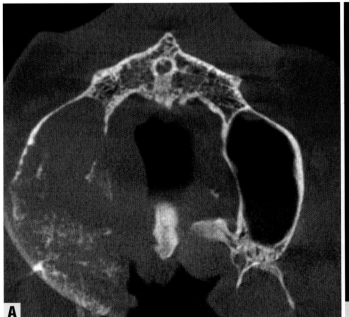

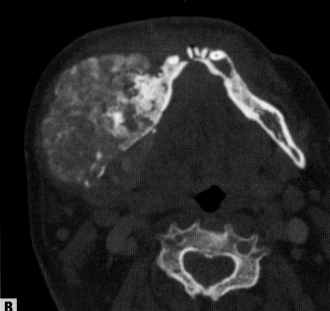

Fig. 7.97 Osteosarcoma of the jaw. **A** Cone-beam CT, axial view, displaying a destructive osteosarcoma of the left maxilla with moderate internal mineralization. **B** Conventional type. CT, axial view, showing a large and densely mineralized tumour expanding and destroying the right mandible.

Chapter 7

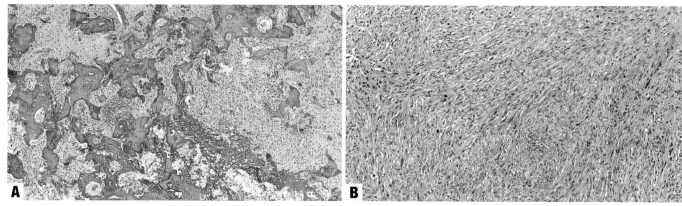

Fig. 7.98 Osteosarcoma of the jaw. **A** Conventional type. Moderately atypical spindle cells displaying an irregular and partly lace-like osteoid formation. **B** Conventional fibroblastic osteosarcoma. Highly pleomorphic spindle cells resembling fibrosarcoma.

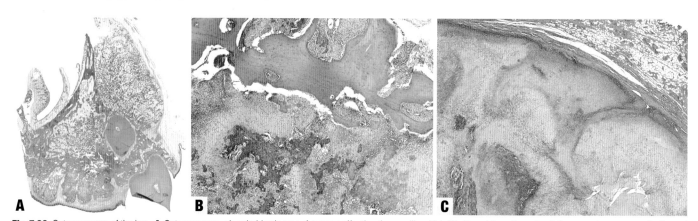

Fig. 7.99 Osteosarcoma of the jaw. **A** Osteosarcoma, chondroblastic type. A tumour affecting the maxilla with infiltration of the adjacent soft tissue and mucosa, on the buccal aspect showing the parallel trabeculae of bone that produce the sunray appearance radiologically. **B** Conventional chondroblastic osteosarcoma. Dense tumour proliferation with lace-like osteoid formation and permeative growth. **C** Conventional chondroblastic osteosarcoma. A well-delineated tumour showing a cambium-like proliferative and hypercellular layer at the periphery, directly adjacent to soft tissue.

Clinical features

The most frequent clinical manifestation is local swelling, which can be associated with pain and ulceration. Other signs include loosening of the adjacent teeth and pathological fracture {3974, 4469}.

Imaging

Presentation depends on the amount of mineralized matrix formed by the tumour. Most osteosarcomas present as mixed radiolucent and sclerotic tumours; high-grade lesions show osteodestructive growth, aggressive periosteal reactions (Codman triangle, sunburst appearance), and soft tissue extension. Widening of the periodontal ligament space of the involved teeth due to tumour infiltration may be observed. CT is particularly useful for assisting biopsy and staging. MRI is important for assessing the intraosseous tumour extension and soft tissue involvement {2737}.

Epidemiology

Osteosarcoma is rare, with an overall incidence of approximately 4–5 cases per 1 million person-years. The jawbones account for approximately 6% of cases and, remarkably, patients are usually 10–20 years older than those developing osteosarcoma in extragnathic sites. There is no sex predilection {377,2533, 4608}.

Etiology

Unknown

Risk factors

Risk factors include local radiotherapy {4005,910,1062}, a history of retinoblastoma, and (very rarely in the jaws) Paget disease of bone {811}.

Genetic factors

Osteosarcoma is associated with Li–Fraumeni syndrome, Werner syndrome, Bloom syndrome, Rothmund–Thomson syndrome, and retinoblastoma syndrome, but the jaws seem extremely rarely involved {1732}.

Pathogenesis

The pathogenesis and cell of origin of osteosarcoma are unknown. Few recurrent mutations have been described; *TP53* and *RB1* are the most commonly mutated genes. The hallmark of osteosarcoma is chromosomal instability resulting in highly complex chromosomal aneuploidy and both intertumoural and intratumoural heterogeneity. It is most likely caused by chromoanagenesis (chromothripsis/chromoplexy) that follows an unknown trigger, probably involving chromosome segregation errors during cell division. Some genes such as *MDM2*, *CDK4*, RAS genes, and *TUG1*, in addition to RNAs such as *ZEB2-AS1*,

CircECE1, and *Circ0085539*, have been implicated. Germline mutations in different RECQs underlie Werner, Bloom, and Rothmund–Thomson syndromes, conferring an increased risk of developing osteosarcoma {2931,3833,1946,4723}.

Macroscopic appearance
Depending on the type, amount, and mineralization of the lesional matrix, osteosarcoma can present with a tan-white and solid cut surface or with a softer, more grey, glistening cut surface. Areas of haemorrhage, necrosis, and cystic change are frequently observed.

Histopathology
Conventional osteosarcoma is the most common and aggressive subtype, whereas periosteal osteosarcoma is of intermediate grade, and low-grade central and parosteal osteosarcomas are low-grade subtypes.

Conventional osteosarcoma is defined by highly atypical cells producing an immature and often lace-like neoplastic osteoid. The extent of matrix can vary significantly, ranging from focal, immature osteoid to heavily mineralized sclerotic bone. The tumours generally show an aggressive and osteodestructive growth permeating marrow spaces. As a result, pre-existing trabeculae become entrapped by tumour infiltrates and neoplastic bone. The periosteum forms a rigid barrier for tumour permeation and may remain as a pseudocapsule around some tumours that have destroyed the cortex. Frequently, fibroblastic components and/or neoplastic cartilage can also be found, and the predominant matrix defines the tumour type as osteoblastic, chondroblastic, or fibroblastic. Chondroblastic osteosarcoma is proportionally more common in the jawbones and can histologically mimic chondrosarcoma, which is far less frequent in the maxillofacial bones {901,3974}. Gnathic osteosarcoma less commonly shows a pleomorphic high-grade morphology, although cytological atypia is nevertheless present but often subtle. Jaw tumours are often well delineated and show a cambium-like proliferative cell layer at the periphery of the lesion. Small cell and telangiectatic subtypes have been reported but are extremely rare.

Periosteal subtypes generally demonstrate a predominant chondroblastic differentiation, with intermediate-grade atypia, but are exceedingly rare in the head and neck region.

Low-grade central and parosteal subtypes generally demonstrate only subtle atypia; mitotic activity can be scarce. They consist of either irregular or interlacing bone trabeculae embedded in a fibroblastic stroma. The stromal component can predominate and is of low to moderate cellularity.

Giant cell–rich osteosarcoma is a morphological subtype that should be kept in mind and distinguished from other giant cell–rich lesions affecting the jaws.

Chemotherapy-related changes can mask original tumour morphology and extent and include frankly necrotic tumour; partly degenerate cells; a framework of tumour osteoid and chondroid matrix with empty lacunae; interlacing trabeculae of reactive bone and loose, sparsely cellular, collagenous tissue with scattered capillaries; and chronic inflammatory cells.

Immunohistochemistry
Positive staining with antibodies against MDM2 and CDK4 might aid in distinguishing low-grade osteosarcoma from benign fibro-osseous mimics {4948,1197}. SATB2 immunohistochemistry may be useful to detect osteoblastic differentiation, but despite its sensitivity it is not specific {1038,2762}.

Cytology
Although there are some studies showing the utility of FNAC in osteosarcomas, core or open biopsy is the gold-standard method for diagnosis {1759}.

Diagnostic molecular pathology
Most low-grade osteosarcomas show *MDM2* and *CDK4* amplification by FISH {3833}.

Essential and desirable diagnostic criteria
Essential: consistent imaging features; tumour cells producing immature and often lace-like neoplastic osteoid; permeative invasion; entrapment of host bone.
Desirable: necrosis; atypical mitosis; pleomorphism; high cellularity.

Staging
Staging follows the eighth edition of the Union for International Cancer Control (UICC) / American Joint Committee on Cancer (AJCC) TNM staging system for craniofacial osteosarcoma. Other systems based on anatomical location (intracompartmental versus extracompartmental; the Musculoskeletal Tumor Society [MSTS] system; and the less-known Spanier system, based on periosteal breach) are not commonly used in jaws, although periosteal breach is prognostically significant {711}.

Prognosis and prediction
Osteosarcomas of the jaws metastasize far less frequently (in 6–21% of cases) and later in the course of disease than do their axial or appendicular skeletal counterparts. Extragnathic osteosarcomas of the skull or facial bones behave as aggressively as tumours of the axial or appendicular skeleton. Histological grade of malignancy and stage of the disease are the most important prognostic factors. Surgical resection with clear margins is the treatment of choice. Low-grade osteosarcomas can be cured by complete resection without additional treatment modalities. The role of (neo)adjuvant treatment for osteosarcomas of the jawbones is controversial. However, a recent meta-analysis showed that chemotherapy might improve survival in patients with positive margins, high-grade tumours, and recurrent tumours {901,3421,2061,1698,1679,4399,377,3974,2636}.

The prognosis for osteosarcoma secondary to irradiation is much worse {4811}.

The chondrosarcoma family of tumours

Baumhoer D
Jay A
Triantafyllou A

Definition
Conventional chondrosarcoma is a malignant bone neoplasm that produces cartilaginous matrix.

ICD-O coding
9222/3 Chondrosarcoma, grade 1
9220/3 Chondrosarcoma, grade 2
9220/3 Chondrosarcoma, grade 3
9221/3 Periosteal chondrosarcoma
9243/3 Dedifferentiated chondrosarcoma
9242/3 Clear cell chondrosarcoma

ICD-11 coding
2B50.Z & XH6LT5 Chondrosarcoma of bone and articular cartilage of unspecified sites & Chondrosarcoma, grade 2
2B50.Z & XH0Y34 Chondrosarcoma of bone and articular cartilage of unspecified sites & Chondrosarcoma, grade 3

Related terminology
None

Subtype(s)
Conventional chondrosarcoma (grade 1, grade 2–3); periosteal chondrosarcoma; dedifferentiated chondrosarcoma; clear cell chondrosarcoma

Localization
Conventional chondrosarcoma affects the maxilla and the nasal septum more frequently than the mandible, but it may occur in any maxillofacial bone {3811,2347}.

Clinical features
Symptoms are nonspecific and depend upon location. Involvement of the nose can result in nasal obstruction. At other sites, asymptomatic or painful swelling is the most common presentation {913}.

Imaging
Imaging shows an osteolytic tumour, ranging from well defined to aggressively destructive, with varying opacity producing a stippled pattern or irregular masses best seen on CT. Dedifferentiation may produce a purely lytic area or soft tissue extension best localized on MRI. Chondrosarcoma has a high T2-weighted signal intensity.

Epidemiology
Maxillofacial chondrosarcoma is almost exclusively of conventional type and accounts for only 3–4% of all chondrosarcomas {3811,1239,4539}. All age groups can be affected, but there is a slight predilection for middle-aged men {2347}.

Etiology
Unknown

Genetic factors
Chondrosarcomas in the maxillofacial skeleton as manifestations of Ollier disease and Maffucci syndrome are exceedingly rare {1982}.

Pathogenesis
Conventional, periosteal, and dedifferentiated chondrosarcomas, but not clear cell chondrosarcoma, harbour somatic mutations in *IDH1* and *IDH2* {157,2256,159}.

Macroscopic appearance
Chondrosarcoma is a lobular tumour with a glistening blue-grey or white, solid cut surface. The dedifferentiated subtype also shows a fleshy component.

Histopathology
Chondrosarcoma generally has a lobular morphology and osteodestructive growth with entrapment of pre-existing trabecular bone and/or cortical permeation. Well-differentiated tumours

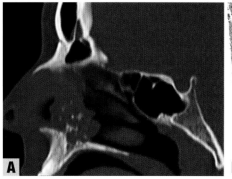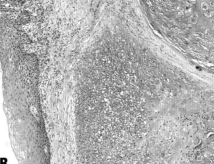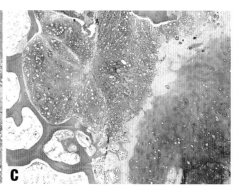

Fig. 7.100 Chondrosarcoma. **A** Grade 1. A tumour of the nasal septum containing the typical cartilaginous popcorn calcifications. CT, sagittal reconstruction. **B** Grade 2. Lobules of neoplastic cartilage infiltrating the submucosal soft tissues. **C** Grade 2. Cartilaginous tumour formation showing permeative and osteodestructive growth.

resemble hyaline cartilage with oval to polygonal cells in lacunar spaces surrounded by basophilic matrix. The nuclei are small and uniform, with round to oval outlines and evenly distributed dense chromatin. With increasing grade, the nucleoli become discernible due to open chromatin. Nuclear pleomorphism, increased cellularity with irregular distribution, decreased volume of cytoplasm, myxoid background, and mitoses are also associated with higher tumour grade {1298}.

Subtypes

Conventional chondrosarcoma is a malignant bone neoplasm that arises in the medullary cavity and produces cartilaginous matrix. Periosteal chondrosarcoma develops on the surface of bone. Dedifferentiated chondrosarcoma shows abrupt transition into a high-grade, non-cartilaginous sarcoma. Clear cell chondrosarcoma is a low-grade malignancy of lobules of cells with abundant clear cytoplasm.

Immunohistochemistry

Immunohistochemistry has limited diagnostic value. The tumour cells usually stain for S100, SOX9, ERG, and podoplanin {3255}.

Differential diagnosis

Because chondromas in the maxillofacial bones are extremely rare, tumours with pure cartilaginous differentiation should always be considered to be chondrosarcoma until proved otherwise. Chondroblastic osteosarcoma is far more common than chondrosarcoma, especially in the jawbones, requiring a thorough search to exclude small foci of neoplastic osteoid formation. Accordingly, a diagnosis of maxillofacial chondrosarcoma should not be made solely on a core needle biopsy. The high-grade component of dedifferentiated chondrosarcoma most frequently resembles undifferentiated pleomorphic sarcoma, but it can vary. Clear cell chondrosarcoma shows lobules of cells with abundant pale (attributable to glycogen) or slightly eosinophilic cytoplasm and frequently includes woven bone formation. In the temporomandibular joint, synovial chondromatosis / calcified chondroid mesenchymal neoplasms are much more common {2686A}.

Cytology

Not clinically relevant

Diagnostic molecular pathology

Detection of *IDH1/2* mutations can be helpful in distinguishing conventional, periosteal, and dedifferentiated chondrosarcoma from chondroblastic osteosarcoma in selected cases but is generally not required {157,2256}. Detection of *IDH1/2* mutation may be less likely in chondrosarcomas of the facial skeleton, whereas the skull base tumours reportedly have a higher detection rate {4348}.

Essential and desirable diagnostic criteria

Essential: consistent imaging features; a malignant tumour with cartilaginous matrix; entrapped pre-existing bone; a lack of neoplastic bone or osteoid formation.

Staging

Staging follows the eighth edition of the Union for International Cancer Control (UICC) / American Joint Committee on Cancer (AJCC) TNM staging system for craniofacial chondrosarcoma {913}.

Prognosis and prediction

Surgical resection is the treatment of choice in the maxillofacial bones. Histological grade and complete resection are the most important prognostic factors. The prognosis of dedifferentiated chondrosarcoma is usually poor.

Mesenchymal chondrosarcoma

Bell D
Baumhoer D
Neville BW
Triantafyllou A

Definition

Mesenchymal chondrosarcoma (MCS) is a high-grade, biphasic, malignant cartilaginous neoplasm characterized by sheets of small blue round to spindle-shaped cells interspersed with well-differentiated lobules of hyaline cartilage.

ICD-O coding

9240/3 Mesenchymal chondrosarcoma

ICD-11 coding

2B50.Z & XH8X47 Chondrosarcoma of bone and articular cartilage of unspecified sites & Mesenchymal chondrosarcoma

Related terminology

None

Subtype(s)

None

Localization

The most common sites in the head and neck are the jaws (the mandible more frequently), followed by the skull {3152,1974,433, 784,3451,1223}. Within the sinonasal tract, the maxillary sinus is most commonly affected, followed by the ethmoid and nasal cavity {2341}.

Clinical features

Patients present with swelling, pain, and possible pathological fracture.

Imaging

An aggressive lytic and destructive mass is seen radiologically, sometimes with soft tissue extension and calcifications.

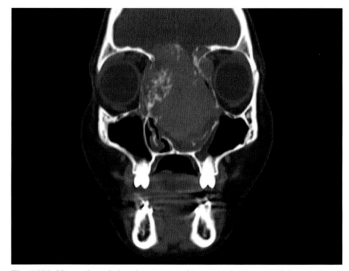

Fig. 7.101 Mesenchymal chondrosarcoma. An aggressive tumour of the nasal cavity infiltrating the surrounding structures, with cortical destruction and patchy internal mineralization. CT, coronal reconstruction.

Epidemiology

MCSs account for 2–10% of all chondrosarcomas, and 20–30% of cases arise in the head and neck {2642}. The peak incidence is in the third decade of life (age range: 7–80 years) {1510A}. There is no sex predilection {1473,3927}.

Etiology

Unknown

Pathogenesis

Almost all cases harbour a specific *HEY1::NCOA2* fusion gene, or (much more rarely) *IRF2BP2::CDX1*. Small-cell areas show

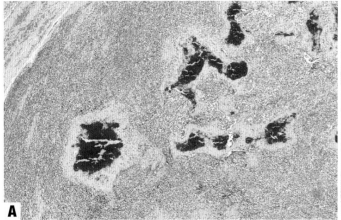 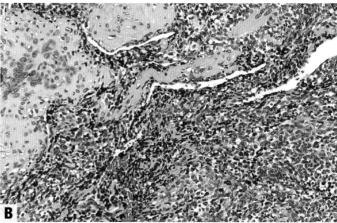

Fig. 7.102 Mesenchymal chondrosarcoma. **A** At low magnification, the characteristic histological feature is small, uniform, round to spindle-shaped cells that resemble Ewing sarcoma, with a perivascular haemangiopericytoma–like pattern, necrosis, and mineralization in cartilage islands. **B** The characteristic histological feature is a bimorphic pattern: small, uniform, round to spindle-shaped cells with a perivascular haemangiopericytoma–like pattern and admixed cartilaginous tissue.

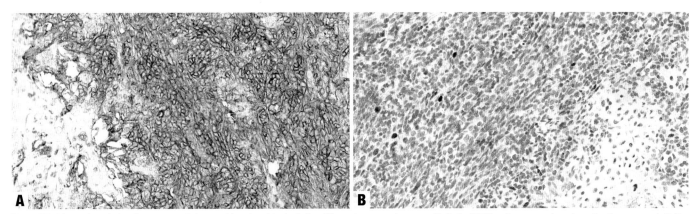

Fig. 7.103 Mesenchymal chondrosarcoma. **A** Immunohistochemistry includes diffuse strong membrane positivity for CD99 on the mesenchymal small cell component. **B** Nuclear SOX9 immunoreactivity has a patchy distribution in both the small cell and chondroid components.

TP53 loss, RB1 pathway alterations, and homozygous loss of CDKN2A {2927,4580}.

Macroscopic appearance
MCS is a grey, grey-white, or pink tumour and can be soft, firm, or hard with nodules of cartilage and bone.

Histopathology
MCS has a characteristic biphasic pattern. Large areas are composed of small, uniform, round to spindle-shaped cells, which resemble those of Ewing sarcoma, often with a perivascular arrangement and haemangiopericytoma-like pattern, necrosis, and frequent mitoses. Admixed lobules of highly differentiated cartilage may be limited or extensive and can exhibit calcification and immature ossification.

Immunohistochemistry
Immunohistochemistry shows positivity for membranous CD99 and nuclear SOX9. NKX3-1 {4949} has been suggested to be highly specific; there may be aberrant muscle marker expression.

Cytology
Cytology shows small cells with high N:C ratios, singly and in clumps, in a basophilic extracellular matrix.

Diagnostic molecular pathology
HEY1::NCOA2 recurrent translocation is present in almost all MCSs {4705,3154}; IRF2BP2::CDX1 is reported much more rarely {3253}. IDH1 and IDH2 mutations do not occur {157, 3609}.

Essential and desirable diagnostic criteria
Essential: a sarcoma with a prominent primitive component of round to spindled cells punctated with islands of mature cartilage.
Desirable: HEY1::NCOA2 fusion (in selected cases).

Staging
Staging follows the eighth edition of the Union for International Cancer Control (UICC) / American Joint Committee on Cancer (AJCC) TNM staging system.

Prognosis and prediction
MCS has a high local recurrence rate, with metastasis potentially occurring after a long disease-free interval. MCS in general has 5- and 10-year survival rates of 51% and 43% respectively, depending on the site, surgical resectability, and the type and duration of therapy {3927}. Jaw tumours generally have a better prognosis {992,1974,1003}.

Rhabdomyosarcoma with *TFCP2* rearrangement

Le Loarer F
Koutlas IG

Definition

Rhabdomyosarcoma with *TFCP2* rearrangement (TFCP2-RMS) is a high-grade rhabdomyosarcoma characterized by the fusion of *TFCP2* to *EWSR1* or *FUS*.

ICD-O coding

8900/3 Rhabdomyosarcoma with *TFCP2* rearrangement

ICD-11 coding

2B66.Y & XH0GA1 Other specified malignant neoplasms of other and unspecified parts of mouth & Rhabdomyosarcoma, NOS

Related terminology

None

Subtype(s)

None

Localization

TFCP2-RMSs arise mostly in bone, and less frequently in soft tissue {2500,4889}. There is a striking predilection for craniofacial bones (in decreasing order of frequency: the mandible, maxilla, and skull bones), from where TFCP2-RMS commonly infiltrates into the soft tissues of the mouth, nose, and neck.

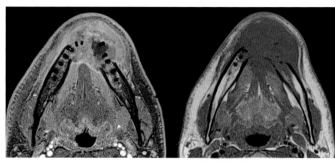

Fig. 7.104 Rhabdomyosarcoma with *TFCP2* rearrangement. T1-weighted (left) and T2-weighted (right) MRI showing an osteolytic mass of the mandible with soft tissue extension.

Clinical features

Patients present with a large, rapidly growing swelling, with pain and signs related to compression. Tumour size varies widely (median diameter: 60 mm) {2500}.

Imaging

Imaging shows large, poorly defined, infiltrating and destructive masses, commonly centred on bones and invading soft tissue.

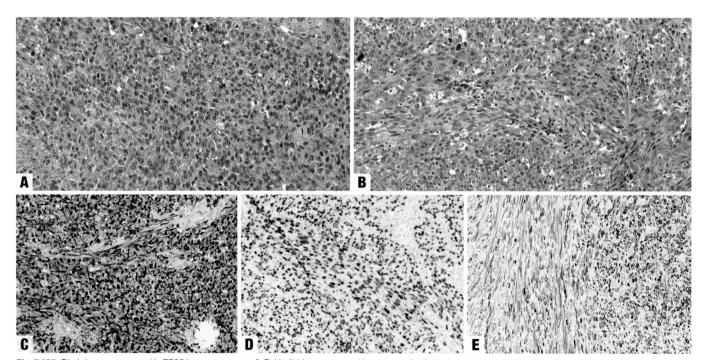

Fig. 7.105 Rhabdomyosarcoma with *TFCP2* rearrangement. **A** Epithelioid component with tumour cells displaying abundant eosinophilic cytoplasm along with large vesicular nuclei. **B** Mixed spindle cell and epithelioid components showing tumour cells with abundant eosinophilic cytoplasm, either globoid or elongated, forming short fascicles. **C** Diffuse expression of keratin by tumour cells (AE1/AE3 immunohistochemistry). **D** Diffuse nuclear expression of MYOD1 by tumour cells (MYOD1 immunohistochemistry). **E** Strong expression of ALK by tumour cells. Detection is variable between antibody clones and this example is stained with the 1A4 clone.

Epidemiology

TFCP2-RMS typically affects young adults (median age: 25 years, range: 11–86 years) {2500,4889}; 30% of cases arise in patients aged < 18 years. Both sexes are equally affected.

Etiology

Unknown

Pathogenesis

TFCP2-RMSs are defined by *TFCP2* rearrangement, fused at the 5′ end to either *FUS* or *EWSR1*, producing expression profiles distinct from those of other rhabdomyosarcomas {4745}. The translocation may be unbalanced. *TFCP2*, located at 12q13.12, encodes the transcription factor LSF, which regulates the expression of an enzyme involved in the regulation of DNA synthesis {4308}. The breakpoint occurs at the 5′ end of exon 2 of *TFCP2*, preserving the DNA-binding domain (DBD) of the protein {4745}. TFCP2-RMS harbour complex, commonly aneuploid genomic profiles {1034,4839} with multiple copy-number alterations across their genomes. Homozygous deletions of *CDKN2A* are present in virtually all cases. *TERT* overexpression has been observed {1034,4745}. Occasional alterations include *MDM2* amplification {2500}, mutations of *TP53* {4889}, and chromothripsis in 1p and 3p {1034,4839}. Intragenic deletions of *ALK* are present in roughly half of all cases, preserving the kinase domain of the protein, and correlate with ALK upregulation at the transcript and protein levels. These alterations may lead to ALK activation through alternative transcription initiation {4818}.

Macroscopic appearance

Nonspecific, solid, white-grey tumour with necrosis

Histopathology

TFCP2-RMSs are usually biphasic, with spindle cell and epithelioid areas in solid sheets or fascicles with scant accompanying stroma. More rarely, TFCP2-RMSs are composed purely of epithelioid, spindle, or round cells. Tumour nuclei are large, displaying brisk mitotic activity and dotted with conspicuous nucleoli. Overall, tumour nuclei are monotonous but may show focal hyperchromatism and pleomorphism. Necrosis is common.

Immunohistochemistry

Virtually all cases are positive for cytokeratins (AE1/AE3) and desmin. All, by definition, express myogenin and/or MYOD1, MYOD1 being more sensitive. There is occasional expression of ALK, p63, CK7, SATB2, p53, CD30, CD4, S100, caldesmon, and SMA; SMARCB1 (INI1) expression is retained {1034,2379, 887,4889}.

Differential diagnosis

Particularly in older adults, the differential diagnosis includes metastatic carcinoma because of the keratin expression and epithelioid features {4327}. Alveolar rhabdomyosarcoma commonly expresses cytokeratins and ALK but harbours *FOXO1* fusions. Malignant peripheral nerve sheath tumour with rhabdomyoblastic differentiation (Triton tumour) or anaplastic lymphoma may be suspected when S100 is positive, especially if the tumour is purely epithelioid. Sarcomas with *PATZ1* fusions are rare and have a variable appearance; they often express myogenin, MYOD1, and S100 but are associated with *PATZ1* translocations.

Cytology

Unknown

Diagnostic molecular pathology

The diagnosis can be confirmed by molecular testing using FISH with a break-apart probe for *TFCP2* or by sequencing.

Essential and desirable diagnostic criteria

Essential: a high-grade epithelioid, spindle cell, or mixed tumour; MYOD1 or myogenin expression.

Desirable: location in bone; *TFCP2* rearrangement or typical immunophenotype with coexpression of AE1/AE3 and ALK.

Staging

None

Prognosis and prediction

TFCP2-RMSs are aggressive and associated with a poor outcome, presenting at a locally advanced stage with bone and soft tissue destruction {2500,4889}. Distant metastasis is present at diagnosis or follow-up in 65% of cases, usually to bone, lungs, or lymph nodes {2500}. The estimated median survival time is 14 months, but follow-up data are limited {2500,4889}.

Most TFCP2-RMSs recur after surgery and progress despite aggressive multimodal therapy. Evaluation of chemotherapy regimens is ongoing {2500,887}. ALK inhibitors have proved ineffective alone but have some effect with combined irradiation {2583,605}.